POCKET COMPANION TO

CECIL TEXTBOOK of MEDICINE

POCKET COMPANION TO

CECIL TEXTBOOK of MEDICINE

21st Edition

Lee Goldman, M.D.
Julius Krevans Distinguished Professor and Chairman
Department of Medicine
Associate Dean for Clinical Affairs
School of Medicine
University of California, San Francisco
San Francisco, California

J. Claude Bennett, M.D.
Distinguished University Professor Emeritus
University of Alabama at Birmingham
Formerly President, Spencer Professor of Medicine, and Chairman, Department of Medicine
University of Alabama at Birmingham
Birmingham, Alabama

W.B. SAUNDERS COMPANY
A Harcourt Health Sciences Company
Philadelphia ▪ London ▪ New York ▪ St. Louis ▪ Sydney ▪ Toronto

W.B. Saunders Company
A Harcourt Health Sciences Company

The Curtis Center
Independence Square West
Philadelphia, Pennsylvania 19106

Library of Congress Cataloging-in-Publication Data

Pocket companion to Cecil textbook of medicine/
[edited by] Lee Goldman, J. Claude Bennett.

p. cm.

ISBN 0–7216–8972–8

1. Internal medicine—Handbooks, manuals, etc. I. Goldman, Lee.
II. Bennett, J. Claude. III. Cecil, Russell L. (Russell La Fayette), 1881–1965. Cecil textbook of medicine.

RC46.C423 1996b suppl.

616—dc21 00-34506

Acquisitions Editor: Lisette Bralow

Project Manager: Evelyn Adler

Production Manager: Frank Polizzano

Illustration Specialist: Peg Shaw

POCKET COMPANION TO CECIL TEXTBOOK OF MEDICINE ISBN 0–7216–8972–8

Printed in the United States of America.

Last digit is the print number: 9 8 7 6 5 4 3 2 1

PREFACE

The *Cecil Textbook of Medicine* has been the definitive, authoritative, comprehensive medical textbook since 1927, and *Cecil Essentials of Medicine* has been the preferred textbook for medical students since 1986. Now, we are pleased to add the newest member of the Cecil family, the *Pocket Companion,* to these keystone texts.

This work is designed to be a readily accessible, easy to read, condensed source of authoritative medical information. The *Pocket Companion* focuses on issues most important to daily practice, with special emphasis on tables and flow diagrams that will help guide bedside diagnosis and therapy. The *Pocket Companion* is an ideal source of quick information for students, trainees, and practitioners because it includes the key information you will need to help you think on your feet.

In preparing the *Pocket Companion to Cecil Textbook of Medicine,* the editors are especially grateful to the many Cecil authors who contributed to the parent book. We also thank our associate editors—Jeffrey M. Drazen, Gordon N. Gill, Robert C. Griggs, Juha P. Kokko, Gerald L. Mandell, Don W. Powell, and Andrew I. Schafer—who have carefully reviewed the book's contents to be sure that we have captured the most important aspects of the *Cecil Textbook of Medicine* and have updated it to include key advances since the publication of the parent text.

LEE GOLDMAN, M.D.
J. CLAUDE BENNETT, M.D.

NOTICE

Medicine is an ever-changing field. Standard safety precautions must be followed, but as new research and clinical experience broaden our knowledge, changes in treatment and drug therapy become necessary or appropriate. Readers are advised to check the product information currently provided by the manufacturer of each drug to be administered to verify the recommended dose, the method and duration of administration, and contraindications. It is the responsibility of the treating physician, relying on experience and knowledge of the patient, to determine dosages and the best treatment for the patient. Neither the publisher nor the editor assumes any responsibility for any injury and/or damage to persons or property.

THE PUBLISHER

CONTENTS

CHAPTER 1

CLINICAL ETHICS AND CARE OF THE DYING PATIENT

DECISION MAKING BY COMPETENT PATIENTS

Most clinical decisions are reached by a shared decision-making process in which physicians provide information and guidance that allow competent adult patients to base decisions on their own preferences, values, and goals. Competent adult patients have an ethical and legal right to accept or refuse medical care, including life-sustaining treatments.

INFORMED CONSENT AND DISCLOSURE. *Informed consent* is defined as voluntary acceptance by a competent patient of a plan for medical care after the physician adequately discloses the proposed plan, its risks and benefits, and alternative approaches. Legal and ethical standards of informed consent are not satisfied merely by obtaining the patient's signature on a consent form but require a process of effective communication and education between physician and patient. If the patient lacks decision-making capacity, the physician should seek consent from the appropriate substitute decision maker.

Disclosure must include proposed diagnostic tests and treatments and their risks, benefits, and alternatives. Patients must also be told of unfavorable diagnoses, such as metastatic cancer, and their prognoses.

DECISION-MAKING CAPACITY AND COMPETENCE. Decision-making capacity is the ability to understand relevant information and appreciate the consequences of a decision. Competence is the parallel legal concept. Patients who have been determined to have decision-making capacity should make their own health care decisions, based on the principle of autonomy; patients who have been determined to lack it should be protected from making bad and sometimes irreversible decisions, based on the principle of beneficence.

The most appropriate person to make a substitute decision is someone designated by the patient while still competent, either orally or through a written proxy or advance directive. Other substitute decision makers, in order of priority, include the spouse, an adult child, parent, sibling, and any other relative or concerned friend. In some jurisdictions a public official may serve if no one else is available. The standards for making substitute decisions are the patient's explicit wishes, values and beliefs, and best interests.

For more information about this subject, see the corresponding chapters in *Cecil Textbook of Medicine,* 21st edition. Philadelphia, W.B. Saunders Company, 2000. Part II: Social and Ethical Issues in Medicine, pages 5–12.

Proxy directives or durable power of attorney authorizes another to make treatment decisions if the patient cannot. Instruction directives, or living wills, state what treatment the person would want or not want in various situations

END-OF-LIFE DECISIONS

Patients may refuse all medical interventions, including life-sustaining treatment such as cardiopulmonary resuscitation, mechanical ventilation, dialysis, and artificial nutrition and hydration, even if such a decision results in the patient's death. A patient's decision to discontinue (withdraw) or not to initiate (withhold) life-sustaining treatment is not considered the moral or legal equivalent of suicide. These decisions may be made by the patient or a designated decision maker. However, euthanasia and physician-assisted suicide are, at this writing, prohibited in most legal systems, except in the state of Oregon.

FUTILITY

Sometimes families or patients wish to initiate or continue treatments that physicians believe are futile. Physicians should strive to establish consensus within the health care team and communicate with the patient and family to reach consensus on a treatment plan.

PALLIATIVE CARE

Palliative care aims to improve the quality of life when treatment to cure disease or prolong life is no longer realistic. The main symptoms associated with terminal illness may include pain, the anorexia-cachexia syndrome, weakness and fatigue, dyspnea and cough, nausea and vomiting, mouth problems, skin problems, lymphedema, ascites, confusion, dementia, and anxiety. Because symptoms may change rapidly, frequent reevaluation is essential (see Table 1–1).

COMMUNICATION ISSUES AND FAMILY CARE

Integrating "bad news" is usually a process, not an event. Discussions should be positive, yet reality-oriented. Family meetings may help to prevent crises, clarify misunderstandings, and build bridges for support. The bereaved are a high-risk population with increased incidence of impaired function, medical illness, psychological distress, and even death.

LOCATION OF DYING

Although most patients prefer to die at home, not all expressing this wish will be able to live in comfort at home until death. Effective palliative care involves a team. A trusted physician is essential. Careful planning and prompt response to requests for emergency assistance can avoid unnecessary hospitalization as clinical crises increase.

Table 1–1 ■ GUIDELINES FOR SYMPTOM CONTROL

1. "Nothing matters more than the bowels" (Saunders). Daily assessment needed.
2. Control of one symptom improves control of all symptoms.
3. Most symptoms are caused by multiple factors. Psychological distress may augment all symptoms.
4. "Assessment must precede treatment" (Twycross).
5. Rule out correctable factors underlying each symptom.
6. Clarify who is bothered by the symptoms: patient, family, or staff.
7. Give a simple explanation for each symptom to the patient and family. Diagrams helpful.
8. Consider the anticipated prognosis, functional status, and the patient's goals in determining appropriate treatment.
9. Discuss treatment options with patient and family and involve them in treatment planning when practical.
10. Determine what was helpful in the past.
11. Use a total-care approach employing nondrug, environmental, and other supportive measures.
12. If needed, use combinations of pharmacologic agents when differing mechanisms of action and toxicity permit.
13. Prescribe drugs prophylactically in individually optimized, regular doses for persistent symptoms.
14. Never say "Nothing more can be done." Consult or refer if comfort is not achieved.

CHAPTER 2

GERIATRICS

The process of aging produces important physiologic changes in the central nervous system, including neuroanatomic, neurotransmitter, and neurophysiologic changes. These processes in turn result in age-related symptoms and manifestations (Table 2–1) for many older persons. However, these physiologic changes develop at dramatically different rates in different older persons, the decline being modified by factors such as diet, environment, lifestyle, genetic predisposition, disability, disease, and the side effects of drugs.

Neuropsychiatric disorders, the leading cause of disability in older persons, account for nearly 50% of functional incapacities. Severe neuropsychiatric conditions have been estimated to occur in 15 to 25% of older adults worldwide. Alzheimer's disease and related dementias occur in approximately 10% of those aged 65 years and older and in up to 40% of those older than 85 years. Delirium occurs in 5 to 10% of all persons 65 years and older, usually in the setting of acute illness and hospitalization. Severe

Table 2–1 ■ NEUROPSYCHIATRIC MANIFESTATIONS OF AGE-RELATED PHYSIOLOGIC CHANGES

SYSTEM	MANIFESTATIONS
Cognition	Forgetfulness
	Processing speed declines throughout adult life
	Neuropsychological declines: selective attention, verbal fluency, retrieval, complex visual perception, logical analysis
Reflexes	Stretch reflexes lose sensitivity
	Decreased or absent ankle reflexes
	Decreased autonomic and righting reflexes; postural instability
Sensory	Presbycusis (high-frequency hearing loss), tinnitus
	Deterioration of vestibular system, vertigo
	Presbyopia (decreased lens elasticity)
	Slowed pupil reactivity, decreased upgaze
	Olfactory system deterioration
	Decreased vibratory sensation
Gait, balance	Gait stiffer, slowed, forward-flexed
	Increased body sway and mild unsteadiness
Sleep	Decreased sleep efficiency, fatigue
	Increased awakenings, insomnia
	Decrease in sleep stages 3 and 4
	Sleep duration more variable, more naps

For more information about this subject, see the corresponding chapters in *Cecil Textbook of Medicine,* 21st edition. Philadelphia, W.B. Saunders Company, 2000. Part III: Aging and Geriatric Medicine, pages 13–25.

depression occurs in approximately 5% of older people, with as many as 15% having significant depressive symptoms. Anxiety disorders occur in 10% of older people.

MENTAL STATUS EXAMINATION

For depression screening, scores of 6 or more on the 15-item short-form Geriatric Depression Scale (Table 2–2) indicate substantial depressive symptoms requiring further evaluation. For cognitive testing, the most widely used instrument is the Mini-Mental State Examination, a 19-item, 30-point scale that can be completed in 10 minutes (Table 2–3).

FUNCTIONAL ASSESSMENT

The functional assessment should include an assessment of the patient's ability to carry out basic self-care activities of daily living, as well as higher-level activities needed for independent living. Performance of activities of daily living reflects the ability of the patient to maintain basic self-care activities, including feeding, grooming, bathing, dressing, toileting, transferring, and walking. Performance of instrumental activities of daily living reflects the ability of the patient to handle more complex tasks, including shopping, meal preparation, managing finances, housekeeping, using the telephone, taking medications, driving, and using transportation.

Table 2–2 ■ GERIATRIC DEPRESSION SCALE—SHORT FORM

1. Are you basically satisfied with your life?	yes/**NO**
2. Have you dropped many of your activities and interests?	**YES**/no
3. Do you feel that your life is empty?	**YES**/no
4. Do you often get bored?	**YES**/no
5. Are you in good spirits most of the time?	yes/**NO**
6. Are you afraid that something bad is going to happen to you?	**YES**/no
7. Do you feel happy most of the time?	yes/**NO**
8. Do you feel helpless?	**YES**no
9. Do you prefer staying home rather than going out and doing new things?	**YES**/no
10. Do you feel you have more problems with memory than most?	**YES**/no
11. Do you think it is wonderful to be alive now?	yes/**NO**
12. Do you feel pretty worthless the way you are now?	**YES**/no
13. Do you feel full of energy?	yes/**NO**
14. Do you feel that your situation is hopeless?	**YES**/no
15. Do you think that most people are better off than you?	**YES**/no

Scoring: Answers indicating depression are in **boldface capital letters;** six or more **boldface** answers indicate depressive symptoms.

Adapted from Yesavage J, Brink T, Rowe T, et al: Development and validation of a geriatric depression screening scale: A preliminary report. J. Psychiatr Res 17:37, 1983.

Table 2–3 ■ MINI-MENTAL STATE EXAMINATION

COGNITIVE DOMAIN	MAXIMUM SCORE
Orientation	
What is the (year) (season) (date) (day) (month)?	5
Where are we (city) (state) (county) (hospital) (floor)?	5
Registration	
Name 3 objects: 1 sec to say each. Ask the patient for all 3 after you have said them. Give 1 point for each correct answer. Repeat them until all 3 are learned. Count the trials and record the number.	3
Attention and Calculation	
Serial 7s backward from 100 (stop after 5 answers). Alternatively, spell WORLD backward.	5
Recall	
Ask for the 3 objects repeated above. Give 1 point for each correct answer.	3
Language and Praxis	
Show a pencil and watch, and ask the patient to name them.	3
Ask the patient to repeat the following: "No ifs, ands, or buts."	1
Three-stage command: "Take this paper in your right hand, fold it in half, and put it on the floor."	3
"Read and obey the following: Close your eyes."	1
"Write a sentence."	1
"Copy this design" (interlocking pentagons).	1

A score of 25 or greater signifies intact cognitive function.

Adapted from Folstein MF, Folstein SE, McHugh PR: "The Mini-Mental State": A practical method for grading the cognitive state of patients for the clinician. J Psychiatr Res 12:189, 1975.

PSYCHOACTIVE EFFECTS OF DRUGS IN OLDER PERSONS

Iatrogenic complications occur in 29 to 38% of older hospitalized patients, with a three- to fivefold increased risk in older as compared with younger patients. Nearly every class of drugs has the potential to cause delirium in a vulnerable patient, but specific drugs have been most commonly implicated (Table 2–4). When drug therapy is required in the elderly, physicians should choose the drug with the least toxic potential and emphasize drugs that have been well tested in elderly populations (Table 2–5).

EVALUATION OF MENTAL STATUS CHANGE IN THE OLDER PATIENT

Mental status change, one of the most common presenting symptoms in the acutely ill older population, is estimated to account for up to 30% of emergency evaluations for older patients. A broad range of medical, neurologic, and psychiatric conditions can lead to mental status changes, and a systematic approach aids in the evalu-

Table 2–4 ■ DRUGS WITH PSYCHOACTIVE EFFECTS

Sedative-hypnotics
- Benzodiazepines (especially flurazepam, diazepam)
- Barbiturates
- Sleeping medications (chloral hydrate)

Narcotics (especially meperidine)

Anticholinergics
- Antihistamines (diphenhydramine, hydroxyzine)
- Antispasmodics (belladonna, diphenoxylate-atropine [Lomotil])
- Heterocyclic antidepressants (amitriptyline, imipramine, doxepin)
- Neuroleptics (chlorpromazine, haloperidol, thioridazine)
- Antiparkinsonian (benztropine, trihexyphenidyl)
- Atropine, scopolamine

Cardiac
- Digitalis glycosides
- Antiarrhythmics (quinidine, procainamide, lidocaine)
- Antihypertensives (β-blockers, methyldopa)

Gastrointestinal
- H_2-antagonists (cimetidine, ranitidine, famotidine, nizatidine)
- Metoclopramide (Reglan)

Miscellaneous
- Non-steroidal anti-inflammatory drugs
- Corticosteroids
- Anticonvulsants
- Levodopa
- Lithium

Over-the-counter drugs
- Cold, sinus preparations (antihistamines, pseudoephedrine)
- Sleep aids (diphenhydramine, alcohol-containing elixirs)
- Stay Awake (caffeine)
- Nausea, gastrointestinal (attapulgite [Donnagel], meclizine, H_2-antagonists, loperamide)

ation of suspected mental status change in an older patient (Fig. 2–1).

DELIRIUM

Delirium, a clinical syndrome characterized as an acute disorder of attention and cognitive function, is the most frequent complication of hospitalization in older patients and a potentially devastating problem. Delirium is often unrecognized despite sensitive methods for its detection (Table 2–6). The development of delirium usually involves a complex interrelationship between a vulnerable patient with pertinent predisposing factors and exposure to noxious insults or precipitating factors.

Medications contribute to delirium in up to 40% of cases. Other causes include renal or hepatic failure, hypoxemia, hypercarbia, myocardial ischemia or heart failure, dehydration, occult infections, and a variety of metabolic disorders, including hypernatremia or hyponatremia, hypercalcemia, and thyroid or adrenal disorders.

The cardinal features of delirium include acute onset and inattention. Patients are inattentive, that is, they have difficulty focusing, maintaining, and shifting attention. They appear easily distracted and may have difficulty with simple repetitive tasks, digit spans,

Table 2–5 ■ GUIDELINES FOR DRUG THERAPY IN THE ELDERLY

General principles:

Remember that the elderly are highly sensitive to the psychoactive effects of all drugs.

Know the pharmacology of the drugs you prescribe. Know a few drugs well.

Recommended approach:

1. Use non-pharmacologic approaches whenever possible.
2. Avoid routine use of "as needed" drugs for sleep, anxiety, pain.
3. Choose the drug with the least toxic potential.
4. Substitute less toxic alternatives whenever possible (antacid or sucralfate for an H_2-blocker, Metamucil or Kaopectate for Lomotil, scheduled acetaminophen or choline magnesium salicylate regimen for pain management).
5. Reduce the dosage.
6. "Start low and go slow." Start with 25–50% of the standard dose of psychoactive drugs in the elderly. Titrate the drug slowly. Set realistic end points: titrate to improvement, not elimination of symptoms.
7. Keep the regimen cycle.
8. Regularly reassess the medication list. Have the patient bring in all bottles and review what is being taken.
9. Reevaluate chronic drug use since the patient is changing.
10. Review over-the-counter medication use.

and recitation of months backward. The cornerstone of evaluation of delirium is a comprehensive history and physical examination (Table 2–7).

In general, non-pharmacologic approaches should be used in all delirious patients and they will usually be successful for symptom management. Neuroleptics are the preferred agents of treatment, with haloperidol and thioridazine being the most widely used agents. The recommended starting dose is haloperidol 0.5 to 1.0 mg orally or parenterally or thioridazine 10 to 25 mg orally, and then, after the vital signs have been rechecked, repeat dose every 30 minutes until sedation has been achieved. The end point should be an awake but manageable patient.

Non-pharmacologic management techniques recommended for every delirious patient include encouraging the presence of family members, using "sitters" to be orienting influences, or transferring a disruptive patient to a private room or closer to the nurse's station for increased supervision. Interpersonal contact and communication, including verbal reorientation strategies, simple instructions and explanations, and frequent eye contact, are vital. The most effective intervention strategy to reduce delirium and its associated complications is primary prevention of delirium before it occurs (Table 2–8).

DRUGS AND RISKS

In general, the loading dose of medications should not be altered in the presence of renal dysfunction, but subsequent doses, especially medications that have narrow therapeutic-to-toxic ratios and are eliminated by the kidney, such as digoxin and aminoglycosides,

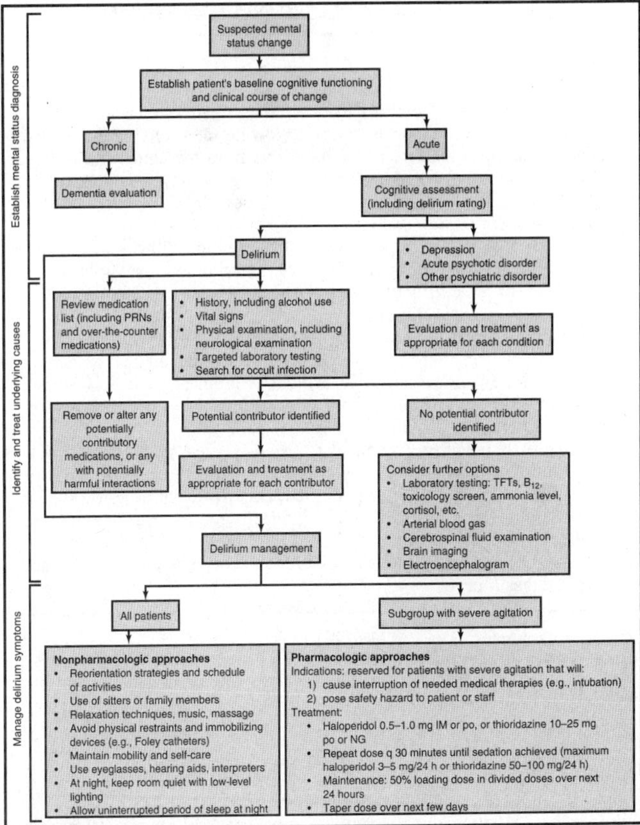

FIGURE 2–1 ■ Algorithm for evaluation of suspected mental status change in an older patient. TFTs = thyroid function tests.

must be adjusted according to actual renal function for any medication. Formulas such as

$$\text{Creatinine clearance} = \frac{\text{weight (kg)} \times (140 - \text{age})}{72 \times \text{serum creatine (mg/dL)}}$$

(for women, multiply result by 0.85) for rapid estimation of glomerular filtration rate (GFR) have been validated in subgroups of elderly patients and should be used when dosing decisions are rapidly needed. Serum drug levels should be obtained to guide dosing of drugs with a narrow therapeutic-to-toxic ratio.

BOWEL AND BLADDER PROBLEMS

An important consequence of constipation is fecal impaction, which may be manifested as fever, altered mental status, agitation, urinary retention, or paradoxical diarrhea caused by leakage around

Table 2–6 ■ DIAGNOSTIC CRITERIA FOR DELIRIUM

The CAM Diagnostic Algorithm

Feature 1. Acute onset and fluctuating course

This feature is usually obtained from a family member or nurse and is shown by positive responses to the following questions: Is there evidence of an acute change in mental status from the patient's baseline? Did the (abnormal) behavior fluctuate during the day, i.e., tend to come and go, or increase and decrease in severity?

Feature 2. Inattention

This feature is shown by a positive response to the following question: Did the patient have difficulty focusing attention, e.g., being easily distracted, or have difficulty keeping track of what was being said?

Feature 3. Disorganized thinking

This feature is shown by a positive response to the following question: Was the patient's thinking disorganized or incoherent, such as rambling or irrelevant conversation, unclear or illogical in flow of ideas, or unpredictable and switching from subject to subject?

Feature 4. Altered level of consciousness

This feature is shown by any answer other than alert to the following question: Overall, how would you rate this patient's level of consciousness (alert [normal], vigilant [hyperalert], lethargic [drowsy, easily aroused], stuporous [difficult to arouse], or comatose [unarousable])?

The diagnosis of delirium by CAM requires the presence of features 1 and 2 and either 3 or 4.

CAM = Confusion Assessment Method.

From Inouye SK, van Dyck CH, Alessi CA, et al: Clarifying confusion: The Confusion Assessment Method. A new method for detection of delirium. Ann Intern Med 113:941, 1990.

the impaction. Fetal impaction can usually be treated with suppositories, enemas, or manual disimpaction, but in extreme cases mechanical bowel obstruction may require surgical intervention. Prevention consists of strict attention to the patient's bowel habits, adequate hydration, adequate but not excessive dietary fiber, avoidance of constipating medications when possible, and judicious use of laxatives.

Urinary incontinence affects 10 to 30% of the community-residing elderly (Table 2–9). The most common cause of urinary incontinence in elderly men and women is overactivity of the bladder detrusor. In this condition (called "detrusor instability"), the detrusor muscle contracts in response to inappropriately small volumes of urine, often preceded by a sense of urgency. The symptoms of detrusor instability—frequency and urge incontinence—may be ameliorated by "bladder training," which consists of prolonging the interval between voidings by using behavioral techniques or by antispasmodics such as oxybutynin.

In elderly women, post-menopausal stress incontinence typically occurs immediately after a cough or a sneeze; it may respond to treatment with exogenous estrogens. Chronic indwelling catheters should not be used in the management of incontinence, even in patients with decubitus ulcers, because urinary tract infection develops in virtually 100% of chronically catheterized patients, and chronic antibiotic suppression merely leads to the production of resistant strains of organisms.

Table 2–7 ■ EVALUATION OF DELIRIUM IN ELDERLY PATIENTS

1. Cognitive testing and determination of baseline cognitive functioning. Establish the diagnosis of delirium
2. Comprehensive history and physical examination, including careful neurologic examination for focal deficits and search for occult infection
3. Review the medication list: discontinue or minimize all psychoactive medications. Check the side effects of all medications
4. Laboratory evaluation (tailored to the individual): complete blood count, electrolytes, blood urea nitrogen, creatinine, glucose, calcium, phosphate, liver enzymes, oxygen saturation
5. Search for occult infection: physical examination, urinalysis, chest radiography, selected cultures (as indicated)
6. When no obvious cause is revealed from the above steps, further targeted evaluation is considered in selected patients:
   - Laboratory tests: magnesium, thyroid function tests, vitamin B_{12} level, drug levels, toxicology screen, ammonia level
   - Arterial blood gas: indicated in patients with dyspnea, tachypnea, any acute pulmonary process, or history of significant respiratory disease
   - Electrocardiogram: indicated in patients with chest or abdominal discomfort, shortness of breath, or cardiac history
   - Cerebrospinal fluid examination: indicated when meningitis or encephalitis is suspected
   - Brain imaging: indicated in patients with new focal neurologic signs or with a history or signs of head trauma
   - Electroencephalogram: useful in diagnosing occult seizure disorder and differentiating delirium from non-organic psychiatric disorders

FALLS AND FRACTURES

Approximately one third of people 75 years and older fall at least once annually. Falls are most commonly caused by acute or chronic neurologic disease, arthritis, musculoskeletal impairments, poor balance, postural instability, cardiac arrhythmias, generalized weakness from acute or chronic medical illness (including acute myocardial infarction), orthostatic hypotension, or impaired coordination hampering the ability to fall "well."

The probable cause of the fall can be ascertained in 95% of cases with a careful history and physical examination alone. Further diagnostic work-up should be guided by this initial evaluation.

FLUID BALANCE AND ELECTROLYTE DISORDERS

Geriatric patients may become easily dehydrated after a variety of insults such as excessive environmental heat, diarrhea, or febrile illness. Even more common is hyponatremia caused by an exaggerated release of arginine vasopressin after an osmotic stimulus and by a decreased ability to excrete a water load, in part related to the reduced GFR.

PRESSURE SORES

Pressure sores develop when extrinsic pressure on the skin exceeds the mean capillary pressure (32 mm Hg). Typical sites in-

Table 2–8 ■ DELIRIUM RISK FACTORS AND POTENTIAL INTERVENTIONS

RISK FACTOR	INTERVENTIONS
Cognitive impairment	Therapeutic activities program Reality orientation program (reorienting techniques, communication)
Sleep deprivation	Noise reduction strategies Scheduling of nighttime medications, procedures, and nursing activities to allow uninterrupted period of sleep
Immobilization	Early mobilization (e.g., ambulation or bedside exercises) Minimizing immobilizing equipment (e.g., bladder catheters)
Psychoactive medications	Restricted use of "as needed" sleep and psychoactive medications (e.g., sedative-hypnotics, narcotics, anticholinergic medications) Non-pharmacologic protocols for management of sleep and anxiety
Vision impairment	Provision of vision aids (e.g., magnifiers, special lighting) Provision of adaptive equipment (e.g., illuminated phone dials, large-print books)
Hearing impairment	Provision of amplifying devices Repair of hearing aids
Dehydration	Early recognition and volume repletion

clude dependent areas possessing minimal subcutaneous fat, and bony prominences such as the sacrum, greater trochanter, scapula, lateral malleolus, thoracic spine, and heels. The hallmark of prevention is avoidance of pressure.

Uncomplicated blisters should be managed without débridement or dressing. Ulcers involving subcutaneous tissue may generate substantial necrotic tissue, which should be débrided. Ulcer craters should not be treated with topical antibiotics, which promote antimicrobial resistance without enhancing wound healing.

Table 2–9 ■ COMMON FORMS OF URINARY INCONTINENCE IN THE ELDERLY

TYPE	CAUSE OR ASSOCIATION
Urge (detrusor instability)	Postmenopause, old age, CNS disease
Stress	Increased intra-abdominal pressure superimposed on
"True"	Incompetent urethral sphincter
Reflex	Overdistended bladder
Mixed urge and stress	See above
Overflow	Incomplete bladder outlet obstruction (e.g., BPH), bladder atony (e.g., long-standing diabetes)
Pseudoincontinence	Inability to toilet, confusional states

CNS = central nervous system; BPH = benign prostatic hypertrophy.

Foam "egg crate" pads and mattresses redistribute pressure, and sheepskin padding absorbs moisture. Air-fluidized beds (warm air flowing through silicon beads) and alternating air pressure mattresses redistribute and reduce extrinsic pressure.

CHAPTER 3

PREVENTIVE HEALTH CARE

THE PREVENTIVE HEALTH EXAMINATION

The American College of Physicians, the Canadian Task Force, and the U.S. Preventive Services Task Force (USPSTF) have developed guidelines for the preventive health examination. The widely used USPSTF recommendations have been intentionally limited to procedures with adequate supportive evidence and are a minimum set of guidelines that are likely to increase as further evidence accumulates and new approaches are introduced. Other organizations, especially those with a specific disease or professional focus, generally recommend more intensive or aggressive examinations (Table 3–1).

DIET

Dietary recommendations aimed at reducing the disease risk of the entire population can be of major benefit for the nation's health because even a relatively small reduction in risk in a large number of people at moderate risk could lead to greater benefit for the total population than a large reduction in risk for a small number of people at high risk (Table 3–2).

PHYSICAL ACTIVITY

The physical activity prescription can take the traditional vigorous exercise approach or follow the recommendation for daily moderate physical activity. Both provide significant health benefits (Table 3–3).

TOBACCO

Currently, about 45 million people in the United States are cigarette smokers, including 28% of men and 23% of women. Tobacco use is motivated primarily by the desire for nicotine.

Tobacco is a major cause of death from cancer, cardiovascular disease, and pulmonary disease. Smoking, the single largest preventable cause of cancer, is responsible for about 30% of cancer deaths. Lung cancer is the leading cause of cancer deaths in the United States and is predominantly attributable to cigarette smoking. Smokeless tobacco is addictive and is associated with an increased risk of oral cancer at the site where the tobacco is usually placed. Considerable evidence indicates that exposure to environ-

---

For more information about this subject, see the corresponding chapters in *Cecil Textbook of Medicine,* 21st edition. Philadelphia, W.B. Saunders Company, 2000. Part IV: Preventive Health Care, pages 26–76.

Table 3–1 ■ U.S. PREVENTIVE SERVICES TASK FORCE PERIODIC EXAMINATION RECOMMENDATIONS: SCREENING HISTORY, PHYSICAL EXAMINATION, AND LABORATORY WORK—AGES 19 AND OLDER

Schedule every 1–3 yr at age 19–64 yr and every year if 65 or older

The recommended schedule applies only to the periodic visit itself. The frequency of the individual preventive services is left to clinical discretion except as indicated. The table indicates recommended ages and high-risk (HR) groups for whom the recommendations are made. Recommendations are applicable to age groups indicated in parentheses

HISTORY	PHYSICAL EXAMINATION
Dietary intake (≥19) Physical activity (≥19) Tobacco/alcohol/drug use (≥19) Sexual practices (19–64) Functional status (≥65)	**Height and weight (≥19)** **Blood pressure (≥19)** **Visual acuity (≥65)** **Hearing (≥65)** **Clinical breast exam (≥50)** and 19–49 **HR**—Annually >50, women ≥35 with a family history of premenopausally diagnosed breast cancer in a first-degree relative **Testicular exam (HR 19–39)**—Men with a history of cryptorchidism, orchiopexy, or testicular atrophy **Symptoms of TIA (≥65)** **Complete skin exam (HR ≥19)**—Persons with a family or personal history of skin cancer, increased occupational or recreational exposure to sunlight, or clinical evidence of precursor lesions (e.g., dysplastic nevi, certain congenital nevi) **Thyroid for nodules (HR ≥19)**—Persons with a history of upper body irradiation **Auscultation for carotid bruits (HR ≥40)**—Persons with risk factors for cerebrovascular or cardiovascular disease (e.g., hypertension, smoking, coronary disease, atrial fibrillation, diabetes) or those with neurologic symptoms (e.g., TIAs or a history of cerebrovascular disease) **Complete oral cavity exam (HR ≥19)**—Persons with exposure to tobacco or excessive amounts of alcohol or those with suspicious symptoms or lesions detected through self-examination

LABORATORY WORK

Nonfasting total cholesterol (≥19)

Papanicolaou smear (19–64, HR ≥65)—Pap smear every 1–3 yr. At ≥65, only women who have not had previous documented screening in which smears have been consistently negative

Fasting glucose (HR ≥19)—The markedly obese, persons with family history of diabetes, or women with a history of gestational diabetes

Rubella antibodies (HR 19–39)—Women lacking evidence of immunity

VDRL (HR 19–64)—Prostitutes, persons who engage in sex with multiple partners in areas in which syphilis is prevalent, or contacts of persons with active syphilis

Urinalysis for bacteremia (HR 19–64)—Persons with diabetes

Table continued on following page

Table 3–1 ■ U.S. PREVENTIVE SERVICES TASK FORCE PERIODIC EXAMINATION RECOMMENDATIONS: SCREENING HISTORY, PHYSICAL EXAMINATION, AND LABORATORY WORK—AGES 19 AND OLDER *Continued*

LABORATORY WORK
Dipstick urinalysis (≥65)
Mammography (HR 35–49; ≥50)—Women ≥35 with a family history of premenopausally diagnosed breast cancer in a first-degree relative; otherwise every 1–2 yr beginning at age 50. See text
Chlamydial testing (HR 19–64)—Persons who attend clinics for sexually transmitted diseases, attend other high-risk health care facilities (e.g., adolescent and family planning clinics), or have other risk factors for chlamydial infection (e.g., multiple sexual contacts or a sexual partner with multiple sexual contacts, age <20 yr)
Gonorrhea culture (HR 19–64)—Prostitutes, persons with multiple sexual partners or a sexual partner with multiple contacts, sexual contacts of persons with culture-proven gonorrhea, or persons with a history of repeated episodes of gonorrhea
Counseling and testing for HIV infection (HR 19–64)—Persons seeking treatment for sexually transmitted disease; homosexual and bisexual men; past or present IV drug users; persons with a history of prostitution or multiple sexual partners; women whose past or present sexual partners were HIV-infected, bisexual, or IV drug users; persons with long-term residence or birth in an area with high prevalence of HIV infection; or persons with a history of transfusion between 1978 and 1985
Hearing (HR 19–64)—Persons exposed regularly to excessive noise
PPD (HR ≥19)—Household members of persons with tuberculosis or others at risk for close contact with the disease (e.g., staff of tuberculosis clinics, shelters for the homeless, nursing homes, substance abuse treatment facilities, dialysis units, correctional institutions); recent immigrants or refugees from countries in which tuberculosis is common, migrant workers; residents of nursing homes, correctional institutions, or homeless shelters; or persons with certain underlying medical disorders (e.g., HIV infection)
Fecal occult blood/sigmoidoscopy (HR)—Persons ≥50 who have first-degree relatives with colorectal cancer; a personal history of endometrial, ovarian, or breast cancer; or a previous diagnosis of inflammatory bowel disease, adenomatous polyps, or colorectal cancer
Colonoscopy (HR 19–39)—Persons with a family history of familial polyposis coli or cancer family syndrome
Fecal occult blood/colonoscopy (≥40)—Persons with a family history of familial polyposis coli or cancer family syndrome
Fecal occult blood/sigmoidoscopy (≥50)—See text
Bone mineral content (HR 40–64)—Premenopausal women at increased risk for osteoporosis (e.g., white race, bilateral oophorectomy before menopause, slender build) and for whom estrogen replacement therapy would otherwise not be recommended
Electrocardiogram (≥19)—Persons who would endanger public safety were they to experience sudden cardiac events, e.g., commercial airline pilots. Men >40 with 2 or more cardiac risk factors (high blood cholesterol, hypertension, cigarette smoking, diabetes mellitus, family history of coronary artery disease) or sedentary or high-risk persons planning to begin a vigorous exercise program
Thyroid function tests (women ≥65)
Glaucoma testing by eye specialist (≥65)

TIA = transient ischemic attack; HIV = human immunodeficiency virus; PPD = purified protein derivative.
From U.S. Preventive Services Task Force: Guide to Clinical Preventive Services, 2nd ed. Alexandria, VA, International Medical Publishing, 1996.

Table 3–2 ■ DIETARY GUIDELINES

Weight control	Keep body mass index (weight in kg ÷ ht^2 in meters) <25
Fat	<25% of calories as total fat, <7% of calories as saturated fat, <300 mg/d of dietary cholesterol
Carbohydrate	>55% of calories as carbohydrates
Salt	<6 g/d
Protein	<2–3 servings/d of high protein foods
Dairy	Up to 2–3 servings/d of low-fat dietary products
Alcohol	≤1 oz/d (2 drinks)

mental tobacco smoke (ETS) (i.e., passive smoking) is harmful to the health of non-smokers.

Cigarette smoking accounts for about 20% of cardiovascular deaths in the United States. Although the risk of cardiovascular

Table 3–3 ■ THE EXERCISE PRESCRIPTION

Type of Physical Activity

Continuous or intermittent
Primarily aerobic
Stretching for flexibility
Resistance exercise for strength

Intensity

Moderate (40–60% relative to capacity, "brisk walk")
OR
Vigorous (>60% relative to capacity)

Duration

20–60 min/d
150–300 kcal/d

Frequency

Daily for intermittent moderate activity
Three or more times per week for continuous, vigorous activity

Session

For planned exercise:
- Warm-up, 3–5 min
- Conditioning, 15–40 min
- Cool-down, 2–5 min

For lifestyle activity: incorporate activity into the daily routine; "pulses" of activity should be at least 10 min long and at an intensity equal to brisk walking

Progression

Increase duration, intensity, and frequency gradually
Evaluate progress each visit

Warning signs

Severe musculoskeletal pain
Claudication
Chest pressure, pain, or discomfort
Unusual shortness of breath
Dizziness, nausea, vomiting

disease is roughly proportional to cigarette consumption, the risk persists at levels as low as one to two cigarettes per day.

More than 80% of chronic obstructive lung disease in the United States is attributable to cigarette smoking. Cigarette smoking also increases the risk of respiratory infection, including pneumonia.

Cigarette smoking increases the risk of duodenal and gastric ulcers and is also associated with esophageal reflux symptoms. Cigarette smoking is a risk factor for osteoporosis and is a major cause of reproductive problems resulting in approximately 4600 infant deaths annually in the United States.

A person who quits smoking before age 50 has half the risk of dying in the next 15 years of a continuing smoker. After quitting, smokers gain an average of 5 to 7 lb.

Among smokers, spontaneous quit rates are about 1% per year. Simple physician advice increases the quit rate to 3%. Minimal-intervention programs increase quit rates to 5 to 10%, whereas more intensive treatments, including smoking cessation clinics, can yield quit rates of 25 to 30%.

Currently, two medications have been approved for smoking cessation: nicotine and bupropion. Nicotine replacement medications include 2- and 4-mg nicotine polacrilex gum, transdermal nicotine patches, nicotine nasal spray, and nicotine inhalers. Bupropion is dosed at 150 to 300 mg/day for 7 days prior to stopping smoking and then at 300 mg/day for the next 6 to 12 weeks. Bupropion can also be used in combination with a nicotine patch.

IMMUNIZATION

Immunization is one of the most cost-effective means of preventing morbidity and mortality from infectious diseases (Table 3–4).

ALCOHOLISM AND ALCOHOL ABUSE

A recent U.S. survey found the 12-month prevalence of alcohol abuse and alcoholism to be 2.5% and 7.2%, respectively; the lifetime prevalence was 9.4% and 14.1%. At least twice as many men are alcoholic as women.

Ethanol is absorbed completely from the gastrointestinal tract and is detected in the blood within minutes of ingestion. About 25% enters the bloodstream from the stomach and 75% from the intestine. Ninety to 98% is removed in the liver, and the remainder is excreted by the kidneys, lungs, and skin. Elimination proceeds at a constant rate, independent of the blood alcohol concentration (zero-order kinetics); a 70-kg man can metabolize 5 to 10 g ethanol per hour. In a non-alcoholic, intoxication occurs at blood alcohol levels of 50 to 150 mg/dL (Table 3–5).

Alcoholics often obtain 50% of their calories from ethanol. Serious nutritional deficiencies, particularly protein, thiamine, folate, and pyridoxine deficiency, are frequent (Table 3–6).

When drinking is abruptly reduced or discontinued, physical dependence is manifested by a hyperexcitable *alcohol withdrawal syndrome* (Fig. 3–1). Generalized tonic-clonic seizures develop in about one third of alcoholics, most often within 12 to 24 hours after reducing or stopping drinking. Delirium tremens occurs in

Table 3–4 ■ SELECTED IMMUNIZING AGENTS INDICATED FOR ADULTS*

DISEASE	MAJOR INDICATIONS	COMMENTS AND PRECAUTIONS
Diphtheria	All adults	
Hepatitis A	Travelers to highly or intermediately endemic countries; men who have sex with men; illegal drug users (injectors and non-injectors); persons who work with virus-infected primates or do research with the virus; persons with chronic liver disease; recipients of clotting factors	
Hepatitis B	Adolescents; health care and public safety workers potentially exposed to blood; clients and staff of institutions for the developmentally disabled; hemodialysis patients; men who have sex with men; users of illicit injectable drugs; recipients of clotting factors; household and sexual contacts of HBV carriers; inmates of long-term correctional facilities; heterosexuals treated for sexually transmitted diseases or with multiple sexual partners; travelers with close contact for ≥6 mo with populations with high prevalence of HBV carriage	
Influenza	All adults ≥65 yr; other adults with high-risk conditions; adults caring for persons with high-risk conditions, including medical personnel (see text); women who will be in 2nd or 3rd trimester of pregnancy during influenza season	Anaphylactic hypersensitivity to eggs is a contraindication
Lyme disease	Primarily persons who live, work, or visit areas at high or moderate risk for Lyme disease	
Measles	All adults born after 1956 without history of live vaccine on or after 1st birthday	Altered immunity is a contraindication
Meningococcal disease	Terminal complement component deficiencies, anatomic or functional asplenia	

Table continued on following page

Table 3–4 ■ SELECTED IMMUNIZING AGENTS INDICATED FOR ADULTS* *Continued*

DISEASE	MAJOR INDICATIONS	COMMENTS AND PRECAUTIONS
Mumps	All adults born after 1956 without history of live vaccine on or after 1st birthday	Altered immunity is a contraindication
Pneumococcal disease	Adults with cardiovascular disease, pulmonary disease, diabetes mellitus, alcoholism, cirrhosis, cerebrospinal fluid leaks, splenic dysfunction or anatomic asplenia, Hodgkin's disease, lymphoma, multiple myeloma, chronic renal failure, nephrotic syndrome, immunosuppression, HIV infection; high-risk populations such as certain Native Americans and *all* adults ≥65 yr	
Poliomyelitis	Certain adults who are at greater risk of exposure to wild poliovirus than the general population	OPV: immunodeficiency diseases are a contraindication
Rabies	High-risk persons	Further doses needed following exposure
Rubella	Adults, particularly women of childbearing age, who lack history of rubella vaccine and detectable rubella-specific antibodies in serum	Women should be counseled to avoid pregnancy for 3 mo; pregnancy and altered immunity are contraindications
Tetanus	All adults	
Varicella	Persons who have contact with patients at high risk of complications from varicella	Immunocompromise and pregnancy are contraindications

HBV = hepatitis B virus; HIV = human immunodeficiency virus; OPV = live virus trivalent oral polio vaccine.

*See the package inserts and more comprehensive sources, including *Cecil Textbook of Medicine,* 21st ed, for a full list of indications, schedules, precautions, and contraindications.

about 5% of alcoholics. It consists of agitated arousal, global confusion and disorientation, insomnia, and vivid, often threatening hallucinations and delusions.

Diagnosis and Treatment

Simple screening questionnaires such as the CAGE outperform laboratory measures in detecting excessive alcohol consumption (Fig. 3–2). Mild-to-moderate ethanol intoxication requires no specific therapy. Gastric lavage may be performed if obtundation is due to recent and massive alcohol consumption, but it must be

Table 3–5 ■ BLOOD ETHANOL LEVELS AND SYMPTOMS

BLOOD ETHANOL LEVELS (mg/dL)	SYMPTOMS	
	Sporadic Drinkers	**Chronic Drinkers**
50–100	Euphoria, gregariousness, incoordination	Minimal or no effect
100–200	Slurred speech, ataxia, labile mood, drowsiness, nausea	Sobriety or incoordination Euphoria
200–300	Lethargy, combativeness Stupor, incoherent speech Vomiting	Mild emotional and motor changes
300–400	Coma	Drowsiness
>500	Respiratory depression, death	Lethargy, stupor, coma

preceded by endotracheal intubation. Hemodialysis should be considered if the blood alcohol concentration exceeds 500 mg/dL or when methanol or ethylene glycol has been ingested concurrently.

Treatment of alcohol withdrawal includes managing delirium and autonomic stability and preventing seizures. Patients with mild

Table 3–6 ■ ALCOHOL-RELATED MEDICAL DISORDERS

AFFECTED ORGAN OR SYSTEM	DISORDERS
Nutrition	Deficiencies of Vitamins: folate, thiamine, pyridoxine, niacin, riboflavin Minerals: magnesium, zinc, calcium Protein
Metabolites and electrolytes	Hypoglycemia, ketoacidosis, hyperlipidemia, hyperuricemia, hypomagnesemia, hypophosphatemia
Gastrointestinal tract	Liver: fatty liver, hepatitis, cirrhosis Gut: esophagitis, gastritis Pancreatitis
Nervous system	Brain: hepatic encephalopathy, Wernicke-Korsakoff syndrome, central pontine myelinolysis Neuromuscular: neuropathy, myopathy Amblyopia
Cardiovascular	Heart: arrhythmia, cardiomyopathy Hypertension
Bone marrow	Macrocytosis, anemia, thrombocytopenia, leukopenia
Endocrine	Pseudo–Cushing's syndrome, testicular atrophy, amenorrhea
Other	Traumatic injury Aerodigestive neoplasms Osteopenia Fetal alcohol syndrome

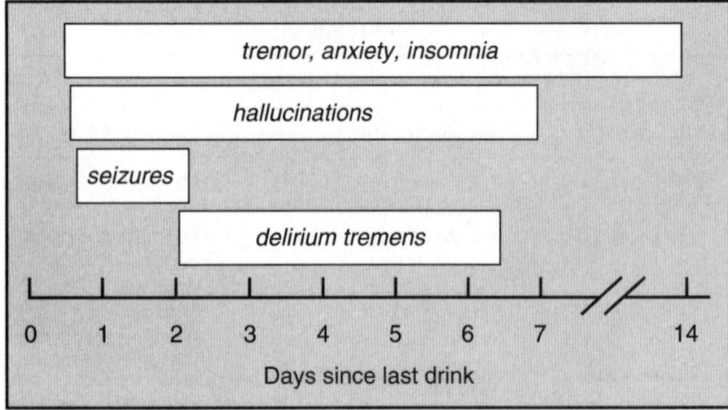

FIGURE 3–1 ■ Time course of alcohol withdrawal.

tremulousness and few associated symptoms usually respond to oral diazepam 5 to 10 mg every 4 to 6 hours. The dosage is then reduced by 20 to 25% on successive days or increased if symptoms of withdrawal return. β-Blockers are useful ancillary therapy. If withdrawal is more severe, patients may require hourly medication at doses that would be fatal in non-tolerant persons. Benzodiazepines should not be given intramuscularly because of inconsistent absorption. Alcohol withdrawal seizures can often be managed with intravenous benzodiazepines such as diazepam or lorazepam.

Delirium tremens requires hospitalization and vigorous management in an intensive care setting. The goal is to control behavior and suppress symptoms. Five to 10 mg or more of diazepam is given intravenously every 5 to 15 minutes until the patient is calm, and maintenance therapy is continued every 1 to 4 hours, as needed.

Alcoholics stop drinking for many reasons, including serious alcohol-related medical, surgical, or psychiatric conditions. Hence symptoms or signs of trauma, infection, liver disease, gastritis, pancreatitis, arrhythmia, or electrolyte disturbance should be sought. Thiamine 100 mg should be given intravenously to all patients to prevent or treat Wernicke's encephalopathy.

Heavy drinkers should be counseled. Diverse psychosocial interventions are equally effective, and a successful outcome is related more to interested personal intervention than to psychotherapy. Disulfiram can be helpful in carefully selected patients. The opiate antagonist naltrexone (ReVia), the only other agent currently approved by the Food and Drug Administration (FDA) for the treatment of alcoholism, appears to decrease the relapse rate in abstinent alcoholics.

DRUG ABUSE AND DEPENDENCE

Heroin and Other Opioids

In the United States, an estimated 2.5 million people have reported prior use of heroin, and more than 100,000 addicts are enrolled in over 700 methadone maintenance programs. Heroin may

3

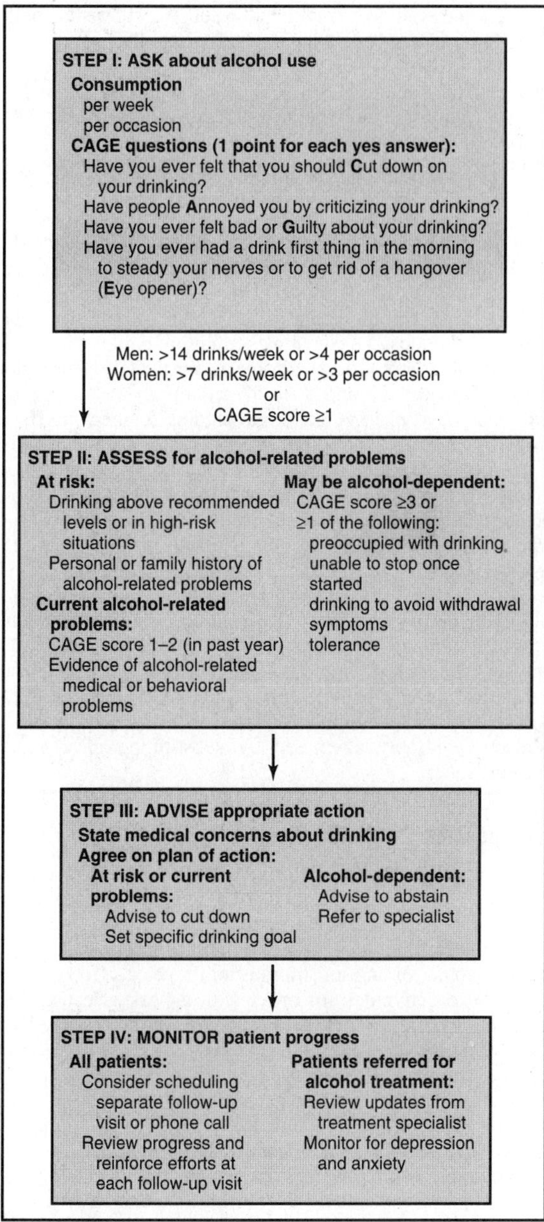

STEP I: ASK about alcohol use
Consumption
per week
per occasion
CAGE questions (1 point for each yes answer):
Have you ever felt that you should Cut down on your drinking?
Have people Annoyed you by criticizing your drinking?
Have you ever felt bad or Guilty about your drinking?
Have you ever had a drink first thing in the morning to steady your nerves or to get rid of a hangover (Eye opener)?
Men: >14 drinks/week or >4 per occasion
Women: >7 drinks/week or >3 per occasion
or
CAGE score ≥1
STEP II: ASSESS for alcohol-related problems
At risk:
Drinking above recommended levels or in high-risk situations
Personal or family history of alcohol-related problems
Current alcohol-related problems:
CAGE score 1–2 (in past year)
Evidence of alcohol-related medical or behavioral problems
May be alcohol-dependent:
CAGE score ≥3 or
≥1 of the following:
preoccupied with drinking
unable to stop once started
drinking to avoid withdrawal symptoms
tolerance
STEP III: ADVISE appropriate action
State medical concerns about drinking
Agree on plan of action:
At risk or current problems:
Advise to cut down
Set specific drinking goal
Alcohol-dependent:
Advise to abstain
Refer to specialist
STEP IV: MONITOR patient progress
All patients:
Consider scheduling separate follow-up visit or phone call
Review progress and reinforce efforts at each follow-up visit
Patients referred for alcohol treatment:
Review updates from treatment specialist
Monitor for depression and anxiety

FIGURE 3–2 ■ Screening and brief intervention for alcohol problems in clinical practice.

be injected intravenously or subcutaneously, snorted, smoked, or ingested. High levels of tolerance develop rapidly.

From the patient's perspective, withdrawal from heroin is a dreaded clinical condition, but it is not life-threatening. The acute withdrawal syndrome will peak in intensity after 36 to 72 hours and resolve over a period of 5 to 7 days.

Most opioid-related medical complications occur as a result of the spread of infectious agents by injection drug use among heroin addicts. The major cardiac complication is bacterial endocarditis, and the most common pulmonary complication is bacterial pneumonia. Renal complications include acute diseases (myoglobinuria, necrotizing angiitis, glomerulonephritis associated with endocarditis or hepatitis) and chronic diseases (nephrotic syndrome, renal failure, renal amyloidosis). The most common pathologic finding in heroin-associated nephrotic syndrome is focal and diffuse glomerulosclerosis. Between 50 and 90% of patients in methadone maintenance clinics have positive serologic studies for hepatitis B and C. Seizures, most often generalized, are the most common non-infectious neurologic complication. Other neurologic complications include transverse myelitis, brachial and lumbosacral plexitis, peripheral neuropathies, and myopathies.

Pharmacologic treatment of opioid abuse can be approached in three ways: agonist substitution, antagonist treatment, or symptomatic treatment. With detoxification, the goal is amelioration of the symptoms of heroin or other opioid withdrawal by methadone (agonist substitution) with a slow taper over a period of 1 to 6 months, by clonidine (symptomatic treatment) for 5 to 7 days, or by a combination of clonidine and naltrexone (antagonist treatment) for 3 to 5 days. Prevention of relapse to active heroin abuse has been most commonly attempted by substitution of a safer drug (e.g., methadone).

Cocaine and Other Psychostimulants

In 1996 an estimated 1.7 million Americans, 0.8% of the population aged 12 years and older, had used cocaine in the prior month. Cocaine can be smoked, orally ingested, applied to mucous membranes, or injected intravenously. The onset of action varies according to the route of administration: oral, peak effect in 1 hour; intranasal, 3 to 5 minutes for onset with a peak effect in 30 to 60 minutes; intravenous, onset in 12 to 16 seconds, with 10 to 20 minutes' duration of effect; and smoked, onset in 6 to 8 seconds with 5 to 10 minutes' duration of effect.

The acute effects of cocaine include intense euphoria, increased energy and self-confidence, enhanced mental acuity and sensory awareness (including sexual), decreased appetite, and sympathomimetic symptoms. Withdrawal symptoms are the inverse of the acute effects. Chronic users become tolerant to its acute effects.

Cocaine use leads to ischemia and myocardial infarction as a result of increased myocardial demand because of tachycardia and hypertension, to diffuse and local coronary spasm in normal or atherosclerotic arteries, and to a propensity to thrombus formation. Other cardiac complications include supraventricular and ventricular arrhythmias, cardiomyopathy, and myocarditis. Other complications of cocaine use include vascular headaches, rhabdomyolysis with acute renal failure, chronic rhinitis, perforated nasal septum, pulmonary edema, and sexual dysfunction. Cocaine abuse is treated by psychotherapy, behavioral therapy, and 12-step programs.

ELECTRICAL INJURY

Tissue damage associated with electrical injury occurs when electrical energy is converted to thermal energy and causes a thermal burn. Cardiopulmonary arrest is common in patients with high-voltage electrical injuries, particularly lightning injury. In patients who survive to be admitted to the hospital, the electrical burn itself becomes a major focus of treatment. Underlying injury to major muscle compartments is accompanied by edema formation, signs of vessel and nerve compression, loss of sensation, pain, and decreased pulses. Because extremities sustain the majority of direct electrical injuries, associated peripheral nerves are most often damaged at the time of contact. Such injuries are usually permanent and may determine the ultimate salvageability of the extremity.

Patients in whom cardiac arrest has occurred frequently respond to cardiopulmonary resuscitation, particularly after lightning injury. Fluid loss into damaged tissue is replenished with lactated Ringer's solution sufficient to maintain a urinary output of 50 to 75 mL/hour. Wound care involves treating both the cutaneous and deep soft tissue injuries.

HEAVY METAL POISONING

Lead

The major toxic effects of lead are referable to the abdomen, the blood, and the nervous system. The crampy, diffuse, often intractable abdominal pain may be accompanied by nausea, vomiting, anorexia, constipation, or occasionally diarrhea. Anemia is frequent in severe acute lead poisoning; it may be normocytic normochromic but usually is microcytic hypochromic. The red blood cell abnormalities include punctate basophilic stippling. The central nervous system symptoms include irritability, incoordination, memory lapses, labile affect, sleep disturbances, restlessness, listlessness, paranoia, headache, lethargy, and dizziness. Wristdrop and footdrop occur.

Blood lead levels and a careful examination of the peripheral blood for basophilic stippling establish the diagnosis. Three agents promote lead's biologic inactivation and elimination from tissues: dimercaprol (BAL, British antilewisite), calcium disodium edetate (Calcium Disodium Versenate), and D-penicillamine.

Mercury

The greatest exposure to metallic mercury is in industry. Heavy aerosol exposure to mercury produces chills, fever, cough, chest pain, and hemoptysis; radiographs show diffuse pulmonary infiltrates. In contrast, ingesting even large amounts of metallic mercury usually produces no clinical disturbance. Exposure to the salts of mercury causes proteinuria, granular casts in the urinary sediment, the nephrotic syndrome, and pyuria from tubular damage.

Arsenic

Elemental arsenic is not toxic even if ingested in substantial amounts. Arsine gas poisoning is usually overwhelming and frequently fatal. Arsenic salt ingestion can be insidious or overwhelming with cramping abdominal pain, diarrhea, nausea, vomiting, dysphagia, cyanosis, headache, hematuria, and weakness. Hyperesthesia, muscle cramps, conjunctivitis, syncope, excessive thirst, periorbital swelling, epistaxis, and tinnitus may also occur. The most prominent manifestation after the first week of illness is symmetrical polyneuropathy. Chronic exposure is associated with cutaneous lesions, particularly hyperpigmentation (arsenic melanosis) and hyperkeratoses located primarily on the palms and soles.

If the diagnosis is suspected, arsenic concentrations can be measured in blood, urine, hair, or nails. The treatment of choice is dimercaprol given within the first 24 hours after exposure.

CHAPTER 4

PRINCIPLES OF EVALUATION AND MANAGEMENT

Although modern medicine has shifted attention toward the laboratory, even today most of the diagnostic process is accomplished through history taking and physical examination (Table 4–1). The physical examination should follow a standard order and be performed in a systematic manner.

The impact of information from tests is often expressed as *probabilities* (Table 4–2). It is often useful to use *odds* to quantify uncertainty instead of probability. Odds of 1:2 suggest that the likelihood of an event is only half the likelihood that the event will not occur. The relationship between odds and probability is ex-

Table 4–1 ▪ THE PATIENT'S MEDICAL HISTORY

Description of patient
  Age, sex, race, occupation, and, for women, parity
Chief complaint
  Four or 5 words, preferably quoting the patient, stating the purpose of the visit and the duration of the complaint; occasionally the patient states the visit and the duration of the complaint; occasionally the patient states a request (e.g., "I need a flu shot") instead of a complaint
Other physicians involved in the patient's care
  Name, address, telephone number, and relationship to the patient
History of the present illness
  For each major symptom, what, where, when, how much, chronologic course, what makes the symptom better or worse, past medical care, questions to narrow diagnostic possibilities
Past medical history
  Previous illnesses and hospitalizations, immunization, medications the patient takes, allergies, and alcohol, tobacco, and drug habits
Social and occupational history
  Description of a typical day in the patient's life and how the present illness affects it, social supports (family, friends, and colleagues) available to the patient, and occupational history
Family history
  History of genetically related diseases in the patient's family and longevity and cause of death of family members
Review of systems
  Systematic review of major organ systems: skin, hematopoietic system (including lymph nodes), head, eyes, ears, nose, mouth, throat, neck, breasts, and respiratory, cardiovascular, gastrointestinal, genitourinary, musculoskeletal, nervous, endocrine, and psychiatric systems

---

For more information about this subject, see the corresponding chapters in *Cecil Textbook of Medicine,* 21st edition. Philadelphia, W.B. Saunders Company, 2000. Part V: Principles of Evaluation and Management, pages 77–125.

Table 4–2 ■ KEY DEFINITIONS*

Probability = A number between 0 and 1 that expresses an estimate of the likelihood of an event.
Odds = The ratio of [the probability of an event] to [the probability of the event not occurring].

Test Performance Characteristics

Sensitivity = Percentage of patients with disease who have an abnormal test result.
Specificity = Percentage of patients without disease who have a normal test result.
Positive predictive value (PV+) = Percentage of patients with an abnormal test result who actually have disease.
Negative predictive value (PV−) = Percentage of patients with a normal test result who do not have disease.

Bayesian Analysis

Pre-test (or prior) probability = The probability of a disease before the information is acquired.
Post-test (or posterior) probability = The probability of an event after new information is acquired.

$$\text{Pre-test (or prior) odds} = \frac{\text{Pre-test probability of disease}}{(1 - \text{pre-test probability of disease})}$$

$$\text{Likelihood ratio} = \frac{\text{Probability of result in diseased persons}}{\text{Probability of result in non-diseased persons}}$$

*Note that *disease* can mean a condition, such as coronary artery disease, or an outcome, such as postoperative cardiac complications.

pressed in the formula:

$$\text{Odds} = p/(1 - p)$$

where p is the probability of an event.

To calculate the post-test odds of disease, pre-test odds are multiplied by the *likelihood ratio* (LR) for a specific test result. The mathematical presentation of this form of Bayes' theorem is as follows:

$$\text{Post-tests odds} = (\text{Pre-test odds}) \times (\text{LR})$$

Post-test odds can be converted to post-test probabilities according to the following formula:

$$\text{Probability} = \text{Odds}/(1 + \text{odds})$$

Before ordering a test, clinicians should therefore consider whether that test result could change the choice of management strategies (Table 4–3). This approach is called the threshold approach to medical decision making, and it requires the physician to be able to estimate the threshold probability at which one strategy will be chosen over another.

Because resources available for health care are limited, decisions must be made as to which of the many competing "investments"

Table 4–3 ■ PRINCIPLES OF TEST ORDERING AND INTERPRETATION

1. The interpretation of test results depends on what is already known about the patient.
2. No test is perfect; clinicians should be familiar with their diagnostic performance (see Table 4–2) and never believe that a test "forces" them to pursue a specific management strategy.
3. Tests should be ordered if they may provide *additional* information beyond that already available.
4. Tests should be ordered if there is a reasonable chance that the data will influence patient care.
5. Two tests that provide similar information should not both be ordered.
6. When choosing between two tests that provide similar data, use the test that has lower costs and/or causes less discomfort and inconvenience to the patient.
7. Clinicians should seek all of the information provided by a test, not just a positive or negative result.
8. The cost-effectiveness of strategies using non-invasive tests should be considered in a manner similar to that of therapeutic strategies.

should be chosen. Cost-effectiveness analyses can provide important insights into the relative attractiveness of different management strategies and can also help guide policymakers to determine which technologies to make available.

PRINCIPLES OF DRUG THERAPY

To obtain the desired concentration over time in the presence of kidney disease, adjustments can be made by decreasing the dose while maintaining the dose interval, by maintaining the dose but increasing the interval between doses, or by a combination of both (Table 4–4). Any adjustment of drug dose in kidney disease can use the creatinine clearance to calculate the dose needed because renal drug clearance is proportional to creatinine clearance.

Decreased cardiac output or hypotensive conditions lead to decreased perfusion of the organs, including those responsible for eliminating drugs. As with primary kidney disease, the dose can be adjusted for decreased renal perfusion by using the creatinine clearance. For drugs that have a high hepatic extraction (e.g., lidocaine), decreased hepatic blood flow suggests a need to reduce doses. Unlike renal disease, no useful laboratory test is available on which to base dose adjustments in patients with liver disease.

There are two basic types of drug interaction: pharmacokinetic drug interactions, caused by a change in the amount of drug or active metabolite at the site of action; and pharmacodynamic drug interactions (without a change in pharmacokinetics), due to a change in drug effect. For a detailed listing see standard pharmacology tests.

PAIN

Pain is the most common symptom for which patients seek medical evaluation. The physician's task is twofold: to discover

Table 4–4 ■ ADJUSTMENT OF DRUG DOSAGE IN RENAL FAILURE

DRUG	TYPE OF ELIMINATION	HALF LIFE (hr)		Method*	ADJUSTMENT FOR RENAL FAILURE: GFR (mL/min)			Removed by Dialysis†
		Normal	End-Stage Renal		>50	10–50	<10	
Amikacin	Renal	2–3	30	DD	60–90%	30–70%	20–30%	Yes
				II	12 hr	12–18	24 hr	
Aspirin	Hepatic (renal)	2–19	Unchanged	II	4 hr	4–6 hr	Avoid	Yes
Carbamazepine	Hepatic (renal)	35	?	DD	Unchanged	Unchanged	75%	No
Digoxin	Renal (non-renal) 15–40%)	36–44	80–120	DD	Unchanged	25–75%	10–25%	No
				II	24 hr	36 hr	48 hr	
Disopyramide	Renal + hepatic	5–8	10–18	II	Unchanged	12–24 hr	24–40 hr	No
Ethosuximide	Hepatic, renal	55	60	DD	Unchanged	Unchanged	75%	Yes
Gentamicin sulfate	Renal	2	24–48	DD	60–90%	30–70%	20–30%	Yes
				II	8–12 hr	12 hr	24 hr	
Lidocaine	Hepatic (renal <20%)	1.2–2.2	1.3–3.0	DD	Unchanged	Unchanged	Unchanged	No
Lithium carbonate	Renal	14–28	Prolonged	DD	Unchanged	50–75%	25–50%	Yes

Mexiletine	Hepatic (renal)	8–13	16	DD	Unchanged	Unchanged	50–75%	Yes
Penicillin G	Renal (hepatic)	0.5	6–20	DD	Unchanged	75%	25–50%	Yes
				II	6–8 hr	8–12 hr	12–16 hr	
Phenobarbital	Hepatic (renal 30%)	60–150	117–160	II	Unchanged	Unchanged	12–16 hr	Yes
Phenytoin	Hepatic (renal)	24	8	DD	Unchanged	Unchanged	Unchanged	No
Primidone	Hepatic (renal <20%)	8	12	II	8 hr	8–12 hr	12–24 hr	Yes
Procainamide	Renal (hepatic 7–24%)	2.5–4.9	5.3–5.9	II	4 hr	6–12 hr	8–24 hr	Yes
Quinidine sulfate	Hepatic (renal 10–50%)	5.0–7.2	4–14	II	Unchanged	Unchanged	Unchanged	Yes
Theophylline	Hepatic	3–12	?	DD	Unchanged	Unchanged	Unchanged	Yes
Tobramycin	Renal	2.5	56	DD	60–90%	30–70%	20–30%	Yes
				II	8–12 hr	12 hr	24 hr	
Valproic acid	Hepatic	Biphasic I and 12	10	DD	Unchanged	Unchanged	Unchanged	No
Vancomycin	Renal	6–8	200–250	II	24–72 hr	72–240 hr	240 hr	No

GFR = glomerular filtration rate.
*Method: DD (alone)—decrease dose (maintain same interval); II (alone)—increase interval between doses (maintain dose); DD and II (together)—combination of both approaches.
†Dialysis refers to hemodialysis.

and treat the cause of the pain and to treat the pain itself (Table 4–5). No patient should be evaluated inadequately because of a significant pain problem.

Analgesic drugs can be divided into three groups. The *non-opioid analgesics,* such as aspirin and acetaminophen, and the non-steroidal anti-inflammatory drugs (NSAIDs) act both peripherally and, in some instances, centrally, through inhibition of various enzyme systems. The *opioid agonist* drugs activate opioid receptors in the central and peripheral nervous systems. The *adjuvant analgesic* drugs produce analgesia in certain pain states (e.g., amitriptyline, paroxetine, and gabapentin in neuropathic pain) or potentiate the opioid analgesics.

Non-opioid analgesics have a ceiling effect, and their long-term use is compromised by gastrointestinal and hematologic side effects (Table 4–6). Effective use of opioid analgesics requires balancing the desirable effects of pain relief against the undesirable side effects of nausea, vomiting, mental clouding, sedation, tolerance, and physical dependence (Table 4–7). Combining drugs enables the physician to improve pain relief without escalating the opioid dose. Several combinations have proved effective, including an opioid plus a non-opioid (aspirin, acetaminophen, or ibuprofen), an opioid plus an amphetamine (dextroamphetamine 10 mg), and an opioid plus an antihistamine (hydroxyzine 100 mg intramuscularly).

Patient-controlled analgesia (PCA) is a useful approach to treat both acute pain associated with mental illness (postoperative pain, sickle cell pain) and chronic cancer-related pain (Tables 4–8 and 4–9). The management of cancer pain attempts to integrate assessment techniques, drug therapy, and anesthetic, neurosurgical, and behavioral approaches, as well emphasizing continuity of care.

Table 4–5 ■ CLINICAL ASSESSMENT OF PAIN

1. Believe the patient's complaint of pain
2. Take a careful history of the pain complaint to place it temporally in the patient's history
3. Assess the characteristics of each pain, including site, referral pattern, and aggravating and relieving factors
4. Clarify the temporal aspects of the pain: acute, subacute, chronic, episodic, intermittent, breakthrough, or incident
5. List and prioritize each pain complaint
6. Evaluate the response to previous and current analgesic therapies
7. Evaluate the psychological state of the patient
8. Ask if the patient has a past history of alcohol or drug dependence
9. Perform a careful medical and neurologic examination
10. Develop a series of diagnosis-related hypotheses
11. Order and personally review the appropriate diagnostic procedures
12. Design the diagnostic and therapeutic approach to suit the individual
13. Provide continuity of care from evaluation to treatment to ensure patient compliance and to reduce patient anxiety
14. Reassess the patient's response to pain therapy
15. Discuss advance directives for managing pain of dying patients

Table 4–6 ■ EFFECTS OF COMMONLY USED ANALGESIC AND ANTIPYRETIC AGENTS

	ACETYLSALICYLIC ACID						
	Low Dose*	Intermediate Dose*	High Dose*	SODIUM SALICYLATE	TRADITIONAL NSAIDs	SELECTIVE COX-2 INHIBITORS	ACETAMINOPHEN
Antipyretic	0	+	+	+	+	+	+
Analgesic	0	+	+	+	+	+	+
Anti-inflammatory	0	0	+	+	+	+	0
Inhibit prostaglandin synthesis of platelets	+	+	+	0	+	0	0
Inhibit prostaglandin synthesis systemically	0	+	+	±	+	+	0
Inhibit colon cancer	?	+	?	?	+	?	0
Retard Alzheimer's disease	?	+	?	?	+	?	0
Prevent coronary, cerebral thrombosis	+	+	?	?	?	0	0

NSAIDs = non-steroidal anti-inflammatory drugs.
*Low dose, 80 to 325 mg/d; intermediate dose, 650 mg to 3 g/d; high dose > 3 g/d.

Table 4–7 ■ GUIDELINES FOR THE USE OF ANALGESICS IN THE MANAGEMENT OF PAIN

1. Start with a specific drug for a specific type of pain
2. Individualize the choice of drug, dose, timing, and route of administration
3. Know the pharmacology of the drug prescribed
   a. Relative potency of the drug
   b. Duration of the analgesic effect
   c. Pharmacokinetics of the drug
   d. Equianalgesic doses of the drug and its route of administration
4. Administer analgesics on a regular basis
5. Use a combination of drugs to provide additive analgesia
   a. Opioid plus non-opioid (e.g., aspirin, acetaminophen, and NSAIDs)
   b. Opioids plus adjuvants (e.g., hydroxyzine and dextroamphetamine)
6. Gear the route of administration to the patient's needs:

Oral	Transdermal
Buccal	Subcutaneous
Sublingual	Intravenous
Transmucosal	Intrathecal
Intranasal	Intraventricular
Rectal	

7. Anticipate and treat side effects:

Sedation	Constipation
Respiratory depression	Multifocal myoclonus
Nausea and vomiting	Seizures

8. Know the differences among tolerance, physical dependence, and psychological dependence
9. Prevent and treat acute withdrawal
10. Know how to manage the tolerant patient:
    a. Use combinations of non-opioid and opioid drugs
    b. Use combinations of drug therapy, anesthetic, and neurosurgical procedures
    c. Switch to an alternative opioid analgesic starting with one-fourth to one-half the equianalgesic dose and titrate to analgesia
    d. Use epidural local anesthetics alone or in combination with opioids
11. Reassess the nature of the pain
12. Do not use placebos to assess pain

NSAIDs = non-steroidal anti-inflammatory drugs.

GLUCOCORTICOSTEROIDS IN RELATION TO INFLAMMATORY DISEASE

The variety of glucocorticosteroid preparations available for systemic use differ in their relative anti-inflammatory potency, potential for sodium retention, and plasma and biologic half-lives (Table 4–10). The decision to implement therapy with glucocorticosteroids must be derived from a precise understanding of these agents and the often formidable adverse reactions that accompany their use (Table 4–11).

Therapy is usually initiated as a single oral morning dose of prednisone 0.5 to 1.0 mg/kg. The once-daily regimen is maintained until the disease is stable and clinical improvement is recognized or deemed unlikely or side effects develop. Tapering should not be

4

Table 4–8 ■ OPIOID ANALGESIC DRUGS

DRUG	EQUIANALGESIC DOSE
Codeine	32–65*
Oxycodone	5*
Meperidine	50*
Propoxyphene HCl (Darvon)	65–130*
Pentazocine	50*
Butorphanol tartrate (Stadol)	2*
Morphine (MSIR, MS Contin, Roxanol, Kadian)	10–60†
Hydromorphone HCl (Dilaudid)	1.5–8.0†
Methadone HCl (Dolophine)	10–20†
Levorphanol tartrate (Levo-Dromoran)	2–4†
Fentanyl (Duragesic)	NA
Oxycodone (OxyContin)	15/30†
Oxymorphone	1/10 PR

NA = not applicable; PR = per rectum.
*Equianalgesic doses for mild to moderate pain compared with 650 mg aspirin.
†Equianalgesic doses by IM/oral routes for severe pain compared with 10 mg IM morphine standard.

undertaken until the disease process is clinically quiescent, at which time reduction to an alternate-day regimen should be initiated with the goal of administering enough prednisone on the high-dose, or "on," day to suppress disease activity on the low-dose, or "off," day.

The possibility of hypothalamic-pituitary-adrenal suppression in patients receiving chronic glucocorticosteroid therapy is problematic, particularly around times of stress, such as surgery. The amount of supplemental glucocorticosteroids required during surgery can be estimated by ascertaining the "amount" of stress (minor, moderate, or severe) anticipated in the perioperative period, with an upward adjustment of daily hydrocortisone (25 mg for minor stress; 50–75 mg for moderate stress, 100–150 mg for major stress) for up to 3 days.

Topical and ophthalmic glucocorticosteroid preparations can often control cutaneous and ocular disease. Glucocorticosteroids administered nasally for allergic rhinitis, by inhalation for asthma or lower airway disease, and intra-articularly or by soft tissue injection for musculoskeletal inflammatory conditions may control the underlying disease. When local glucocorticosteroid therapy and even systemic daily oral treatment are inadequate to control the underlying disease, intermittent, short-term, high-dose intravenous methylprednisolone can be used in inflammatory and immunologically mediated diseases, using 3- to 5-day regimens at 20 mg/kg/day or 1 g/m^2/day.

Table 4–9 ■ GUIDELINES FOR MANAGING CHRONIC OPIOID THERAPY FOR NON-MALIGNANT PAIN

1. Opioid therapy should be considered only after all other reasonable attempts at analgesia have failed.
2. A history of substance abuse, severe character disorder, and chaotic home environment should be viewed as relative contraindications.
3. A single practitioner should take primary responsibility for treatment.
4. Patients should give informed consent before the start of therapy; points to be covered include recognition of the low risk of true addiction as an outcome, potential for cognitive impairment with the drug alone and in combination with sedative-hypnotics, likelihood that physical dependence will occur (abstinence syndrome possible with acute discontinuation), and understanding by female patients that children born when the mother is on opioid maintenance therapy will likely be physically dependent at birth.
5. After drug selection, doses should be given around the clock; several weeks should be agreed on as the period of initial dose titration; and although improvement in function should be continually stressed, all should agree to at least partial analgesia as the appropriate goal of therapy.
6. Failure to achieve at least partial analgesia at relatively low initial doses in the non-tolerant patient raises questions about the potential treatability of the pain syndrome with opioids.
7. Emphasis should be given to attempts to capitalize on improved analgesia by gains in physical and social function; opioid therapy should be considered complementary to other analgesic and rehabilitative approaches.
8. In addition to the daily dose determined initially, patients should be permitted to escalate the dose transiently on days of increased pain; 2 methods are acceptable: (a) prescription of an additional 4–6 "rescue doses" to be taken as needed during the month; (b) instruction that 1 or 2 extra doses may be taken on any day but must be followed by an equal reduction of dose on subsequent days.
9. Initially, patients must be seen and drugs prescribed at least monthly. When stable, less frequent visits may be acceptable.
10. Exacerbations of pain not effectively treated by transient, small increases in dose are best managed in the hospital, where dose escalation, if appropriate, can be observed closely and a return to baseline doses can be accomplished in a controlled environment.
11. Evidence of drug hoarding, acquisition of drugs from other physicians, uncontrolled dose escalation, or other aberrant behaviors must be carefully assessed. In some cases, tapering and discontinuing opioid therapy is necessary. Other patients may appropriately continue therapy within rigid guidelines. Consideration should be given to consulting with an addiction specialist.
12. At each visit, assessment should specifically address:
    a. Comfort (degree of analgesia)
    b. Opioid-related side effects
    c. Functional status (physical and psychosocial)
    d. Existence of aberrant drug-related behaviors
13. Use of self-report instruments may be helpful but should not be required.
14. Documentation is essential; and the medical record should specifically address comfort, function, side effects, and the occurrence of aberrant behaviors repeatedly during the course of therapy.

From Portenoy RK: Opioid therapy for chronic nonmalignant pain: Current status. *In* Fields HL, Liebeskind JC (eds): Progress in Pain Research and Management, vol 1. Seattle, IASP Press, 1994, p 247.

Table 4–10 ■ GLUCOCORTICOSTEROID PREPARATIONS

	ANTI-INFLAMMATORY POTENCY	EQUIVALENT DOSE (mg)	SODIUM-RETAINING POTENCY	PLASMA HALF-LIFE (min)	BIOLOGIC HALF-LIFE (hr)
Hydrocortisone	1	20	2+	90	8–12
Cortisone	0.8	25	2+	30	8–12
Prednisone	4	5	1+	60	12–36
Prednisolone	4	5	1+	200	12–36
Methylprednisolone	5	4	0	180	12–36
Triamcinolone	5	4	0	300	12–36
Betamethasone	20–30	0.6	0	100–300	36–54
Dexamethasone	20–30	0.75	0	100–300	36–54

From Garber EK, Targoff C, Paulus HE: *In* Paulus HE, Furst DE, Droomgoole SH (eds): Drugs for Rheumatic Diseases. New York, Churchill Livingstone, 1987, p 446.

Table 4–11 ■ SIDE EFFECTS OF GLUCOCORTICOSTEROID THERAPY

Characteristic early in therapy: essentially unavoidable
- Insomnia
- Emotional lability
- Enhanced appetite or weight gain or both

Common in patients with underlying risk factors or other drug toxicities
- Hypertension
- Diabetes mellitus
- Peptic ulcer disease
- Acne vulgaris

Anticipated with use of sustained and intense treatment: minimize risk by conservative dosing regimens and steroid-sparing agents when possible
- Cushingoid habitus
- Hypothalamic-pituitary-adrenal suppression
- Infection diathesis
- Osteonecrosis
- Myopathy
- Impaired wound healing

Insidious and delayed: likely dependent on cumulative dose
- Osteoporosis
- Skin atrophy
- Cataracts
- Atherosclerosis
- Growth retardation
- Fatty liver

Rare and unpredictable
- Psychosis
- Pseudotumor cerebri
- Glaucoma
- Epidural lipomatosis
- Pancreatitis

From Boumpas DT, Chrousos GP, Wilder RL, et al: Glucocorticoid therapy for immune-mediated diseases: Basic and clinical correlates. Ann Intern Med 119:1198, 1993.

CHAPTER 5

CARDIOVASCULAR DISEASES

5

APPROACH TO THE PATIENT WITH POSSIBLE CARDIOVASCULAR DISEASE

History

Chest discomfort or pain is the cardinal manifestation of myocardial ischemia due to coronary artery disease or any condition that causes myocardial ischemia. New, acute, often ongoing pain may indicate an acute myocardial infarction (MI), unstable angina, or aortic dissection; a pulmonary cause such as acute pulmonary embolism or pleural irritation; a musculoskeletal condition of the chest wall, thorax, or shoulder; or a gastrointestinal abnormality such as esophageal reflux or spasm, peptic ulcer disease, or cholecystitis (Table 5–1). Functional status should be assessed using standardized approaches (Table 5–2).

In cardiovascular conditions, dyspnea is usually caused by increases in pulmonary venous pressure due to left ventricular (LV) failure or valvular heart disease. Orthopnea, which is an exacerbation of dyspnea when the patient is recumbent, is due to increased work of breathing because of either increased venous return to the pulmonary vasculature or loss of gravitational assistance in diaphragmatic effort. Paroxysmal nocturnal dyspnea is severe dyspnea that awakens a patient at night and forces the assumption of a sitting or standing position to achieve gravitational redistribution of fluid.

Palpitations may be caused by any arrhythmia with or without important underlying structural heart disease. The feeling associated with a premature atrial or ventricular contraction, often described as a "skipped beat" or a "flip-flopping of the heart," must be distinguished from the irregularly irregular rhythm of atrial fibrillation (AF) and the rapid but regular rhythm of supraventricular tachycardia. Associated symptoms of chest pain, dyspnea, lightheadedness, dizziness, or sweating suggest an important effect on cardiac output and mandate further evaluation (Table 5–3).

Lightheadedness or syncope can be caused by any condition that decreases cardiac output (e.g., bradyarrhythmia, tachyarrhythmia, obstruction of left or right ventricular inflow or outflow, cardiac tamponade, aortic dissection, or severe pump failure), by reflex-mediated vasomotor instability (e.g., vasovagal, situational, or carotid sinus syncope), or orthostatic hypotension. The history, physical examination, and electrocardiogram (ECG) are often diagnostic.

For more information about this subject, see the corresponding chapters in *Cecil Textbook of Medicine,* 21st edition. Philadelphia, W.B. Saunders Company, 2000. Part VII: Cardiovascular Diseases, pages 160 to 378.

Table 5–1 ■ CAUSES OF CHEST PAIN

CONDITION	LOCATION	QUALITY	DURATION	AGGRAVATING OR RELIEVING FACTORS	ASSOCIATED SYMPTOMS OR SIGNS
Cardiovascular Causes					
Angina	Retrosternal region; radiates to or occasionally isolated to neck, jaw, epigastrium, shoulder, or arms—left common	Pressure, burning, squeezing, heaviness, indigestion	<2–10 min	Precipitated by exercise, cold weather, or emotional stress; relieved by rest or nitroglycerin; atypical (Prinzmetal's) angina may be unrelated to activity, often early morning	S_3, or murmur of papillary muscle dysfunction during pain
Rest or unstable angina	Same as angina	Same as angina but may be more severe	Usually <20 min	Same as angina, with decreasing tolerance for exertion or at rest	Similar to stable angina, but may be pronounced; transient cardiac failure can occur
Myocardial infarction	Substernal and may radiate like angina	Heaviness, pressure, burning, constriction	Sudden onset ≥30 min but variable	Unrelieved by rest or nitroglycerin	Shortness of breath, sweating, weakness, nausea, vomiting
Pericarditis	Usually begins over sternum or toward cardiac apex and may radiate to neck or left shoulder; often more localized than the pain of myocardial ischemia	Sharp, stabbling, knifelike	Lasts many hours to days; may wax and wane	Aggravated by deep breathing, rotating chest, or supine position; relieved by sitting up and leaning forward	Pericardial friction rub
Aortic dissection	Anterior chest; may radiate to back	Excruciating, tearing, knifelike	Sudden onset, unrelenting	Usually occurs in setting of hypertension or predisposition such as Marfan syndrome	Murmur of aortic insufficiency, pulse or blood pressure asymmetry; neurologic deficit

Noncardiac Causes					
Pneumonia with pleurisy; pulmonary embolism	Localized over involved area	Pleuritic; localized	Brief or prolonged	Painful breathing	Dyspnea, cough, fever, dull to percussion, bronchial breath sounds, rales, occasional pleural rub; signs of acute right ventricular failure, and pulmonary hypertension with large emboli; hemoptysis with pulmonary infarction
Musculoskeletal disorders	Variable	Aching	Short or long duration	Aggravated by movement; history of muscle exertion or injury	Tender to pressure or movement
Esophageal reflux	Substernal, epigastric	Burning, visceral discomfort	10–60 min	Aggravated by large meal, postprandial recumbency; relief with antacid	Water brash
Peptic ulcer	Epigastric, substernal	Visceral burning, aching	Prolonged	Relief with food, antacid	
Gallbladder disease	Epigastric, right upper quadrant	Visceral	Prolonged	May be unprovoked or follow meals	Right upper quadrant tenderness may be present
Anxiety states	Often localized over precordium	Variable; location often moves from place to place	Varies; often fleeting	Situational	Sighing respirations, often chest wall tenderness

From Andreoli TE, Bennett JC, Carpenter CCJ, Plum F: Evaluation of the patient with cardiovascular disease. *In Cecil Essentials of Medicine,* 4th ed. Philadelphia, WB Saunders, 1997, pp 11–12.

Table 5–2 ■ THREE METHODS OF ASSESSING CARDIOVASCULAR DISABILITY

CLASS	NEW YORK HEART ASSOCIATION FUNCTIONAL CLASSIFICATION	CANADIAN CARDIOVASCULAR SOCIETY FUNCTIONAL CLASSIFICATION	SPECIFIC ACTIVITY SCALE
I	Patients with cardiac disease but without resulting limitations of physical activity. Ordinary physical activity does not cause undue fatigue, palpitation, dyspnea, or anginal pain.	Ordinary physical activity, such as walking and climbing stairs, does not cause angina. Angina with strenuous or rapid or prolonged exertion at work or recreation.	Patients can perform to completion any activity requiring ≥ 7 metabolic equivalents, e.g., can carry 24 lb up 8 steps; carry objects that weigh 80 lb; do outdoor work (shovel snow, spade soil); do recreational activities (skiing, basketball, squash, handball, jog/walk 5 mph).
II	Patients with cardiac disease resulting in slight limitation of physical activity. They are comfortable at rest. Ordinary physical activity results in fatigue, palpitations, dyspnea, or anginal pain.	Slight limitation of ordinary activity. Walking or climbing stairs rapidly, walking uphill, walking or stair climbing after meals, in cold, in wind, or when under emotional stress, or only during the few hours after awakening. Walking more than 2 blocks on the level and climbing more than 1 flight of ordinary stairs at a normal pace and in normal conditions.	Patient can perform to completion any activity requiring ≥ 5 metabolic equivalents but cannot and does not perform to completion activities requiring ≥ 7 metabolic equivalents, e.g., have sexual intercourse without stopping, garden, rake, weed, roller-skate, dance fox trot, walk at 4 mph on level ground.

III	Patients with cardiac disease, resulting in marked limitation of physical activity. They are comfortable at rest. Less than ordinary physical activity causes fatigue, palpitations, dyspnea, or anginal pain.	Marked limitation of ordinary physical activity. Walking 1–2 blocks on the level and climbing more than 1 flight in normal conditions.	Patient can perform to completion any activity requiring ≥ 2 metabolic equivalents but cannot and does not perform to completion any activities requiring ≥ 5 metabolic equivalents, e.g., shower without stopping, strip and make bed, clean windows, walk 2.5 mph, bowl, play golf, dress without stopping.
IV	Patient with cardiac disease resulting in inability to carry on any physical activity without discomfort. Symptoms of cardiac insufficiency or of the anginal syndrome may be present even at rest. If any physical activity is undertaken, discomfort is increased.	Inability to carry on any physical activity without discomfort—anginal syndrome *may be* present at rest.	Patient cannot or does not perform to completion activities requiring ≥ 2 metabolic equivalents. *Cannot* carry out activities listed above (Specific Activity Scale, Class III).

From Goldman L, et al: Comparative reproducibility and validity of systems for assessing cardiovascular functional class: Advantages of a new specific activity scale. Circulation 64: 1227, 1981. Reproduced by permission of the American Heart Association.

Table 5–3 ■ AHA/ACC GUIDELINES FOR USE OF DIAGNOSTIC TESTS IN PATIENTS WITH PALPITATIONS*

Ambulatory Electrocardiography	
Class I	Palpitations, syncope, dizziness
Class II	Shortness of breath, chest pain, or fatigue (not otherwise explained, episodic and strongly suggestive of an arrhythmia as the cause because of a relation of the symptom with palpitation)
Class III	Symptoms not reasonably expected to be due to arrhythmia
Electrophysiologic Study	
Class I	1. Patients with palpitations who have a pulse rate documented by medical personnel as inappropriately rapid and in whom electrocardiographic recordings fail to document the cause of the palpitations 2. Patients with palpitations preceding a syncopal episode
Class II	Patients with clinically significant palpitations, suspected to be of cardiac origin, in whom symptoms are sporadic and cannot be documented; studies are performed to determine the mechanisms of arrhythmias, to direct or provide therapy, or to assess prognosis
Class III	Patients with palpitations documented to be due to extracardiac causes (e.g., hyperthyroidism)
Echocardiography	
Class I	Arrhythmias with evidence of heart disease Family history of genetic disorder associated with arrhythmias
Class II	Arrhythmias commonly associated with, but without evidence of, heart disease Atrial fibrillation or flutter
Class III	Palpitation without evidence of arrhythmias Minor arrhythmias without evidence of heart disease

AHA/ACC = American Heart Association/American College of Cardiology.

*Class I, general agreement the test is useful and indicated; class II, frequently used, but there is a divergence of opinion with respect to its utility; class III, general agreement the test is not useful.

Modified from Goldman L, Braunwald E (eds): Primary Cardiology. Philadelphia, WB Saunders, 1998, p 126.

Physical Examination

The external jugular veins help in assessment of mean right atrial pressure, which normally varies between 5 and 10 cm H_2O. The height (in centimeters) of the central venous pressure is measured by adding 5 cm to the height of the observed jugular venous distention above the sternal angle of Louis. Abnormalities of the jugular veins are found in heart failure, pericardial disease, and tricuspid or pulmonic valve disease.

The carotid pulse should be examined for volume and contour. The carotid pulse may be increased in amplitude in patients with a higher stroke volume due to aortic regurgitation, arteriovenous fistula, hyperthyroidism, fever, or anemia. In aortic regurgitation or arteriovenous fistula, the pulse may have a bisferiens quality. The carotid upstroke is delayed in patients with valvular aortic stenosis and has a normal contour but diminished amplitude in any cause of reduced stroke volume.

Low-frequency phenomena such as systolic heaves or lifts from the LV (at the cardiac apex) or right ventricle (RV) (parasternal in the third or fourth intercostal space) are best felt with the heel of the palm. The LV apex is more diffuse and may sometimes be frankly dyskinetic in patients with advanced heart disease. The distal palm is best for feeling thrills.

The first heart sound (S_1) is produced by closure of the mitral and—to a lesser extent—the tricuspid valves. The second heart sound (S_2) is caused primarily by closure of the aortic valve, but closure of the pulmonic valve is also commonly audible; with expiration the two sounds are virtually superimposed, whereas with inspiration the increased stroke volume of the RV commonly leads to a discernible delay and hence splitting of S_2. This splitting may be fixed in patients with an atrial septal defect or a right bundle branch block. The split may be paradoxical in patients with left bundle branch block or other causes of delayed LV emptying.

Early systolic ejection sounds are related to forceful opening of the aortic or pulmonic valve. Midsystolic or late systolic clicks are most commonly caused by mitral valve prolapse.

The third heart sound (S_3) corresponds to rapid ventricular filling during early diastole. After about age 40 years, an S_3 should be considered abnormal. An LV S_3 gallop is best heard at the apex, whereas the RV S_3 gallop is best heart at the fourth intercostal space at the left parasternal border. A fourth heart sound (S_4) is rarely heard in young persons but is common in adults older than 40 or 50 years because of reduced ventricular compliance during atrial contraction (Fig. 5–1).

Heart murmurs may be classified as systolic, diastolic, or continuous. Murmurs are graded by intensity on a scale of 1 to 6. Grade 1 is faint and appreciated only by careful auscultation; 2, readily audible; 3, moderately loud; 4, loud and associated with a palpable thrill; 5, loud and audible with the stethoscope only partially placed on the chest; 6, loud enough to be heard without the stethoscope on the chest. Maneuvers such as inspiration, expiration, standing, squatting, and handgripping can be especially useful in the differential diagnosis of a murmur; however, echocardiography will commonly be required to make a definitive diagnosis of both cause and severity (Tables 5–4 and 5–5).

The most common cause of hepatomegaly in patients with heart disease is engorgement from elevated right-sided pressures associated with RV failure of any cause. Hepatojugular reflux is elicited by pressing on the liver and showing an increase in the jugular venous pressure; it indicates advanced RV failure or obstruction to RV filling.

The extremities should be evaluated for peripheral pulses, edema, cyanosis, and clubbing. Diminished peripheral pulses suggest peripheral arterial disease. Delayed pulses in the legs are consistent with coarctation of the aorta and are also seen after aortic dissection.

All patients with known or suspected cardiac disease should have an ECG and chest radiograph. Echocardiography is the most useful test to analyze valvular and ventricular function. Using Doppler

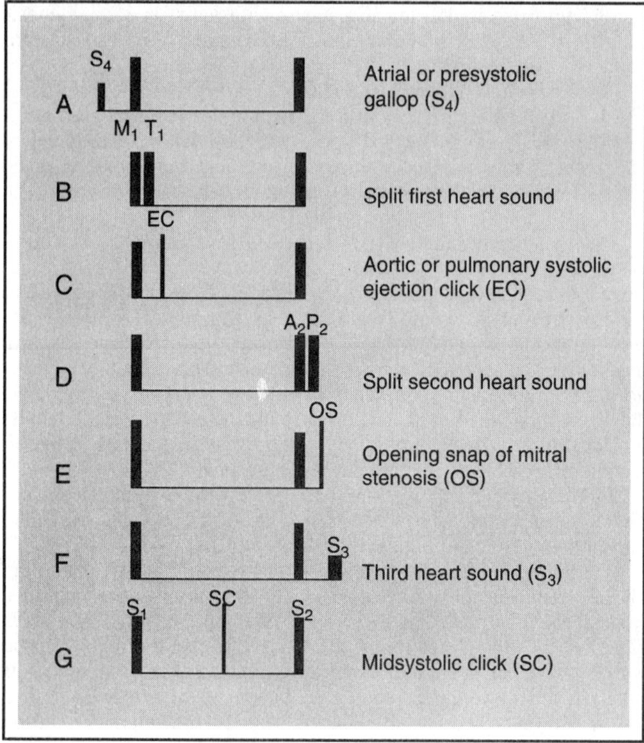

FIGURE 5–1 ■ Timing of the different heart sounds and added sounds. (Modified and reproduced, with permission, from Wood P: *Diseases of the Heart and Circulation,* 3rd ed. Philadelphia, JB Lippincott, 1968.)

flow methods, both stenotic and regurgitant lesions can be quantified.

For more information about this subject, see *Cecil Textbook of Medicine,* 21st edition. Philadelphia, W.B. Saunders Company, 2000. Chapter 38, Approach to the Patient with Possible Cardiovascular Disease, pages 160 to 167.

CARDIAC FUNCTION AND CIRCULATORY CONTROL

Cardiac performance depends on four fundamental factors: (1) preload, (2) afterload, (3) ventricular contractility, and (4) heart rate.

Preload, which refers to the degree to which sarcomeres are stretched just before the onset of systole, is generally defined for the ventricle as either end-diastolic pressure or end-diastolic volume. An increase in preload leads to an increase in ventricular pressure and flow generation.

Afterload refers to the physical forces that must be overcome for myocytes to shorten and for the ventricle to eject blood. In the

Table 5–4 ■ SOME COMMON CAUSES OF HEART MURMURS

	USUAL LOCATION	COMMON ASSOCIATED FINDINGS
SYSTOLIC		
Holosystolic		
Mitral regurgitation (MR)	Apex → axilla	↑ With handgrip; S_3 if marked MR; LV dilation common
Tricuspid regurgitation (TR)	LLSB	↑ With inspiration; RV dilation common
Ventricular septal defect (VSD)	LLSB → RLSB	Often with thrill
Early-Midsystolic		
Aortic valvular stenosis (AS)	RUSB	
Fixed supravalvular or subvalvular	RUSB	Ejection click if mobile valve; soft or absent A_2 if valve immobile; later peak associated with more severe stenosis
Dynamic infravalvular	LLSB → apex + axilla	Hypertrophic obstructive cardiomyopathy; murmur louder if LV volume lower or contractility increased, softer if LV volume increased*; can be later in systole if obstruction delayed
Pulmonic valvular stenosis (PS)	LUSB	↑ With inspiration
Infravalvular (infundibular)	LUSB	↑ With inspiration
Supravalvular	LUSB	↑ With inspiration
"Flow murmurs"	LUSB	Anemia, fever, increased flow of any cause†
Mid-Late Systolic		
Mitral valve prolapse (MVP)	LLSB or apex → axilla	Preceded by click; murmur lengthens with maneuvers that ↓ LV volume
Papillary muscle dysfunction	Apex → axilla	Ischemic heart disease

Table continued on following page

Table 5–4 ■ SOME COMMON CAUSES OF HEART MURMURS *Continued*

	USUAL LOCATION	COMMON ASSOCIATED FINDINGS
DIASTOLIC		
Early Diastolic		
Aortic regurgitation (AR)	RUSB, LUSB	High-pitched, blowing quality; endocarditis, diseases of the aorta, associated AS; signs of low peripheral vascular resistance
Pulmonic valve regurgitation (PR)	LUSB	Pulmonary hypertension as a causative factor
Mid-Late Diastolic		
Mitral stenosis (MS), tricuspid stenosis (TS)	Apex, LLSB	Low-pitched; in rheumatic heart disease, opening snap commonly precedes murmur; can be due to increased flow across normal valve†
Atrial myxomas	Apex (L), LLSB (R)	"Tumor plop"
CONTINUOUS		
Venous hum	Over jugular or hepatic vein or breast	Disappears with compression of vein or pressure of stethoscope
Patent ductus arteriosus (PDA)	LUSB	
Arteriovenous (AV) fistula		
Coronary	LUSB	
Pulmonary, bronchial, chest wall	Over fistula	
Ruptured sinus of Valsalva aneurysm	RUSB	Sudden onset

LUSB = left upper sternal border (2nd–3rd intercostal spaces); RUSB = right upper sternal border (2nd–3rd intercostal spaces); LLSB = left lower sternal border (4th intercostal space); RLSB = right lower sternal border (4th intercostal space); LV = left ventricular; RV, right ventricular.

*Left ventricular volume is decreased by standing or during prolonged, forced expiration against a closed glottis (Valsalva maneuver); it is increased by squatting or by elevation of the legs; contractility is increased by adrenergic stimulation or in the beat after a post-extrasystolic beat

†Including a left-to-right shunt through an atrial septal defect for tricuspid or pulmonic flow murmurs and a ventricular septal defect for pulmonic or mitral flow murmurs.

Table 5–5 ■ BEDSIDE MANEUVERS IN THE IDENTIFICATION OF SYSTOLIC MURMURS

MANEUVER	RESPONSE	MURMUR
Inspiration	↑	RS
Expiration	↓	RS
Valsalva maneuver	↑	HC
Squat to stand	↑	HC
Stand to squat	↓	HC
Leg elevation	↓	HC
Handgrip	↓	HC
Handgrip	↑	MR, VSD
Transient arterial occlusion	↑	MR, VSD

RS = right-sided; HC = hypertrophic cardiomyopathy; MR = mitral regurgitation; VSD = ventricular septal defect.

Modified with permission from Lembo NJ, Dell'Italia LJ, Crawford MH, et al.: Bedside diagnosis of systolic murmurs. N Engl J Med 318:1572–1578, 1988.

absence of LV outflow obstruction, arterial pressure is an appropriate index for quantifying myocyte afterload.

Contractility refers to the intrinsic strength of the cardiac muscle (*myocardial contractility*) or the ventricle (*ventricular contractility*), independent of external conditions imposed by either preload or afterload.

The importance of *heart rate* in determining cardiac performance is readily appreciated by noting that cardiac output measured in liters per minute is equal to the amount of blood ejected at each heartbeat (stroke volume in liters per beat) multiplied by the number of beats per minute.

Oxygen consumption for the entire body during strenuous exercise increases approximately 18-fold. Two thirds of this increase in oxygen consumption results from greater cardiac output and the remaining third from an increase in oxygen extraction from arterial blood. Arterial oxygen saturation usually remains near 100%, whereas venous oxygen saturation decreases from approximately 75 to 25%.

For more information about this subject, see *Cecil Textbook of Medicine,* 21st edition. Philadelphia, W.B. Saunders Company, 2000. Chapter 40, Cardiac Function and Circulatory Control, pages 170 to 177.

ELECTROCARDIOGRAPHY

ECG paper is graph paper with horizontal and vertical lines at 1-mm intervals with a heavier line every 5 mm. Time is measured along the horizontal lines with 1 mm = 0.04 second. Voltage is measured along the vertical lines and is expressed as millimeters (10 mm = 1 mV). In routine clinical practice, the recording speed is 25 mm/sec (Fig. 5–2).

The *P wave* is the deflection produced by atrial depolarization; it is normally 0.12 second long or less and is directed leftward and inferiorly in the frontal plane. An abnormally long P wave signifies an interatrial conduction delay. The QRS complex represents ven-

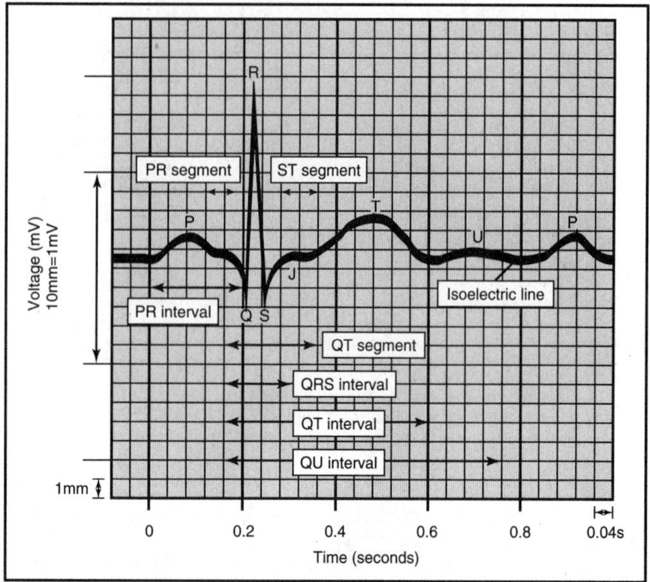

FIGURE 5-2 ■ Schematic illustration of the ECG grid and normal complexes, intervals, and segments. (Adapted from Goldschlager N, Goldman MJ: Principles of Clinical Electrocardiography, 13th ed. Norwalk, CT, Appleton & Lange, 1989.)

tricular depolarization. Capital letters (Q, R, S) refer to waves over 5 mm; lowercase letters (q, r, s) refer to waves under 5 mm. The *Q(q) wave* is the initial negative deflection resulting from the onset of ventricular depolarization; the *R (r) wave* is the first positive deflection resulting from ventricular depolarization; and the *S (s) wave* is the negative deflection of ventricular depolarization that follows the first positive (R) wave. A *QS wave* signifies a negative deflection that does not rise above the baseline. An *R′ (r′) wave* is a second positive deflection and follows an S wave; a negative deflection that follows the r′ is termed the *s′ wave;* if an s wave does not follow the initial R wave, the second positive deflection is still termed an *R′ (r′) wave,* and the QRS complex is described as an R′ (rR′) complex. The *T wave* is the deflection produced by ventricular repolarization. The *U wave* is the (usually positive) deflection following the T wave and preceding the subsequent P wave.

The *PR segment* is measured from the end of the P wave to the onset of the QRS complex. It should be 0.12 to 0.20 second. The *ST segment* begins at the J point and ends at the onset of the T wave.

The *RR interval* is the interval between two consecutive R waves. The *QRS interval* represents ventricular depolarization time. The upper limit of normal is 0.11 second. The *QT interval* represents total ventricular repolarization time.

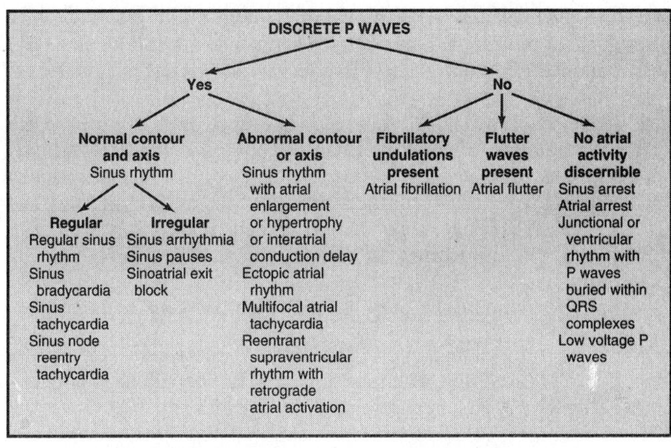

FIGURE 5–3 ■ An approach to interpretation of the ECG.

Steps in Analyzing an ECG

1. Identify the atrial rhythm and measure its rate. If atrial and ventricular rates are different from each other, their rates must be determined separately (Fig. 5–3).
2. Determine the P wave axis, duration, and morphology to provide information about the focus or origin of the atrial rhythm and whether the atria are being depolarized antegradely or retrogradely (Fig. 5–4).
3. Identify the ventricular rate and whether it is regular or irregular. Ascertain whether it is associated with the atrial rhythm

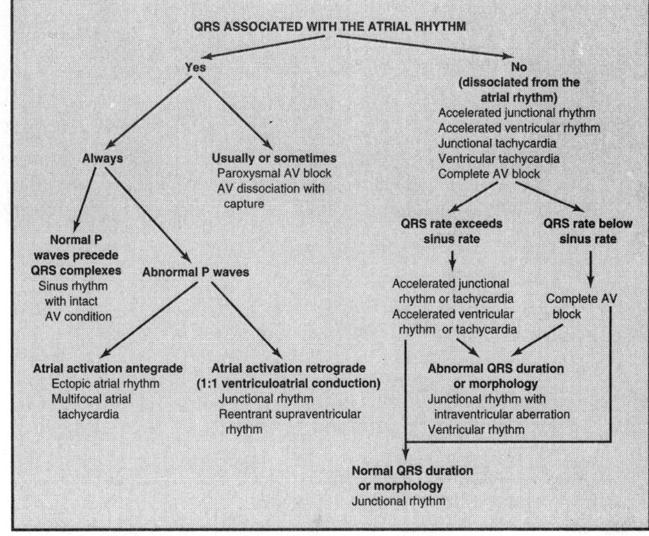

FIGURE 5–4 ■ The QRS rhythm.

and what their relationships are: Is there one P wave for each QRS complex? Do the P waves precede or follow the QRS complexes? What is the PR interval? Is it constant or does it change?

4. Determine the QRS axis and duration, and describe QRS morphology. Rhythms originating above the ventricles usually use the normal His-Purkinje system to activate ventricular muscle, and the resulting QRS complexes are narrow and normal-appearing unless bundle branch block is present. QRS complexes originating from ventricular tissue, however, are broad and bizarre.
5. Finally, compare the present ECG with previous records.

For more information about this subject, see *Cecil Textbook of Medicine,* 21st edition. Philadelphia, W.B. Saunders Company, 2000. Chapter 42, Electrocardiography, pages 185 to 191.

CATHETERIZATION AND ANGIOGRAPHY

Cardiac catheterization is most commonly performed to determine the nature and extent of a suspected cardiac problem in a symptomatic patient in whom surgical or interventional therapy is anticipated (Table 5–6). It is also used to exclude the presence of significant disease when findings from other modalities, such as stress testing or echocardiography, are equivocal or when the patient continues to be severely symptomatic and a definitive diagnosis is important in the patient's management.

The measurement of intracardiac pressure is one essential component (Table 5–7). Cardiac output can be measured by the direct Fick method, by indicator dilution methods, or by angiographic techniques. The formula for calculating Fick cardiac output is:

$$\frac{\text{Oxygen consumption (mL } O_2\text{/min)}}{\text{Arterial-venous oxygen difference (vol \% } \times 10)}$$

where the arterial-venous oxygen difference = 1.39 (O_2 carrying capacity of blood) X hemoglobin (g/dL) × (arterial-oxygen saturation difference). The indicator dilution method is based on the Stewart-Hamilton equation, in which cardiac output is determined by the following formula:

$$\text{Cardiac output} = \frac{\text{I} \times 60}{\text{cm} \times \text{t}}$$

where I = amount of indicator injected, 60 = sec/min, cm = mean indicator concentration (mg/L), and t = total indicator circulatory time in seconds.

For more information about this subject, see *Cecil Textbook of Medicine,* 21st edition. Philadelphia, W.B. Saunders Company, 2000. Chapter 46, Catheterization and Angiography, pages 204 to 207.

Table 5–6 ■ INDICATIONS FOR CARDIAC CATHETERIZATION AND ANGIOGRAPHY

I. Coronary artery disease
  A. Asymptomatic or symptomatic
    1. High risk for adverse outcome based on non-invasive testing
    2. After resuscitation from cardiac arrest or sustained ventricular tachycardia
  B. Symptomatic
    1. Severe angina on medical therapy
    2. Unstable angina (high or intermediate risk)
    3. Acute myocardial infarction
      a. Primary reperfusion with angioplasty
      b. Recurrent ischemic episodes during hospitalization
      c. Shock or hemodynamic instability
      d. Mechanical complications such as mitral regurgitation or ventricular septal defect
    4. Chest pain of uncertain origin and non-invasive testing is equivocal
    5. High-risk patients undergoing non-cardiac surgery
II. Valvular heart disease
  A. Aortic valve disease
    1. Symptomatic patients (angina, heart failure, syncope) with suspected severe aortic stenosis or aortic regurgitation
    2. Asymptomatic patients with aortic regurgitation but with progressive cardiac enlargement or reduction of ejection fraction
  B. Mitral valve disease
    1. Symptomatic patients (dyspnea, heart failure, emboli) with suspected severe mitral stenosis or regurgitation
III. Other
  A. Congenital heart disease
    1. Before cardiac surgery or percutaneous correction
  B. Pericardial disease
    1. Symptomatic patients with suspected constrictive pericarditis or tamponade
  C. Vascular disease
    1. Aortic dissection or aneurysm with suspected concomitant coronary disease
  D. Heart failure
    1. New onset
    2. Suspected to be secondary to coronary artery disease
  E. Hypertrophic cardiomyopathy
    1. Angina
  F. Cardiac transplantation
    1. Presurgical and postsurgical evaluation

Adapted from American College of Cardiology/American Heart Association Ad Hoc Task Force on Practice Guidelines: ACC/AHA Guidelines for Coronary Angiography. J Am Coll Cardiol 34:890–911, 1999.

HEART FAILURE

Heart failure is a syndrome that may result from many cardiac and systemic disorders (Table 5–8). Until the recent widespread use of non-invasive assessments of LV function, heart failure with preserved systolic function was considered unusual in the absence of valvular abnormalities or other specific and uncommon causes. However, it is now recognized that 20 to 40% of heart failure patients have normal ejection functions (Table 5–9).

Table 5–7 ■ NORMAL HEMODYNAMIC MEASUREMENTS

	NORMAL RANGE
Pressures (mm Hg)	
Right heart	
Right atrium (mean, a wave, v wave)	0–5, 1–7, 1–7
Right ventricle (peak systole, end-diastole)	17–32, 1–7
Pulmonary artery (peak systole, diastole, mean)	17–32, 4–13, 9–19
Pulmonary capillary wedge (mean)	4–12
Left heart	
Left atrium (mean, a wave, v wave)	4–12, 4–15, 4–15
Left ventricle (peak systole, end-diastole)	90–140, 5–12
Aorta (peak systole, diastole, mean)	90–140, 60–90, 70–105
Cardiac Output and Resistances	
Cardiac index (L/min/m^2)	2.8–4.2
Arteriovenous oxygen difference (vol %)	3.5–4.8
Systemic vascular resistance (dyne · sec · cm^{-5})	900–1400
Pulmonary vascular resistance (dyne · sec · cm^{-5})	40–120
Oxygen consumption (mL/min)	115–140

Many patients with chronic heart failure maintain a stable course and then abruptly present with acutely or subacutely worsening symptoms (Table 5–10). The common symptoms of heart failure are dyspnea, orthopnea, paroxysmal nocturnal dyspnea, exercise intolerance, fatigue, and edema. Some patients develop sleep disorders, congestive hepatomegaly, poor intestinal function, and cardiac cachexia.

Physical Findings

The physical findings associated with heart failure generally reflect elevated ventricular filling pressures and, to a lesser extent, reduced cardiac output. Either an elevated jugular venous pressure or abnormal abdominal-jugular reflux has been reported in 80% of patients with advanced heart failure.

Rales, representing alveolar fluid, are a hallmark of heart failure; when present in patients without accompanying pulmonary disease, they are highly specific for the diagnosis. However, in chronic heart failure they are usually absent, even in patients known to have pulmonary capillary wedge pressures above 20 mm Hg (normal $<$ 12 mm Hg).

Assessment of the point of the LV maximal impulse may provide information concerning the size of the heart (enlarged if lateral to the midclavicular line) and its function (abnormal if sustained beyond one third of systole or palpable over two interspaces). An apical S_3 gallop is a strong indicator of significant LV dysfunction but is present only in a minority of patients with low ejection fractions and elevated LV filling pressures. An S_4 is not a specific indicator of heart failure, but it is usually present in patients with diastolic dysfunction. An S_3 at the lower left or right sternal border or below the xiphoid indicates RV dysfunction.

Table 5–8 ■ PATHOGENESIS OF HEART FAILURE

I. Impaired systolic (contractile) function
  A. Ischemic damage or dysfunction
    1. Myocardial infarction
    2. Persistent or intermittent myocardial ischemia
    3. Hypoperfusion (shock)
  B. Chronic pressure overload
    1. Hypertension
    2. Obstructive valvular disease
  C. Chronic volume overload
    1. Regurgitant valvular disease
    2. Intracardiac left-to-right shunting
    3. Extracardiac shunting
  D. Non-ischemic dilated cardiomyopathy
    1. Familial/genetic disorders
    2. Toxic/drug-induced damage
    3. Immunologically mediated necrosis
    4. Infectious agents
    5. Metabolic disorders
    6. Infiltrative processes
    7. Idiopathic conditions
II. Diastolic function (restricted filling, increased stiffness)
  A. Pathologic myocardial hypertrophy
    1. Primary (hypertrophic cardiomyopathies)
    2. Secondary (hypertension)
  B. Aging
  C. Ischemic fibrosis
  D. Restrictive cardiomyopathy
    1. Infiltrative disorders (amyloidosis, sarcoidosis)
    2. Storage diseases (hemochromatosis, genetic abnormalities)
  E. Endomyocardial disorders
III. Mechanical abnormalities
  A. Intracardiac
    1. Obstructive valvular disease
    2. Regurgitant valvular disease
    3. Intracardiac shunts
    4. Other congenital abnormalities
  B. Extracardiac
    1. Obstructive (coarctation, supravalvular aortic stenosis)
    2. Left-to-right shunting (patent ductus)
IV. Disorders of rate and rhythm
  A. Bradyarrhythmias (sinus node dysfunction, conduction abnormalities)
  B. Tachyarrhythmias (ineffective rhythms, chronic tachycardia)
V. Pulmonary heart disease
  A. Cor pulmonale
  B. Pulmonary vascular disorders
VI. High output states
  A. Metabolic disorders
    1. Thyrotoxicosis
    2. Nutritional disorders (beri-beri)
  B. Excessive blood flow requirements
    1. Chronic anemia
    2. Systemic arteriovenous shunting

Table 5–9 ■ CAUSES OF (AND ALTERNATIVE EXPLANATIONS FOR) HEART FAILURE WITH PRESERVED SYSTOLIC FUNCTION (LEFT VENTRICULAR EJECTION FRACTION >45–50%)

Inaccurate diagnosis of heart failure (e.g., pulmonary diseases, obesity)
Inaccurate measurements of ejection fraction
Systolic function overestimated by ejection fraction (e.g., mitral regurgitation)
Episodic, unrecognized systolic dysfunction
- Intermittent ischemia
- Arrhythmia
- Severe hypertension
- Alcoholic cardiomyopathy

Diastolic dysfunction
- Abnormalities of myocardial relaxation
  - Ischemia
  - Hypertrophy
- Abnormalities of myocardial compliance
  - Hypertrophy
  - Aging
  - Fibrosis
  - Diabetes
  - Infiltrative diseases (amyloidosis, sarcoidosis)
  - Storage diseases (hemochromatosis)
  - Endomyocardial diseases (endomyocardial fibrosis, radiation, anthracyclines)

Pericardial diseases (constriction, tamponade)

The size, pulsatility, and tenderness of the liver should be evaluated for evidence of passive congestion and tricuspid regurgitation. Ascites and edema should be sought and quantified.

Radiographic Findings

Cardiomegaly (a cardiothoracic ratio above 0.50) is a strong indicator of heart failure. However, nearly 50% of heart failure

Table 5–10 ■ FACTORS THAT MAY PRECIPITATE ACUTE DECOMPENSATION OF CHRONIC HEART FAILURE

Discontinuation of therapy (patient non-compliance or physician-initiated)
Initiation of medications that worsen heart failure (calcium antagonists; β-blockers; non-steroidal, anti-inflammatory drugs; antiarrhythmic agents)
Iatrogenic volume overload (transfusion, fluid administration)
Dietary indiscretion
Alcohol consumption
Increased activity
Pregnancy
Exposure to high altitude
Arrhythmias
Myocardial ischemia or infarction
Worsening hypertension
Worsening mitral or tricuspid regurgitation
Fever or infection
Anemia

patients do not have this high a cardiothoracic ratio, and there are many other causes of cardiomegaly (Fig. 5–5). Most patients with acute heart failure, but only a minority of those with chronic heart failure, will have upper lobe redistribution, enlarged pulmonary veins, haziness of the central vascular shadows, increased central interstitial lung markings, or perihilar or patchy peripheral infiltrates.

Routine Diagnostic Assessment

Routine testing should include a complete blood cell count (to detect anemia and systemic diseases with hematologic manifestations); measurement of renal function and electrolytes, including

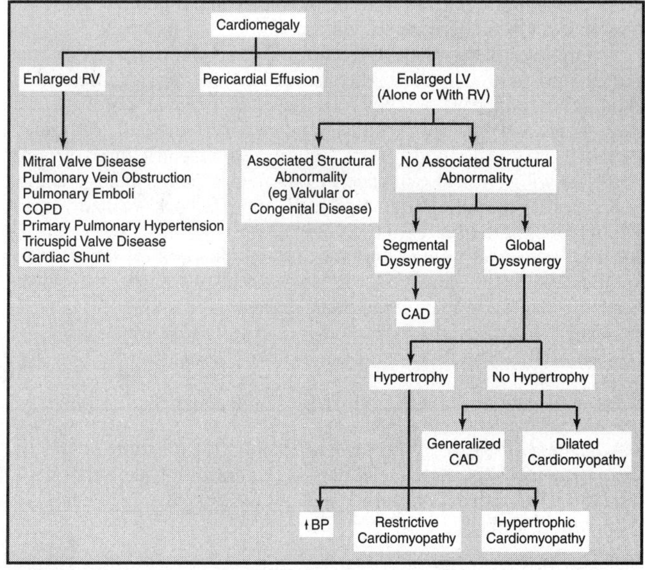

FIGURE 5–5 ■ Echocardiographic approach to cardiomegaly. The initial step in the evaluation of a patient with evidence of cardiomegaly involves examining the echocardiogram to determine whether the enlargement is due to pericardial effusion or whether it involves the right ventricle (RV) or left ventricle (LV) alone or in combination. If isolated right ventricular enlargement is present, the potential causes are enumerated. If left ventricular enlargement is found, the physician must next determine whether there are associated structural abnormalities such as valvular or congenital heart disease. If no associated anatomic abnormalities are present, the observation of segmental dyssynergy points strongly toward underlying coronary artery disease. If generalized global dyssynergy is present, the echocardiogram should distinguish the presence or absence of increased wall thickening. Conditions associated with increased wall thickening include infiltrative processes associated with restrictive cardiomyopathy and hypertrophy associated with hypertension or hypertrophic cardiomyopathy. A dilated left ventricle with global dyssynergy in the absence of hypertrophy may represent dilated cardiomyopathy or generalized left ventricular dysfunction due to widespread coronary artery disease (CAD) (sometimes referred to as ischemic cardiomyopathy). COPD = chronic obstructive pulmonary disease.

magnesium (to exclude renal failure and to provide a baseline for subsequent therapy); liver enzyme tests (to exclude accompanying liver abnormalities and provide a baseline); and blood sugar and lipid testing (to diagnose diabetes and dyslipidemia, both of which should be managed aggressively in heart failure patients). Many guidelines recommend thyroid function tests in all patients, or at least in the elderly and in those with AF. Hemochromatosis is a potentially treatable cause of heart failure; particularly, if there is accompanying diabetes of hepatic disease, serum ferritin levels are indicated.

Additional Diagnostic Evaluation

The transthoracic echocardiogram provides clues to the cause of heart failure as well as a quantitative assessment of LV function. It should be obtained at the time of diagnosis and whenever there are substantive changes in the patient's condition.

Quantitative assessment of exercise capacity provides additional insight into prognosis. The exercise test or exercise or stress scintigraphy or echocardiography can detect coexistent coronary disease, which may affect prognosis and require treatment. A prudent approach is to subdivide heart failure patients into three groups: (1) those with clinical evidence of ongoing ischemia (active angina or a possible ischemic equivalent), (2) those who have had a prior MI but do not currently have angina, and (3) those who may or may not have underlying coronary disease. There is no rationale for routine myocardial biopsy in patients with heart failure, even in the subgroup without apparent coronary disease.

Management

Each of the four phases of heart failure (Fig. 5–6) requires a specific therapeutic approach (Fig. 5–7). The goals of outpatient management of heart failure due to systolic dysfunction of the LV are (1) control of fluid retention; (2) control of neurohormonal activation (to reduce morbidity and mortality); and (3) control of symptoms and disability (Fig. 5–8).

Control of Fluid Retention

Diuretics are generally initiated in low doses (Table 5–11), and the dose is increased until signs and symptoms of fluid retention are alleviated. The principal adverse effects of diuretics include (1) electrolyte depletion, (2) neurohormonal activation, and (3) hypotension and azotemia.

Control of Neurohormonal Activation

Three types of neurohormonal antagonists are (1) angiotensin-converting enzyme (ACE) inhibitors, which interfere with the actions of the renin-angiotensin system; (2) β-adrenergic receptor blockers, which interfere with the actions of the sympathetic nervous system; and (3) aldosterone antagonists.

ACE inhibitors relieve dyspnea, prolong exercise tolerance, and reduce the need for emergency care for worsening heart failure. These benefits are seen in patients with mild, moderate, and severe symptoms, whether or not they are treated with digitalis. In addition, ACE inhibitors can reduce the risk of death and retard the

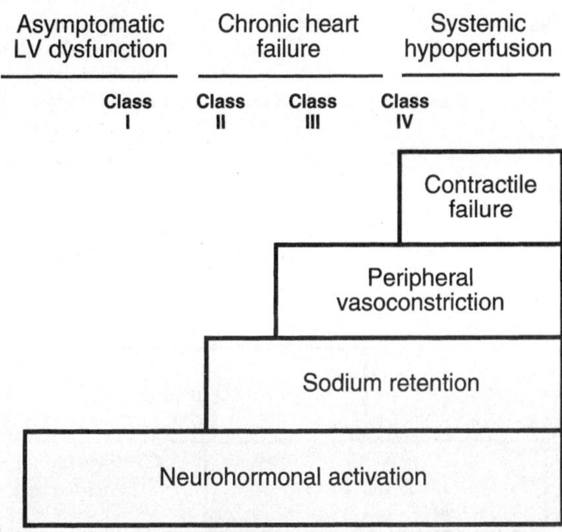

FIGURE 5–6 ■ Mechanisms contributing to the development of heart failure at each stage of the disease. This diagram should be used in conjunction with Figure 5–7; see text for details. The classes designated at the top of the page refer to the functional classification developed by the New York Heart Association. According to this classification system, patients may have symptoms at rest (Class IV), on less than ordinary exertion (Class III), on ordinary exertion (Class II), or only at levels that would cause symptoms in normal individuals (Class I) (see Table 5–2).

progression of heart failure. However, ACE inhibitors should not be used before (or instead of) diuretics in patients with a history of fluid retention. ACE inhibitors produce greater effects on survival than a combination of direct-acting vasodilators (e.g., hydralazine and isosorbide dinitrate). The available data do not justify withholding ACE inhibitors from any specific subset of patients, even patients with low blood pressure or impaired renal function. Treatment is generally maintained even in patients who do not experience symptomatic benefits. Because fluid retention can attenuate the effects of ACE inhibitors, the dose of diuretics must be optimized before initiating treatment. Decreases in blood pressure or increases in blood urea nitrogen or in the potassium level may be seen. Most patients with hypotension, azotemia, or hyperkalemia can be managed with a dose reduction without the withdrawal of the ACE inhibitor.

In patients who are intolerant of ACE inhibitors, angiotensin II receptor antagonists (e.g., losartan, valsartan, irbesartan, eprosartan, cardesartan) interfere with the actions of the renin-angiotensin system by blocking the interaction of angiotensin II with its receptor. Angiotensin II receptor antagonists should not be used for the treatment of heart failure in patients who have no prior exposure to ACE inhibitors, and these drugs should not be substituted for ACE inhibitors in patients who are tolerating ACE inhibitors without difficulty. Angiotensin II receptor antagonists may be used in patients who cannot tolerate an ACE inhibitor because of cough or

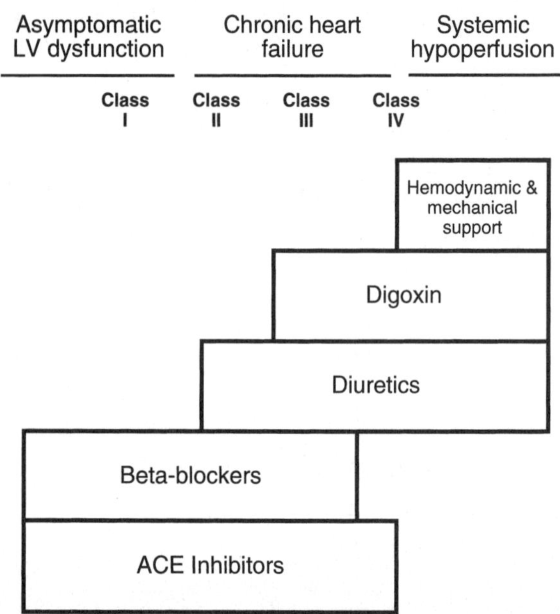

FIGURE 5–7 ■ Treatment strategies appropriate to each stage of heart failure. This diagram should be used in conjunction with Figure 5–6; see text for details. The classes designated at the top of the page refer to the functional classification developed by the New York Heart Association (see Table 5–2). ACE = angiotensin-converting enzyme.

angioedema. A combination of isosorbide dinitrate and hydralazine has been reported to reduce the risk of death in patients with heart failure receiving digitalis and diuretics. However, when compared with ACE inhibitors, the nitrate-hydralazine combination is associated with a higher risk of death, despite greater benefits on exercise fraction and exercise tolerance.

β-Blockers can produce important clinical benefits in heart failure. β-Blockers relieve symptoms, improve clinical status, reduce the risk of death, and retard the progression of heart failure in patients with mild-to-moderate and moderate-to-severe symptoms, regardless of whether heart failure has an ischemic or non-ischemic cause, whether or not they are treated with digitalis. β-Blockers are generally used together with ACE inhibitors.

Patients with Class II or Class III heart failure due to LV systolic dysfunction should receive a β-blocker unless they have a contraindication to or are unable to tolerate treatment with the drug. Treatment is generally maintained even in patients who do not experience symptomatic benefits. However, there are insufficient data on the efficacy and safety of β-blocker use in patients with Class IV symptoms or those receiving intravenous (IV) drugs for heart failure to justify the use of these drugs in those with end-stage disease. β-Blockers can produce hypotension, fluid retention, bradycardia, and heart block. These adverse reactions occur during initiation of therapy but are generally mild in severity, can be

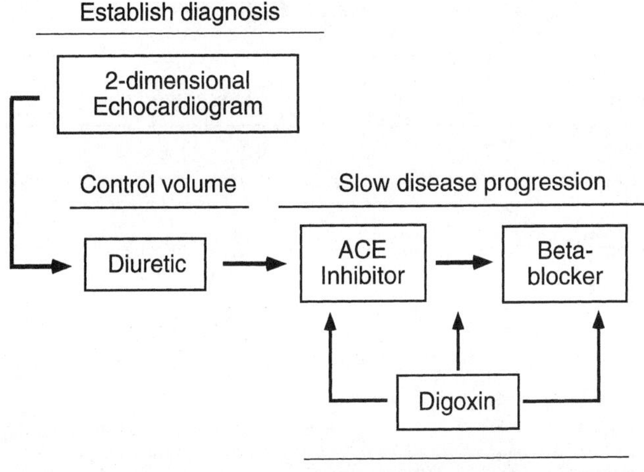

5

FIGURE 5-8 ■ Algorithm for the management of chronic heart failure. *Step 1: Establish the diagnosis.* A two-dimensional echocardiogram can quantify the type and magnitude of ventricular dysfunction and can identify disorders of the valves, pericardium, or great vessels that may be corrected surgically. *Step 2: Control volume with the use of diuretics.* The dose of diuretic should be adjusted until there is no evidence of fluid retention, as reflected either by resolution of peripheral edema or normalization of jugular venous pressure. *Step 3: Slow disease progression with the use of ACE inhibitors and β-blockers.* Even if symptoms are controlled with a diuretic, ACE inhibitors and β-blockers should be used together to reduce the risk of death and hospitalization. (There is little information about the use of β-blockers in patients with Class IV symptoms.) *Step 4: Treat any residual symptoms with digoxin.* Some physicians prescribe digoxin to all symptomatic patients with systolic dysfunction receiving a diuretic, whereas others reserve digoxin for patients who remain symptomatic despite the use of a diuretic, ACE inhibitor, and β-blocker.

managed by changes in concomitant therapy, usually subside after several days or weeks of treatment, and thus infrequently lead to the withdrawal of treatment.

The addition of low doses of spironolactone (12.5–25 mg/day) to patients with current or recent Class IV symptoms receiving ACE inhibitors decreased the risk of death by 25 to 30% and the risk of hospitalization for heart failure by approximately 35% in the Randomized Aldactone Evaluation Study (RALES) trial. Although this result has not yet been replicated, the use of low doses of spironolactone merits consideration in patients with advanced heart failure. Such use, however, is not currently approved by the Food and Drug Administration (FDA) at the time of this writing.

Relief of Symptoms and Disability

Controlled studies have shown that digoxin can improve symptoms, quality of life, and exercise tolerance in patients with mild-to-moderate heart failure. However, in a long-term controlled clinical trial, digoxin did not reduce the risk of death and was associated with only a modest reduction in the combined risk of

Table 5-11 ■ DRUGS RECOMMENDED FOR GENERAL USE IN CHRONIC HEART FAILURE

DRUG	STARTING DOSE	SUBSEQUENT DOSES
Diuretics		
Furosemide	20–40 mg once or twice daily	Titrate to achieve dry weight (up to 200 mg/d)
Torsemide	10–20 mg once or twice daily	Titrate to achieve dry weight (up to 200 mg/d)
Bumetanide	0.5–1.0 mg once or twice daily	Titrate to achieve dry weight (up to 10 mg/d)
Angiotensin-Converting Enzyme Inhibitors		
Captopril	6.25 mg twice daily	Titrate to target dose (50 mg three times daily)
Enalapril	2.5 mg twice daily	Titrate to target dose (10–20 mg twice daily)
Lisinopril	2.5–5.0 mg/d	Titrate to target dose (20–35 mg twice daily)
Quinapril	10 mg twice daily	Target dose not established (should not exceed 40 mg twice daily)
Fosinopril	5–10 mg/d	Target dose not established (should not exceed 40 mg/d)
Ramipril	1.25–2.5 mg/d	Titrate to target dose (5 mg twice daily)
β-Receptor Blockers		
Carvedilol	3.125 mg twice daily	Titrate to target dose (25–50 mg twice daily)
Metoprolol* (sustained release)	12.5–25 mg/d	Titrate to target dose (200 mg/d)
Bisoprolol*	1.25 mg/d	Titrate to target dose (10 mg/d)
Aldosterone Antagonists		
Spironolactone*	12.5–25 mg/d	Titrate to target dose (25 mg/d)
Digitalis Glycosides		
Digoxin	0.125–0.25 mg/d	Target dose not established (should not exceed 0.5 mg/d)

*Drugs not approved by the U.S. Food and Drug Administration for use in the management of chronic heart failure, January 1999.

death and hospitalization. The principal adverse effects of digoxin include (1) cardiac arrhythmias (e.g., ectopic and re-entrant cardiac rhythms and heart block); (2) gastrointestinal symptoms (e.g., anorexia, nausea, vomiting); and (3) neurologic complaints (e.g., visual disturbances, disorientation, and confusion). These side effects are commonly associated with serum digoxin levels greater than

2 mg/mL, but digitalis toxicity may occur with lower digoxin levels, particularly if hypokalemia or hypomagnesemia coexist.

Treatment of Coexistent Cardiac Disorders

Most patients with heart failure have frequent and complex ventricular arrhythmias, but when asymptomatic these do not presage or contribute to the occurrence of sudden death and thus do not require therapy. The agent most likely to suppress atrial arrhythmias in patients with heart failure is amiodarone, but the substantial toxicity of the drug has justifiably discouraged its widespread use. In patients who have immediate life-threatening ventricular arrhythmias (sustained ventricular tachycardia [VT] or ventricular fibrillation [VF]) or who have been resuscitated from sudden death, use of an implantable cardioverter-defibrillator may reduce the risk of a lethal recurrence. Anticoagulation is recommended primarily for patients with a previous embolic event or AF.

Drugs to Be Avoided

Most patients with heart failure should not receive non-steroidal anti-inflammatory agents. Whether the recommendation to avoid inhibitors of prostaglandin synthesis applies to aspirin remains controversial. Clinicians should not use calcium channel blockers for the treatment of heart failure, and most calcium channel blockers should be avoided in the treatment of angina, AF, or hypertension in patients with heart failure. Of the available agents, only amlodipine has strong evidence supporting its safety in patients with advanced disease. Deleterious responses have been observed with most types of antiarrhythmic agents, including class I (encainide, flecainide, and mexiletine) and class III (sotalol) drugs.

Treatment of Patients Hospitalized for Heart Failure

The major syndromes requiring hospitalization include (1) fluid overload resistant to orally administered diuretics (e.g., refractory peripheral edema); (2) severe respiratory distress with or without hypoxemia (e.g., acute pulmonary edema); and (3) refractory symptoms with poor end-organ perfusion requiring IV therapy.

Fluid Overload Refractory to Oral Diuretics

A frequent cause of this syndrome is non-compliance with diet or medications. Diuretics acting on the loop of Henle (e.g., furosemide) should be administered IV. If the patient fails to respond to large doses, a second diuretic with a different renal tubular site of action (e.g., metolazone) may be added. Every effort should be made to achieve dry weight, even if this goal requires a prolonged hospitalization.

Pulmonary Congestion (Pulmonary Edema)

Pulmonary congestion may be the first evidence of heart failure in patients without a history of cardiac disease; it may appear in patients who are already hospitalized for an acute cardiac disorder (e.g., MI), or it may complicate the course of a patient with long-standing heart failure. If severe, abrupt, and accompanied by clinical evidence of sympathetic overactivity (tachycardia, diaphoresis, and vasoconstriction), the syndrome is designated as acute pulmonary edema. Every effort should be made to identify an underlying precipitating factor, because its correction is often critical to the success of treatment. Because of the critical role of peripheral vasoreconstruction in the pathogenesis of pulmonary edema, pharmacologic dilation of peripheral vessels represents the key element in management. This goal can be achieved with the use of (1) morphine; (2) loop diuretic drugs (e.g., furosemide); and (3) direct-acting vasodilators (e.g., nitroglycerin and nitroprusside). Morphine is administered in intermittent doses of 2 to 4 mg IV (up to 10–15 mg) until dyspnea is relieved and diaphoresis subsides. In patients who have not received loop diuretics, treatment is usually begun with low doses (40–80 mg IV), whereas patients who have received long-term therapy may require large doses of the drug (120–200 mg IV). Nitroprusside or nitroglycerin is usually initiated as a continuous low-dose IV infusion, the rate of which is increased to achieve specific hemodynamic or clinical goals. Nitroglycerin is preferred in patients with underlying ischemic heart disease, while nitroprusside is preferred in patients with severe hypertension or valvular regurgitation.

Refractory Symptoms with Systemic Hypoperfusion

The most serious presentation of heart failure in the hospitalized patient is the syndrome of refractory heart failure, which is characterized by hemodynamic instability and systemic hypotension. The central feature is a deterioration of cardiac performance to a level incompatible with adequate perfusion of peripheral organs. The most important therapeutic measures in the treatment of refractory heart failure are (1) fluid management; (2) IV positive inotropic agents; (3) IV vasoconstrictor agents; and (4) surgical interventions. Patients should be maintained at dry weight as long as this goal can be achieved without compromising peripheral perfusion. A combination of dobutamine and milrinone may be particularly useful in selected patients, but such a regimen should be used cautiously. Dobutamine is administered as a continuous IV infusion, initially at a rate of 3 to 6 μg/kg/minute (without a bolus), and the rate may be increased up to 10 to 15 μg/kg/minute. Milrinone is generally initiated with a bolus dose of 0.5 μg/kg, followed by a continuous infusion at a rate of 0.375 to 0.75 μg/kg/minute.

Two vasoconstrictor agents are commonly used to support systemic blood pressure in patients with refractory heart failure: dopamine and levarterenol. Dopamine in low doses (<2 μg/kg/minute) dilates the renal and splanchnic circulations. Moderate doses (2–5 μg/kg/minute) increase cardiac output but produce little change in pulmonary wedge pressure, heart rate, or systemic vascular resistance. High doses (>5 μg/kg/minute) increase pulmonary wedge pressure, blood pressure, and heart rate and may reduce renal blood flow. Levarterenol is generally infused in doses ranging from 0.03 to 0.12 μg/kg/minute. If pharmacologic interventions fail to stabilize the patient with refractory heart failure, intra-aortic balloon counterpulsation, an LV assist device, or cardiac transplantation may be effective (Table 5–12).

For more information about this subject, see *Cecil Textbook of Medicine,* 21st edition. Philadelphia, W.B. Saunders Company, 2000. Chapter 47, Pathophysiology of Heart Failure, and Chapter 48, Management of Heart Failure, pages 207 to 226.

Table 5–12 ■ INDICATIONS FOR CONSIDERATION FOR CARDIAC TRANSPLANTATION (CONSIDER REFERRAL TO CARDIAC TRANSPLANT CENTER)

- Irremediable cardiac disease with estimated mortality of more than 25–30% at 1 yr; survival without transplantation is estimated from heart disease etiology, disease duration, hemodynamics, functional capacity, and presence or absence of cardiac arrhythmias
- Unacceptable quality of life primarily due to cardiac disease limitations
- Acceptable social and financial support
- Acceptable neurocognitive function
- Absence of significant psychological or pathologic disorders or substance abuse
- Transplantation surgical risk acceptable from a technical standpoint
- Absence of co-morbid conditions that would significantly limit post-transplantation survival or significantly worsen post-transplantation quality of life, including advanced physiologic age, coexistent systemic illness with poor prognosis, irreversible pulmonary hypertension, acute pulmonary thromboembolism, severe peripheral and/or cerebrovascular disease, irreversible renal or liver disease, active peptic ulcer, active diverticulosis, diabetes mellitus with significant end-organ disease, severe obesity, severe osteoporosis, and active severe infection

ARRHYTHMIAS

Bradyarrhythmias

Bradyarrhythmias (Table 5–13) can be broadly classified into sinus node disease (SND) and atrioventricular (AV) block. Rates less than 60 beats per minute are usually described as bradycardia. *Sinus bradycardia* of clinical significance is usually defined as persistent rates less than 45 beats per minute while awake. Because SND often represents atrial disease processes (e.g., fibrosis, degeneration, and inflammation), bradycardia often coexists with atrial tachyarrhythmias (bradycardia-tachycardia syndrome).

Table 5–13 ■ BRADYCARDIAS

- Sinus node dysfunction
- Sinus bradycardia <45/min
- Sinoatrial exit block
  - First-degree
  - Second-degree
  - Third-degree
- Sinus arrest
- Bradycardia-tachycardia syndrome
- Atrioventricular block
  - First-degree
  - Second-degree
    - Mobitz type I (Wenckebach phenomenon)
    - Mobitz type II
    - Higher degree (e.g., 2:1, 3:1)
  - Third-degree
    - Atrioventricular node
    - His-Purkinje system

Sudden disappearance of P waves could be due to either sinoatrial (SA) exit block or cessation of sinus node pacemaker function. SA exit block and sinus arrest must be distinguished from blocked premature atrial contractions (PACs) and sinus arrhythmia. Blocked PACs are likely to distort the ST–T segment and reset the sinus node so that the PP cycle with a blocked PAC is less than two PP intervals.

AV block is defined when some impulses do not reach the ventricle during normal sinus rhythm or sinus tachycardia. In first-degree AV block, there is prolonged AV conduction (PR interval) with a 1 : 1 P-QRS relationship. In second-degree AV block (intermittent AV conduction), some P waves fail to produce a QRS complex. In type I, also called Mobitz type I or Wenckebach phenomenon, there is a progressive increase in the PR interval, despite a constant PP rate, until a P wave blocks and the cycle is repeated. Type II AV, or Mobitz type II, block causes a sudden, unexpected block of a P wave without a discernible change in the PR interval before the AV block. Mobitz type I second-degree AV block is usually caused by AV nodal disease, while Mobitz II block is commonly caused by abnormalities at or below the bundle of His. A 2 : 1, 3 : 1, or higher AV ratio of AV block may be noted with progression of either Mobitz I or II block to third-degree AV block.

In third-degree (complete) AV block (no AV conduction), complete failure of impulse propagation along the AV conduction system necessitates emergence of a subsidiary intrinsic pacemaker distal to the site of block to depolarize the ventricles. AV dissociation occurs when the atria and ventricles are driven by different and unrelated pacemakers.

Clinical Features of Bradycardias

Aside from medications such as digitalis, antiarrhythmic drugs, and vagal influences, the most common causes of SND are muscle degeneration, fibrosis with advanced age, and/or cardiac disease such as coronary artery disease. Acute inferior wall myocardial ischemia or MI associated with disease of the proximal right coronary artery may cause transient SND. AV nodal blocks can be caused by digitalis, antiarrhythmic drugs, vagal influences, and involvement of the AV junctional area with any inflammatory or other disease process.

Sinus bradycardia and various degrees of AV nodal blocks are also noted during sleep even in otherwise healthy people. Persistent second- and third-degree AV nodal block during the waking hours and during activity is abnormal and is often associated with symptoms, including dizziness, fatigue, exertional dyspnea, aggravation of heart failure, near-syncope, or syncope.

Therapy for Bradycardias

Asymptomatic SND or AV nodal block require no therapy. Acute management of symptomatic SND and second- and third-degree AV block includes administration of IV atropine 1.0 mg or isoproterenol, usually a 1 to 2-μg/minute infusion to increase heart rate. Temporary cardiac pacing may be needed. Temporary pacemaker leads generally are inserted percutaneously into an internal jugular or subclavian vein, or by cutdown into a brachial vein, then positioned under fluoroscopic guidance in the RV apex and attached to an external generator. For all forms of persistent symptomatic SND or second- or third-degree AV block, permanent pacing is the therapy of choice (Tables 5–14 and 5–15).

Supraventricular Tachyarrhythmias

Supraventricular tachyarrhythmias can occur either as isolated premature complexes or in the form of non-sustained or sustained tachycardias. With premature atrial complexes, the P wave always precedes the QRS complex. If the P wave encounters the absolute refractory period of the AV node or the His-Purkinje system, it will be blocked and not be followed by a QRS complex.

Sinus tachycardia is usually due to enhanced automaticity due to increased adrenergic drive. In sinus node re-entry, the P wave morphology is similar to sinus rhythm but the underlying mechanism is re-entry in the region of the sinus node. Unlike physiologic sinus tachycardia, which has a gradual onset and termination, sinus node re-entry starts and ends abruptly.

Sustained supraventricular tachyarrhthmias can be atrial or AV junctional (Table 5–16). Atrial tachycardias (ATs) are usually independent of AV nodal conduction; with effective vagal maneuvers (e.g., carotid sinus massage, Valsalva maneuver), AV block occurs, but the atrial process continues. Conversely, most AV junctional tachycardias require propagation through the AV node; the tachycardia generally terminates if vagal maneuvers induce AV nodal block.

Atrial Tachycardias

Any tachycardia that arises above the AV junction and has a P wave configuration different from sinus rhythm is called atrial

Table 5–14 ■ CLASS I INDICATIONS FOR IMPLANTATION OF A PERMANENT PACEMAKER*

I. Atrioventricular (AV) block
   A. Third-degree AV block associated with symptoms
   B. Third-degree AV block with pauses ≥3 sec or with an escape rate <40 beats per minute in awake patients
   C. Postoperative AV block that is not expected to resolve
   D. Second-degree AV block associated with symptoms
   E. Chronic bifascicular or trifascicular block with intermittent third-degree AV block or type II second-degree AV block

II. AV block associated with myocardial infarction
   A. Second- or third-degree AV block in the His-Purkinje system
   B. Transient second- or third-degree infranodal AV block and associated bundle branch block
   C. Persistent, symptomatic second- or third-degree AV block

III. Sinus node dysfunction
   A. Symptomatic sinus bradycardia or sinus pauses
   B. Symptomatic chronotropic incompetence

IV. Carotid sinus syndrome: recurrent syncope or near-syncope due to carotid sinus syndrome

*Class I indications are conditions for which there is general agreement that a pacemaker is indicated.

Based on the recommendations of the Committee on Pacemaker Implantation, American College of Cardiology/American Heart Association Task Force on Practice Guidelines. J Am Coll Cardiol 31:1175–1209, 1998.

Table 5–15 ■ CLASS II INDICATIONS FOR IMPLANTATION OF A PERMANENT PACEMAKER*

I. Atrioventricular (AV) block
   A. Asymptomatic third-degree AV block with an escape rate ≥40 beats per minute
   B. Asymptomatic Mobitz II second-degree AV block
   C. Asymptomatic Mobitz I second-degree AV block in the His-Purkinje system
   D. Bifascicular or trifascicular block and syncope without identifiable cause
   E. His–ventricular interval >100 ms
   F. Pacing-induced block in the His-Purkinje system
II. AV block associated with myocardial infarction: persistent second- or third-degree AV block at the level of the AV node
III. Sinus node dysfunction: heart rate ≤40 beats per minute, without clear association between symptoms and bradycardia
IV. Neurocardiogenic syncope: recurrent neurocardiogenic syncope associated with significant bradycardia reproduced by tilt-table testing.

*Class II indications are conditions for which pacemakers are often used, without unanimous agreement among experts that a pacemaker is necessary.

Based on the recommendations of the Committee on Pacemaker Implantation. American College of Cardiology/American Heart Association Task Force on Practice Guidelines. J Am Coll Cardiol 31:1175–1209, 1998.

tachycardia. ATs can result from enhanced normal automaticity, abnormal automaticity, triggered activity, and re-entry. *Multifocal atrial tachycardia* implies three or more different P wave morphologies. Atrial rates range between 100 and 250 beats per minute.

Atrial flutter causes regular atrial rates ranging from 250 to 350 beats per minute with "sawtooth" appearance in leads II, III, and a V_F. The ventricular response is usually 2:1 or 4:1.

Atrial fibrillation is the most common sustained arrhythmia in adults. The atria have disorganized, rapid, irregular electrical activity exceeding 400 beats per minute. The ventricular response is also irregular and quite variable (irregularly irregular). The atria do not contract effectively, so intra-atrial clot formation is promoted. With subsequent resumption of atrial contraction, embolism can occur. In the absence of accessory pathways, the average ventricular response via the AV node–His-Purkinje system is seldom more than 200 and generally less than 150 beats per minute.

AV Junctional Tachycardias

The vast majority of AV junctional tachycardias requiring long-term management are re-entrant. AV re-entry in the Wolff-Parkinson-White (WPW) syndrome is the classic form and is usually (>90%) initiated by an atrial and/or ventricular premature complex. A combination of a short PR interval and initial slurring of the QRS is termed *ventricular pre-excitation.* In a typical case of WPW syndrome, however, the impulse reaches the ventricle first through the accessory pathway and starts the QRS earlier, resulting in a shorter PR interval.

The most common sustained arrhythmia in patients with WPW syndrome is orthodromic AV re-entry, in which the impulse propagates to the ventricles by means of the normal pathway and retrograde to the atria through the accessory pathway; during the tachy-

Table 5–16 ■ SUPRAVENTRICULAR TACHYCARDIAS

Atrial Tachycardias
Sinus tachycardia
Sinus node re-entry
Atrial tachycardia
Unifocal
Mutlifocal
Atrial flutter
Atrial fibrillation
Atrioventricular (AV) Junctional Tachycardia
AV re-entry (Wolff-Parkinson-White syndrome)
Orthodromic
Antidromic
AV nodal re-entry
Common
Uncommon
Non-paroxysmal junctional tachycardia
Automatic junctional tachycardia

cardia, there is no evidence of ventricular pre-excitation. In rare instances, the circuit of re-entry may be reversed (antidromic). The second most common arrhythmia and frequently the most serious is AF. If the accessory pathway conducts rapidly during AF, a very fast ventricular rate may occur and cause severe hypotension and/or syncope and precipitate VF.

In the absence of ventricular pre-excitation, the most common AV junctional tachycardia is AV nodal re-entry (AVNR). The entire re-entry circuit is localized to the region of the AV node. AV re-entry accounts for more than 75% of cases frequently labeled as paroxysmal atrial tachycardia (PAT).

The main difference between automatic junctional tachycardia and non-paroxysmal junctional tachycardia is the rate. In the automatic variety, rates are faster (range, 130–200 beats per minute), while in non-paroxysmal junctional tachycardia, ventricular rates seldom exceed 150 beats per minute.

Clinical Features of Supraventricular Tachycardia

Sinus tachycardia is caused by increased metabolic demands from high adrenergic states such as fever, physical exertion, hypovolemia, heart failure, sympathomimetic or parasympatholytic medications, thyrotoxicosis, and pheochromocytoma. All other supraventricular tachycardias represent abnormalities of rhythm and commonly produce tachycardia-related symptoms, including palpitation, dizziness, shortness of breath, chest discomfort, presyncope, and sometimes frank syncope.

Atrial dilation, fibrosis, and acute or chronic inflammatory states involving the atrial myocardium or pericardium may cause ATs. Multifocal AT is relatively frequent in the presence of chronic pulmonary disease. AF is often associated with aging, hypertension, valvular and pulmonary diseases, acute and chronic coronary disease, hyperadrenergic states, and metabolic abnormalities such as thyrotoxicosis. Lone AF may also be noted in the absence of any detectable cardiac disorder.

Re-entrant tachycardias have an abrupt onset and an abrupt ending, particularly when terminated with vagal maneuvers or IV medications. Non-paroxysmal AV junctional tachycardia is frequently seen with high adrenergic drive.

Therapy for Supraventricular Tachyarrhythmias

Isolated premature beats do not warrant aggressive therapy. Conversely, sustained or prolonged repeated episodes of non-sustained supraventricular tachycardia generally require effective therapy (Table 5–17). An acute episode of junctional tachycardia from either AVNA or AV re-entry can be terminated with vagal maneuvers. In most ATs adenosine and/or vagal stimulation produces enough AV block to unmask the atrial origin of the tachycardia.

For sustained control of the ventricular rate during AT, AF, or atrial flutter-fibrillation, IV esmolol and diltiazem are quite effective. If the ventricular response during AF is through a rapidly conducting accessory pathway, IV digitalis and calcium channel blockers are contraindicated; procainamide is a better choice.

When ATs, including atrial flutter or AF, persist, or if rapid conversion is needed, direct-current cardioversion is usually required. An initial energy level of 50 J is appropriate for cardioversion of atrial flutter. In AF, in which cardioversion usually is performed on an elective basis, an initial shock of 100 to 200 J is appropriate.

For symptomatic patients with sustained AV junctional re-entry, control can sometimes be achieved with digitalis, β-blockers, and calcium channel blockers or with class I or class III drugs. However, radiofrequency ablation is now the preferred therapy.

Table 5–17 ■ DRUGS AND DOSES USED TO TREAT SUPRAVENTRICULAR TACHYCARDIAS

DRUG	IV BOLUS	IV INFUSION	ORAL DOSE
Digoxin	0.5–1.0 mg		0.125–0.5 mg/d
Adenosine	6–12 mg		
β-Blockers			
Esmolol	5 μg/kg/min	3 μg/kg/min	
Propranolol	1–3 mg		10–40 mg tid
Calcium channel blockers			
Verapamil	5–15 mg		80–120 mg tid/qid
Diltiazem	15–25 mg	15 mg/hr	120 mg bid/tid
Class IA			
Procainamide	10–15 mg/kg	5 mg/kg	750–1500 mg qid
Quinidine			300–600 mg qid
Disopyramide			100–200 mg tid
Class IC			
Flecainide			50–200 mg bid
Propafenone			150–300 mg tid
Class III			
Ibutilide	1–2 mg		
Sotalol			80–160 mg bid
Amiodarone	2–3 mg/kg	0.5–1.0 mg/min	800–1600 mg/d for 7- to 10-day loading dose, then 100–400 mg/d

In patients with AT, atrial flutter, or AF, ventricular rate control is possible by means of relative AV nodal block using digitalis, β-blockers, and calcium channel blockers. For termination or prevention of atrial tachyarrhythmias, class Ia, Ic, or III drugs are usually needed. Sotalol and amiodarone are currently the most effective drugs for long-term control of AF and flutter.

In patients with drug-refractory AF associated with an uncontrolled ventricular rate, either radiofrequency ablation or modification of the AV node can improve symptoms, functional capacity, and LV function. In AV node ablation, third-degree AV block is intentionally induced; the success rate is 100%, and all patients require a permanent pacemaker. In the AV node modification procedure, the intent is to slow the ventricular rate without creating the need for a pacemaker. Two other ablation procedures that can be helpful in patients with AF are the creation of linear lesions in the right and/or left atrium to eliminate AF and ablation of a focal source of paroxysmal AF, usually within one of the pulmonary veins.

Anticoagulation therapy with warfarin is recommended for all patients with AF who are older than 65 years of age or who have risk factors for thromboembolism and have no contraindication to anticoagulation. The international normalized ratio (INR) goal is 2.0 to 3.0, unless mitral stenosis is present, in which case the target is an INR of 2.5 to 3.5. Aspirin may be better than no treatment for patients who cannot tolerate warfarin.

Ventricular Arrhythmias

Premature ventricular complexes (PVCs) are ubiquitous arrhythmias that are recognized on the ECG by their wide (generally >120 ms) and bizarre QRS morphology, occurring independently of P waves. Most PVCs are followed by a "compensatory pause." Two consecutive PVCs are termed a *couplet.* Three or more consecutive PVCs at a rate of 100 beats per minute or more are termed *ventricular tachycardia.* A given patient may manifest PVCs with two or more different morphologies, in which case the ectopy is termed *multiform.*

PVC frequency and complexity have no prognostic significance for patients who do not have structural heart disease. Among patients with heart disease, both frequent (>10 PVCs per hour) and complex ventricular ectopy are associated with an increased risk of death, but this risk is strongly concentrated in patients with depressed LV function.

Because there is no evidence that treatment directed at suppressing PVCs improves overall mortality, the primary indication for treatment is to relieve symptoms. Most patients with symptomatic PVCs in the absence of structural heart disease can be managed with a β-blocker. An alternative is radiofrequency catheter ablation of the arrhythmogenic focus.

Ventricular parasystole results when an automatic focus arises from the ventricles and fires independently of supraventricular impulses conducted through the AV node. Although generally benign, parasystolic rhythms may result in PVCs at a critical point during repolarization (R on T) and precipitate VF.

Accelerated idioventricular rhythm (AIVR) describes an ectopic ventricular rhythm characterized by three or more consecutive

PVCs occurring at a rate faster than the normal ventricular escape rate of 30 to 40 beats per minute but slower than VT. AIVR has a gradual onset, acceleration ("warm-up"), and deceleration before termination. AIVR occurs most often in the setting of acute MI. AIVR is usually brief and asymptomatic, and it generally requires no specific treatment. If patients with LV dysfunction do not tolerate AIVR, increasing the atrial rate with atropine or by pacing suppresses AIVR.

VT originates below the bundle of His at a rate greater than 100 beats per minute. It is a wide complex rhythm that may be monomorphic (uniform) or polymorphic with beat-to-beat changes in the QRS configuration. Sustained VT persists for 30 seconds or more or requires termination because of hemodynamic instability. Sustained polymorphic VT is usually unstable and often degenerates into VF. Sustained monomorphic VT may be stable for long periods of time or, in the setting of faster rates or myocardial ischemia, may degenerate into polymorphic VT or VF. Torsades de pointes, a particular form of polymorphic VT, has a characteristic morphology ("twisting around a point") and is associated with prolongation of the QT interval on the ECG.

It is important to distinguish monomorphic VT from supraventricular tachycardia with aberrant conduction, because both present as wide complex tachycardias (Table 5–18). Most VT is insensitive to vagal maneuvers such as carotid sinus massage and Valsalva, as well as to adenosine, whereas most forms of supraventricular tachycardia terminate or persist with transient high-grade AV block in response to these maneuvers.

For minimally symptomatic patients without hypotension (systolic blood pressure >90 mm Hg), pharmacologic therapy should be initiated. IV lidocaine is often chosen as a first-line agent because it can be administered rapidly (bolus dose of 1.0–1.5 mg/kg, followed by additional boluses of 0.5–0.75 mg/kg at 5- to 10-minute intervals, up to a maximal dose of 3 mg/kg) and maintained with an infusion (1–4 mg/minute). If lidocaine is ineffective, alternatives include IV procainamide (maximal dose 17 mg/kg), at an infusion rate up to 20 to 30 mg/minute, or IV amiodarone 15 mg/minute over 10 minutes followed by 1 mg/minute over the next 6 hours and then 0.5 mg/minute over 18 hours. If pharmacologic therapy is unsuccessful for hemodynamically stable VT, synchronized cardioversion with a direct-current shock may be required, beginning with 50 to 100 J and increasing to 360 J if necessary. For patients with severe signs or symptoms during VT, immediate synchronous cardioversion is indicated.

Ventricular flutter is an extremely rapid, hemodynamically unstable VT that typically progresses to VF. With rare exceptions, VF occurs in patients with underlying structural heart disease, especially ischemic heart disease with LV systolic dysfunction. Treatment of VF always is emergent, and a 200-J shock should be delivered as quickly as possible, followed by one or more 360-J shocks if necessary.

Long QT Syndrome

Patients with the long QT syndrome are at risk for torsades de pointes, which may result in syncope or sudden cardiac death. The *acquired* long QT syndrome predisposes to torsades de pointes and

Table 5–18 ■ ELECTROCARDIOGRAPHIC CHARACTERISTICS OF VENTRICULAR TACHYCARDIA

Atrioventricular Relationship

- Atrioventricular dissociation
- Sinus capture beats
- Fusion beats

QRS Width

- Left bundle branch block: >160 ms
- Right bundle branch block: >140 ms

QRS Axis

- Extreme left axis (-90 to $-180°$)
- Right-axis deviation in the presence of left bundle branch block ($+90$ to $+180°$)

QRS Morphology

- Right bundle branch block
  - Morphology in V_1
    - Monophasic R wave
    - Biphasic (QR or RS)
    - Triphasic with $R > R'$
  - Morphology in V_6
    - R/S ratio <1
- Left bundle branch block
  - Morphology in V_1
    - Broad R wave (>30 ms)
    - Onset of R wave to nadir of S wave >60 ms
    - Notched downstroke in lead V_1
  - Morphology in V_6
    - QR or QS complex
- Onset of R wave to nadir of S wave >100 ms in any precordial lead
- Absence of RS wave in any precordial lead
- Positive or negative precordial concordance

is usually related to electrolyte abnormalities such as hypokalemia and hypomagnesemia; tricyclic antidepressants; phenothiazines; non-sedating antihistamines such as terfenadine and astemizole; macrolide antibiotics such as erythromycin; other drugs such as pentamidine, probucol, and cisapride; and class IA and class III antiarrhythmic medications.

Therapy for the acquired long QT syndrome is directed at reversing the metabolic abnormalities or withholding the offending medication. Infusion of magnesium and temporary pacing decrease the QT interval and prevent pause-dependent arrhythmias, whereas isoproterenol is a temporizing measure to increase the sinus rate. Class IB antiarrhythmic medications, which tend to shorten the action potential duration and decrease the QT interval, may also be used.

Sudden Cardiac Death

Most survivors of sudden cardiac death (SCD) or cardiac arrest have structural heart disease. VF may be the first manifestation in as many as 25% of patients with ischemic heart disease. Dilated cardiomyopathy accounts for 10 to 15% of survivors of SCD. Other causes include valvular heart disease, hypertrophic cardiomyopathy, arrhythmogenic RV dysplasia, the long QT syndrome, anomalous origin of the coronary arteries, WPW syndrome, and repair of congenital cardiac anomalies. In a small subset of patients, no structural heart disease is detected. Although SCD is not usually associated with an acute Q wave MI, transient ischemia often precedes SCD.

The most important factor that determines the outcome of cardiac arrest is the time to defibrillation. Another significant factor is the initial rhythm identified. VT is associated with the best prognosis, followed by VF; patients with asystole or electromechanical dissociation rarely survive.

In assessing prognosis and planning a treatment strategy, it is useful to classify SCD as either primary (without a clear trigger) or secondary. A primary episode has a 10 to 30% 1-year recurrence rate, whereas most secondary episodes are associated with recurrence rates of less than 2%. Most patients should undergo comprehensive evaluation of myocardial function and coronary anatomy. Echocardiography is useful for excluding hypertrophic cardiomyopathy and valvular heart disease, magnetic resonance imaging (MRI) for diagnosing arrhythmogenic RV dysplasia, and myocardial biopsy for identifying infiltrative diseases such as myocarditis, amyloidosis, hemochromatosis, and sarcoidosis. Coronary angiography should be performed to assess coronary occlusive disease and to exclude coronary artery anomalies.

Implantable cardioverter-defibrillators (ICDs) are first-line therapy in patients who have survived VF not associated with an acute MI or who have had hemodynamically significant, sustained VT. They also reduce mortality in MI survivors who have a low ejection fraction and either non-sustained VT or inducible sustained VT that is not suppressed with procainamide. Regardless of whether or not residual ischemia is present, initial therapy in all post-MI patients without contraindications should include a β-blocker, which consistently reduces SCD (30–45%) as well as total mortality (25–60%) in survivors of MI.

Amiodarone reduces arrhythmic deaths in MI survivors who have an ejection fraction of 40% or less with either frequent PVCs or non-sustained VT, and amiodarone and β-blockers may be synergistic in their benefits. However, amiodarone does not appear to improve overall mortality. In non-ischemic cardiomyopathy, amiodarone appears to reduce total mortality, SCD, and deaths due to heart failure. It does not, however, confer benefit in patients with heart failure due to ischemic cardiomyopathy. Other antiarrhythmic drugs do not improve survival.

Diagnostic Approach to Palpitations, Dizziness, and Syncope (Table 5–19)

Palpitations are usually due to atrial or ventricular extrasystoles and usually do not require further evaluation. When pre-syncope accompanies the palpitations, evaluation is necessary. Antiarrhythmic drug therapy is inappropriate except for very frequent and highly symptomatic ectopy or more advanced forms of arrhythmia.

Table 5–19 ■ DIAGNOSTIC APPROACH TO PALPITATIONS, DIZZINESS, AND SYNCOPE

CONDITION	MOST COMMON CAUSES	ORDER OF DIAGNOSTIC TESTING
Palpitations	PACs, PVCs, SVTs including AF, VT, AVB, psychiatric disorder	History and examination > Holter or event monitor, depending on frequency of symptoms > exercise stress test if exercise-related > EPS if symptoms suggest sustained arrhythmia
Dizziness	Cardiac arrhythmia, medications, vestibular disorder, cerebellar disease, psychiatric disorder	History and examination > Holter or event monitor, depending on frequency of symptoms > ENT or neurologic consultations > tilt test > EPS if symptoms are severe and arrhythmia has not been excluded
Syncope	Cardiac arrhythmia, neurocardiogenic reflex, medications, psychiatric disorder	History and examination > event monitor > tilt test > EPS if arrhythmia still suspected > neurologic or psychiatric evaluation

PACs = premature atrial contractions; PVCs = premature ventricular contractions; SVT = supraventricular tachycardia; AF = atrial fibrillation; VT = ventricular tachycardia; AVB = atrioventricular block; EPS = electrophysiologic study; ENT = ear, nose, and throat.

Most syncopal spells have a cardiovascular cause. The most common cardiovascular causes are arrhythmia and neurocardiogenic syncope (in essence, an exaggerated vasovagal response). Patients with SND usually experience pre-syncope rather than syncope. When patients experience true syncope, they usually have several seconds of warning symptoms before fainting. Drop attacks associated with His-Purkinje disease, or Morgagni-Stokes-Adams attacks, are usually more abrupt. Tachyarrhythmic syncope may occur with or without warning, depending on the rhythm (see pages 684–687).

Neurocardiogenic syncope is usually heralded by dizziness and other symptoms but may be very abrupt. Often the event is preceded by a change in posture to sitting or standing, a prolonged period of standing with little movement, or an inciting incident such as venipuncture.

Holter monitoring has only a secondary role in the evaluation of syncope and is likely to be helpful only in patients with daily episodes. Event monitoring is more useful. In difficult cases, especially patients who experience severe spells less frequently than monthly, an electrophysiologic study or an implantable loop recorder may be the only means of diagnosis.

Antiarrhythmic Drugs

Of the many available antiarrhythmic agents, none is completely effective for all patients, and every agent can cause serious toxicity (Fig. 5–9).

Antiarrhythmic Drug Actions

Vaughn-Williams Class		Drug	Channels: Na	Ca	K	Receptors: α	β	ACh	Ado	Clinical effects: Pro-Arrhy	LV Fx	Heart rate	Extra cardiac	ECG changes
I	A	Quinidine	Moderate		High	Low		Moderate		High			Moderate	A
		Procainamide	Moderate		Moderate					Moderate			High	
		Disopyramide (Norpace)	Moderate		Moderate			Moderate		Low	↓↓		Moderate	
	B	Lidocaine (Xylocaine)	Low							Low			Moderate	B
		Mexiletine (Mexitil)	Low							Low			Moderate	
	C	Propafenone (Rythmol)	High				Moderate			Moderate	↓↓	↓	Low	C
		Flecainide (Tambocor)	High							High	↓↓		Low	
II		β adrenergic antagonists					High			Low	↓	↓↓	Low	
III		Bretylium (Bretylol)			High	▲	▲			Low		↓	Low	
		Sotalol (Betapace)			High		High			High	↓	↓	Low	
		Amiodarone (Cordarone)	Low	Low	High	Moderate	Moderate	Moderate		Low		↓	High	
		Ibutilide (Corvert)	△		High					High			Low	
IV		Verapamil (Calan, Isoptin)		High						Low	↓↓	↓	Low	
		Diltiazem (Cardizem)		Moderate						Low	↓	↓	Low	
Misc		Adenosine (Adenocard)							△	Low		↓	Low	

Antagonist Relative Potency: ○Low ◍Moderate ●High

△ = Agonist

▲ = Agonist/Antagonist

FIGURE 5–9 ■ This figure is a modification of the Sicilian Gambit drug classification system and includes designation by the Vaughan Williams system. The sodium channel blockers are subdivided into the A, B, and C subgroups based on their relative potency. The targets of antiarrhythmic drugs, listed across the columns, are the ion channels (sodium, calcium, and potassium) and the receptors (α-adrenergic, β-adrenergic, cholinergic [ACh], and adenosinergic [Ado]). The next columns compare the drugs' clinical actions. These include proarrhythmic potential (Pro-Arrhy), effect on left ventricular function (LV Fx), effects on heart rate (Heart rate), and potential for extracardiac side effects (Extra cardiac). The ECG tracings indicate the changes that are caused by usual dosages of the drug (i.e., PR interval, QRS interval, and QT interval). The drugs are listed in rows with their brand names shown in parentheses. The symbols in the table indicate the drugs' relative potency as agonists or antagonists. The solid triangle indicates the biphasic effects of bretylium initially to release norepinephrine and act as an agonist and subsequently to block further release and act as an antagonist of adrenergic tone. The number of arrows and their direction indicate the magnitude and direction of effect of the drugs on heart rate and left ventricular function (i.e., inotropy).

Lidocaine (Xylocaine) is often the drug of first choice for the acute suppression of ventricular arrhythmias. For a stable patient, a total loading dose of lidocaine should be 3 to 4 mg/kg administered as a series of doses over 20 to 30 minutes. At the time of initiation of the loading regimen, a maintenance infusion, designed to replace ongoing losses due to drug elimination, should be started, usually in a range of 20 to 60 μg/kg/min. CNS symptoms are the most frequent side effects.

Mexiletine (Mexitil) is used in the treatment of ventricular arrhythmias. With normal renal function, the recommended initial oral mexiletine dosage is 200 mg every 8 hours. All patients with renal failure should be given low initial doses. Adverse reactions are most often dose-related and include tremor, visual blurring, dizziness, dysphoria, and nausea.

Procainamide (Pronestyl-SR, Procan SR) is effective against both supraventricular and ventricular arrhythmias. When administered IV, procainamide can be given as a constant 25-minute loading infusion of 275 μg/kg/minute or by a series of doses (100 mg delivered over 3 minutes) given every 5 minutes up to a total dose of 1 g. If the loading infusion is well tolerated with no hypotension and less than 25% QRS or QT widening, the maintenance IV infusion is 20 to 60 μg/kg/minute. With normal renal and cardiac function, the initial recommended oral maintenance dose is 50 mg/kg/day in the sustained-release form every 6 to 8 hours. Because the electrophysiologic effects of procainamide and its active metabolite *N*-acetyl procainamide (NAPA) are quite different, monitoring of patients receiving procainamide should include measurement of plasma concentrations of both agents to determine their relative concentrations. Up to 40% of patients discontinue procainamide in the first 6 months due to adverse reactions. Arrhythmia may be aggravated, and 15 to 20% of patients develop a lupus-like syndrome. Procainamide can cause agranulocytosis, so a white blood cell count should be obtained every 2 weeks for the first 3 months.

Disopyramide (Norpace) (class IA) is effective against a broad range of supraventricular and ventricular arrhythmias. The usually effective dosage for disopyramide is 100 to 400 mg two to four times daily, to a maximal dose of 800 mg/day. Its negative inotropic and anticholinergic actions frequently limit its usefulness.

Quinidine (class IA) is used for a variety of supraventricular and ventricular arrhythmias. The usually effective dosage of quinidine sulfate ranges from 800 to 2400 mg/day, with the maximum recommended single dose being 600 mg. Marked prolongation of the QT interval can occur with usual or even low doses.

Propafenone (Rythmol) (class IC) is used for supraventricular arrhythmias. Effective dosages range from 300 to 900 mg/day in two to four divided doses. Combination with β-blockers should be avoided.

Flecainide (Tambocor) (class IC) is very effective in suppressing a variety of ventricular and supraventricular tachycardias. Patients with supraventricular tachycardia should receive 50 mg every 12 hours as a starting dose; after 3 to 4 days, the dose can be adjusted up to 100 to 150 mg every 12 hours. Flecainide can induce proarrhythmic events even when prescribed as recommended.

β-Blockers are effective for a variety of supraventricular and ventricular tachyarrhythmias. The dosages are generally similar to those required for treatment of hypertension or angina.

Bretylium (Bretylol) (class III) is effective acute therapy for VT and/or VF. The usual IV dosage for bretylium is 5 mg/kg given by rapid injection into a central IV line. Many patients experience nausea and vomiting

Sotalol (Betapace) is effective in suppressing a variety of supraventricular and ventricular arrhythmias, but it increases instability in patients with ventricular arrhythmias after an MI. The recommended initial dose of sotalol is 80 mg every 12 hours. In patients who do not respond and have QT intervals less than 500 ms, the dosage may be increased to 160 mg twice daily and, if necessary, to 240 mg twice daily. Torsades de pointes occurs with an overall incidence of approximately 2%.

Amiodarone (Cordarone) is officially approved only for life-threatening ventricular arrhythmias refractory to other available forms of therapy, but numerous trials describe its efficacy in the conversion and slowing of AF, AVNR tachycardia, and tachycardias associated with the WPW syndrome. Without a loading dose, amiodarone requires several weeks to months before producing its antiarrhythmic action. Large IV (150 mg over 10 minutes, followed by 360 mg over the next 6 hours, followed by 0.5 mg/minute for 18 hours) or oral (600–800 mg/day for 14 days) loading dosages can hasten the onset of therapeutic effects. The usual maintenance dose varies from 200 to 600 mg/day. The most serious adverse reaction is lethal interstitial pneumonitis. Thirty per cent or more of patients have abnormally elevated serum hepatic enzyme levels.

Calcium channel blockers (verapamil and diltiazem) are useful in the management of supraventricular tachycardia. The usual dosages for verapamil are 2.5 to 5.0 mg IV over 2 to 4 minutes, with another 5 to 10 mg if necessary 15 to 30 minutes later to a maximum total dose of 20 mg. For diltiazem the recommendation is either an IV bolus of 0.25 mg/kg (about 20 mg) over 2 minutes, with a second dose of 0.35 mg/kg if necessary, or a continuous infusion at 5 to 10 mg/hour with maximum dose of 15 mg/hour and maximum duration of 24 hours. Oral doses are similar to those used for angina.

Adenosine (Adenocard) is very effective for the acute conversion of paroxysmal supraventricular tachycardia caused by re-entry involving the AV node. For adults, the initial dose is 6 mg injected over 1 to 2 seconds. If the arrhythmia persists, a 12-mg dose can be injected 1 to 2 minutes later. Adenosine is contraindicated in patients with sick sinus syndrome or second- or third-degree heart block. Less frequent side effects include nausea, lightheadedness, headache, sweating, palpitations, hypotension, and blurred vision.

For more information about this subject, see *Cecil Textbook of Medicine,* 21st edition. Philadelphia, W.B. Saunders Company, 2000. Chapter 49, Principles of Electrophysiology; Chapter 50, Electrophysiologic Diagnostic Procedures; Chapter 51, Cardiac Arrhythmias with Supraventricular Origin; Chapter 52, Ventricular Arrhythmias and Sudden Death; Chapter 53, Electrophysiologic Interventional Procedures and Surgery; and Chapter 54, Antiarrhythmic Drugs, pages 226 to 258.

ARTERIAL HYPERTENSION

Blood pressure (BP) is based on the average of two or more readings taken at each of two or more visits after an initial screening (Table 5–20). Optimal BP with respect to cardiovascular risk is less than 120/80 mm Hg, but unusually low readings should be evaluated for their clinical significance. *Isolated systolic hypertension* is defined as systolic BP greater than 140 mm Hg and diastolic BP less than 90 mm Hg and staged appropriately (e.g., 170/82 mm Hg is defined as stage 2 isolated systolic hypertension).

The *medical history* should focus on identifying known, remediable causes of high BP, establishing the presence or absence of target organ disease and cardiovascular disease, and identifying other cardiovascular risk factors or co-morbid conditions that might affect prognosis or treatment. The *physical examination* should include height; weight; fundoscopic examination; verification of hypertension in the contralateral arm; a careful examination of the

Table 5–20 ■ CLASSIFICATION OF BLOOD PRESSURE FOR ADULTS

	BLOOD PRESSURE (mm Hg)		
CATEGORY	Systolic		Diastolic
Optimal	<120	*and*	<80
Normal	<130	*and*	<85
High-normal	130–139	*or*	85–89
Hypertension			
Stage 1	140–159	*or*	90–99
Stage 2	160–179	*or*	100–109
Stage 3	≥180	*or*	≥110

From Joint National Committee on Prevention, Detection, Evaluation, and Treatment of High Blood Pressure: The Sixth Report of the Joint National Committee on Prevention, Detection, Evaluation, and Treatment of High Blood Pressure (JNC VI). Arch Intern Med 157:2413, © 1997, American Medical Association.

neck, abdomen, and extremities for bruits; neurologic assessment; and if coarctation of the aorta is suspected, BP measurement in the leg. Pre-treatment laboratory tests can be restricted to those generally performed as part of a routine medical evaluation. Clues from the medical history, physical examination, initial laboratory evaluation, and clinical course help identify the 5% of hypertensive patients with specific causes for the disorder (Table 5–21 and Fig. 5–10).

In any given patient, the decision to initiate therapy is governed by the risk of cardiovascular disease, which is determined by the extent of the BP elevation and the presence or absence of target organ disease (LV hypertrophy, angina, prior MI, prior coronary revascularization, heart failure, stroke or transient ischemic attack, nephropathy, peripheral arterial disease, or retinopathy) and/or additional cardiovascular risk factors, including smoking, dyslipidemia, diabetes mellitus, age older than 60 years, sex (men or postmenopausal women), and a family history of cardiovascular disease (women ≤ age 65 or men ≤ age 55 years). For example, a patient with diabetes and a BP of 142/94 mm Hg plus LV hypertrophy should be classified as having stage 1 hypertension with target organ disease (LV hypertrophy) and with another major risk factor (diabetes). This patient would be categorized as a stage 1, risk group C, and be recommended for immediate initiation of pharmacologic treatment. Consensus guidelines stratify hypertensive patients into risk groups for therapeutic decisions (Table 5–22).

Non-pharmacologic interventions (lifestyle modifications) are generally beneficial in reducing a variety of cardiovascular risk factors, including high BP, and in promoting good health, and should therefore be used in all hypertensive patients, either as definitive treatment or as an adjunct to drug therapy (Fig. 5–11). Monotherapy with antihypertensive drugs effectively controls BP in fewer than 50% of patients. Non-adherence to prescribed therapy is a major problem.

For many hypertensive patients, especially those without co-morbid conditions, target organ damage, or concomitant cardiovascular risk factors, drug therapy should begin with a diuretic or a β-blocker.

Table 5–21 ■ CAUSES OF SECONDARY HYPERTENSION

Systolic and Diastolic Hypertension

Renal

- Renal parenchymal disease: acute glomerulonephritis, chronic nephritis, collagen-vascular disease, diabetic nephropathy, hydronephrosis, polycystic disease
- Renal vascular disease
- Renal transplantation
- Renin-secreting tumors

Endocrine

- Adrenal: Primary aldosteronism; overproduction of 11-deoxycorticosterone (DOC), 18-OH-DOC, and other mineralocorticoids; congenital adrenal hyperplasia; Cushing's syndrome; pheochromocytoma
- Extra-adrenal chromaffin tumors
- Hyperparathyroidism
- Acromegaly
- Pregnancy-induced hypertension
- Sleep apnea
- Coarctation of the aorta

Neurologic disorders

- Dysautonomia
- Increased intracranial pressure
- Quadriplegia
- Lead poisoning
- Guillain-Barré syndrome
- Postoperative hypertension

Drugs and chemicals

- Amphetamines
- Antidepressants
- Appetite suppressants
- Cocaine
- Cyclosporine
- Erythropoietin
- Ethanol
- Glucocorticoids
- Mineralocorticoids, including licorice and carbenoxolone
- Monoamine oxidase inhibitors
- Nasal decongestants
- Non-steroidal anti-inflammatory agents
- Oral contraceptives
- Phenothiazines
- Tyramine

Isolated Systolic Hypertension

Aging, with associated aortic rigidity

Increased cardiac output

- Thyrotoxicosis
- Anemia
- Aortic valvular insufficiency

Decreased peripheral vascular resistance

- Arteriovenous shunts
- Paget's disease of bone
- Beri-beri

From Oparil S, Calhoun DA: High blood pressure. *In* Dale DC, Federman DD (eds): Scientific American Medicine, vol. 1. New York, Scientific American, 1997, sect 1, subsect 3, pp 1–14.

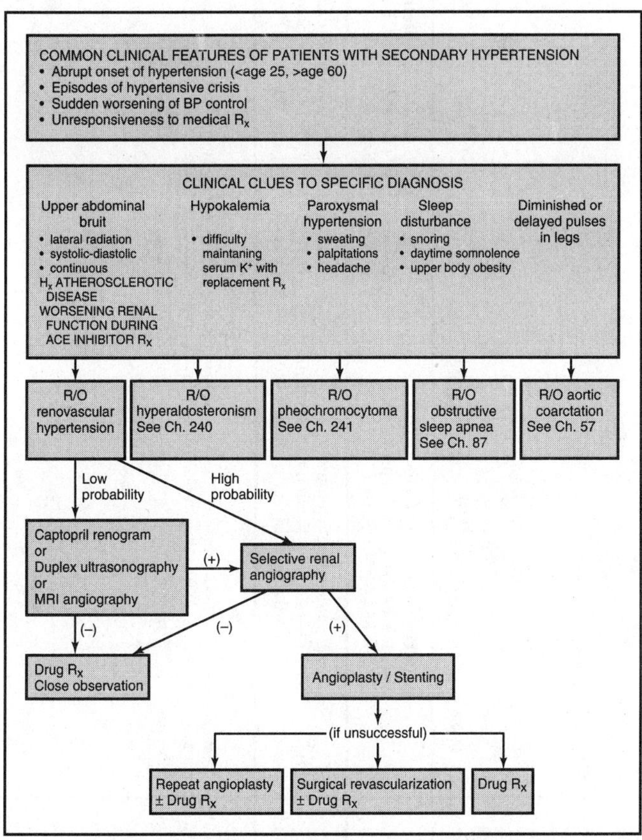

FIGURE 5–10 ■ Algorithm for identifying patients for evaluation of secondary causes of hypertension. R/O = rule out.

For some patients, however, co-morbid conditions may dictate the choice of another class of drug (Table 5–23). Data from one recent study suggest that α-blockers increase the risk of heart failure compared with other hypertensive medications and should not be a first-choice option. When monotherapy is unsuccessful, a second agent, usually of a different class, should be added (Table 5–24). Step-down therapy, that is, withdrawing antihypertensive medication under close monitoring, should be attempted in patients with stage 1 or stage 2 hypertension whose BP has been adequately controlled for a year or more.

BP above 200/120 mm Hg in the presence of neurologic, cardiovascular, or renal deterioration and fundoscopic abnormalities is a hypertensive crisis. Usually the cause of any particular hypertensive crisis is not known, and therapy must be empiric. Patients typically require parenteral antihypertensive therapy administered in an intensive care setting (Tables 5–25 and 5–26). The goal is a prompt but gradual reduction in BP to just above normotensive levels.

For more information about this subject, see *Cecil Textbook of*

Table 5–22 ■ TREATMENT STRATEGIES AND RISK STRATIFICATION

BLOOD PRESSURE STAGE (mm Hg)	RISK GROUP A (NO RISK FACTORS, NO TOD/CCD)	RISK GROUP B (AT LEAST ONE RISK FACTOR, NOT INCLUDING DIABETES; NO TOD/CCD)	RISK GROUP C (TOD/CCD AND/OR DIABETES, WITH OR WITHOUT OTHER RISK FACTORS)
High-normal (130–139/85–89)	Lifestyle modification	Lifestyle modification	Drug therapy; lifestyle modification
Stage 1 (140–159/90–99)	Lifestyle modification (up to 12 mo)	Lifestyle modification (up to 6 mo)	Drug therapy; lifestyle modification
Stages 2 and 3 (≥160/≥100)	Drug therapy; lifestyle modification	Drug therapy; lifestyle modification	Drug therapy; lifestyle modification

TOD/CCD = target organ disease/clinical cardiovascular disease.

From Joint National Committee on Prevention, Detection, Evaluation, and Treatment of High Blood Pressure: The Sixth Report of the Joint National Committee on Prevention, Detection, Evaluation, and Treatment of High Blood Pressure (JNC VI). Arch Intern Med 157:2413, © 1997, American Medical Association.

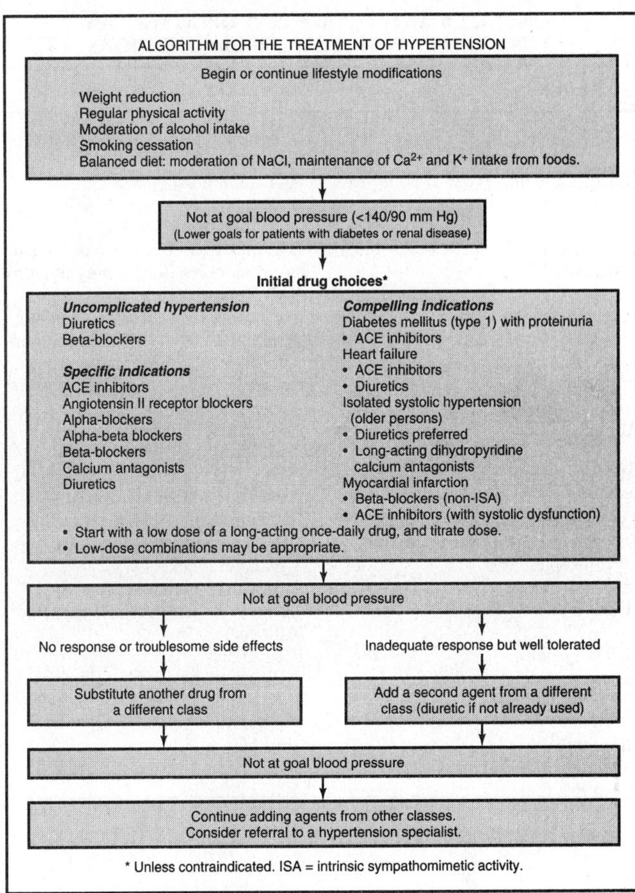

ALGORITHM FOR THE TREATMENT OF HYPERTENSION
Begin or continue lifestyle modifications
Weight reduction
Regular physical activity
Moderation of alcohol intake
Smoking cessation
Balanced diet: moderation of NaCl, maintenance of Ca2+ and K+ intake from foods.
Not at goal blood pressure (<140/90 mm Hg)
(Lower goals for patients with diabetes or renal disease)
Initial drug choices*
Uncomplicated hypertension
Diuretics
Beta-blockers
Specific indications
ACE inhibitors
Angiotensin II receptor blockers
Alpha-blockers
Alpha-beta blockers
Beta-blockers
Calcium antagonists
Diuretics
Compelling indications
Diabetes mellitus (type 1) with proteinuria
• ACE inhibitors
Heart failure
• ACE inhibitors
• Diuretics
Isolated systolic hypertension
(older persons)
• Diuretics preferred
• Long-acting dihydropyridine
calcium antagonists
Myocardial infarction
• Beta-blockers (non-ISA)
• ACE inhibitors (with systolic dysfunction)
• Start with a low dose of a long-acting once-daily drug, and titrate dose.
• Low-dose combinations may be appropriate.
Not at goal blood pressure
No response or troublesome side effects
Inadequate response but well tolerated
Substitute another drug from
a different class
Add a second agent from a different
class (diuretic if not already used)
Not at goal blood pressure
Continue adding agents from other classes.
Consider referral to a hypertension specialist.
* Unless contraindicated. ISA = intrinsic sympathomimetic activity.

FIGURE 5–11 ■ Treatment algorithm for patients with essential hypertension. If the goal blood pressure is not achieved in response to a given intervention, the additional interventions indicated in the lower boxes are added. ACE = angiotensin-converting enzyme. (Adapted from Joint National Committee on Prevention, Detection, Evaluation, and Treatment of High Blood Pressure: The Sixth Report of the Joint National Committee on Prevention, Detection, Evaluation, and Treatment of High Blood Pressure [JNC VI]. Arch Intern Med 157:2413, Copyright 1997, American Medical Association.)

Medicine, 21st edition. Philadelphia, W.B. Saunders Company, 2000. Chapter 55, Arterial Hypertension, pages 258 to 273.

PULMONARY HYPERTENSION

Pulmonary hypertension may be acute or chronic. RV failure may develop in either setting as a result of the increase in RV pressure work.

Pulmonary hypertension can be divided into three classes based

Text continued on page 88

Table 5–23 ■ ANTIHYPERTENSIVE DRUG THERAPY FOR PATIENTS WITH CO-MORBID CONDITIONS

INDICATION	DRUG THERAPY
	Compelling Indications unless Contraindicated
Diabetes mellitus (type I) with proteinuria	ACE inhibitors
Heart failure	ACE inhibitors, diuretics
Isolated systolic hypertension (older patients)	Diuretics (preferred), calcium channel blockers (long-acting dihydropyridine)
Myocardial infarction	β-Blockers (non-intrinsic sympathomimetic activity), ACE inhibitors (with systolic dysfunction)
	Favorable Effects on Co-Morbid Conditions
Angina	β-Blockers, calcium channel blockers (long-acting)
Atrial tachycardia and fibrillation	β-Blockers, calcium channel blockers (non-dihydropyridine)
Cyclosporine-induced hypertension	Calcium channel blockers
Diabetes mellitus (types I and II) with proteinuria	ACE inhibitors (preferred), calcium channel blockers
Essential tremor	β-Blockers (non-cardioselective)
Heart failure	Carvedilol, angiotensin II receptor blockers*
Hyperthyroidism	β-Blockers
Migraine	β-Blockers (non-cardioselective), calcium channel blockers (non-dihydropyridine)
Osteoporosis	Thiazides
Benign prostatic hyperplasia	α-Blockers
Renal insufficiency (except in renovascular hypertension and creatinine ≥265.2 mmol/L [3 mg/dL])	ACE inhibitors
	Potential Unfavorable Effects on Co-Morbid Conditions
Bronchospastic disease	β-Blockers
Depression	β-Blockers, central α-antagonists, reserpine
Diabetes mellitus (types I and II) or marked hypertriglyceridemia	β-Blockers, high-dose diuretics
Gout	Diuretics
Second- and third-degree heart block	β-blockers, diltiazem, verapamil
Heart failure	β-Blockers (except in low doses), calcium channel blockers (except amlodipine, felodipine)
Liver disease	Labetalol, methyldopa
Pregnancy	ACE inhibitors, angiotensin II receptor blockers*
Renal insufficiency	Potassium-sparing agents
Renovascular disease	ACE inhibitors, angiotensin II receptor blockers*

ACE = angiotensin-converting enzyme.

*Angiotensin II receptor blockers may be useful in the same clinical settings as ACE inhibitors, but this has not yet been demonstrated in controlled clinical trials.

From Joint National Committee on Prevention, Detection, Evaluation, and Treatment of High Blood Pressure: The Sixth Report of the Joint National Committee on Prevention, Detection, Evaluation, and Treatment of High Blood Pressure (JNC VI). Arch Intern Med 157:2413, © 1997, American Medical Association.

Table 5–24 ■ COMMON ANTIHYPERTENSIVE DRUGS IN AMBULATORY TREATMENT OF HYPERTENSION

GENERIC NAME	TRADE NAME	ADULT MAINTENANCE DOSE (mg/d)	FREQUENCY OF ADMINISTRATION (times per day)	DURATION OF ACTION (hr)
β-Adrenergic Blockers				
Acebutolol	Sectral	400–1200	1 or 2	12–24
Atenolol	Tenormin	50–100	1	24
Bisoprolol	Zebeta	2.5–20	1	24
Metoprolol	Lopressor	100–450	2	12
Nadolol	Corgard	40–320	1	24
Propranolol	Inderal	40–640	2	6–12
α-Adrenergic Blockers				
Doxazosin	Cardura	2–16	1	24
Terazosin	Hytrin	1–20	1	24
Diuretics				
Chlorthalidone	Thalitone	15–50	1	24–72
Hydrochlorothiazide	HydroDIURIL	12.5–50	1–2	12–18
Potassium-Sparing Diuretics				
Amiloride	Midamor	5–20	1	24
Triamterene	Dyrenium	50–300	1–2	3–6

Table continued on following page

Table 5–24 ■ COMMON ANTIHYPERTENSIVE DRUGS IN AMBULATORY TREATMENT OF HYPERTENSION *Continued*

GENERIC NAME	TRADE NAME	ADULT MAINTENANCE DOSE (mg/d)	FREQUENCY OF ADMINISTRATION (times per day)	DURATION OF ACTION (hr)
Angiotensin-Converting Enzyme Inhibitors				
Benazepril	Lotensin	10–80	1 or 2	12–24
Captopril	Generic	75–450	2–3	4–8
Enalapril	Vasotec	5–40	1 or 2	12–24
Lisinopril	Prinivil, Zestril	10–40	1	24
Angiotensin II Antagonist				
Valsartan	Diovan	80–320	1	24
Calcium Channel Antagonists				
Nifedipine	Procardia XL, Adalat CC	30–90	1	24
Nicardipine	Generic	60–120	2	12
Diltiazem	Cardizem SR	120–360	2	12
	Cardizem CD	120–360	1	24
Verapamil	Covera-HS	180–480	1 (at bedtime)	24
	Isoptin SR	120–480	1 or 2	12–24

Table 5-25 ■ HYPERTENSIVE EMERGENCIES AND TREATMENT RECOMMENDATIONS

EMERGENCY	RECOMMENDED TREATMENT
Hypertensive encephalopathy	Nitroprusside, labetalol, fenoldopam, nicardipine
Subarachnoid hemorrhage	Nimodipine, nitroprusside, fenoldopam, labetalol
Ischemic stroke	Nitroprusside, fenoldopam, labetalol
Intracerebral hemorrhage	No treatment, nitroprusside, fenoldopam, labetalol
Myocardial ischemia/infarction	IV nitroglycerin, labetalol, calcium antagonists, nitroprusside
Left ventricular failure	Nitroprusside, IV nitroglycerin
Aortic dissection	β-Antagonist with nitroprusside; trimethaphan, labetalol
Hyperadrenergic states (cocaine overdose, clonidine withdrawal, pheochromocytoma, diet pills, amphetamines)	Phentolamine, labetalol, nitroprusside, clonidine (for clonidine withdrawal only)
Acute renal insufficiency	Fenoldopam, nitroprusside, nicardipine, labetalol
Eclampsia	Magnesium sulfate, hydralazine, labetalol, calcium antagonists
Postoperative crisis	Labetalol, fenoldopam, nitroglycerin, nicardipine, nitroprusside

Table 5-26 ■ ANTIHYPERTENSIVE DRUGS FOR MANAGEMENT OF HYPERTENSIVE EMERGENCY

DRUGS	SINGLE DOSE*	CONTINUOUS INFUSION
Sodium nitroprusside (Nipride)	—	0.5–10 μg/kg/min
Fenoldopam (Corlopam)	—	0.1–0.8 μg/kg/min
Nicardine (Cardene)	5 mg/hr initially, titrated upward by 1.0–2.5 mg/hr every 15 min as needed up to 15 mg/hr	—
Phentolamine (Regitine)	5–15 mg (rapid injection essential)	—
Labetalol	20 mg initially over 2 min, then 40–80 mg at 10-min intervals as needed up to 300 mg total	2 mg/min to a total dose of 300 mg

*Start with the lowest dose shown. Subsequent doses and intervals of administration should be adjusted according to blood pressure response. Constant surveillance is mandatory.

Table 5–27 ■ PATHOPHYSIOLOGY OF PULMONARY HYPERTENSION

MECHANISM	DISEASE ENTITIES
Increased pulmonary blood flow	Congenital heart disease with left-to-right shunts; marked increase in cardiac output (e.g., severe anemia); severe bronchiectasis with systemic-to-pulmonary shunts
Abnormalities in the pulmonary arteries; increased resistance to flow or loss of cross-sectional area	Pulmonary embolism; pulmonary fibrosis; sarcoidosis; scleroderma; extensive pulmonary resection; severe COPD; thoracic deformities (e.g., kyphoscoliosis, severe pectus excavatum); schistosomiasis; extensive neoplastic or inflammatory infiltration
Abnormalities in the pulmonary arterioles: vasoconstriction, obliteration	Hypoxia (e.g., altitude); COPD, hypoventilation syndromes (e.g., sleep apnea); acidosis; toxic substances; primary pulmonary hypertension
Abnormalities in pulmonary veins or venules; elevated pulmonary venous pressure and vascular resistance	Left atrial hypertension (e.g., mitral stenosis, left ventricular failure); pulmonary venous thrombosis; pulmonary veno-occlusive disease; mediastinitis (e.g., methysergide-induced sclerosing mediastinitis)
Increased blood viscosity	Polycythemia vera; leukemia with very high leukocyte counts
Increased intrathoracic pressure	COPD; mechanical ventilation, especially with positive end-expiratory pressure

COPD = chronic obstructive pulmonary disease.

on the location of the abnormal increase in pulmonary vascular resistance: precapillary, passive, and reactive (Table 5–27). Patients with increased pulmonary arteriolar and/or arterial resistance are classified as having *precapillary pulmonary hypertension.* Pulmonary arterial pressure is increased, but pulmonary capillary wedge and pulmonary venous pressures are normal. The gradient between the mean pulmonary arterial pressure and the pulmonary capillary or pulmonary venous pressure is greater than 12 mm Hg. Individuals with increased pulmonary venous pressure secondarily causing pulmonary arterial hypertension have *passive pulmonary hypertension.* Pulmonary arterial, capillary, and venous pressures are all elevated. The gradient between the mean pulmonary arterial pressure and the pulmonary capillary or pulmonary venous pressures is less than or equal to 12 mm Hg. In *reactive pulmonary hypertension,* patients have elevated pulmonary venous pressure as well as pulmonary arteriolar vasoconstriction. The gradient between the mean pulmonary arterial pressure and the pulmonary capillary or pulmonary venous pressures is greater than 12 mm Hg.

Patients with mild to moderate pulmonary hypertension are often

Table 5–28 ■ COMMONLY USED CLINICAL CUES SUGGESTING THE DIAGNOSIS OF PULMONARY HYPERTENSION

Increased loudness of the pulmonic component of S_2
Right ventricular enlargement on physical exam: left parasternal impulse or lift
Signs of right ventricular failure present on physical exam: jugular venous distention, right ventricular S_3, hepatomegaly, ascites, hepatojugular reflux, peripheral edema
Right ventricular hypertrophy on ECG
Enlargement of the right ventricle and/or pulmonary arteries on the chest radiograph, echocardiogram, radionuclide ventriculogram, or CT/MRI
Pulmonary arterial systolic blood pressure >30 mm Hg by Doppler echocardiography or catheterization

asymptomatic. Individuals with more severe pulmonary hypertension usually complain of dyspnea on exertion. Physical examination usually reveals one or more signs (Table 5–28). The ECG and chest film help differentiate the causes of pulmonary hypertension (Table 5–29).

Primary pulmonary hypertension (PPHT) is a disease of unknown cause. The differential diagnosis of PPHT includes mitral stenosis, recurrent pulmonary embolism, congenital cardiac defects with severe pulmonary vascular disease, sickle cell anemia, collagen-vascular disease, and rare entities such as cor triatriatum. Any disease that causes LV failure with resultant left atrial hypertension is accompanied by pulmonary hypertension.

Because a variety of disease entities with varying pathophysiologic abnormalities lead to pulmonary hypertension, it is impossible to recommend one specific remedy (Fig. 5–12).

For more information about this subject, see *Cecil Textbook of Medicine,* 21st edition. Philadelphia, W.B. Saunders Company, 2000. Chapter 56, Pulmonary Hypertension, pages 273 to 279.

CONGENITAL HEART DISEASE IN ADULTS

Patients may be unoperated or surgically palliated or may have undergone physiologic repair. Congenital heart lesions can be classified as *acyanotic* or *cyanotic. Palliative* interventions serve either to increase or decrease pulmonary blood flow while allowing a mixed circulation and cyanosis to persist. *Physiologic* repair applies to procedures that provide total or nearly total anatomic and physiologic separation of the pulmonary and systemic circulations in complex cyanotic lesions and result in patients who are acyanotic.

Eisenmenger's physiology is used to designate the physiologic response of shunt lesions in which a right-to-left shunt occurs in response to an elevation in pulmonary vascular resistance. The term *Eisenmenger's syndrome* should be reserved for patients in whom pulmonary vascular obstructive disease is present and pulmonary vascular resistance is fixed and irreversible. These findings in combination with the absence of left-to-right shunting render the patient inoperable. The clinical manifestations of Eisenmenger's syndrome include dyspnea on exertion, syncope, chest pain, congestive heart failure, and symptoms related to erythrocytosis and hyperviscosity. On physical examination, central cyanosis and digital clubbing are

Table 5–29 ■ LABORATORY FINDINGS IN PATIENTS WITH PULMONARY HYPERTENSION

DISEASE ENTITY	ECG	CHEST X-RAY	OTHER USEFUL TESTS	CATHETERIZATION
Precapillary Pulmonary Hypertension				
PPHT	RVH	↑ ↑ RA, ↑ RV, clear lungs with tapered periph arteries	PFTs nl; lung scan nl or min abn	PAP ↑ ↑, nl PCWP, ↑ RAP, PAgram nl
Pulmonary embolism	nl or acute cor pulmonale ($S_1Q_3T_3$ or new IRBBB or RBBB)	nl or infiltrate, unilateral pleural effusion	abnl ABGs; ↓ Po_2, ↑ pH, ↓ Pco_2, lung scan: seg perf defects, nl ventil scan	PAP ↑, nl PCWP, RAP nl or ↑; + PAgram
Disorders of ventilation	nl or RVH	Specific abnl in various entities	ABGs, PFTs abnl	PAP ↑, PCWP nl, RAP nl or ↑
Congenital heart disease	RVH	Clear lungs, ↑ ↑ PA, ↑ RV, tapered distal arteries, specific abnl in various entities	Cardiac echo: specific abnl in various entities	↑ ↑ PAP, nl PCWP, RA ↑ or nl, ↓ PaO_2

Passive Pulmonary Hypertension				
Mitral stenosis	AF or NSR, LAE, RVH, or no VH	pulm congestion, ↑ LA, ↑ RV	Echo: LAE, abnl MV, nl LV	Gradient across MV, PAP ↑ PCW ↑, RAP nl or ↑
Left ventricular failure	abnl depends on specific entity: LVH, MI, BBB	↑ ↑ or ↑ LV, ↑ LA, ↑ or nl RV, pulm congestion	Echo: abnl LV function, LAE	abnl LV function, ↑ LVEDP, ↑ PCW, ↑ PAP
Reactive Pulmonary Hypertension				
Long-standing mitral stenosis	AF, RVH	↑ ↑ PA, ↑ ↑ RV, ↑ ↑ LA, pulm congestion	Echo: very abnl MV, ↑ ↑ RV, ↑ ↑ LA	MV gradient, PCW ↑ ↑, ↑ ↑ PAP, ↑ RAP
Pulmonary veno-occlusive disease	RVH	↑ ↑ PA, ↑ ↑ RV	Lung scan: nl or minor defects	Absent MV gradient, PCW ↑ or nl, LAP nl, LVP nl

PPHT = primary pulmonary hypertension; PA = pulmonary artery; RV = right ventricle; RA = right atrium; LV = left ventricle; LA = left atrium; PAP = pulmonary artery pressure; RAP = right atrial pressure; LVP = left ventricular pressure; PCWP = pulmonary capillary wedge pressure; LAP = left atrial pressure; nl = normal; abnl = abnormal or abnormality; pulm = pulmonary; ABGs = arterial blood gases; PFTs = pulmonary function tests; seg = segmental; PAgram = pulmonary angiogram; RVH = right ventricular hypertrophy; LVH = left ventricular hypertrophy; NSR = normal sinus rhythm; VH = ventricular hypertrophy; LAE = left atrial enlargement; AF = atrial fibrillation; MI = myocardial infarction; BBB = bundle branch block; IRBBB = incomplete right bundle branch block; RBBB = right bundle branch block; LVEDP = left ventricular end-diastolic pressure; min = minimal; MV = mitral valve; periph = peripheral; perf = perfusion; ventil = ventilation; + = positive; ↑ ↑ = markedly increased; ↑ = increased; ↓ = decreased.

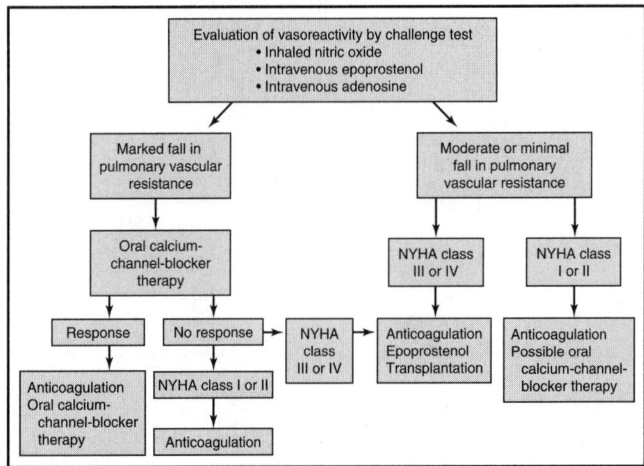

FIGURE 5–12 ■ Algorithm for the management of primary pulmonary hypertension. NYHA = New York Heart Association. (From Rubin LJ: Primary pulmonary hypertension. N Engl J Med 336:116, 1997. Copyright © 1997. Massachusetts Medical Society. All rights reserved.)

hallmark findings, as are signs of pulmonary hypertension (see Table 5–28).

Atrial Septal Defect (ASD)

An *ostium secundum* ASD occurs in the central portion of the interatrial septum as a result of an enlarged foramen ovale. Abnormal development of embryologic endocardial cushions results in the *ostium primum* location, typically accompanied by a cleft mitral valve and mitral regurgitation. The *sinus venosus* defect, which accounts for 2 to 3% of all interatrial communications, is located superiorly at the junction of the superior vena cava and right atrium and is generally associated with anomalous drainage of the right-sided pulmonary veins into the superior vena cava or right atrium.

Right atrial and RV dilation occur as shunt size increases with pulmonary-to-systemic flow ratios (Qp/Qs) greater than 1.5:1.0. Stroke can result from paradoxical emboli, atrial arrhythmias, or both. Pulmonary hypertension is unusual before 20 years of age, but is seen in 50% of patients older than 40 years.

On auscultation, the hallmark of an ASD is the wide and fixed splitting of S_2. A soft midsystolic murmur generated by the increased flow across the pulmonary valve is usually heard in the second left interspace. The ECG characteristically shows an incomplete right bundle branch pattern. Cardiac ultrasound is diagnostic. Closure of a significant asymptomatic shunt is generally indicated up to age 40.

Ventricular Septal Defect (VSD)

The pathophysiology and clinical course of VSDs depend on the size of the defect and the status of the pulmonary vascular bed.

Approximately half of all native VSDs are small, and more than half of them will close spontaneously. Patients who have a small defect with trivial or mild shunts are defined as those with a Qp/Qs of less than 1.5 and normal pulmonary artery pressure and vascular resistance.

Minimal or mild defects usually cause no significant hemodynamic or physiologic abnormality. A moderate or severe defect will cause left atrial and ventricular dilation consistent with the degree of left-to-right shunting. A thrill may be palpable at the left sternal border. A grade 4 or louder, widely radiating, high-frequency, pansystolic murmur is heard maximally in the third or fourth intercostal space. Echocardiography can identify the defect and determine the significance of the shunt.

All patients with a VSD of any size require endocarditis prophylaxis. Patients with a defect of moderate or greater physiologic significance should have surgical closure unless contraindicated by high pulmonary vascular resistance. Patients with Eisenmenger's syndrome have pulmonary vascular resistance that prohibits surgery.

Patent Ductus Arteriosus (PDA)

A small PDA has continuous flow throughout the entire cardiac cycle without left-sided heart dilation, pulmonary hypertension, or symptoms. In the presence of a continuous aortopulmonary gradient, the classic "machinery" murmur of a PDA can be heard at the first or second left intercostal space below the left clavicle. Patients with a small PDA remain at risk for infectious endarteritis, which usually develops on the pulmonary side of the duct. Ductal closure should be considered even when the PDA is small. In patients with Eisenmenger's physiology, a right-to-left shunt from the pulmonary artery to the descending aorta results in cyanosis and clubbing that is most prominent in the toes.

Pulmonary Arteriovenous Fistulas

Pulmonary arteriovenous fistulas can occur as isolated congenital disorders or as part of generalized hereditary hemorrhagic telangiectasia (Osler-Weber-Rendu syndrome). The most common finding is an abnormal opacity on the chest radiograph. Shunting is typically small and not significant enough to result in dilation of the left atrium and ventricle. Hemoptysis can result if a fistula ruptures into a bronchus.

Valvar Pulmonary Stenosis

On physical examination, an expiratory systolic ejection click is characteristic if the leaflets are still mobile. In moderate or severe stenosis, a grade 3 or louder systolic murmur can be heard and felt in the second left interspace. Survival at 25 years with valvar pulmonary stenosis is greater than 96% but is worse in those with severe stenosis and peak systolic gradients greater than 80 mm Hg. For gradients less than 50 mm Hg, conservative management is indicated and exercise should not be limited. For gradients of 50 to 80 mm Hg, intervention is generally recommended, particularly in symptomatic patients.

Coarctation of the Aorta

Aortic coarctation typically occurs just distal to the left subclavian artery at the site of the aortic ductal attachment or its residual ligamentum arteriosum. The most common complications are systemic hypertension and secondary LV hypertrophy with heart failure. Coarctation should always be considered in adolescents and young adult males with unexplained upper extremity hypertension.

BP measurements should be obtained in each arm and one leg; an abnormal measurement is an increase in popliteal systolic BP of less than 10 mm Hg compared with arm systolic BP. The coarctation itself generates a systolic murmur heard posteriorly in the midthoracic region. On the chest radiograph, bilateral rib notching is seen on the posterior of the third to eighth ribs. Repair is considered in patients with gradients greater than 30 mm Hg.

Sinus of Valsalva Aneurysms

A weakness in the wall of the sinus can result in aneurysm formation with or without rupture. Rupture typically occurs into the right side of the heart at the right atrial or ventricular level. A previously asymptomatic young man typically has chest pain and rapidly progressive shortness of breath. The classic murmur is loud and continuous, often with a thrill. The echocardiogram is diagnostic.

Coronary Artery Fistulas

Fistulas arise from the right or left coronary arteries and drain into the RV, the right atrium, or the pulmonary artery. Angina can occur as the fistula creates a coronary steal by diverting blood away from the myocardium. Heart failure is seen with large fistulas. A continuous murmur is heard. The echocardiogram, especially the transesophageal echocardiogram (TEE), is diagnostic.

Anomalous Origin of the Coronary Arteries

Isolated ectopic or anomalous origins of the coronary arteries are seen in 0.6 to 1.5% of patients undergoing coronary angiography. Risks of ischemia, MI, and death are increased and depend on the specific lesion. For an anomalous coronary artery that originates from the pulmonary artery, surgical reimplantation into the aorta is preferred. For an anomalous artery that courses between the pulmonary artery and aorta, a bypass graft to the distal vessel is preferred.

Tetralogy of Fallot

The tetrad is pulmonary stenosis, VSD, aortic override, and RV hypertrophy. Examination of unrepaired patients reveals central cyanosis and clubbing. The RV impulse is prominent. The S_2 is single and represents the aortic closure sound with an absent or inconspicuous pulmonic second sound (P_2). Typically, little or no systolic murmur is heard across the pulmonary valve because the more severe the obstruction, the more right-to-left shunting occurs and the less blood flows across a diminutive RV outflow tract.

Complete surgical repair consists of patch closure of the VSD and relief of the RV outflow tract obstruction. Complete repair in childhood yields a 90 to 95% 10-year survival rate with good functional results; 30-year survival rates may be as high as 85%.

After repair, residual pulmonary stenosis, proximal or distal, with an RV pressure greater than 50% of systemic occurs in up to 25% of patients. Residual VSDs can be found in up to 20% of patients. Ventricular arrhythmias are common following repair, with an incidence of sudden death as high as 5%.

Right-Sided Ebstein's Anomaly

5

In right-sided Ebstein's anomaly of the tricuspid valve, the right side of the heart consists of three anatomic components: right atrium proper, true RV, and the atrialized portion of the RV between the two. Surgical options include replacement or repair of the tricuspid valve.

Anomalous Venous Connections

In *partial anomalous pulmonary venous return,* one or more but not all four pulmonary veins are not connected to the left atrium. The most common pattern has the right pulmonary veins connected to the superior vena cava, usually with a *sinus venosus* ASD.

For more information about this subject, see *Cecil Textbook of Medicine,* 21st edition. Philadelphia, W.B. Saunders Company, 2000. Chapter 57, Congenital Heart Disease in Adults, pages 279 to 291.

ANGINA PECTORIS

Stable angina is usually reproducible in an individual patient and is consistent over time. In most patients, it is precipitated by effort, relieved by rest, and related to fixed stenoses of one or more epicardial coronary arteries. *Unstable angina* is diagnosed clinically when a patient has new-onset angina (by definition, any patient with new-onset angina has a brief interval of instability), increasing angina (angina that is more frequent, more prolonged, or precipitated by less effort than before), or angina occurring at rest. Most commonly, unstable angina is caused by a clot superimposed on a fixed coronary obstruction, although the definition of unstable angina remains clinical and is not based on specific pathophysiology.

Stenoses of more than 75% of the cross-sectional area (corresponding to more than 50% of the luminal diameter by coronary angiography [Fig. 5–13]) can result in ischemia when the energy requirements are high, as in physical exercise in stable effort angina. In *syndrome X,* patients with normal epicardial coronary arteries develop true myocardial ischemia.

The cardinal manifestation of effort angina is chest pain triggered by exercise and promptly relieved by rest. Chest pain is variably described but is typically a tightness, squeezing, or constriction; however, some patients describe an ache, a feeling of dull discomfort, indigestion, or burning pain. The discomfort is most commonly midsternal and radiates to the neck, left shoulder, and left arm. It can also be precordial or radiate to the jaw, teeth, right arm, back, and, more rarely, to the epigastrium. Episodes of discomfort that are less than 1 minute or more than 30 minutes in duration are unlikely to be stable angina, but prolonged episodes

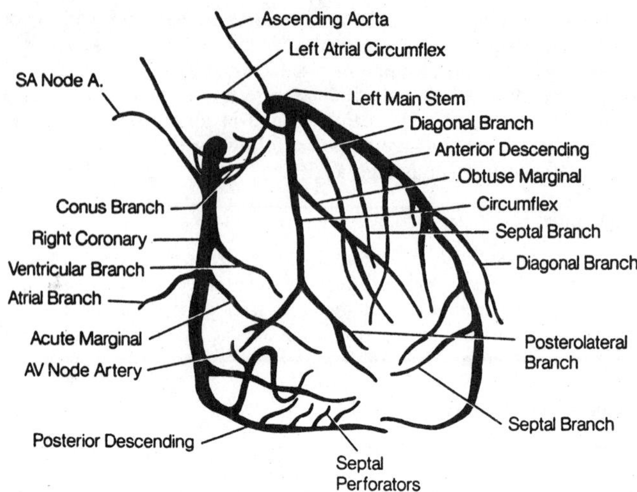

FIGURE 5–13 ■ The coronary vessels are shown in the right anterior oblique (RAO) view. The major arteries are the left main, left anterior descending, circumflex, and right coronary arteries. (From Yang SS, Bentivoglio LG, Maranhao V, Goldberg H [eds]: From Cardiac Catheterization Data to Hemodynamic Parameters, © 1988. Used by permission of Oxford University Press, Inc.)

can be consistent with unstable angina. When discomfort is considered clinically typical for angina, about 80% of patients will have demonstrable coronary artery disease. The probability of coronary artery disease varies by age range, sex, and characteristics of symptoms (Table 5–30).

Unstable angina covers a wide spectrum of clinical severity and is considered an intermediary syndrome between stable angina and MI (Table 5–31). The clinical presentation of a non–Q wave MI is often indistinguishable from unstable angina, and treatment of the two conditions is generally similar.

Prinzmetal's variant angina is associated with transient ST segment elevation, occurring most often at rest. Prinzmetal's variant angina is caused by an occlusive spasm, typically in a normal or minimally diseased coronary artery.

Nocturnal angina is true myocardial ischemia and may occur soon after a patient lies down, because of an increase in venous return that increases myocardial oxygen demand beyond the capacity of supply, or several hours later, related to increases in myocardial oxygen demand or vasospasm. Non-cardiac precipitants of myocardial ischemia include anemia, thyrotoxicosis, hypoxemia, and severe pulmonary disease (see Table 5–1).

Atypical angina describes symptoms that are suggestive of angina but unusual with regard to location, characteristics, triggers, or duration. In patients with atypical angina symptoms, the prevalence of underlying coronary artery disease ranges from 20 to 50%.

Table 5–30 ■ PROBABILITY OF CORONARY ARTERY DISEASE BY AGE, SEX, AND SYMPTOMS

AGE (yr)*	SEX	TYPICAL/DEFINITE ANGINA PECTORIS†	ATYPICAL/PROBABLE ANGINA PECTORIS†	NONANGINAL CHEST PAIN†	ASYMPTOMATIC†
30–39	Men	Intermediate	Intermediate	Low	Very low
	Women	Intermediate	Very low	Very low	Very low
40–49	Men	High	Intermediate	Intermediate	Low
	Women	Intermediate	Low	Very low	Very low
50–59	Men	High	Intermediate	Intermediate	Low
	Women	Intermediate	Intermediate	Low	Very low
60–69	Men	High	Intermediate	Intermediate	Low
	Women	High	Intermediate	Intermediate	Low

*No data exist for patients <30 or >69 years, but it can be assumed that the prevalence of coronary artery disease increases with age. In a few cases, patients with ages at the extremes of the decades listed may have probabilities slightly outside the high or low range.

†High indicates $>90\%$; intermediate 10–90%; low, $<10\%$; and very low, $<5\%$.

From Gibbons RJ, Balady GJ, Beasley JW, et al: ACC/AHA guidelines for exercise testing: Executive summary. A report of the American College of Cardiology/American Heart Association Task Force on Practice Guidelines (Committee on Exercise Testing). Circulation 96:345–354, 1997.

Table 5–31 ■ CLASSIFICATION OF UNSTABLE ANGINA

Severity	
Class I	New-onset, severe, or accelerated angina Patients with angina of <2-mo duration, severe or occurring ≥3 times per day, or angina that is distinctly more frequent and precipitated by distinctly less exertion; no rest pain in the last 2 mo
Class II	Angina at rest; subacute Patients with 1 or more episodes of angina at rest during the preceding month but not within the preceding 48 hr
Class III	Angina at rest; acute Patients with one or more episodes at rest within the preceding 48 hr
Clinical Circumstances	
Class A	Secondary unstable angina A clearly identified condition extrinsic to the coronary vascular bed that has intensified myocardial ischemia (e.g., anemia, infection, fever, hypotension, tachyarrhythmia, thyrotoxicosis, hypoxemia secondary to respiratory failure)
Class B	Primary unstable angina
Class C	Post-infarction unstable angina (within 2 wk of documented myocardial infarction)
Electrocardiogram	
Without/with transient ST segment deviations or T wave changes	
Intensity of Treatment	
1. Absence of treatment or minimal treatment	
2. Occurring in presence of standard therapy for chronic stable angina (conventional doses of oral β-blockers, nitrates, and calcium antagonists)	
3. Occurring despite maximally tolerated doses of all three categories of oral therapy, including intravenous nitroglycerin.	

Adapted from Braunwald E: Unstable angina: A classification. Circulation 80:410, 1989.

Diagnosis

The cardiopulmonary physical examination may be totally normal in patients with stable angina, even during an anginal attack. During ischemia, however, pulmonary rales, a transient S_4 or S_3 gallop, a sustained or dyskinetic LV impulse, a transient mitral regurgitation murmur caused by papillary muscle dysfunction, or paradoxical splitting of S_2 may be appreciated. The physical examination may also help diagnose other causes of chest discomfort, including costochondritis and pulmonary disorders, as well as nonischemic causes of cardiac chest pain, including aortic dissection or pericarditis (see Table 5–1).

The laboratory evaluation should include a complete blood cell count, thyroid function tests, and assessment of renal function. Enzyme markers (troponin T, troponin I, creatine kinase MB band [CK-MB]) help distinguish unstable angina from a non–Q wave MI. Patients should be routinely evaluated for coronary risk factors. The resting ECG obtained at times other than during episodes of chest pain has limited value.

The exercise ECG is most likely to indicate ischemia when the ST changes are horizontal or down-sloping, are more than 1 mV, occur during the early stages of exercise or at a low workload, persist for several minutes after exercise, and are accompanied by symptoms consistent with angina. False-positive results are most common in patients with underlying LV hypertrophy or interventricular conduction abnormalities on the resting ECG, such as the WPW syndrome, electrolyte abnormalities, or digitalis use. The sensitivity of the exercise ECG for detecting coronary artery disease is about 70%, and its specificity for excluding coronary artery disease is about 75% (Table 5–32). The sensitivity and specificity of perfusion scintigraphy using either the planar or the single-photon emission computed tomographic (SPECT) imaging techniques are generally somewhat better (Table 5–33).

Echocardiography with exercise has a sensitivity and specificity at least equivalent to those of exercise ECG. *Continuous ECG monitoring* allows detection of otherwise clinically silent ischemia. The choice among provocative tests depends on the patient's characteristics (Table 5–34).

Treatment

Stable Angina

Management of angina targets control of symptoms, prevention of the complications of MI and death, as well as corrective measures to control the underlying atherosclerotic process, halt its progression, and promote its regression (Table 5–35). Nitroglycerin (Table 5–36) produces immediate vasodilation. Long-acting nitrates administered orally or transdermally are effective in preventing angina and improving tolerance to exercise. A period of the day free of exposure is recommended to avoid tachyphylaxis.

β-Blocker therapy (Table 5–37) helps reduce heart rate at rest and during exercise and reduce blood pressure. Calcium channel antagonists (Table 5–38) are potent vasodilators to relieve coronary artery spasm. A controversy exists over the possible deleterious effects on mortality of calcium antagonists, particularly short-acting

Table 5–32 ■ APPROXIMATE SENSITIVITIES AND SPECIFICITIES OF COMMON TESTS TO DIAGNOSE CORONARY ARTERY DISEASE

	SENSITIVITY	SPECIFICITY
Exercise electrocardiography		
>1 mV ST depression	0.70	0.75
>2 mV ST depression	0.33	0.97
>3 mV ST depression	0.20	0.99
Perfusion scintigraphy		
Planar	0.83	0.88
SPECT	0.86–0.88	0.60–0.68
Echocardiography		
Exercise	0.83–0.87	0.74–0.80
Pharmacologic stress	0.86–0.96	0.66–0.95

SPECT = single-photon emission computed tomography.

Table 5–33 ■ RADIONUCLIDE TESTING TO DIAGNOSE ISCHEMIC HEART DISEASE

INDICATION	TEST	CLASS*
1. Diagnosis of symptomatic and selected patients at high risk for asymptomatic myocardial ischemia	Exercise or pharmacologic myocardial perfusion imaging, including PET*†	I
2. Assessment of ventricular performance (rest or exercise)	Exercise RNA	IIa
	RNA‡	I
3. Assessment of myocardial viability in patients with left ventricular dysfunction in planning revascularization	Gated Tc-99m sestamibi imaging	IIb
	Rest-distribution Tl-201 imaging	I
	Stress-redistribution-reinjection Tl-201 imaging	I
	PET imaging with FDG	I
	Dobutamine RNA	IIb
	Post-exercise RNA	IIb
	Post-NTG RNA	IIb
4. Planning PTCA—identifying lesions causing myocardial ischemia, if not otherwise known	Exercise or pharmacologic myocardial perfusion imaging	I
	Exercise RNA	IIa
5. Risk stratification before noncardiac surgery	Pharmacologic or exercise perfusion imaging	I
6. Screening of asymptomatic patients with low likelihood of disease	All tests	III

FDG = ^{18}F-2-deoxyglucose; RNA = radionuclide angiography; NTG = nitroglycerin; PTCA = percutaneous transluminal coronary angioplasty.

*Class I = usually appropriate and considered useful; class II = acceptable but usefulness less well established; class IIa = weight of evidence in favor of usefulness; class IIb = can be helpful but not well established by evidence; class III = generally not appropriate.

†The relative cost of positron emission computed tomography (PET), thallium (Tl)-201 or technetium (Tc)-99m agents and lesser availability of PET must be considered when selecting this technique.

‡RNA can be accomplished by first-pass imaging of a technetium-based myocardial perfusion agent.

Adapted with permission from Ritchie JL, Bateman TM, Bonow RO, et al: Guidelines for clinical use of cardiac radionuclide imaging. Report of the American College of Cardiology/American Heart Association Task Force on Assessment of Diagnostic and Therapeutic Cardiovascular Procedures (Committee on Radionuclide Imaging), developed in collaboration with the American Society of Nuclear Cardiology. J Am Coll Cardiol 25:521–547, 1995.

Table 5–34 ■ SUGGESTED NON-INVASIVE TESTS IN DIFFERENT TYPES OF PATIENTS WITH STABLE ANGINA

Exertional angina, mixed angina, walk-through angina, postprandial angina with or without prior myocardial infarction

A. Normal resting ECG: treadmill exercise ECG test
B. Abnormal uninterpretable resting ECG: exercise myocardial perfusion scintigraphy (thallium-201 sestamibi)
C. Unsuitable for exercise, unable to exercise adequately: dipyridamole or adenosine myocardial perfusion scintigraphy, dobutamine stress echocardiography

Atypical chest pain with normal or borderline abnormal resting ECG or with nondiagnostic stress ECG, particularly in women: exercise myocardial perfusion scintigraphy

Vasospastic angina: ECG during chest pain, ST segment depressed during ambulatory ECG

Dilated ischemic cardiomyopathy with typical angina or for assessment of the extent of hibernating myocardium: assessment of regional and global ejection fraction by radionuclide ventriculography or two-dimensional echocardiography, radionuclide myocardial perfusion scintigraphy; in selected patients, flow and metabolic studies with positron emission tomography

Syndrome X: initially treadmill exercise stress ECG (after demonstration of presence of normal coronaries, coronary blood flow reserve can be assessed non-invasively by positron emission tomography)

Known severe aortic stenosis or severe hypertrophic cardiomyopathy with stable angina: exercise stress tests are contraindicated; dipyridamole or adenosine myocardial perfusion scintigraphy in selected patients; coronary angiography is preferred and should be done if surgery is planned

Mild aortic valvular disease or hypertrophic cardiomyopathy with typical exertional angina: treadmill myocardial perfusion scintigraphy under strict supervision or dipyridamole or adenosine myocardial perfusion scintigraphy

ECG = electrocardiogram

From Goldman L, Braunwald E: Primary Cardiology. Philadelphia, WB Saunders, 1998, p 242.

nifedipine. Diltiazem and verapamil are contraindicated in patients with LV dysfunction occurring after MI.

Percutaneous transluminal coronary angioplasty (PTCA) and coronary artery bypass grafting (CABG) result in immediate relief of the obstruction to blood flow and are indicated to treat unacceptable symptoms in patients with stable angina. Catheter-based revascularization using balloon dilatation, atherectomy devices, and stents when indicated can successfully dilate about 84% of lesions with a 1% risk of death, 2% risk of non-fatal MI, and about 0.2% risk of emergency CABG. The risk of re-stenosis in the next year is 10 to 15%.

For single-vessel disease, both PTCA and CABG can provide substantial symptomatic relief, but neither has been documented to improve survival. In patients with multivessel disease, PTCA and CABG appear to have equivalent results in terms of death and MI, with PTCA allowing patients to return to work sooner and CABG being associated with fewer symptoms and better exercise tolerance. CABG is usually preferred over PTCA in patients with diabetes mellitus. A substantial proportion of PTCA procedures is ac-

Table 5–35 ■ THERAPEUTIC APPROACH FOR STABLE ANGINA

General medical therapy—cessation of smoking: control of hypertension, diabetes, and hyperlipidemia: regular exercise and reduction of weight; aspirin if not contraindicated

Medical therapy in patients with stable angina in the absence of specific indications for revascularization to improve prognosis and prevent symptoms (β-blockers); pre-exercise prophylaxis (nitroglycerin); add long-acting nitrates and then calcium channel blockers as needed; goal is acceptable exercise capacity and quality of life and prevention of frequent or severe ischemia; revascularization therapy (catheter-based revascularization or surgical revascularization procedure depending on anatomic considerations) unless contraindications for refractory angina, frequent or severe symptomatic ischemia, unacceptable quality of life, or intolerable side effects of medications

Indications for revascularization therapy to improve prognosis in the absence of other major life-limiting diseases

- Significant left main coronary artery stenosis → coronary artery bypass surgery
- Significant 3-vessel coronary artery disease with or without associated left main coronary artery stenosis and with or without normal left ventricular ejection fraction → coronary artery bypass surgery, including internal mammary arteries as conduits
- Double-vessel coronary artery stenosis, including proximal left anterior descending coronary artery stenosis → coronary artery bypass surgery or catheter-based revascularization
- Other single- or double-vessel coronary artery stenosis → catheter-based revascularization or coronary artery bypass surgery

In elderly (>75 yr) patients, patients with other life-limiting diseases, or patients needing urgent noncardiac surgery, catheter-based revascularization may be preferable when either type of revascularization is reasonable from a coronary perspective

In patients with moderately to severely depressed left ventricular ejection fraction with angina or angina equivalent with or without signs of heart failure → surgical revascularization if feasible

From Goldman L, Braunwald E: Primary Cardiology. Philadelphia, WB Saunders, 1998, p 255.

companied by stent placement, which improves long-term patency and outcomes. Transmyocardial laser revascularization is an experimental surgery that has shown promise for treatment of refractory angina.

Unstable Angina

For unstable angina, IV or sublingual nitroglycerin (up to three sublingual nitroglycerin tablets at 5-minute intervals) is administered for the relief of chest pain and is followed by an IV infusion of nitroglycerin beginning at 5 to 10 μg/minute and increasing by up to 10 μg/minute every 5 minutes as needed and tolerated. Aspirin should be started immediately at an initial dose of 160 to 325 mg followed by 80 to 160 mg/day. For patients who cannot tolerate aspirin, clopidogrel 75 mg/day or ticlopidine 250 mg twice daily is an appropriate alternative. Heparin should be started on all patients at high or intermediate risk immediately and be continued for 2 to 5 days until the patient has been free of chest pain for at least 24 hours or a coronary intervention procedure is performed. The recommended dose for regular heparin is 80 U/kg

Table 5–36 ■ CLINICAL USE OF NITROGLYCERIN AND NITRATES

COMPOUND	DOSE	CLINICAL EFFECTS	USE
Nitroglycerin			
Sublingual or buccal spray	0.15–1.5 mg	Relief of angina within 2 min	Before or at onset of pain
Ointment	7.5–15 mg	Antianginal benefit for 8–12 hr	Prophylaxis of pain
Transdermal	>50 mg/24 hr applied for 12 hr	Effective 8–16 hr	Patch on for 12 hr, then off
Intravenous	5–800 μg/min for 24–48 hr	Ongoing: increasing dose may be required	Unstable angina
Isosorbide dinitrate			
Sublingual	2.5–15 mg	Same as nitroglycerin sublingual but slower	Before onset of pain
Oral	5–80 mg/d	Antianginal effect for 10–12 hr	Prophylaxis
Isosorbide-5-mononitrate			
Oral	20 mg bid	Antianginal effect for 8–12 hr	Prophylaxis
Slow release	60–240 mg/d	Antianginal effect for 12–18 hr	Prophylaxis

Table 5–37 ■ CLINICAL USE OF β-BLOCKERS

COMPOUND	INTRINSIC SYMPATHOMIMETIC ACTIVITY*	HALF-LIFE (hr)	CLEARANCE	USE
Non-cardioselective				
Propranolol	–	1–6	Liver	40–80 mg bid–qid
Propranolol long-acting	–	8–11	Liver	80–360 mg/d
Nadolol	–	20–40	Kidney	40–240 mg/d
Sotalol	–	7–18	Kidney	40–160 mg bid
Timolol	–	4–5	Liver-kidney	10–15 mg bid
Cardioselective				
Acebutolol	++	8–13	Liver-kidney	200–600 mg bid
Atenolol	–	6–7	Kidney	50–200 mg/d
Metoprolol	–	3–7	Liver	50–200 mg bid

*Pressure commonly associated with maintenance or increase in heart rate; absence associated with decrease in heart rate.

Table 5–38 ■ PROPERTIES OF CALCIUM CHANNEL BLOCKING DRUGS IN CLINICAL USE

DRUG	VASCULAR SELECTIVITY*	USUAL DOSE	PLASMA HALF-LIFE	SIDE EFFECTS
Dihydropyridines				
Nifedipine	3.1	Immediate release: 20–40 mg 3 tid Slow release: 30–180 mg daily	4 hr	Hypotension, dizziness, flushing, nausea, constipation, edema
Amlodipine	†	5–10 mg once daily	30–50 hr	Headache, edema
Felodipine	5.4	5–10 mg once daily	11–16 hr	Headache, dizziness
Isradipine	7.4	2.5–10 mg bid	8 hr	Headache, fatigue
Nicardipine	17.0	20–40 mg tid	2–4 hr	Headache, dizziness, flushing, edema
Nisoldipine	†	20–40 mg once daily	2–6 hr	Similar to nifedipine
Nitrendipine	14.4	20 mg once or twice daily	5–12 hr	Similar to nifedipine
Other				
Bepridil	‡	200–400 mg once daily	24–40 hr	Arrhythmias, dizziness, nausea
Diltiazem	0.3	Immediate release: 30–80 mg qid Slow release: 120–320 mg once daily	3–4 hr	Hypotension, dizziness, flushing, bradycardia
Verapamil	1.3	Immediate release: 80–160 mg tid Slow release: 120–480 mg once daily		Hypotension, myocardial depression, heart failure, edema

*Numerical data give the ratio of vascular potency to cardiac potency; higher numbers indicate greater vascular, less cardiac potency.
†Significant degree of vasodilation greater than myocardial depression.
‡Myocardial depression greater than vasodilation.
Adapted from Katzung BG, Chatterjee K: Vasodilators and the treatment of angina. *In* Katzung BG (ed): Clinical Pharmacology. Norwalk, CT, Appleton & Lange, 1994, pp. 171–187. Appeared in Goldman L, Braunwald E: Primary Cardiology. Philadelphia, WB Saunders, 1998.

as an IV bolus followed by 8 U/kg/minute by infusion. Low-molecular-weight heparin, however, administered subcutaneously appears to be preferable to regular heparin and avoids the need for monitoring.

IV glycoprotein IIb/IIIa antagonists such as abciximab, eptifibatide, and tirofiban provide incremental benefits. Optimal antithrombotic therapy of unstable angina and non–ST elevation MI is achieved with a combination of aspirin, heparin, and a glycoprotein IIb/IIIa antagonist.

β-Blockers are indicated in patients at high risk for adverse events unless contraindications coexist. Therapy is begun IV in patients with evolving pain and is followed by oral therapy to a target of 50 to 60 beats per minute: metoprolol 5 mg by slow IV bolus repeated every 5 minutes for a total initial dose of 15 mg followed in 1 to 2 hours by 25 to 100 mg orally every 12 hours; propranolol 0.5 to 1.0 mg IV followed in 1 to 2 hours by 40 to 80 mg orally every 6 to 8 hours; atenolol as two 5-mg IV doses 5 minutes apart followed by 50 to 100 mg/day orally; or esmolol in an IV infusion of 0.1 mg/kg/minute titrated by 0.05 mg/kg/minute every 10 to 15 minutes until the desired response has been achieved or a maximum dose of 0.2 mg/kg/minute is given.

Patients with poorly controlled symptoms should generally be revascularized with PTCA or CABG. A randomized trial has suggested that the rates of death or MI are reduced by a routine aggressive management strategy as compared with a conservative strategy in patients whose unstable angina presents with electrocardiographic ischemia or macromolecular markers of myocardial damage. For other patients, a conservative strategy appears to be equally good provided that angiography followed by indicated intervention is performed in patients who have persistent or recurrent ischemia, heart failure, LV ejection fraction below 50%, malignant ventricular arrhythmias, or a clearly high-risk, positive, non-invasive study.

General Issues

For all patients with angina, prevention of future events includes smoking cessation; control of blood cholesterol, blood sugar, and hypertension; physical fitness; and perhaps lowering of homocysteine levels.

For more information about this subject, see *Cecil Textbook of Medicine,* 21st edition. Philadelphia, W.B. Saunders Company, 2000. Chapter 59, Angina Pectoris, pages 296 to 304.

ACUTE MYOCARDIAL INFARCTION

A seminal precipitating factor of acute coronary syndromes, including unstable angina, SCD, and acute MI, is hemorrhagic rupture or fissuring of a fat-laden, unstable atheroma with consequent thrombosis. *ST elevation MIs* (previously called *Q wave* or *transmural*) appear to result when occlusive thrombi persist. *Non–ST elevation MIs* (previously called *non–Q wave* or *subendocardial*) result from incomplete or spontaneously or therapeutically recanalized thrombotic occlusions after ischemia that are persistent enough to elicit necrosis.

Risk factors for MI include diabetes mellitus, hypertension, truncal obesity, smoking, increased levels of low-density lipoprotein (LDL) cholesterol, decreased levels of high-density lipoprotein (HDL) cholesterol, elevated levels of plasma homocysteine, and positive family history for atherosclerosis. Rare causes of acute MI include coronary arterial emboli, coronary thrombosis caused by trauma or by use of oral contraceptives in women, vasculitis, and vasospasm (idiopathic or associated with cocaine or amphetamine abuse).

Signs and Symptoms

5

MI may be manifested by prodromal symptoms of fatigue, chest discomfort, or malaise in the days preceding the event, or it may occur suddenly, without warning. Typical pain is intense, severe, unremitting for 30 to 60 minutes, and retrosternal, often radiating down the ulnar aspect of the left arm and into the neck, to the left shoulder, jaw, or teeth. The pain is classically described as crushing or squeezing, but it also may be described as an ache, burning, indigestion, or a feeling of fullness or "gas." Decreased systolic ventricular performance accounts for impaired perfusion of vital organs and reflex-mediated compensatory responses to hypotension, such as restlessness and impaired mentation, pallor, cutaneous vasoconstriction and sweating, tachycardia, and prerenal failure. MI also may be clinically silent (in as many as 25% of elderly patients, a population in whom 50% of MIs occur), with the diagnosis established only retrospectively by ECG criteria.

Physical Findings

Heart rate is often increased secondary to sympathoadrenal discharge, but bradyarrhythmias may be present and attributable to impaired sinus node function, AV nodal block, or infranodal block. With RV MI or severe LV dysfunction, hypotension occurs.

Rales or wheezes secondary to pulmonary venous hypertension are common with extensive LV MI. Lateral displacement of the apex impulse, dyskinesis, a palpable S_4 gallop, and a soft S_1 sound may indicate diminished contractility of the compromised LV. Accentuated S_4 and S_3 gallops may reflect increased LV volume. A mitral regurgitation murmur may be indicative of either papillary muscle dysfunction or rupture. A systolic murmur and thrill indicative of ventricular septal rupture may be heard, and a pericardial friction rub may be evident.

ECG and Laboratory Findings

The diagnosis can be established with certainty when typical ST elevation persists for hours and is followed by inversion of T waves within the first few days and by development of Q waves. However, initial ST depression or T wave inversion is difficult to differentiate from that seen with ischemia without MI or in unrelated conditions (Table 5–39). Detection of elevated concentration in plasma of macromolecules released from irreversibly injured myocardium has become the definitive diagnostic criterion of MI (Table 5–40).

Differential Diagnosis

Without the aid of laboratory tests and cardiac imaging, differentiation from ischemia without MI and from pericarditis may be

Table 5–39 ■ CONDITIONS ASSOCIATED WITH ELECTROCARDIOGRAPHIC CHANGES THAT MAY OBSCURE OR SIMULATE THOSE INDICATIVE OF ACUTE MYOCARDIAL INFARCTION

ABNORMALITY	EXAMPLE
Intraventricular conduction abnormalities	Left bundle branch block, left anterior superior fascicular block, infranodal arborization block, right ventricular transvenous or epicardial pacing
Electrolyte disturbances	Hypokalemia or hyperkalemia, hypocalcemia
Pre-excitation	
Early repolarization	
Cerebrovascular accident	
Myocarditis	Inflammatory, infiltrative, viral, or collagen-vascular disorders; pheochromocytoma, cardiac allograft rejection, neuromuscular disorders such as muscular dystrophy and Friedreich's ataxia
Left ventricular hypertrophy	Hypertrophic cardiomyopathy, dilated cardiomyopathy, valvular heart disease, hypertension
Right ventricular hypertrophy	Cor pulmonale, acute pulmonary embolus, pneumothorax
Cardiac tumors	
Pericarditis	

difficult (see Table 5–1). A critical differential diagnostic consideration is aortic dissection, which should be suspected whenever pain is severe yet atypical, radiates to the back, is accompanied by pulse or BP inequalities in the arms or legs, or is not associated with ECG changes typical of MI.

In the initial evaluation, definitive diagnosis often cannot be made immediately, and definitive immediate diagnosis is less important than appropriate assessment (Fig. 5–14), interim management, and rapid triage (Table 5–41).

Table 5–40 ■ SERUM MARKERS OF ACUTE MYOCARDIAL INFARCTION

	CARDIAC TROPONINS		
	cTnI	cTnT	CK-MB
First detectable (hr)	2–4		3–4
100% sensitivity (hr)	8–12		8–12
Peak (hr)	10–24		10–24
Duration (d)	5–10	5–14	2–4

cTnI = cardiac-specific troponin I; cTnT = cardiac-specific troponin T; CK-MB = creatine kinase MB band.

Adapted with permission from Adams J, Abendschein D, Jaffe A: Biochemical markers of myocardial injury: Is MB creatine kinase the choice for the 1990s? Circulation 88:750–763, 1993.

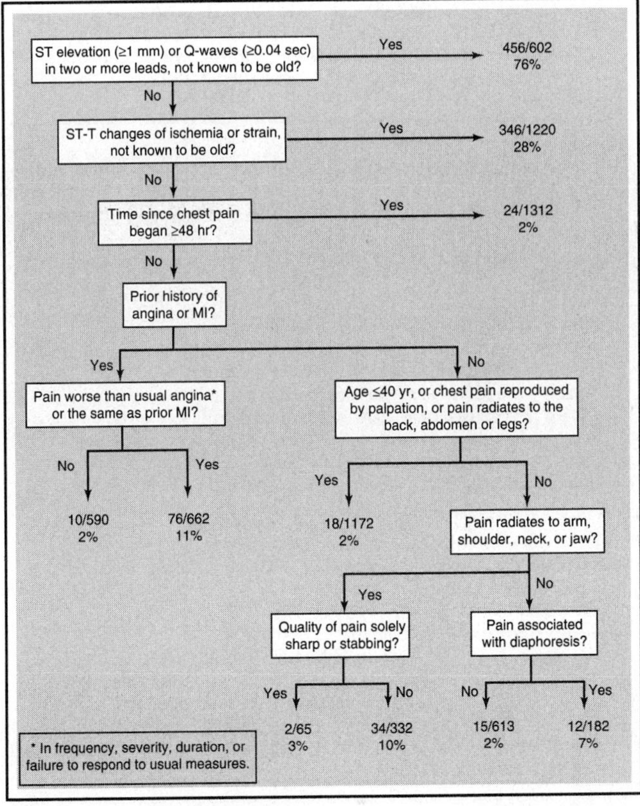

FIGURE 5–14 ■ Flow diagram for estimating the risk of acute myocardial infarction (MI) in emergency settings in patients with acute chest pain. For each clinical subset, the numerator is the number of patients with the set of presenting characteristics who developed an MI, whereas the denominator represents the total number of patients presenting with that characteristic or set of characteristics. (Adapted from Pearson SD, Goldman L, Garcia TB, et al: Physician response to a prediction rule for the triage of emergency department patients with chest pain. J Gen Intern Med 9:241–247, 1994. Reprinted by permission of Blackwell Science, Inc.)

Treatment

All patients with suspected MI immediately should be given 160 to 325 mg of aspirin to chew unless a documented aspirin allergy is present. Refractory or severe pain should be treated symptomatically with morphine, given as IV doses of 4 to 8 mg at intervals of 5 to 15 minutes.

Relative hypotension may be treated with elevation of the lower extremities or administration of fluids, except in patients with concomitant pulmonary congestion, in whom treatment for cardiogenic shock may be required. Atropine may increase blood pressure if hypotension reflects bradycardia or excess vagal tone.

Table 5–41 ■ RECOMMENDED TRIAGE STRATEGIES FOR PATIENTS WITH ACUTE CHEST PAIN WHO DO NOT OTHERWISE REQUIRE INTENSIVE CARE BECAUSE OF THE NEED TO TREAT ONGOING LIFE-THREATENING CONDITIONS*

Intensive Care

1. Major ischemic electrocardiographic (ECG) changes in ≥2 leads, not known to be old:
   a. ST elevation of 1 mm or more or Q waves of 0.04 sec or more
   or
   b. ST depression of 1 mm or more or T wave inversion consistent with ischemia
   or
2. Any two of the following, with or without major ECG changes:
   a. Unstable known coronary disease (in terms of frequency, duration, intensity, or failure to respond to usual measures)
   b. Systolic blood pressure <110 mm Hg
   c. Major new arrhythmias (new-onset atrial fibrillation, atrial flutter, sustained supraventricular tachycardia, second-degree or complete heart block, or sustained or recurrent ventricular arrythmias)
   d. Rales above the bases

Intermediate Care/Step-down Unit

Patients who do not meet criteria for intensive care but who either:

1. Have one unstable characteristic:
   a. Unstable known coronary disease
   b. Systolic blood pressure <110 mm Hg
   c. Rales above the bases
   d. Major new arrhythmias (new-onset atrial fibrillation, atrial flutter, sustained supraventricular tachycardia, second-degree or complete heart block, or sustained or recurrent ventricular arrhythmias)
2. A patient with new onset of very typical ischemic heart disease that meets the clinical criteria for unstable angina and that is occurring now at rest or with minimal exertion

Evaluation/Observation Unit

1. Other patients with new-onset symptoms that may be consistent with ischemic heart disease but that are not associated with ECG changes or a convincing diagnosis of unstable ischemic heart disease at rest or with minimal exertion
2. Some patients with known coronary disease whose presentation does not suggest a true worsening but for whom further observation is thought to be beneficial

Home with Office Follow-up in 7–10 Days to Determine Whether Further Testing Is Needed

Other patients

*Except in patients in whom other serious noncoronary causes of chest pain are being considered, such as possible aortic dissection or pulmonary embolism, where the triage will be dictated by the appropriate evaluation for these other possible diagnoses.

For patients with probable MI who are appropriate candidates for reperfusion because of 1 mm or more of new ST elevation in two or more leads, or presumably new bundle branch block in the setting of a typical clinical syndrome, plans should be made for prompt treatment to induce recanalization even while the patient is in the emergency department. Alternative methods of coronary recanalization include IV thrombolytic agents or catheter-based ap-

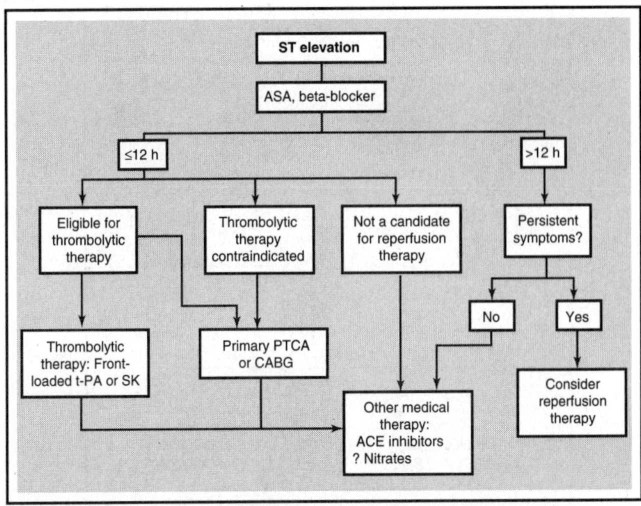

FIGURE 5–15 ■ Recommendations for management of patients with ST elevation. All patients with ST segment elevation on the ECG should receive aspirin (ASA). β-adrenergic blockers (in the absence of contraindications), and an antithrombin (particularly if tissue-type plasminogen activator [t-PA] is used for thrombolytic therapy). Whether heparin is required in patients receiving streptokinase (SK) remains a matter of controversy; the small additional risk for intracranial hemorrhage may not be offset by the survival benefit afforded by adding heparin to SK therapy. Patients treated within 12 hours who are eligible for thrombolytics should expeditiously receive either front-loaded t-PA or an alternative such as reteplase, anistreplase, or SK or be considered for primary percutaneous transluminal coronary angioplasty (PTCA). Primary PTCA is also to be considered when thrombolytic therapy is absolutely contraindicated. Coronary artery bypass graft (CABG) may be considered if the patient is seen in less than 6 hours from the onset of symptoms. Individuals treated after 12 hours should receive the initial medical therapy noted above and, on an individual basis, may be candidates for reperfusion therapy or angiotensin-converting enzyme (ACE) inhibitors (particularly if left ventricular function is impaired). (Modified from Antman EM: Medical therapy for acute coronary syndromes: An overview. *In* Califf RM [ed]: Atlas of Heart Diseases, VIII. Philadelphia. Current Medicine, 1996.)

proaches (Fig. 5–15) in ST elevation MI and an emphasis on antiplatelet agents and heparin for non–ST elevation MI (Fig. 5–16). Plasminogen activators should not be given to patients with active internal bleeding or a bleeding diathesis, suspected aortic dissection, recent trauma, intracranial neoplasm, or hypertensive crisis; relative contraindications include prolonged or traumatic cardiopulmonary resuscitation, peptic ulcer disease, remote cerebrovascular accident, and hepatic failure.

β-Adrenergic blockers are part of routine therapy unless contraindicated by hypotension, bradyarrhythmias, or severe obstructive lung disease. Regimens include IV atenolol 5 to 10 mg followed by 50 to 100 mg/day orally, or metoprolol 5 mg IV repeated for a total of three doses followed by 50 to 100 mg/day given orally.

Hemodynamic observations are critical in guiding therapy (Table 5–42). ACE inhibitors appear to benefit patients who have no

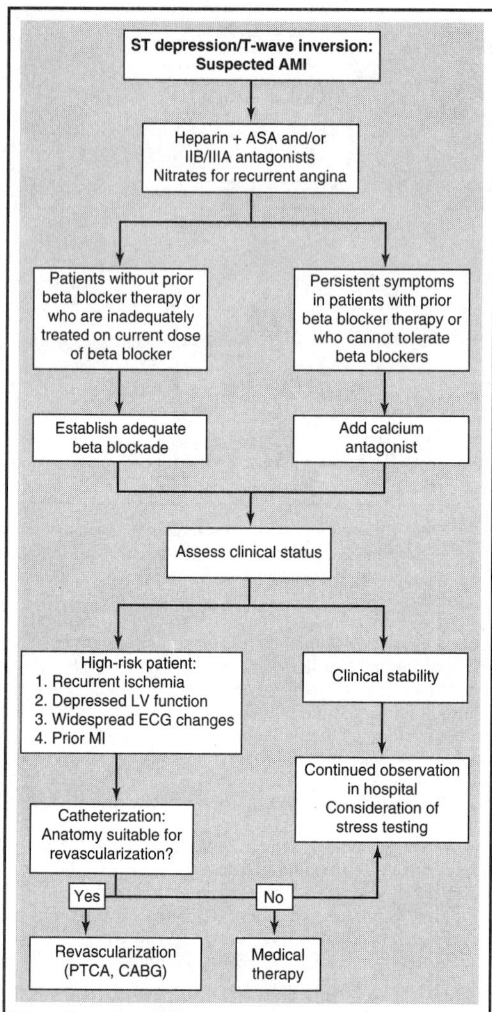

FIGURE 5–16 ■ Recommendations for management of patients with acute myocardial infarction (MI) without ST elevation. All patients without ST elevation should be treated with an antithrombin and aspirin (ASA). Nitrates should be administered for recurrent episodes of angina. Adequate β-adrenergic blockade should then be established; when this is not possible or contraindications exist, a calcium antagonist can be considered. High-risk patients should be triaged to cardiac catheterization with plans for revascularization if they are clinically suitable; patients who are clinically stable can be treated more conservatively, with continued observation in the hospital and consideration of a stress test to screen for myocardial ischemia. LV = left ventricular; ECG = electrocardiographic; PTCA = percutaneous transluminal coronary angioplasty; CABG = coronary artery bypass graft. (Modified from Antman EM: Medical therapy for acute coronary syndromes: An overview. *In* Califf RM [ed]: Atlas of Heart Diseases, VIII. Philadelphia. Current Medicine, 1996.

Table 5–42 ■ THERAPEUTIC INTERVENTIONS TAILORED TO SPECIFIC HEMODYNAMIC SUBSETS

	HEMODYNAMIC SUBSET	INTERVENTION	REMARKS
I	Normal hemodynamics	None required	
II	Hyperdynamic state	β-Adrenergic blockade	Analgesics and anxiolytic drugs may be helpful.
III	Hypovolemia	Intravenous fluids to augment effective vascular volume	Marked increases in pulmonary artery occlusive pressure reflecting pulmonary venous hypertension and increased left ventricular filling pressure may occur if heart failure is unmasked or exacerbated; manifestations may include dyspnea, hypoxemia, bronchospasm, and rales, as well as radiographic evidence of pulmonary congestion
IV	Left ventricular failure		
	A. Mild	Systemic arterial vasodilators	Diuretics may be useful if failure is refractory
	B. Severe	Systemic arterial vasodilators and diuretics	Cardiotonic agents may be helpful if hypotension supervenes, but their use can exacerbate the imbalance between myocardial oxygen requirements and supply; thus, sympathomimetic and dopaminergic agents may be helpful, but their beneficial effect on hemodynamics is usually only transitory, and their use may exacerbate ischemic injury
V	Cardiogenic shock	Coronary recanalization and circulatory support	
VI	Shock attributable to right ventricular infarction	Augmentation of vascular volume and cardiotonic agents	

Adapted from Forrester JS, et al: Medical therapy of acute myocardial infarction by application of hemodynamic subsets. N Engl J Med 295:1404, 1976.

evidence of hypotension if administration is begun within the first 24 hours after onset of MI. Alternatives include captopril 12.5 to 50 mg given orally twice a day or enalapril 5 to 40 mg given orally daily or twice a day.

Continuing chest pain indicative of ischemia is an indication for cardiac catheterization and revascularization (PTCA or surgery), with the decision to proceed and choice of modality based largely on results of angiography and assessment of ventricular function. IV nitroglycerin, titrated to avoid hypotension (10–200 g/minute), reduces peripheral arterial resistance and ventricular afterload.

Prophylactic lidocaine administration is not indicated. After successful resuscitation from VF, lidocaine should be administered by continuous infusion (20–50 μg/kg of body weight per minute), particularly in the presence of frequent, closely coupled, multiform, or repetitive PVCs or VT. Treatment of arrhythmias is the same as that used when they occur under other circumstances.

Pericarditis occurs in up to 20% of patients after Q wave MI, usually between 1 day and about 6 weeks after the acute event. Rupture of a papillary muscle, which causes acute mitral (and rarely tricuspid) regurgitation, or of the ventricular septum, which causes an acute left-to-right shunt, leads to acute hemodynamic compromise. Rupture of the free wall of the LV usually presents with pericardial tamponade and cardiovascular collapse.

Step-down Care

Patients with uncomplicated MI require critical care unit (CCU) care generally for no more than 48 to 72 hours. Subsequent care is often facilitated by 1 to 3 days in a step-down unit equipped with telemetry for continuous ECG monitoring; however, with entirely uncomplicated MI treated with effective reperfusion, patients may be discharged directly from the CCU.

Risk Stratification, Convalescence, and Rehabilitation

Before hospital discharge all post-MI patients should have a functional assessment of cardiac performance (Fig. 5–17). Unless there are contraindications, all MI patients should receive aspirin, a β-blocker, interventions to reduce LDL cholesterol levels to <130 mg/dL, and (for anterior MI or ejection fractions <40%) an ACE inhibitor. Other long-term interventions are similar to those in patients with angina.

For more information about this subject, see *Cecil Textbook of Medicine,* 21st edition. Philadelphia, W.B. Saunders Company, 2000. Chapter 60, Acute Myocardial Infarction, pages 304 to 320.

VALVULAR HEART DISEASE

When aortic or mitral valve disease is severe, the associated hemodynamic burdens can lead to ventricular dysfunction, heart failure, and sudden death (Table 5–43). In almost every instance, the definitive therapy for severe valvular heart disease is mechanical restoration of valve function.

Aortic Stenosis

Aortic stenosis must be suspected in patients with a systolic murmur, especially if it radiates to the carotid artery. Whenever

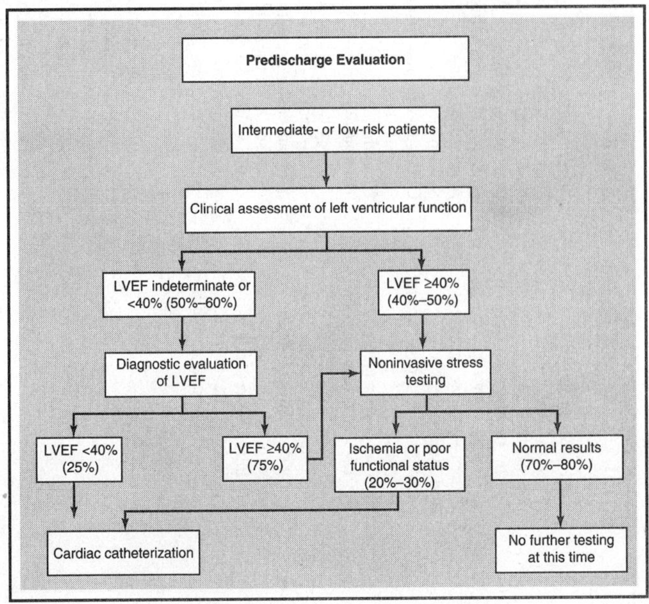

FIGURE 5–17 ■ Flow diagram for predischarge risk stratification. LVEF = left ventricular ejection fraction.

aortic stenosis is suspected (especially if a patient has symptoms of chest pain, dyspnea, or dizziness), evaluation by echocardiography is mandatory.

The only effective therapy for aortic stenosis is aortic valve replacement. Once the valve is replaced, survivorship returns nearly to normal. Even octogenarians benefit from valve replacement unless other co-morbid factors preclude surgery. The only indicated medical therapy is antibiotic prophylaxis to prevent bacterial endocarditis.

Mitral Stenosis

In most patients with *mitral stenosis,* an excellent result can be obtained from percutaneous balloon valvotomy. Patients with pliable valves, little valvular calcification, little involvement of the subvalvular apparatus, and less than moderate mitral regurgitation are ideal candidates.

Mitral Regurgitation

In severe *acute mitral regurgitation,* arterial vasodilators reduce systemic resistance to flow and thereby preferentially increase aortic outflow and simultaneously decrease the amount of mitral regurgitation and left atrial hypertension. Vasodilator therapy is clearly effective in the treatment of acute mitral regurgitation and in chronic aortic regurgitation. However, perhaps because afterload is usually not increased in *chronic* asymptomatic mitral regurgitation,

Table 5–43 ■ SUMMARY OF SEVERE VALVULAR HEART DISEASE

	AORTIC STENOSIS	MITRAL STENOSIS	MITRAL REGURGITATION	AORTIC REGURGITATION
Etiology	Idiopathic calcification of a bicuspid or tricuspid valve Congenital Rheumatic	Rheumatic fever Annular calcification	Mitral valve prolapse Ruptured chordae Endocarditis Ischemic papillary muscle dysfunction or rupture Collagen-vascular diseases and syndromes Secondary to LV myocardial diseases	Annuloaortic ectasia Hypertension Endocarditis Marfan syndrome Ankylosing spondylitis Aortic dissection Syphilis Collagen-vascular disease
Pathophysiology	Pressure overload upon the LV with compensation by LVH As disease advances, reduced coronary flow reserve causes angina Hypertrophy and afterload excess lead to both systolic and diastolic LV dysfunction	Obstruction to LV inflow increases left atrial pressure and limits cardiac output mimicking LV failure; mitral valve obstruction increases the pressure work of the right ventricle Right ventricular pressure overload is augmented further when pulmonary hypertension develops	Places volume overload on the LV; ventricle responds with eccentric hypertrophy and dilation, which allow for increased ventricular stroke volume Eventually, however, LV dysfunction develops if volume overload is uncorrected	*Chronic* Total stroke volume causes hyperdynamic circulation, induces systolic hypertension, and thus causes both pressure and volume overload; compensation is by both concentric and eccentric hypertrophy *Acute* Because cardiac dilation has not developed, hyperdynamic findings are absent; high diastolic LV pressure causes mitral valve pre-closure and potentiates LV ischemia and failure

Symptoms	Angina Syncope Heart failure	Dyspnea Orthopnea PND Hemoptysis Hoarseness Edema Ascites	Dyspnea Orthopnea PND	Dyspnea Orthopnea PND Angina Syncope
Signs	Systolic ejection murmur radiating to neck Delayed carotid upstroke S_4, soft or paradoxical S_2	Diastolic rumble following an opening snap Loud S_1 Right ventricular lift Loud P_2	Holosystolic apical murmur radiates to axilla, S_3 Displaced PMI	*Chronic* Diastolic blowing murmur Hyperdynamic circulation Displaced PMI Quincke pulse DeMusset's sign, etc. *Acute* Short diastolic blowing murmur Soft S_1
ECG	LAE LVH	LAE RVH	LAE LVH	LAE LVH
Chest Radiograph	Boot-shaped heart Aortic valve calcification on lateral view	Straightening of left heart border Double density at right heart border Kerley B lines Enlarged pulmonary arteries	Cardiac enlargement	*Chronic* Cardiac enlargement Uncoiling of the aorta *Acute* Pulmonary congestion with normal heart size
Echocardiographic Findings	Concentric LVH Reduced aortic valve cusp separation Doppler usually shows mean gradient ≥ 50 mm Hg in severe cases	Restricted mitral leaflet motion Valve area ≤ 1.0 cm^2 in most severe cases Tricuspid Doppler may reveal pulmonary hypertension	LV and LAE in chronic severe disease Doppler: large regurgitant jet	*Chronic* LV enlargement Large Doppler jet PHT $<$ 400 ms *Acute* Small LV, mitral valve pre-closure

Table continued on following page

Table 5–43 ■ SUMMARY OF SEVERE VALVULAR HEART DISEASE *Continued*

	AORTIC STENOSIS	MITRAL STENOSIS	MITRAL REGURGITATION	AORTIC REGURGITATION
Catheterization Findings	Increased LVEDP Transaortic gradient $\geq$50 mm Hg AVA $\leq$ 0.7 in most severe cases	Elevated pulmonary capillary wedge pressure Transmitral gradient usually >10 mm Hg in severe cases MVA < 1.0 cm^2	Elevated pulmonary capillary wedge pressure Ventriculography shows regurgitation of dye into left ventricle	Wide pulse pressure Aortography shows regurgitation of dye into LV Usually unnecessary
Medical Therapy	Avoid vasodilators Digitalis, diuretics, and nitroglycerin in inoperable cases	Diuretics for mild symptoms Anticoagulation in atrial fibrillation Digitalis, β-blockers, verapamil or diltiazem for rate control	Vasodilators in acute disease No proven therapy in chronic disease (but vasodilators commonly used)	*Chronic* Vasodilators in chronic asymptomatic disease with normal LV function *Acute* Vasodilators
Indications for Surgery	Appearance of symptoms in patients with severe disease (see text)	Appearance of more than mild symptoms Development of pulmonary hypertension Appearance of persistent atrial fibrillation	Appearance of symptoms EF < 0.60 ESD $\geq$ 45 min	*Chronic* Appearance of symptoms EF < 0.55 ESD $\geq$ 55 min *Acute* Even mild heart failure Mitral valve pre-closure

AVA = aortic valve area; EF = ejection fraction; ESD = end-systolic diameter; LAE = left atrial enlargement; LV = left ventricle; LVEDP = left ventricular end-diastolic pressure; LVH = left ventricular hypertrophy; MS = mitral stenosis; MVA = mitral valve area; PMI = point of maximal impulse; PND = paroxysmal nocturnal dyspnea; PHT = pressure half-time; RVH = right ventricular hypertrophy.

vasodilators have had little effect in reducing LV volume or in improving normal exercise tolerance in chronic mitral regurgitation.

In patients with *symptomatic* mitral regurgitation, ACE inhibitors have been demonstrated to reduce LV volumes and to improve symptoms. However, mitral valve surgery rather than medical therapy usually is preferred in most symptomatic patients with mitral regurgitation. When feasible, mitral valve repair is the preferred operation. In asymptomatic patients, survival is prolonged to or toward normal if surgery is performed before the ejection fraction declines to less than 0.60 or before the LV is unable to contract to an end-systolic dimension of ≤45 mm.

Mitral valve prolapse occurs when one or both of the mitral valve leaflets prolapse into the left atrium superior to the mitral valve annular plane during systole. Most patients are asymptomatic. On physical examination, the mitral valve prolapse syndrome produces characteristic findings of a midsystolic click and a late systolic murmur. Echocardiography is useful to prove that prolapse is present. Most patients with mitral valve prolapse have a benign clinical course. Approximately 10% of patients with thickened leaflets suffer either infective endocarditis, stroke, progression to severe mitral regurgitation, or sudden death. Patients with mitral valve prolapse and its characteristic murmur should observe standard endocarditis prophylaxis. Patients with otherwise normal valve leaflets shown to prolapse during echocardiography with no heart murmur do not require endocarditis precautions. Patients with clearly abnormal valves but no murmur fall into a middle category of endocarditis risk where a firm recommendation about prophylaxis cannot be made. In patients with palpitations and autonomic dysfunction, β-blockers are often effective in relieving symptoms. Low-dose aspirin therapy has been recommended for patients with redundant leaflets, but no large studies are available to support this contention.

Aortic Regurgitation

Because *aortic regurgitation* increases LV afterload, which in turn worsens the aortic regurgitation, afterload-reducing drugs are efficacious in the treatment of asymptomatic patients. Currently, the best prognostic data are for nifedipine, but other vasodilators, including ACE inhibitors and hydralazine, have also demonstrated hemodynamic improvement. In acute aortic regurgitation, once any of the symptoms or signs of heart failure develop, even if mild, medical mortality is high, approaching 75%. Vasodilators, such as nitroprusside, may help improve the patient's condition before surgery. In patients with acute aortic regurgitation caused by bacterial endocarditis, surgery sometimes can be delayed to permit a full or partial course of antibiotics, but persistent, severe aortic regurgitation requires emergency valve replacement.

Patients with clinical aortic regurgitation should undergo aortic valve replacement before symptoms impair lifestyle. It also is clear that asymptomatic patients who manifest evidence of LV dysfunction benefit from surgery. In aortic regurgitation, once ejection fraction falls below 0.55 or end-systolic dimension exceeds 55 mm, postoperative outcome is impaired, presumably because these markers indicate that LV dysfunction has developed. Thus, surgery should intervene before these benchmarks are reached.

Tricuspid Regurgitation

Tricuspid regurgitation is usually secondary to a hemodynamic load on the RV rather than to a structural valve deformity. The symptoms are of right-sided heart failure, including ascites, edema, and occasionally right upper quadrant pain. Tricuspid regurgitation produces jugular venous distention accentuated by a large v wave as blood is regurgitated into the right atrium during systole. The definitive diagnosis is made during echocardiography. The therapy for secondary tricuspid regurgitation is usually aimed at the cause of the lesion. Surgical intervention for the tricuspid valve is rarely entertained in isolation.

Prosthetic Heart Valves

Different types of prosthetic valves have different advantages and disadvantages (Table 5–44). Whenever a patient with a prosthetic heart valve develops a temperature greater than 100° F, endocarditis must be excluded by blood culture; for fever with signs of sepsis, broad-spectrum antibiotics must be begun while awaiting culture results. Endocarditis prophylaxis should be used at the time of procedures that have a high risk for bacteremia.

All patients with a mechanical heart valve require anticoagulation. Recommended INR values range from 2.0 for the young normotensive patient in sinus rhythm with an aortic valve prosthesis to 3.5 for the patient with AF and a mitral valve prosthesis. Aspirin, at doses of 325 mg, is recommended in addition to warfarin to reduce the risk of valve thrombosis in patients with mechanical prosthetic valves at higher risk for thromboembolic complications.

For more information about this subject, see *Cecil Textbook of Medicine,* 21st edition. Philadelphia, W.B. Saunders Company, 2000. Chapter 63, Valvular Heart Disease, pages 327 to 336.

Table 5–44 ■ ADVANTAGES AND DISADVANTAGES OF SUBSTITUTE CARDIAC VALVES

TYPE OF VALVE	ADVANTAGES	DISADVANTAGES
Bioprosthesis (Carpentier-Edwards; Hancock)	Avoid anticoagulation in patients with sinus rhythm	Durability limited to 10–15 yr Relatively stenotic
Mechanical valves (St. Jude; Medtronic-Hall; Starr-Edwards)	Good flow characteristics in small sizes Durable	Require anticoagulation
Homografts and autografts	Anticoagulation not required Durability increased over that of bioprostheses	Surgical implantation technically demanding

MYOCARDIAL DISEASES AND MISCELLANEOUS CONDITIONS OF THE HEART

Once a patient has been recognized to have symptoms or signs consistent with heart failure, the diagnosis can often be established on the basis of physical examination, but it is generally confirmed by echocardiography (Fig. 5–18).

Dilated Cardiomyopathy

5

Dilated cardiomyopathy, which has many causes (Table 5–45), is characterized by increased LV or biventricular dimensions with decreased ventricular ejection fraction (Table 5–46). The history should also include careful questioning to elucidate symptoms indicative of the level of hemodynamic compensation. In dilated cardiomyopathy, the LV impulse is often displaced far laterally, and an S_3 gallop is prominent. For restrictive cardiomyopathy, the

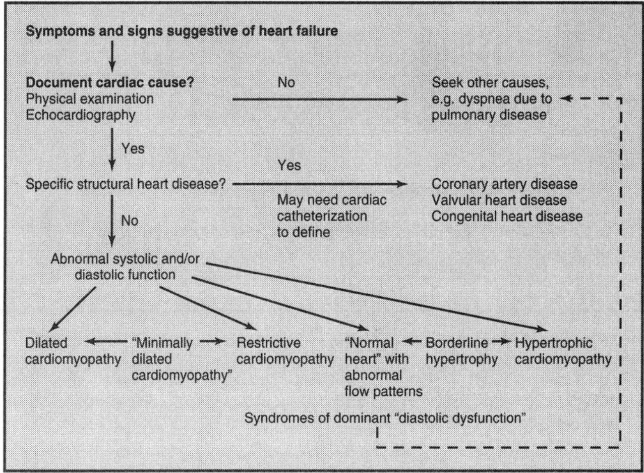

FIGURE 5–18 ■ Initial approach to classification of cardiomyopathy. The evaluation of symptoms or signs consistent with heart failure first includes confirmation that they can be attributed to a cardiac cause. Although this is often apparent from routine physical examination, echocardiography serves to confirm cardiac disease and provides clues to the presence of other conditions, such as focal abnormalities, suggesting primary valve disease or congenital heart disease. Having excluded these conditions, cardiomyopathy is generally considered to be dilated, restrictive, or hypertrophic. Patients with apparently normal cardiac structure and contraction are occasionally found to demonstrate abnormal intracardiac flow patterns consistent with diastolic dysfunction but should also be evaluated carefully for other causes of their symptoms. Most patients with so-called diastolic dysfunction will also demonstrate at least borderline criteria for left ventricular hypertrophy, frequently in the setting of chronic hypertension and diabetes. A moderately decreased ejection fraction without marked dilation or a pattern of restrictive cardiomyopathy is sometimes referred to as "minimally dilated cardiomyopathy," which may represent either a distinct entity or a transition between acute and chronic disease.

Table 5–45 ■ MAJOR CAUSES OF DILATED CARDIOMYOPATHY

Inflammatory

Infectious myocarditis
- Viral
- Rickettsial
- Bacterial
- Mycobacterial
- Spirochetal
- Parasitic
- Fungal

Non-infectious
- Collagen-vascular disease
- Peripartum cardiomyopathy
- Hypersensitivity myocarditis
- Transplant rejection

Granulomatous inflammatory disease
- Sarcoidosis
- Giant cell myocarditis

Toxic

Alcohol
Chemotherapeutic agents: doxorubicin, cyclophosphamide, interferon
Heavy metals: lead, mercury
Occupational exposure: hydrocarbons, arsenicals
Catecholamines: amphetamines, cocaine

Metabolic

Nutritional deficiencies: thiamine, selenium, carnitine
Electrolyte deficiencies: calcium, phosphate, magnesium
Endocrinopathy: thyroid disease, diabetes, pheochromocytoma
Obesity

Familial

Cardiac and skeletal myopathy
Mitochondrial myopathy (e.g., Kearns-Sayre syndrome)
Isolated cardiomyopathy due to dystrophin promoter defect

Overlap with Restrictive Cardiomyopathy

Hemochromatosis
Amyloidosis
Sarcoidosis

Idiopathic

Primary left ventricular or biventricular cardiomyopathy
Arrhythmogenic right ventricular dysplasia

---

impulse is less displaced and is often accompanied by a very prominent S_4. A focused evaluation helps assess both etiology and severity (Table 5–47). Patients with recent-onset cardiomyopathy have almost a 50% chance of substantial recovery. In general, prognosis parallels the functional class. Treatment is as for heart failure.

Restrictive Cardiomyopathies

Most restrictive cardiomyopathies result from deposition of abnormal substances in the myocardium (Table 5–48). Therapy with diuretics is helpful but not curative. The theoretical rationale for

Table 5–46 ■ PROFILES OF SYMPTOMATIC CARDIOMYOPATHY

	DILATED	RESTRICTIVE	HYPERTROPHIC
Ejection fraction (normal ≥55%)	<30%	25–50%	>60%
Left ventricular diastolic dimension (normal <55 mm)	≥60 mm	<60 mm	Often decreased
Left ventricular wall thickness	Decreased	Normal or increased	Markedly increased
Atrial size	Increased	Increased; may be massive	Increased
Valvular regurgitation	Mitral first during decompensation; tricuspid regurgitation in late stages	Frequent mitral and tricuspid regurgitation	Mitral regurgitation
Common first symptoms*	Exertional intolerance	Exertional intolerance	Exertional intolerance; may have chest pain
Congestive symptoms*	Left before right, except right prominent in young adults	Right often exceeds left	Primary exertional dyspnea
Risk for arrhythmia	Ventricular tachyarrhythmia; conduction block in Chagas' disease, giant cell myocarditis, and some families; atrial fibrillation	Ventricular uncommon except in sarcoidosis; conduction block in sarcoidosis and amyloidosis; atrial fibrillation.	Ventricular tachyarrhythmias Atrial fibrillation

*Left-sided symptoms of pulmonary congestion: dyspnea on exertion, orthopnea, paroxysmal nocturnal dyspnea. Right-sided symptoms of systemic venous congestion: discomfort on bending, hepatic and abdominal distention, peripheral edema.

Table 5–47 ■ LABORATORY EVALUATION OF CARDIOMYOPATHY

Routine Initial Evaluation

Electrocardiogram*
Chest radiograph*
Two-dimensional and Doppler echocardiogram*
Chemistry:
Serum sodium,* potassium,* glucose, creatinine, blood urea nitrogen, albumin,* total protein,* liver function tests, serum iron, ferritin, creatine kinase, thyroid-stimulating hormone
Hematology:
Hemoglobin/hematocrit,* white blood cell count with differential, including eosinophils*; erythrocyte sedimentation rate

Initial Evaluation in Selected Patients

Titers for suspected infection:
Acute viral (coxsackievirus, echovirus, influenza virus), human immunodeficiency virus, Epstein-Barr virus, Lyme disease, toxoplasmosis, Chagas' disease
Serologies for active rheumatologic disease
Endomyocardial biopsy

*Included for general initial evaluation of heart failure according to guidelines from Konstam MA, et al: Heart failure: Evaluation and care of patients with left ventricular systolic dysfunction. Agency for Health Care Policy and Research, U.S. Dept. of Health and Human Services, Rockville, MD, 1994.

calcium channel blockers to improve diastolic relaxation has not been confirmed by clinical results.

Hypertrophic Cardiomyopathy

The cardinal features of hypertrophic cardiomyopathy are marked LV hypertrophy not due to other cardiac disease, frequently with asymmetrical involvement of the septum, accompanied by supranormal ejection fraction and decreased LV systolic cavity dimension.

Outflow obstruction, present or inducible in about 25% of patients, is caused by apposition of the anterior mitral valve leaflet to the septum and can elevate filling pressures further and compromise forward output.

Decreased compliance during atrial filling may lead to a palpable and audible S_4 gallop. When present, the murmur is usually best heard at the left lower sternal border, and represents a sum of the outflow murmur and mitral regurgitation. It is typically harsh and increases in intensity with the maneuvers that decrease ventricular size (see Table 5–5).

Echocardiography establishes the diagnosis. Therapy depends on symptoms and on the estimated risk of sudden death (Fig. 5–19).

Miscellaneous Conditions of the Heart

Most primary cardiac tumors are benign, whereas all secondary tumors are malignant (Fig. 5–20). The most common manifestation of blunt trauma is myocardial contusion; new ECG changes or arrhythmias with new regional LV wall motion abnormalities on echocardiography can document myocardial injury.

Table 5–48 ■ CAUSES OF RESTRICTIVE CARDIOMYOPATHIES

Infiltrative
Amyloidosis
Sarcoidosis
Gaucher's disease—glucocerebroside-laden macrophages
Hurler's disease—mucopolysaccharide-laden macrophages
Storage
Hemochromatosis
Fabry's disease
Glycogen storage diseases
Fibrotic
Radiation
Scleroderma
Metabolic
Carnitine deficiency
Defects in fatty acid metabolism
Endocardial
Possibly related diseases
Tropical endomyocardial fibrosis
Hypereosinophilic syndrome (Löffler's endocarditis)
Carcinoid syndrome
Radiation
Doxorubicin
Dilated cardiomyopathy overlap
Early stage ("minimally dilated cardiomyopathy")
Partial recovery from dilated cardiomyopathy
Myocardial metabolic defects
Idiopathic

For more information about this subject, see *Cecil Textbook of Medicine,* 21st edition. Philadelphia, W.B. Saunders Company, 2000. Chapter 64, Diseases of the Myocardium, pages 366 to 347; and Chapter 70, Miscellaneous Conditions of the Heart, pages 372 to 374.

PERICARDIAL DISEASE

The most common clinical pathologic process involving the pericardium is acute pericarditis (Table 5–49). Chest pain symptoms are usually sudden and severe in onset, characteristically with retrosternal or left precordial pain or both; referral to the back and trapezius ridge is common.

Physical examination is most notable for a pericardial friction rub. During the initial few days, diffuse ST segment elevations occur in the absence of reciprocal ST segment depression. After several days, the ST segments normalize and then the T waves become inverted.

In the absence of significant pericardial effusion, treatment is non-steroidal anti-inflammatory agents such as indomethacin 25 to 50 mg three times daily or aspirin (325 to 650 mg three times

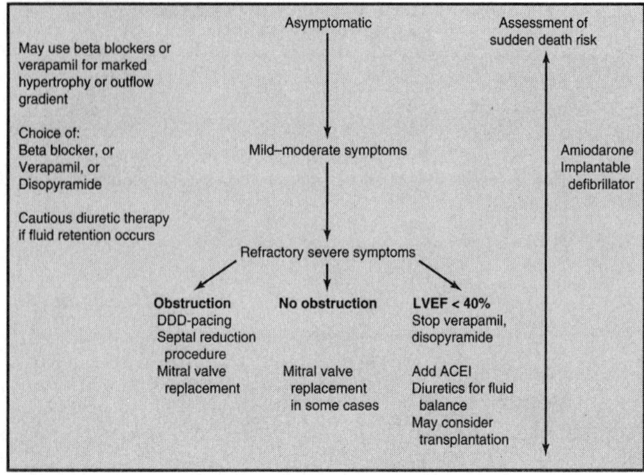

FIGURE 5–19 ■ Approach to therapy of hypertrophic cardiomyopathy according to the severity of symptoms. Risk for sudden death should be considered regardless of symptomatic status. LVEF = left ventricular ejection fraction; ACEI = angiotensin-converting enzyme inhibitor.

daily). Prednisone (20 to 60 mg/day) may be useful for resistant situations.

Pericardial Effusion

Pericardial effusion is often suspected clinically when the patient has symptoms and signs of tamponade physiology, but it may also be suggested by unsuspected cardiomegaly on the chest radiograph

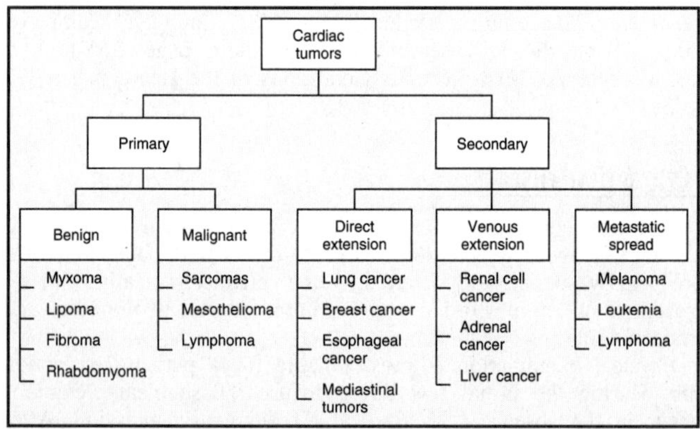

FIGURE 5–20 ■ Classification of the most common primary and secondary tumors. (Adapted from Salcedo EE, Cohen GI, White RD, Davison MG: Cardiac tumors: Diagnosis and management. Curr Probl Cardiol 17:75, 1992.)

Table 5–49 ■ ETIOLOGY OF PERICARDITIS

Infectious Pericarditis
Viral (coxsackievirus A and B, echovirus, mumps, adenovirus, HIV)
Mycobacterium tuberculosis
Bacterial *(Pneumococcus, Streptococcus, Staphylococcus, Legionella)*
Fungal (histoplasmosis, coccidioidomycosis, candidiasis, blastomycosis)
Other (syphilis, parasites)
Non-Infectious Pericarditis
Idiopathic
Neoplasm
Metastatic (lung cancer, breast cancer, melanoma, lymphoma)
Primary (mesothelioma)
Renal failure
Trauma
Irradiation (especially for breast cancer, Hodgkin's disease)
Myocardial infarction
Hypothyroidism
Aortic dissection
Chylopericardium (thoracic duct injury)
Trauma
Postpericardiotomy
Chest wall injury/trauma
Hypersensitivity Pericarditis
Collagen-vascular disease (systemic lupus erythematosus, rheumatoid arthritis, scleroderma, acute rheumatic fever)
Drug-induced (procainamide, hydralazine, isoniazid)
Post myocardial infarction (Dressler's syndrome)

(Fig. 5–21). Two-dimensional transthoracic echocardiography is diagnostic.

Cardiac Tamponade

Accumulation of fluid in the pericardium with a resultant increase in pericardial pressure and impairment of ventricular filling results in cardiac tamponade. Clinical features may mimic heart failure. Typical physical examination includes jugular venous distention, elevated (<10 mm Hg) pulsus paradoxus, and distant heart sounds. Emergency echocardiography is imperative and generally diagnostic. Immediate pericardiocentesis may be life-saving.

Constrictive Pericarditis

With chronic constriction, the pericardium may thicken to 10 mm or greater. Central venous pressue is elevated and displays prominent x and y descents. The pulse pressure is often narrowed, but pulsus paradoxus is usually absent. Increased pericardial thickness is most reliably diagnosed by computed tomography (CT) or MRI. Surgical stripping or removal of both layers of the adherent pericardium is the definitive therapy.

For more information about this subject, see *Cecil Textbook of Medicine,* 21st edition. Philadelphia, W.B. Saunders Company, 2000. Chapter 65, Pericardial Disease, pages 347 to 353.

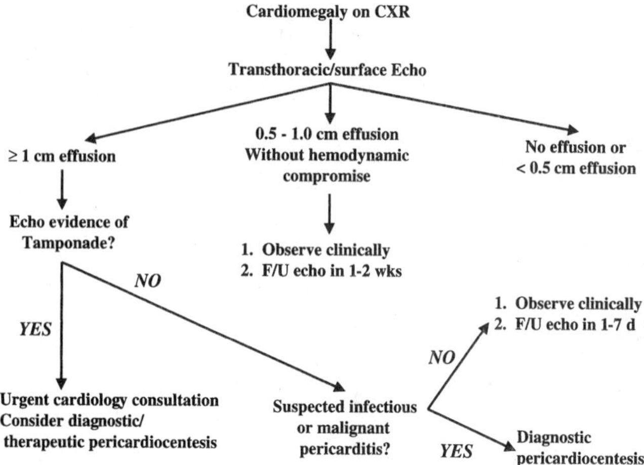

FIGURE 5–21 ■ Schematic for the clinical management of patients with cardiomegaly on chest x-ray (CXR) and suspected pericardial effusion in patients with normal left ventricular systolic function and normal thyroid-stimulating hormone (TSH). F/U = follow up. (Adapted from Lorell BH: Pericardial disease. *In* Goldman L, Braunwald E [eds]: Primary Cardiology. Philadelphia, WB Saunders, 1998, p 440.)

DISEASES OF THE AORTA

Aortic Aneurysm

Atherosclerosis is the major underlying cause of abdominal aortic aneurysms (AAAs). Most AAAs and thoracic aortic aneurysms are asymptomatic when they are discovered on routine physical examination or imaging. Aneurysm expansion or impending rupture may be heralded by new or worsening pain, often of sudden onset. A definitive diagnosis is made by either abdominal ultrasound (US) or CT.

AAAs larger than 6.0 cm should be repaired, as should those larger than 5.0 cm, in good operative candidates. AAAs larger than 4.0 cm should be monitored every 6 months by US or CT. Thoracic aortic aneurysms larger than 6.0 cm should undergo surgical repair, whereas patients with Marfan syndrome should undergo repair when the aneurysm is 5.5 cm or larger because of the high risk of rupture.

Aortic Dissection

Some two thirds of aortic dissections are type A (proximal); the other third are type B (distal). A history of hypertension is present in the large majority of cases without Marfan syndrome. Severe pain may be retrosternal, in the neck or throat, interscapular, in the lower back, abdominal, or in the lower extremities, depending on the location of the aortic dissection. Complications include compromise of a coronary artery, causing myocardial ischemia or MI, or retrograde dissection into the pericardium, causing acute tamponade. Involvement of the brachiocephalic arteries may produce stroke or coma.

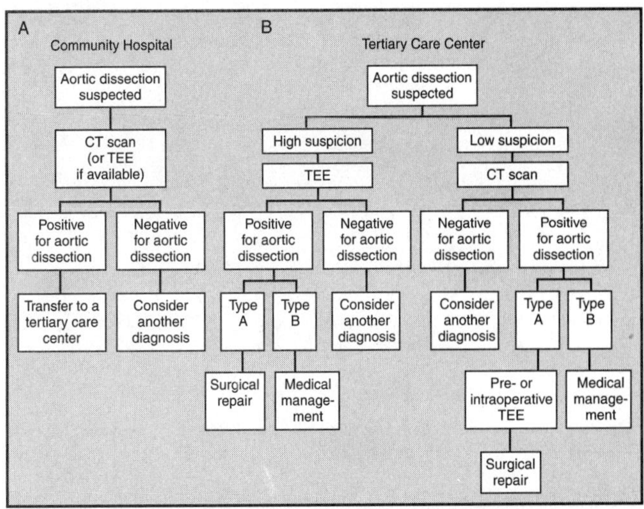

FIGURE 5–22 ■ Suggested algorithms for the evaluation of suspected acute aortic dissection. *A,* Approach used in many community hospitals where cardiac surgery is not performed. *B,* Approach used in many tertiary care centers where transesophageal echocardiography (TEE) and cardiac surgery are both available. CT = computed tomography.

Findings on chest radiography are non-specific and rarely diagnostic. Accurate diagnosis of aortic dissection can be made using CT, MRI, or TEE (Fig. 5–22).

The initial goal of treatment is to reduce systolic blood pressure to 100 to 120 mm Hg, or to the lowest level that maintains cerebral, cardiac, and renal perfusion. IV labetalol may be particularly useful. IV nitroprusside should be added to titrate BP minute by minute. When an acute dissection involves the ascending aorta, surgical repair is indicated. Patients with type B and chronic type A dissections usually can be managed medically.

For more information about this subject, see *Cecil Textbook of Medicine,* 21st edition. Philadelphia, W.B. Saunders Company, 2000. Chapter 66, Diseases of the Aorta, pages 353 to 357.

PERIPHERAL ARTERIAL DISEASE

Chronic arterial insufficiency of the lower extremity causes two very characteristic types of pain, intermittent claudication and ischemic rest pain, often with ulceration or gangrene. Absence of a femoral pulse indicates inflow disease of the iliac arteries. Patients with a palpable femoral pulse but absent pedal pulses have disease confined to the femoropopliteal or infrapopliteal arteries.

The ankle-brachial index (ABI), which is the ankle BP divided by the arm BP as detected by Doppler, helps guide therapy (Fig. 5–23). Cilostazol improves treadmill performance and functional status, as does exercise training. Percutaneous angioplasty or bypass surgery is recommended for rest pain or claudication that unacceptably interferes with lifestyle despite medical management.

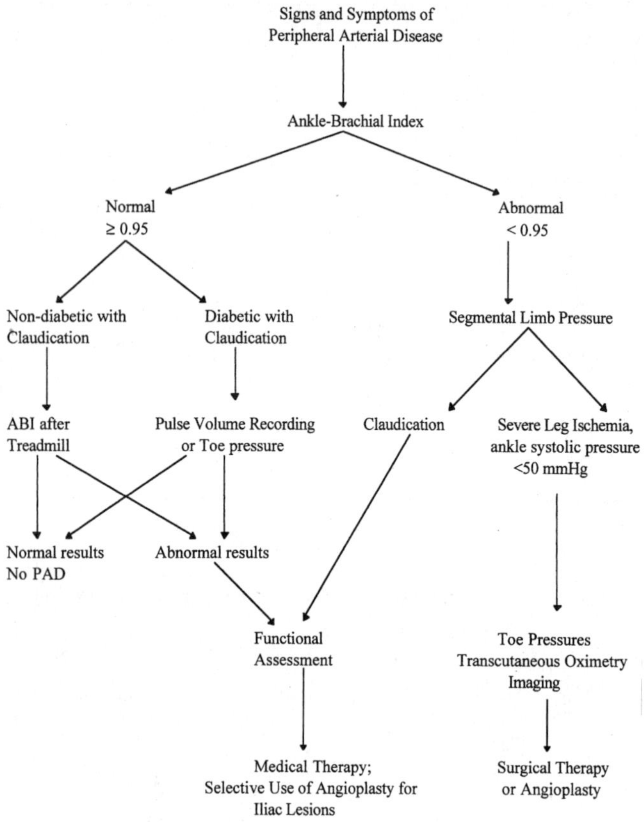

Signs and Symptoms of Peripheral Arterial Disease
Ankle-Brachial Index
Normal ≥ 0.95
Abnormal < 0.95
Non-diabetic with Claudication
Diabetic with Claudication
Segmental Limb Pressure
ABI after Treadmill
Pulse Volume Recording or Toe pressure
Claudication
Severe Leg Ischemia, ankle systolic pressure <50 mmHg
Normal results No PAD
Abnormal results
Functional Assessment
Toe Pressures Transcutaneous Oximetry Imaging
Medical Therapy; Selective Use of Angioplasty for Iliac Lesions
Surgical Therapy or Angioplasty

FIGURE 5–23 ■ Peripheral vascular diagnosis. ABI = ankle-brachial index; PAD = peripheral arterial disease.

The majority of acutely ischemic limbs will be salvageable. The extremity is often pale and cool to palpation; pulses are absent. Initial management requires rapid therapeutic heparin anticoagulation. A vascular surgeon should be consulted immediately.

Atheromatous Embolization

Atheromatous emboli usually originate from ulcerated or stenotic atherosclerotic plaques or aneurysms that are primarily in the thoracic or abdominal aorta, iliac artery, or carotid artery. The most common clinical manifestations include livedo reticularis, purple or blue toes, splinter hemorrhages, gangrenous digits or ulcerations, and nodules in the presence of palpable foot pulses. No single laboratory test is diagnostic. Biopsy remains the most specific way to make the diagnosis, but it is often not required because the clinical findings may be highly suggestive.

Thromboangiitis Obliterans

Thromboangiitis obliterans (Buerger's disease) is a non-atherosclerotic, segmental, inflammatory disease that most commonly affects the small and medium-sized arteries and veins in the upper and lower extremities. The cause is unknown, but there is an extremely strong association with heavy tobacco use. Patients may present with claudication of the foot, legs, and occasionally the arms and hands. The cornerstone of therapy is complete discontinuation of the use of tobacco in any form.

Raynaud's Phenomenon

Primary Raynaud's disease denotes patients who have no underlying cause, whereas secondary Raynaud's phenomenon is associated with other systemic disease processes (Table 5–50). Vasospastic attacks are precipitated by exposure to the cold or emotional stimuli. Serologic evaluation should include a complete blood cell count, multiphasic serologic analysis, urinalysis, sedimentation rate, C-reactive protein, antinuclear antibody, extractable nuclear antigen,

Table 5–50 ■ CONDITIONS ASSOCIATED WITH SECONDARY RAYNAUD'S PHENOMENON

Connective Tissue Diseases	**Trauma**
Scleroderma or CREST syndrome	Vibratory tools, grinders, sanders
Systemic lupus erythematosus	Thermal injury
Rheumatoid arthritis	Electric shock injury
Mixed connective tissue disease	Percussive injury
Polymyositis, dermatomyositis	Hypothenar hammer syndrome
Sjögren's syndrome	**Hematologic Abnormalities**
Arterial Occlusive Diseases	Cryoglobulinemia and cryofibrinogenemia
Vasculitis	Cold agglutinin diseases
Thromboangiitis obliterans (Buerger's disease)	Myeloproliferative diseases
Thromboembolism	Hyperviscosity syndrome
Thoracic outlet syndrome	**Neurologic Disorders**
Atherosclerosis of extremities (rare)	Carpal tunnel syndrome
Drugs and Toxins	Reflex sympathetic dystrophy
β-Adrenergic blocking agents	Stroke
Ergotamine preparations	Intervertebral disk disease
Methysergide	Poliomyelitis
Vinblastine	Syringomyelia
Bleomycin	**Other**
Cisplatin	Hypothyroidism
Polyvinyl chloride	Pulmonary hypertension
Estrogen	Arteriovenous fistula
Heavy metals	Neoplasms
	Renal failure

CREST = *c*alcinosis cutis, *R*aynaud's phenomenon, *e*sophageal dysfunction, *s*clerodactyly, *t*elangiectasia.

anti-DNA, cryoglobulins, complement, anticentromere antibodies, and SCL70 scleroderma antibodies.

Patients should limit exposure to the cold, and smoking should be avoided. Patients may benefit from a short-acting calcium channel blocker such as nifedipine 10 to 20 mg 30 minutes to 1 hour before going out into the cold. When vasospasm occurs more frequently, the extended-release preparations of nifedipine 30 to 90 mg/day, amlodipine 2.5 to 10 mg/day, or diltiazem 120 to 300 mg/day are effective. Prazosin or terazosin can also decrease the severity, frequency, and duration of attacks.

Frostbite

Soon after exposure to the cold, pain develops and gradually progresses to numbness. Frozen tissue should be rapidly rewarmed in a water bath of 40 to 42° C (104–108° F) for 15 to 30 minutes until complete thawing has occurred. With rewarming, the affected parts become hyperemic. Blisters appear within the first 24 hours and are reabsorbed within 1 to 2 weeks, after which a black eschar may persist.

For more information about this subject, see *Cecil Textbook of Medicine,* 21st edition. Philadelphia, W.B. Saunders Company, 2000. Chapter 67 Atherosclerotic Peripheral Arterial Disease, and Chapter 68, Other Peripheral Arterial Diseases, pages 357 to 367.

PERIPHERAL VENOUS DISEASE

Deep vein thrombosis (DVT) usually begins in the deep veins of the calf muscles. DVT may propagate into the proximal venous system, where it becomes a serious and potentially life-threatening disorder. The diagnostic approach to patients with venous thromboembolism (VTE) may involve the lungs or the legs, and prevention of pulmonary embolism is essentially the prevention of DVT.

The clinical features of venous thrombosis include leg pain, tenderness, swelling, a palpable cord, discoloration, venous distention, prominence of the superficial veins, and cyanosis. Upper extremity DVT involving the subclavian, axillary, and brachial veins is often caused by strenuous exercise or central venous catheters.

A number of conditions can mimic venous thrombosis (Table 5–51). US has become the standard technique for the evaluation of patients with clinically suspected DVT. A positive result is highly predictive of acute DVT and warrants anticoagulation, whereas anticoagulant therapy can be safely withheld in symptomatic patients who have negative results by serial US (Fig. 5–24). The combination of a negative D-dimer, a non-diagnostic lung scan, and a low clinical probability of DVT or the combination of a normal D-dimer and normal US may sufficiently exclude DVT so that further diagnostic testing can be safely limited and anticoagulation avoided.

Prevention of Venous Thromboembolism

The primary prophylactic measures most commonly used are low-dose or adjusted-dose unfractionated heparin, low-molecular-

Table 5–51 ■ ALTERNATIVE DIAGNOSES IN PATIENTS WITH CLINICALLY SUSPECTED VENOUS THROMBOSIS AND NEGATIVE VENOGRAMS*

DIAGNOSIS	PATIENTS (%)
Muscle strain	24
Direct twisting injury to the leg	10
Leg swelling in paralyzed limb	9
Lymphangitis, lymphatic obstruction	7
Venous reflux	7
Muscle tear	6
Baker's cyst	5
Cellulitis	3
Internal abnormality of the knee	2
Unknown	26

*The diagnosis was made once venous thrombosis had been excluded by venography.

weight heparin (LMWH), oral anticoagulants (to an INR of 2.0 to 3.0), and intermittent pneumatic leg compression (Table 5–52).

Treatment of Venous Thrombosis

Subcutaneous unmonitored LMWH results in a reduction in major bleeding and mortality when compared with unfractionated heparin. LMWH used out of hospital is as effective and safe as IV unfractionated heparin given in the hospital. The efficacy of heparin therapy depends on achieving an activated partial thromboplastin time (aPTT) 1.5 times the mean of the control value or the upper

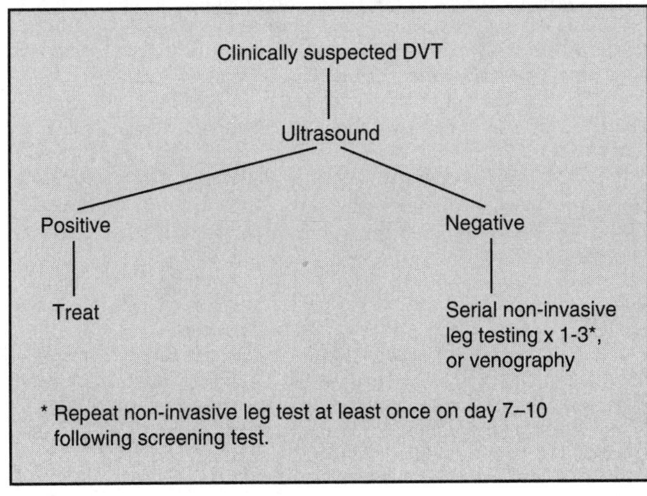

FIGURE 5–24 ■ Algorithm for the diagnosis of deep vein thrombosis (DVT) in patients with no evidence of pulmonary embolism.

Table 5–52 ■ SPECIFIC RECOMMENDATIONS FOR PROPHYLAXIS OF VENOUS THROMBOEMBOLISM FOR VARIOUS CLINICAL RISK CATEGORIES

PATIENT CATEGORY	PROPHYLAXIS RECOMMENDATION
Moderate Risk	
General abdominal, thoracic, gynecologic, or urologic surgery; medical patients	Low-dose unfractionated heparin or LMWH, IPC in patients at high risk of bleeding
Pregnancy with previous DVT	Low-dose heparin or adjusted-dose heparin
Moderate-to-High-Risk	
Neurosurgery	IPC
High Risk	
Elective hip replacement	LMWH, warfarin, IPC
Elective knee replacement	LMWH, IPC
Hip fracture	LMWH, warfarin
Spinal cord injury with paralysis	LMWH, IPC

LMWH = low-molecular-weight heparin; IPC = intermittent pneumatic leg compresssion; DVT = deep vein thrombosis.

limit of the normal aPTT range. In approximately 1 to 2% of patients, heparin-induced thrombocytopenia occurs within 5 to 10 days after heparin treatment has started. Warfarin is administered on the first day of heparin therapy in an initial dose of 5 to 10 mg/day for the first 2 days. The daily dose is then adjusted according to the INR. Heparin therapy is discontinued on the fourth or fifth day after initiation of warfarin therapy, provided that the INR is prolonged into the recommended therapeutic range (INR of 2.0–3.0). All patients with a first episode of VTE should receive warfarin therapy for 3 to 6 months. Warfarin treatment for at least 6 months is indicated for patients who have a continuing risk factor for VTE. The current recommendation is to continue oral anticoagulant therapy for at least 12 months in patients with a first recurrence and indefinitely in those who have more than one recurrence.

Thrombolytic therapy may benefit selected patients with acute massive venous thrombosis. The main indications for the insertion of an inferior vena caval filter for DVT are acute VTE and an absolute contraindication to anticoagulation therapy and the very rare instance of objectively documented recurrent VTE during adequate anticoagulant therapy. Prophylactic vena caval filter placement may be considered in very high-risk patients.

For more information about this subject, see *Cecil Textbook of Medicine,* 21st edition. Philadelphia, W.B. Saunders Company, 2000. Chapter 69, Peripheral Venous Disease, pages 367 to 372; and Chapter 84, Pulmonary Embolism, pages 442 to 449; and Chapter 188, Antithrombotic Therapy, pages 1021 to 1028.

CHAPTER 6

RESPIRATORY DISEASES

APPROACH TO THE PATIENT WITH RESPIRATORY DISEASE

History

6

The five common manifestations of pulmonary disease are cough, shortness of breath or dyspnea, chest pain, a solitary pulmonary nodule, and hemoptysis. Common causes of transient cough are bacterial or viral infections and noxious vapors. For persistent cough, common causes include asthma and regurgitation of acidic gastric contents into the tracheobronchial tree during sleep. An important cause of persistent cough is a tumor in the tracheobronchial tree. Cough is also a complication of angiotensin-converting enzyme (ACE) inhibitor drugs.

The most consistent correlate of dyspnea is increased mechanical work of breathing (Fig. 6–1). Pleuritic pain is sharp and severe, magnified by breathing, and may be associated with a pleural friction rub. A solitary pulmonary nodule on a chest radiograph, especially if it is new, poses the possibility of a malignancy and requires immediate diagnostic evaluation (Fig. 6–2).

The most common cause of hemoptysis is pneumonia or pulmonary infection, including bronchiectasis. The sudden appearance of hemoptysis without other cause must be considered a possible manifestation of lung tumor. A pulmonary embolism that leads to pulmonary infarction may cause hemoptysis. Pulmonary tuberculosis, especially with cavity formation, is a prominent cause of hemoptysis, especially in patients with human immunodeficiency virus (HIV) infection.

A detailed account of the patient's primary symptoms is essential, but other critical information includes the amount of exposure to (1) tobacco smoke; (2) pollutants, such as nitrogen dioxide, beryllium, asbestos, coal, and silica dust; (3) fumes from industrial processes; and (4) animal danders. A family history of emphysema may be present in cases of serum α_1-antitrypsin deficiency. Interstitial pulmonary fibrosis is a complication of therapy with bleomycin, cyclophosphamide, methotrexate, or nitrofurantoin. Bronchospasm may be initiated or exacerbated by β-adrenergic blocking drugs.

Physical Examination and Diagnostic Tests

The physical signs of pulmonary disease are given in Table 6–1. Cyanosis of the tongue and oral mucosa, which is called central cyanosis, provides a crude estimation of the adequacy of arterial

---

For more information about this subject, see *Cecil Textbook of Medicine,* 21st edition. Philadelphia, W.B. Saunders Company, 2000; Part VIII: Respiratory Diseases, pages 379 to 482.

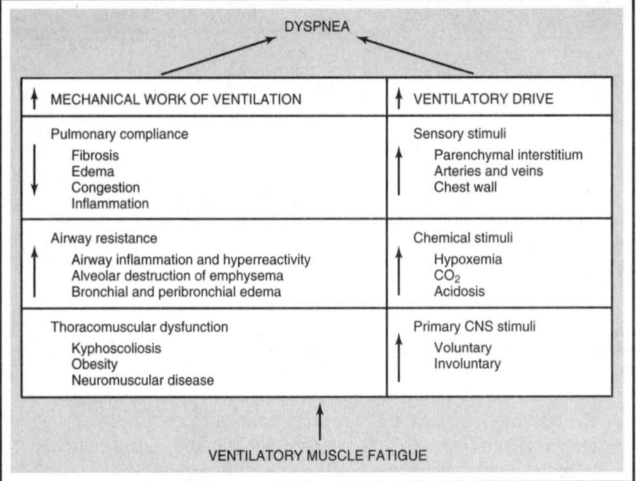

FIGURE 6–1 ■ The symptom of dyspnea can best be related to increases in the mechanical work of breathing and/or increases in ventilatory drive as a result of the effect of different pathogenic factors on ventilatory mechanics and increased ventilatory stimuli. Ventilatory muscle fatigue is an added factor.

oxygenation. Central cyanosis reflects the presence of 3 g/dL or more of reduced, that is, deoxygenated, hemoglobin. However, the blue discoloration also may be caused by dyshemoglobins such as sulfhemoglobin.

Diagnostic investigations include chest radiography, sinus radiography, and computed tomography (CT). When indicated, bronchoscopy and laryngscopy should be performed.

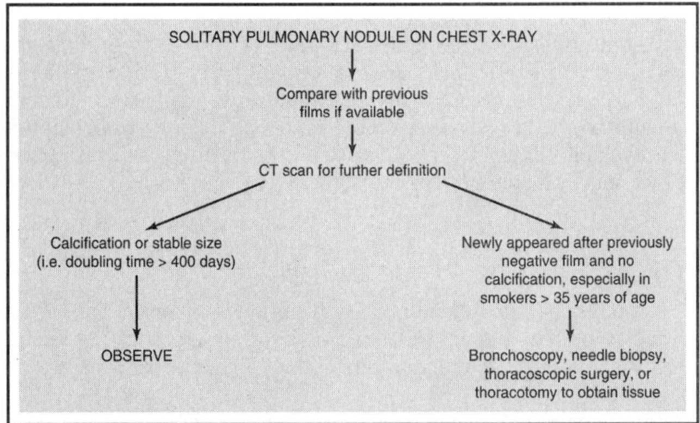

FIGURE 6–2 ■ Steps in the evaluation of the solitary pulmonary nodule.

Table 6–1 ■ PHYSICAL SIGNS OF PULMONARY DISEASE

PATHOGENIC PROCESS	CHEST WALL MOTION AND CONFIGURATION	BREATH SOUNDS	PERCUSSION	FREMITUS
Asthmatic and bronchitic airway obstruction	Increased anteroposterior (AP) diameter, use of accessory muscles of ventilation	May be decreased; prolonged expiration; inspiratory and expiratory wheezes and rhonchi	Hyperresonant	Decreased
Airway obstruction of emphysema	Increased AP diameter, reduced chest wall musculature with general weight loss, use of accessory muscles of ventilation	Markedly diminished; prolonged expiratory phase; rhonchi may be present	Hyperresonant	Decreased
Atelectasis	Inspiratory lag on affected side	Absent over affected area	Dull	Decreased
Consolidation of acute pneumonia	Splinting of chest wall on affected side	Bronchial breath sounds, whispered pectoriloquy, rales, and/or rhonchi	Dull	Increased
Pleural effusion	Lag on affected side	Absent or decreased	Flat	Absent
Pneumothorax	Lag on affected side; tracheal deviation away from affected side	Absent	Hyperresonant	Absent
Diffuse alveolitis or fibrosis	Restricted inspiratory and expiratory excursion	May be increased with diffuse fine rales	Decreased resonance or normal	Increased or normal

Assessment of Arterial Oxygenation

The $PaCO_2$ is used to assess the adequacy of ventilation and to diagnose hypercapneic respiratory failure. At sea level the $PaCO_2$ normally ranges from 35 to 45 mm Hg. Hyperventilation and respiratory alkalosis are said to be present if the $PaCO_2$ is less than 35 mm Hg. Hypoventilation, hypercapnia, and respiratory acidosis are present if the $PaCO_2$ is greater than 45 mm Hg, and ventilatory failure exists when the $PaCO_2$ exceeds 50 mm Hg.

The pH and HCO_3^- concentration measurements can be used to determine whether hypercapnia, hypocapnia, respiratory acidosis, and/or respiratory alkalosis is acute or chronic.

$$pH = 6.1 + \log [HCO_3^-]/0.003\ PaCO_2$$

Acute increases or decreases in $PaCO_2$ cause the pH to fall or rise until the kidneys gradually retain or release HCO_3^- to buffer the fall or rise in pH. The pH normally ranges from 7.35 to 7.45. An acute increase in $PaCO_2$ causes the pH to fall below 7.35, a condition called acute respiratory acidosis. Conversely, an acute decrease in $PaCO_2$ causes the pH to rise above 7.45, creating an acute respiratory alkalosis.

The normal PaO_2 at sea level is approximately 100 mm Hg. However, the PaO_2 is inversely correlated with age:

$$\text{Normal } PaO_2 = 100 \text{ mm Hg} - (0.3) \text{ age in years}$$

The saturation of hemoglobin by O_2 in systemic arterial blood (SaO_2) is related to the PaO_2 by the O_2 hemoglobin dissociation curve (Fig. 6–3).

The arterial-to-alveolar PO_2 ratio (PaO_2/PAO_2) is relatively stable with changing levels of FIO_2 and can be used to predict the expected PaO_2 when the FIO_2 is altered. The normal (PaO_2/PAO_2) is 0.9. The PaO_2-to-FIO_2 ratio (PaO_2/FIO_2) is easier to calculate and is normally 460.

Venous admixture (QVA/QT) is the fraction of mixed venous blood that does not become oxygenated as it courses through the lungs. It can be calculated with the equation

$$QVA/QT = (C'cO_2 - CaO_2) / (C'cO_2 - CvO_2)$$

where QVA is the volume of shunted blood, QT is the cardiac output, and $C'cO_2$, CaO_2, and CvO_2 are the O_2 contents of end-capillary, arterial, and mixed venous blood, respectively. Although end-capillary blood cannot be sampled routinely, the end-capillary O_2 content can be calculated by assuming that the tension of end-capillary blood is the same as PAO_2.

The normal QVA/QT is 0.07 or less; increases in QVA/QT are caused by ventilation-perfusion mismatching or right-to-left intrapulmonary shunting (QS/QT). This equation can be used to calculate QS/QT in patients receiving an FIO_2 of 1.0 because this FIO_2 eliminates areas of ventilation-perfusion mismatch in the lungs. The PaO_2 can rarely be improved by increasing FIO_2 if QS/QT exceeds 0.25.

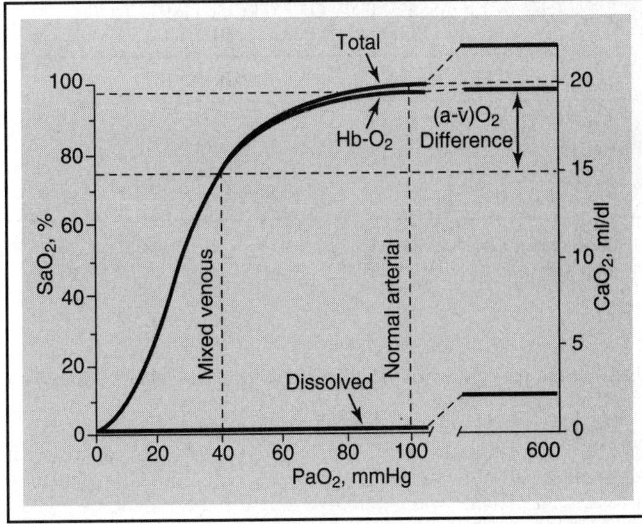

FIGURE 6–3 ■ Normal oxyhemoglobin dissociation curve showing the relationship between the systemic arterial O_2 saturation (SaO_2), tension (PaO_2), and content (CaO_2). See text for further discussion.

6

Pulmonary function tests can provide an objective measurement of lung function (Table 6–2). Spirometry can quantify airway obstruction and determine the response to bronchodilator therapy. Lung volume measurements can diagnose restrictive lung disease. FVC is the maximal volume of air that can be exhaled during a forced exhalation, and FEV_1 is the volume of gas that can be exhaled during the first 1 second of a forced exhalation (Table 6–3). Diffusing capacity (DLCO) can be altered in disorders of

Table 6–2 ■ **PULMONARY FUNCTION TESTS**

Lung Volumes	
TLC	Total lung capacity
FRC	Functional residual capacity
ERV	Expiratory reserve volume
RV	Residual volume
Expiratory Flow	
FEV_1	Forced expiratory volume (in 1 second)
FVC	Forced vital capacity
FEV_1%	FEV_1/FVC ratio (expressed as %)
Diffusing Capacity	
DLCO	Diffusing capacity for carbon monoxide
Arterial Blood Gases	
PaO_2	Arterial O_2 pressure
$PaCO_2$	Arterial CO_2 pressure
pH	

Table 6–3 ■ ASSESSMENT OF EXERCISE LIMITATION IN OBSTRUCTIVE LUNG DISEASE

FEV_1 (L)	IMPAIRMENT*
>3	None
2–3	Mild
1–2	Moderate
<1	Severe

*This assumes a middle-aged person of normal body size having a predicted FEV_1 of close to 4 L. Applying this simple formula commonly requires some adjustment for age and body size.

distribution of ventilation and any disorder that alters pulmonary capillary blood volume.

The primary criterion for airflow obstruction is a reduced FEV_1/FVC%. The hallmarks of restrictive lung diseases are a low total lung capacity (TLC) and a fall in FVC. FEV_1/FVC is generally increased in patients with restrictive lung diseases. Table 6–4 gives the common changes in lung volumes in various classes of restrictive lung diseases.

For more information about this subject, see *Cecil Textbook of Medicine,* 21st edition. Philadelphia, W.B. Saunders Company, 2000. Chapter 72, Approach to the Patient with Respiratory Disease, and Chapter 73, Respiratory Structure and Function, pages 379 to 387.

ASTHMA

Asthma is characterized by recurrent episodes of airway obstruction that resolve spontaneously or as a result of treatment, an exaggerated bronchoconstrictor response to stimuli that have little or no effect in non-asthmatic subjects, and inflammation of the airways. During an asthma attack, shortness of breath is accompanied by cough, wheezing, and anxiety. Dyspnea may occur only with exercise, after aspirin ingestion, after exposure to a specific known allergen, or for no identifiable reason. Variant symptoms include cough, hoarseness, or an inability to sleep through the night when exposed to rapid changes in temperature and humidity.

Table 6–4 ■ LUNG VOLUMES IN RESTRICTIVE LUNG DISEASES

	PULMONARY FIBROSIS	OBESITY (CHEST WALL RESTRICTION)	NEUROMUSCULAR DISORDERS
TLC	↓	↓	↓
FRC	↓	↓	Normal
ERV	↓	↓↓	↓
RV	↓	Normal	↑

For abbreviations, see Table 6–2.

Table 6–5 ■ DIFFERENTIAL DIAGNOSIS OF WHEEZING OTHER THAN ASTHMA

Common

Acute bronchiolitis (infectious, chemical)
Aspiration (foreign body)
Bronchial stenosis
Cardiac failure
Chronic bronchitis
Cystic fibrosis
Eosinophilic pneumonia

Uncommon

Airway obstruction due to masses
- External compression: central thoracic tumors, superior vena cava syndrome, substernal thyroid
- Intrinsic airway: primary lung cancer, metastatic breast cancer

Carcinoid syndrome
Endobronchial sarcoid
Pulmonary emboli
Systemic mastocytosis
Systemic vasculitis (polyarteritis nodosa)

Common features of acute asthma attacks include a rapid respiratory rate (often 25–40 breaths per minute), tachycardia, and pulsus paradoxus (an exaggerated inspiratory fall in the systolic pressure). Patients often use their accessory muscles of ventilation. Percussion of the thorax demonstrates hyperresonance. Auscultation reveals wheezing, which is typical of asthma but does not establish the diagnosis (Table 6–5).

The peak expiratory flow rate (PEFR), the FEV_1, and the maximal midexpiratory flow rate (MMEFR) are all decreased in asthma (Table 6–6). Blood gas analysis need not be undertaken in mild

Table 6–6 ■ RELATIVE SEVERITY OF AN ASTHMATIC ATTACK AS INDICATED BY PEFR, FEV_1, AND MMEFR

TEST	PERCENT OF PREDICTED VALUE	ASTHMA SEVERITY
PEFR	≥80	
FEV_1	≥80	No spirometric abnormalities
MMEFR	≥80	
PEFR	≥80	
FEV_1	≥70	Mild asthma
MMEFR	55–75	
PEFR	≥60	
FEV_1	45–70	Moderate asthma
MMEFR	30–50	
PEFR	<50	
FEV_1	<50	Severe asthma
MMEFR	10–30	

PEFR = peak expiratory flow rate; FEV_1 = forced expiratory volume in 1 second; MMEFR = maximal midexpiratory flow rate.

asthma. In severe asthma, the PaO_2 is usually between 55 and 70 mm Hg and the $PaCO_2$ is between 25 and 35 mm Hg. A normal $PaCO_2$ in a patient with moderate to severe airflow obstruction is reason for concern, as it may indicate that respiratory failure is imminent. Blood eosinophilia is common. The chest radiograph is often normal, but severe asthma is associated with hyperinflation.

Treatment of Chronic Asthma

Patients with *mild intermittent asthma* have normal or near-normal lung function, infrequent asthma symptoms, usually sleep through the night without difficulty, and need to use asthma rescue medications infrequently. The only treatment needed for such patients is an inhaled medium-acting bronchodilator.

Patients with *mild persistent asthma* have normal or near-normal lung function on most occasions but have asthma symptoms daily, have difficulty sleeping 1 or 2 nights a week, and use their asthma rescue medications so frequently that a single 200-μg actuation canister is inadequate to provide a month's treatment. Such patients require a controller agent, such as an inhaled corticosteroid, an antileukotriene agent, or cromolyn sodium, in addition to their rescue treatment. Despite therapy with a single controller agent, patients with *moderate* or *severe persistent asthma* have persistently abnormal lung function, have asthma symptoms more than once daily, and have difficulty sleeping many nights a week. These patients require multiple asthma medications to achieve adequate disease control.

β-Adrenergic agents given by inhalation are the mainstay of bronchodilator treatment for asthma. Patients with mild intermittent asthma should be treated with a moderate-duration β_2-selective inhaler on an as-needed basis. In contrast to medium-acting β-agonists, the only long-acting β-agonist currently available in the United States, salmeterol (Serevent), has a slow onset of action and a duration of action of nearly 12 hours; it is considered a controller rather than a bronchodilator agent. Although ipratropium bromide has a salutary effect on cough in asthma and is useful as an adjunct to inhaled β_2-agonists in chronic stable asthma, it has not been shown to be as effective for the treatment of acute asthmatic bronchospasm as inhaled β_2-agonists.

Inhaled corticosteroids are effective controller treatments for patients with persistent asthma (Table 6–7). Agents with the capacity to inhibit the synthesis or action of the leukotrienes are effective controller medications for the patient with mild or moderate persistent asthma. Treatment with theophylline is recommended only for patients with moderate or severe persistent asthma who are receiving controller medications, such as inhaled steroids or antileukotrienes, but whose asthma is not adequately controlled. Cromolyn sodium and nedocromil sodium are non-steroid inhaled treatments that have proved beneficial in the management of mild-to-moderate persistent asthma. Systemic corticosteroids are effective for the treatment of moderate-to-severe persistent asthma, as well as occasional severe exacerbations of asthma that occur in a patient with otherwise mild asthma. In non-hospitalized patients with asthma refractory to standard therapy, a steroid "pulse" with initial doses

Table 6–7 ■ DOSES OF INHALED CORTICOSTEROIDS AVAILABLE FOR ASTHMA TREATMENT IN THE UNITED STATES

STEROID NAME		DOSAGE		
Generic	**Trade**	**Actuation**	**Starting Dose**	**COMMENTS**
Beclomethasone	Beclovent	42 μg	2 puffs bid	Available in 2 strengths; prescription must indicate strength
Budesonide	Pulmicort	200 μg	2 puffs bid	Available only in the dry powder Turbuhaler
Flunisolide	Aerobid	250 μg	2 puffs bid	
Fluticasone	Flovent	44, 110, or 220 μg	2 puffs bid (44 μg per puff)	Available in 3 strengths; prescription must indicate dose level
Triamcinolone	Azmacort	100 μg	2 puffs bid	

6

of prednisone on the order of 40 to 60 mg/day, tapered to zero over 7 to 14 days, is recommended.

Treatment of Severe Acute Asthma

When a patient with asthma presents for acute emergency care, objective measures of the severity of the attack, including quantification of pulsus paradoxus and measurement of airflow rates (PEFR or FEV_1), should be evaluated in addition to the usual vital signs. When patients have PEFR and FEV_1 values that are greater than 60% of their predicted value on arrival in the emergency department, treatment with inhaled β-agonists alone is likely to result in an objective improvement in airflow rates. If the attack has been prolonged and failed to respond to treatment with bronchodilators and high-dose inhaled steroids before arrival at the emergency department, intravenous steroids (40–60 mg of methylprednisolone) should be administered. Treatment with β-agonists should be repeated at 20- to 30-minute intervals until the PEFR or FEV_1 rises to greater than 40% of the predicted values. If this point is not reached within 2 hours, admission to the hospital for further treatment is strongly advocated.

For patients whose PEFR and FEV_1 values are between 40% and 60% of the values predicted at the time of initial evaluation in the emergency care setting, a plan of treatment varying in intensity between the two cited above is indicated. Failure to respond to treatment by objective criteria (PEFR or FEV_1) within 2 hours of arriving at the emergency department is an indication for more intense therapy.

The asthmatic subject whose PEFR or FEV_1 does not increase to greater than 40% of the predicted value with treatment, whose $Paco_2$ increases without improvement of indices of airflow obstruction, or who develops major complications such as pneumothorax or pneumomediastinum should be admitted to the hospital for close monitoring. Frequent treatments with inhaled β-agonists, intravenous aminophylline (at doses yielding maximal plasma levels), and high-dose intravenous steroids are indicated. For patients whose asthma requires in-hospital treatment but is not considered life-threatening, an initial intravenous bolus of 2 mg/kg of hydrocortisone, followed by continuous infusion of 0.5 mg/kg/hour, has been shown to be beneficial within 12 hours. In attacks of asthma that are considered life-threatening, the use of intravenous methylprednisolone 125 mg every 6 hours has been advocated. In each case, as the patient improves, oral steroids are substituted for intravenous steroids, and the oral dose is tapered over 1 to 3 weeks; addition of inhaled steroids to the regimen when oral steroids are started is strongly recommended. Oxygen should be administered to achieve Sao_2 values between 92% and 94%. If indicated, intubation of the trachea and mechanical ventilation can be instituted.

In some patients, acute exacerbation of asthma may be due to concurrent infection. When infection is suggested, appropriate antibiotics should be used to cover the likely cause.

For more information about this subject, see *Cecil Textbook of Medicine,* 21st edition. Philadelphia, W.B. Saunders Company, 2000. Chapter 74, Asthma, pages 387 to 393.

CHRONIC BRONCHITIS AND EMPHYSEMA

Chronic bronchitis is a clinical diagnosis requiring patients to have a chronic cough productive of sputum for at least 3 months a year for at least 2 consecutive years in the absence of other diseases. Rare patients develop chronic bronchitis with minimal or no history of cigarette smoking.

Emphysema, which is a pathologic diagnosis, consists of enlargement of the terminal air spaces due to destruction of alveolar walls. In centrilobular emphysema, which is usually associated with cigarette smoking, alveolar destruction occurs initially around the respiratory bronchioles. The panlobular variety is often related to α_1-antitrypsin deficiency.

With severe chronic obstructive pulmonary disease (COPD), expiratory flow is so limited that tidal respiration can be achieved only near TLC. Subjects cannot increase ventilation to any significant extent and are unable to accomplish any sustained exercise.

Because COPD does not affect the lung uniformly, ventilation and perfusion distribution is impaired. Areas with low ventilation-perfusion ratios cause arterial hypoxia, which cannot by rectified by increasing ventilation to restore arterial CO_2 to normal.

Diagnosis

Many patients with mild-to-moderate disease and up to 50% reduction in lung function do not complain of shortness of breath. The specificity and sensitivity of chronic cough, mild dyspnea, and even sputum production are low. Patients with excessive secretions may have rhonchi (predominantly expiratory) due to secretions in large airways.

By the time the FEV_1 falls below 50% of predicted, moderate-to-severe disease is present and most patients experience significant symptoms. Patients commonly have an increased respiratory rate, and close inspection reveals use of the strap muscles in their neck during inspiration. Breath sounds may be barely audible, or there may be high-pitched wheezing during expiration. With end-stage emphysema, patients generally lose weight.

If the FEV_1 is reduced much more than the FVC, then the diagnosis is airway obstruction. Routine chest radiographs are remarkably insensitive for diagnosing COPD. In far-advanced COPD, lung peripheral vascular markings are reduced, the diaphragm appears flattened, the rib cage is expanded laterally, and the heart appears small.

Differential Diagnosis

The major challenge in the diagnosis of COPD is not that it is confused with some other condition, but that it is not diagnosed at all. Elderly-onset asthma is differentiated from COPD primarily by CT scan (for emphysema) or by the degree of reversibility in response to therapy. Left ventricular failure can produce dyspnea and even acute onset of wheezing, so-called cardiac asthma; the chest radiograph shows cardiomegaly and pulmonary vascular congestion or pulmonary edema.

Treatment

Current recommendations of the American Thoracic Society include commonly used but controversial treatments for which no good efficacy data exist. Smoking cessation is the most important intervention to alter the clinical course.

Patients who quit smoking in the presymptomatic stage experience only modest improvement in lung function, but thereafter the rate of decline in quitters parallels that in normal individuals. In non-smokers, FEV_1 declines 30 to 40 mL/year. In smokers, the annual decline may be threefold to fourfold greater.

Because many patients with COPD have features of asthma, patients with severe exacerbations are frequently given therapeutic trials of systemic steroids (20–30 mg/day of prednisone). Many physicians prescribe inhaled nonabsorbable steroids chronically for COPD patients, although efficacy has not been demonstrated by well-designed clinical trials.

All COPD patients should have pneumococcal vaccinations and annual influenza vaccinations. In patients with PaO_2 less than 50 mm Hg at rest, continuous oxygen therapy prolongs life. Patients with PaO_2 not justifying continuous O_2 therapy should have overnight O_2 saturation monitored by percutaneous oxymetry; O_2 should be used during sleep if necessary to maintain saturation at 90%. In most COPD patients, O_2 saturation can be restored to near normal by low-flow (1 to 2 L/minute) O_2 delivered by nasal cannula.

For more information about this subject, see *Cecil Textbook of Medicine,* 21st edition. Philadelphia, W.B. Saunders Company, 2000. Chapter 75, Chronic Bronchitis and Emphysema, pages 393 to 401.

CYSTIC FIBROSIS

A variety of mutations of the gene coding the cystic fibrosis (CF) transmembrane conductance regulator (CFTR) cause the disease. The most common CF mutation is a 3-bp deletion that causes the loss of a phenylalanine at position 508 (ΔF508).

Cough is usually intermittent, occurring with what appear to be acute respiratory illnesses. As the disease progresses, the cough becomes productive of thick, purulent, often green sputum. Eventually, exacerbations of cough and sputum production are accompanied by dyspnea, reduced appetite, and weight loss. Lung sounds may be decreased due to hyperinflation. As the disease progresses, rales and rhonchi are common and continuous.

Due to a host defense defect localized to the lung, CF airways become colonized with bacteria, which are virtually impossible to eliminate. Repeated bacterial infections of the airways are the hallmark of CF lung disease. With time, *Pseudomonas aeruginosa* becomes very common. Impaction of mucus and changes consistent with bronchiectasis are observed as the disease progresses.

The PaO_2 tends to decrease with time due to ventilation-perfusion mismatching. Complications include pneumothorax, hemoptysis, digital clubbing, chronic rhinitis, nasal polyps, cor pulmonale, and respiratory failure. Failure of the exocrine pancreas occurs in approximately 85% of patients. Symptoms of pancreatitis occur in a small percentage of adults. More than 95% of males are sterile because of atrophy of wolffian duct structure. Focal biliary cirrhosis may develop as patients live longer.

An increased concentration of Na^+ and Cl^- in sweat is one of the most consistent findings. DNA testing may provide definitive evidence of CF.

The lung disease is progressive, punctuated by exacerbations of lung disease followed by improvement with intensive therapy. Patients with an FEV_1 less than 30% predicted, a PaO_2 less than 55 mm Hg, or a $PaCO_2$ greater than 50 mm Hg have 2-year mortality rates above 50%.

Treatment

Exacerbations of lung disease usually require an intensive course based on sputum cultures. Emergence of antibiotic-resistant organisms is a serious problem. Antibiotics by inhalation are attractive because aerosolized, high-dose tobramycin can reduce the density of *P. aeruginosa* and improve FEV_1. Chest percussion and postural drainage are mainstays of treatment. Beneficial effects of β-adrenergic agonists and anticholinergic agents have been demonstrated in short-term studies. Inhaled, recombinant human deoxyribonuclease can increase the clearance of sputum and decrease the frequency of respiratory exacerbations that require intravenous antibiotics.

Pancreatic enzymes are critical for nutrition. Attention should be paid to adequate salt intake, especially during hot weather.

For more information about this subject, see *Cecil Textbook of Medicine,* 21st edition. Philadelphia, W.B. Saunders Company, 2000. Chapter 76, Cystic Fibrosis, pages 401 to 405.

6

BRONCHIECTASIS

Bronchiectasis is characterized by permanent abnormal dilation and destruction of bronchial walls, with scarring or obstruction from repeated infection. The obstruction often leads to postobstructive pneumonitis. Bronchiectasis requires two factors: an infectious insult; and impairment of drainage, airway obstruction, and/or a defect in host defense.

Patients often report frequent bouts of "bronchitis," purulent phlegm, intermittent hemoptysis, pleurisy, and shortness of breath. Physical findings on chest examination include crackles, rhonchi, and/or wheezing.

Diagnostic Evaluation

Suspicious but not diagnostic radiographic findings include plate-like atelectasis, dilated and thickened airways (tram or parallel lines; ring shadows on cross section), and irregular peripheral opacities that may represent mucopurulent plugs. High-resolution computed tomography (HRCT) of the chest, the defining modality for diagnosis of bronchiectasis, shows airway dilation and bronchial wall thickening. Bronchoscopy is important to examine for obstruction and, in patients with hemoptysis, to help localize bleeding.

Treatment

General therapies include hydration, nebulization with saline solutions and mucolytic agents, mechanical techniques, bronchodilators, and corticosteroids. A cornerstone of therapy is to reduce the microbial load and attendant inflammatory mediators. Antimicrobial agents that are effective against *Streptococcus pneumoniae* and *Haemophilus influenzae* should generally be used for a minimum of 7 to 10 days.

Three organisms that contribute to symptomatic episodes and are particularly problematic include *Pseudomonas aeruginosa, Mycobacterium avium-intracellulare* (MAI), and *Aspergillus* species. *P. aeruginosa* is almost impossible to eradicate in patients with bronchiectasis; ciprofloxacin is currently the only effective oral agent, but resistance often develops. Aerosolized tobramycin or intravenous antibiotics are often needed. For MAI infection, a four-drug regimen of clarithromycin 500 mg twice daily (or azithromycin 250 mg/day), rifampin 600 mg/day, ethambutol 15 mg/kg/day, and streptomycin 15 mg/kg two to three times a week for 8 weeks has been recommended. Therapy is continued until cultures are negative for 12 months. For *Aspergillus,* a prolonged course of itraconazole 400 mg/day improves clinical outcome in some patients.

The major indications and goals for surgery in bronchiectasis include removal of destroyed lung partially obstructed by a tumor or the residue of a foreign body; elimination of bronchiectatic airways causing poorly controlled hemorrhage; or removal of an area suspected of harboring resistant organisms. Lung transplantation should be considered in patients with late-stage disease.

For more information about this subject, see *Cecil Textbook of Medicine,* 21st edition. Philadelphia, W.B. Saunders Company, 2000. Chapter on Bronchiectasis and Localized Airway/Parenchymal Disorders, pages 405 to 409.

INTERSTITIAL LUNG DISEASE

The interstitial lung diseases (ILDs) represent a large and heterogeneous group of lower respiratory tract disorders (Table 6–8). Virtually all ILDs cause breathlessness, exercise intolerance, progressive respiratory insufficiency, and diffuse parenchymal abnormalities on chest radiograph. The pathophysiologic and molecular mechanisms of most ILDs are not known.

Clinical Presentation

Breathlessness is the most prevalent complaint, initially only on exertion. Nonproductive cough and fatigue are also prominent. Pleuritic chest pain should suggest spontaneous pneumothorax. Hemoptysis, which may be the presenting complaint of patients who have diffuse alveolar hemorrhage, should prompt a search for complications such as pulmonary embolus, superimposed infection, or malignancy. Fever and chills are common symptoms in hypersensitivity pneumonitis. If a specific diagnosis is made, it is most often because of information gathered during the history. A detailed, lifelong occupational history must be obtained, because ILDs have long latency periods between occupational exposure and onset of symptoms and radiographic abnormalities.

The physical examination may reveal underlying causes. Velcro-like rales are found in most patients with ILDs. Clubbing of the fingers and toes is a common but nonspecific finding, but the new

Table 6–8 ■ CLINICAL CLASSIFICATION OF INTERSTITIAL LUNG DISEASE (ILD)

Primary Lung Diseases
Idiopathic pulmonary fibrosis*
Sarcoidosis*
Bronchiolitis obliterans with organizing pneumonia*
Lymphocytic interstitial pneumonia
Histocytosis X
Lymphangioleiomyomatosis

ILD Associated with Systemic Rheumatic Disorder
Rheumatoid arthritis*
Systemic lupus erythematosus*
Scleroderma*
Polymyositis-dermatomyositis*
Sjögren's syndrome
Mixed connective tissue disease*
Ankylosing spondylitis

ILD Associated with Drugs or Treatments
Antibiotics (e.g., nitrofurantoin)*
Anti-inflammatory agents
Cardiovascular drugs (e.g., amiodarone)*
Antineoplastic agents (e.g., bleomycin)*
Illicit drugs
Dietary supplements
Oxygen
Radiation
Paraquat

Environment/Occupation–Associated ILD
Organic dusts/hypersensitivity pneumonitis (>40 known agents)
- Farmer's lung*
- Air conditioner–humidifier lung*
- Bird breeder's lung*
- Bagassosis

Inorganic dusts
- Silicosis*
- Asbestosis*
- Coal workers' pneumoconiosis*
- Berylliosis

Gases, fumes, vapors
- Oxides of nitrogen
- Sulfur dioxide
- Toluene diisocyanate
- Oxides of metals
- Hydrocarbons

Alveolar Filling Disorders
Diffuse alveolar hemorrhage
Goodpasture's syndrome
Idiopathic pulmonary hemosiderosis
Pulmonary alveolar proteinosis
Chronic eosinophilic pneumonia*

ILD Associated with Pulmonary Vasculitis
Wegener's granulomatosis
Churg-Strauss syndrome
Hypersensitivity vasculitides
Necrotizing sarcoid granulomatosis
Familial idiopathic pulmonary fibrosis
Neurofibromatosis
Tuberous sclerosis
Gaucher's disease
Niemann-Pick disease
Hermansky-Pudlak syndrome

*Disorders that are the most common causes of ILD or less common conditions in which ILD is a prominent manifestation of disease.

appearance of digital clubbing should prompt a search for a complicating lung malignancy. Cor pulmonale may be noted. Laboratory tests that confirm or suggest a diagnosis include the rheumatoid factor, antinuclear antibodies, serum-precipitating antibodies to inhaled organic antigens, tests for antineutrophil cytoplasmic antibodies (ANCAs), and anti–basement membrane antibodies. The chest radiograph may suggest a specific diagnosis (Table 6–9). A diffuse ground-glass pattern is seen early in the disease. More typically, a chest radiograph demonstrates nodules, linear (reticular) infiltrates, or a combination of these (reticulonodular infiltrates). Cystic areas (honeycomb pattern) appear late in the course. HRCT can detect ILD in subjects with normal chest radiographs in asbestosis, silicosis, sarcoidosis, and scleroderma. The classic physiologic alterations in ILD include reduced DLCO, and a normal or supernormal ratio of FEV_1 to FVC. Arterial blood gas analysis

Table 6–9 ■ RADIOGRAPHIC FEATURES THAT SUGGEST SPECIFIC CAUSES OF INTERSTITIAL LUNG DISEASE

Hilar or Mediastinal Lymphadenopathy

Sarcoidosis
Berylliosis
Silicosis (eggshell calcification)
Lymphocytic interstitial pneumonia
Amyloidosis
Gaucher's disease

Pleural Disease

Asbestosis (pleural effusion, thickening, plaques, mesothelioma)
Systemic rheumatic disorders
Lymphangioleiomyomatosis (chylous effusion)
Nitrofurantoin
Radiation pneumonitis

Pneumothorax

Histiocytosis X
Lymphangioleiomyomatosis
Neurofibromatosis
Tuberous sclerosis

Preserved Lung Volumes or Hyperinflation

Bronchiolitis obliterans organizing pneumonia
Chronic hypersensitivity pneumonitis
Histiocytosis X
Lymphangioleiomyomatosis
Neurofibromatosis
Sarcoidosis
Tuberous sclerosis

Upper Lobe Distribution

Ankylosing spondylitis
Berylliosis
Histiocytosis X
Silicosis
Chronic hypersensitivity pneumonitis
Necrobiotic nodules of rheumatoid arthritis

typically shows mild hypoxemia. Carbon dioxide retention is rare, even late in the course of the disease.

Bronchoscopy should be performed when tissue abnormalities are distributed in the bronchovascular bundle, an alveolar filling disorder is present, or an infectious disease is suspected. Bronchoalveolar lavage (BAL) is diagnostic if an infectious agent or neoplastic cell is noted in the lavage specimen, but BAL usually is nonspecific and is not routinely indicated. Transbronchial biopsy should be performed if sarcoidosis or alveolar filling diseases are likely. An open lung or thoracoscopic biopsy is required to secure a specific diagnosis and accurately stage most cases of ILD.

Therapy

Corticosteroids are the mainstay of therapy. The initial treatment of choice is prednisone 1 mg/kg of ideal body weight per day (maximum, 60 mg/day) given in one dose for 1 month, followed by 40 mg/day given for 2 months. The dose is gradually tapered (5 mg/week) over several months to a maintenance dose of 15 to 20 mg/day. In patients who do not respond to steroid therapy or who cannot tolerate corticosteroids, cyclophosphamide 1 to 2 mg/kg of ideal body weight, may be useful. Oxygen is recommended for patients who have a PaO_2 of less than 55 mm Hg at rest or with exercise. Lung transplantation is now an accepted therapy for patients with end-stage ILD.

Specific Types of Interstitial Lung Disease

IDIOPATHIC PULMONARY FIBROSIS. The mean survival after diagnosis of idiopathic pulmonary fibrosis is 5 to 7 years. Corticosteroids are the mainstay of therapy, although favorable clinical response occurs in only 10 to 20% of patients.

BRONCHIOLITIS OBLITERANS ORGANIZING PNEUMONIA. The distinct onset of a flulike illness with a nonproductive cough is the most common presentation. Chest radiography reveals bilateral diffuse alveolar opacities with normal lung volumes. Infiltrates may be peripheral. Corticosteroid therapy results in recovery in two thirds of patients. Clinical improvement is rapid (days to a few weeks) in some individuals.

ILDs ASSOCIATED WITH SYSTEMIC RHEUMATIC DISORDERS. All systemic rheumatic disorders are associated with ILD (Table 6–10).

RHEUMATOID ARTHRITIS. Pulmonary systems most often follow the onset of arthritis, but simultaneous onset of ILD and arthritis may occur. In one fifth of cases, ILD precedes joint manifestations.

SYSTEMIC LUPUS ERYTHEMATOSUS (SLE). In 50% of patients with acute lupus pneumonitis, the pneumonitis is the presenting manifestation of SLE. Strong consideration should be given to the possibility of pulmonary infections in patients with acute infiltrates, because infections outnumber SLE pneumonitis by a ratio of more than 30:1.

SYSTEMIC SCLEROSIS. Pulmonary symptoms may antedate either cutaneous changes or Raynaud's phenomenon by intervals as long as 14 years. Pulmonary function abnormalities have significant

Table 6–10 ■ PULMONARY MANIFESTATIONS OF SYSTEMIC RHEUMATIC DISORDERS

Rheumatoid Arthritis

Interstitial lung disease (ILD)
Pleural disease (pleuritis with or without effusion, empyema, pyopneumothorax)
Bronchiolitis obliterans with or without organizing pneumonia
Caplan's syndrome
Pulmonary vascular disease
Apical fibrobullous disease
Central airway obstruction secondary to cricoarytenoid arthritis

Systemic Lupus Erythematosus

Pulmonary infection
ILD—acute, chronic
Pleuritis with or without effusion
Pulmonary vascular disease, thromboembolic disease
Bronchiolitis obliterans
Diaphragmatic dysfunction
Central airway obstruction

Systemic Sclerosis (Scleroderma)

ILD
Pulmonary hypertension
Aspiration pneumonia (gastroesophageal reflux)
Bronchogenic carcinoma (scar carcinoma)

Polymyositis/Dermatomyositis

Aspiration pneumonia (pharyngeal/esophageal disorder)
ILD
Bronchiolitis obliterans organizing pneumonia (BOOP)
Respiratory muscle dysfunction (pneumonia, atelectasis, hyperventilation, respiratory failure)
Malignancy (primary, metastatic)

Sjögren's Syndrome

ILD
Lymphocytic interstitial pneumonitis
BOOP
Lymphoma
Chronic bronchitis
Recurrent pneumonia

Mixed Connective Tissue Disease

ILD
Pleuritis with or without effusion
Pulmonary hypertension
Aspiration pneumonia (esophageal disorder)

Ankylosing Spondylitis

Upper lobe fibrobullous disease
Pleural disease (pleural thickening, pneumothorax)
Mycobacterial infections (tuberculous and nontuberculous)
Aspergillomas
Abnormal chest wall mobility
Bronchogenic carcinoma (scar carcinoma)

prognostic implications: patients with normal function have a greater than 90% 5-year survival, whereas those with restrictive spirometry have a 58% 5-year survival.

POLYMYOSITIS AND DERMATOMYOSITIS. Lung disease may precede muscle complaints by months to years or be superimposed on established muscular disease.

DRUG-INDUCED INTERSTITIAL LUNG DISEASE. Most drug-induced ILD is reversible if it is recognized early and the responsible drug is discontinued (Table 6–11).

GOODPASTURE'S SYNDROME. The most common presenting symptoms are hemoptysis, dyspnea, cough, and fatigue. The diagnosis can be confirmed by immunofluorescent studies of renal tissue is some patients. Lung biopsy is seldom necessary.

IDIOPATHIC PULMONARY HEMOSIDEROSIS. Idiopathic pulmonary hemosiderosis is a rare disorder characterized by intermittent, diffuse alveolar hemorrhage without evidence of vasculitis, inflammation, granulomas, necrosis, circulating anti–glomerular basement membrane antibodies, elevated pulmonary venous pressure, or systemic disease. Systemic corticosteroids appear to be beneficial in acute exacerbations.

PULMONARY ALVEOLAR PROTEINOSIS. Approximately half of patients with alveolar proteinosis have been exposed to various dusts or solvents, including silica, asbestos, tin, cadmium, molybdenum, or cement dust. Alveolar proteinosis may present with an abnormal chest radiograph; the abrupt onset of cough, fever, and chest discomfort due to a superimposed infection; or the insidious onset of cough and dyspnea. The clinical course is highly variable.

CHRONIC EOSINOPHILIC PNEUMONIA. Cough, fever (as high as 40° C), dyspnea, weight loss, malaise, and night sweats are the most common symptoms. Wheezing is part of the syndrome in one third to half of patients. Peripheral blood eosinophilia is present in 85%. A classic, almost pathognomonic finding is peripheral, nonsegmental alveolar infiltrates that resolve within 2 to 4 days after treatment with corticosteroids but recur in the same distribution with clinical relapses.

WEGENER'S GRANULOMATOSIS. Wegener's granulomatosis is a systemic disease in which granulomatous, necrotizing vasculitis involves the upper and lower respiratory tracts and kidneys. Patients often have positive tests for ANCA, but a negative ANCA does not exclude Wegener's granulomatosis. An open lung biopsy is the procedure of choice for establishing the diagnosis. Cyclophosphamide 1 to 2 mg/kg/day orally in conjunction with oral corticosteroids (prednisone 60 mg/day) is the standard initial therapy. Trimethoprim-sulfamethoxazole (one double-strength tablet twice a day) can be used to treat early, predominantly granulomatous disease if systemic vasculitis is absent.

For more information about this subject, see *Cecil Textbook of Medicine,* 21st edition. Philadelphia, W.B. Saunders Company, 2000. Chapter 78, Interstitial Lung Disease, pages 409 to 419.

OCCUPATIONAL AND ENVIRONMENTAL LUNG DISEASES

Occupational Pulmonary Disorders

These disorders are primarily the pneumoconioses, or dust diseases of the lung (Table 6–12), and hypersensitivity pneumonitis.

Table 6–11 ■ DRUG-INDUCED INTERSTITIAL LUNG DISEASE

Antibiotics
Nitrofurantoin
Cephalosporins
Sulfonamides
Penicillin
Isoniazid
Anti-Inflammatory Agents
Methotrexate
Gold
Penicillamine
Phenylbutazone
Non-steroidal anti-inflammatory agents
Cardiovascular Drugs
Amiodarone
Tocainide
β-Blockers (propranolol, pindolol, acebutolol)
Hydralazine
Procainamide
Hydrochlorothiazide
Antineoplastic Agents
Bleomycin
Busulfan
Cyclophosphamide
Methotrexate
Nitrosoureas (BCNU, CCNU, methyl-CCNU, DCNU)
Melphalan
Chlorambucil
Mercaptopurine
Mitomycin
Procarbazine
Central Nervous System Drugs
Phenytoin
Carbamazepine
Chlorpromazine
Imipramine
Oral Hypoglycemic Agents
Tolbutamide
Tolazamide
Chlorpropamide
Illicit Drugs
IV use of drugs formulated for oral use
Opiates
Heroin
Propoxyphene
Methadone

BCNU = bis-chloroethyl-nitrosourea (carmustine); CCNU = chloroethyl-cyclohexyl-nitrosourea (lomustine); DCNU = chloroethyl-nitrosoglucosyl urea (chlorozotocin).

Table 6–12 ■ PRINCIPAL PNEUMOCONIOSES CAUSED BY MINERAL DUSTS

AGENT	DISEASE	RADIOGRAPHIC APPEARANCE
Asbestos	Asbestosis	Reticular, basilar predominance
Coat dust	Coal workers' pneumoconiosis	Nodular, upper lobe predominance
Cobalt	Hard metal disease	Reticular, basilar predominance
Silica	Silicosis	Nodular, upper lobe predominance
Talc	Talcosis	Rounded, irregular, or both

Diagnosis of an occupational ILD is based on an appropriate clinical picture and documentation of exposure (Fig. 6–4).

ASBESTOSIS. With the exception of extraordinarily high exposures, manifestations of disease are not usually present until 15 to 20 years have elapsed since first exposure. The chest radiograph shows irregular opacities that are typically most prominent in the lung bases. Pleural disease, particularly in the form of localized and often calcified plaques, is often present as well. No effective treatment is available.

COAL WORKERS' PNEUMOCONIOSIS. The group of lung diseases caused by coal mine dust are commonly referred to as "black lung." The chest radiograph shows the characteristic nodules of progressive massive fibrosis. The nodules may cavitate. No effective treatment is currently available.

SILICOSIS. Accelerated silicosis occurs within 5 to 10 years of exposure and has a clinical picture comparable to that of chronic

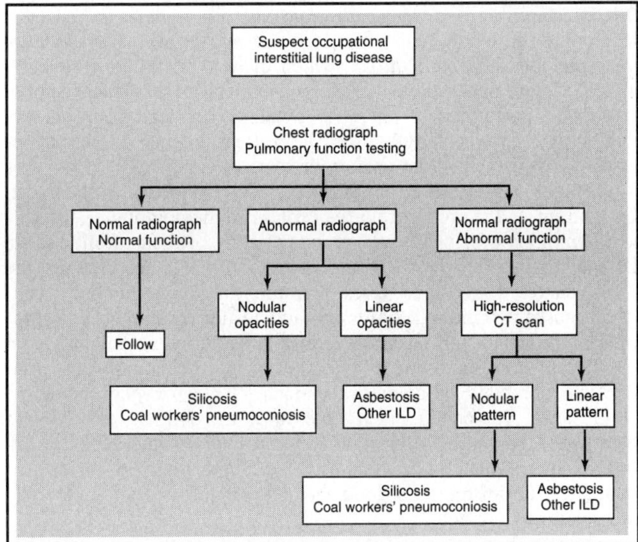

FIGURE 6–4 ■ Diagnostic approach to occupational interstitial lung disease (ILD). CT = computed tomography.

Table 6–13 ■ CURRENT INDUSTRIES USING BERYLLIUM

Aerospace	Foundries
Beryllium extraction, fabrication, smelting	Nuclear reactors
	Nuclear weapons
Ceramics	Plating
Dental alloys and prostheses	Telecommunications
Electronics	Tool and die

silicosis, which develops after a longer latent period. Large numbers of workers in the United States are still exposed to silica. Progressive massive fibrosis can be associated with significant impairment on lung function testing and clinically significant dyspnea. Unless the epidemiologic features of the case make the diagnosis of acute silicosis certain, lung biopsy may be indicated to establish the diagnosis. The prognosis of accelerated and acute silicosis is poor.

BERYLLIUM DISEASE. Beryllium disease is a granulomatous lung disease that results from inhaling beryllium, a rare metal now widely used in high-technology applications (Table 6–13). Patients with beryllium disease may have findings extending from normal to diffuse interstitial infiltrates and hilar adenopathy. Corticosteroid therapy may be beneficial, but lifelong treatment is needed.

Physical, Chemical, and Aspiration Injuries of the Lung

THERMAL INJURIES AND SMOKE INHALATION. Thermal injury to the lung is associated with four groups of complications: (1) *immediate reaction*—direct thermal injury to upper airways leading to upper airway obstruction; (2) carbon monoxide and cyanide poisoning; (3) *acute respiratory distress syndrome* (ARDS), developing 24 to 48 hours after the thermal injury; and (4) *late-onset pulmonary complications,* which include pneumonia, atelectasis, and thromboembolus. Prompt intubation or tracheostomy should be performed if there is evidence of significant airway obstruction. Corticosteroids may help treat edema of the upper airways, but they must be used with caution.

CARBON MONOXIDE POISONING. CO competes with oxygen for binding at the iron-porphyrin centers of hemoglobin. This carboxyhemoglobin (HbCO)-related increase in oxygen affinity shifts the oxyhemoglobin dissociation curve to the left and impairs the release of oxygen to the tissues. Common symptoms include headache, nausea, vomiting, confusion, and visual disturbances. Symptoms of mild CO poisoning generally subside within minutes to a few hours after removing the patient from the noxious environment. In obtunded or comatose patients, 100% oxygen should be administered via endotracheal tube until the HbCO level is less than 5%. Hyperbaric oxygen at 2.5 atm reduces the HbCO half-time to approximately 20 minutes. Neurologic recovery in mild to moderate CO poisoning is good, but the prognosis after severe CO intoxication is variable.

RADIATION LUNG INJURY. The reaction of the lung to radiation injury can be divided into three phases: (1) an *acute phase,* occurring 1 to 2 months after radiation exposure, characterized by vascular damage, congestion, edema, and mononuclear cell infiltration; (2) a *subacute phase,* occurring 2 to 9 months later, and (3) the *chronic* or *fibrotic phase,* which generally occurs more than 9 months after irradiation. Alveolar fibrosis and capillary sclerosis are the predominant histologic features. Radiographic changes generally appear 1 to 3 months after treatment. The affected areas are generally demarcated by a "straight edge" defining the margins of the radiation portal, and they have a ground-glass appearance. Corticosteroids (prednisone 1 mg/kg of body weight) have been advocated for treating severe cases of radiation pneumonitis, but no controlled clinical trials have been undertaken.

ASPIRATION-RELATED INJURIES. Aspiration pneumonitis refers to pulmonary injury caused by acidic stomach contents. The main factors determining the extent of illness are the pH of the aspirate, the presence of food particles, the volume of the aspirate, and the distribution of the aspirate. Acid causes chemical burns of the bronchi, bronchioles, and alveolar walls, with subsequent exudation of fluid into the lungs and imbalance of the normal ventilation-perfusion relationships; hypoxemia is invariably present and is usually severe. Some patients aspirate a large volume of gastric acid and almost immediately become apneic and hypotensive and die. More often, the patient survives the initial crisis but within 1 to 5 hours develops dyspnea, cough, frothy sputum, tachypnea, rales, and rhonchi. Arterial blood gases show hypoxemia. About 50% of patients have radiographic changes consistent with pneumonitis. The airway should be suctioned to remove any particulate matter. Supplemental oxygen is given to maintain a PaO_2 of more than 60 mm Hg. Prophylactic antibiotics and systemic corticosteroids should not be used routinely. Mortality from aspiration pneumonitis is high, reaching 28 to 62%.

NEAR-DROWNING. Drowning can be of two types: (1) "wet" drowning, with initial laryngospasm but early relaxation and subsequent aspiration of copious amounts of fluid; or (2) "dry" drowning, with asphyxiation secondary to intense glottic spasm that persists beyond the point of apnea, so that when the muscles relax, little or no water is aspirated. Cyanosis, coughing, and the production of frothy pink sputum are common. Rales, rhonchi, and, less often, wheezes are heard. Laboratory studies reveal mild hypokalemia, hypernatremia, and hyperchloremia. In freshwater aspiration, the hematocrit may fall slightly in the first 24 hours owing to hemolysis. An isolated increase in serum-free hemoglobin without a change in hematocrit is more common. Oxygen in high concentrations is necessary. Even the patient who quickly becomes apparently normal should be hospitalized for 24 hours to watch for a subsequent clinical picture of ARDS. Bronchospasm should be treated with nebulized β-agonists. Prophylactic antibiotics and corticosteroids have not been shown to be beneficial.

For more information about this subject, see *Cecil Textbook of Medicine,* 21st edition. Philadelphia, W.B. Saunders Company, 2000. Chapter 79, Occupational Pulmonary Disorders, and Chapter 80, Physical, Chemical, and Aspiration Injuries of the Lung, pages 419 to 432.

SARCOIDOSIS

Sarcoidosis is a disease of unknown cause and is characterized by the presence of non-caseating granulomas in one or more organ systems. The peak age incidence of sarcoidosis is in the 20s and 30s, and women are affected slightly more often than men. In the United States, sarcoidosis is more frequent in blacks than whites. Sarcoidosis is notable for its protean manifestations and variable course. Thirty to 60 per cent of patients have no symptoms at the time of presentation, and the disease is identified because of abnormalities on a chest radiograph. Alternatively, patients may present with respiratory systems, such as dyspnea and cough. Ten to 20 per cent of patients present with a syndrome of bilateral hilar adenopathy and erythema nodosum, a constellation of findings that is called *Löfgren's syndrome.*

Respiratory Disease

Both hilar and mediastinal lymph nodes may be affected; involvement of the hilar nodes is usually bilateral and relatively symmetrical. The pulmonary parenchyma demonstrates well-defined, non-caseating granulomas within the pulmonary interstitium. Granulomatous involvement of the airways (i.e, endobronchial sarcoidosis) is common and may lead to bronchostenosis in a small proportion of cases.

Dyspnea and cough, typically non-productive, are the primary symptoms. Examination of the chest is often notable for the paucity or even absence of findings despite the extent of radiographic changes. Pulmonary function tests often demonstrate a pattern of restrictive disease.

Skin Disease

A variety of lesions can be seen, including papules, plaques, and nodules. Erythema nodosum commonly occurs in combination with bilateral hilar adenopathy as part of Löfgren's syndrome.

Eye Disease

Anterior uveitis, the most common form of ocular sarcoidosis, is often associated with the relatively acute onset of a red eye, photophobia, and ocular discomfort. *Heerfordt's syndrome,* or uveoparotid fever, is a form of sarcoidosis in which anterior uveitis is accompanied by parotid gland enlargement and often fever and facial palsy. Conjunctival involvement can produce small, pale-yellow nodules that demonstrate granulomatous inflammation on biopsy.

Cardiac and Neurologic Disease

Five to 10% of patients have significant cardiac involvement, including conduction defects (e.g., first-, second-, or third-degree heart block or a bundle branch block), ventricular or supraventricular arrhythmias, and heart failure. Five to 10% of patients with sarcoidosis develop neurologic complications, including unilateral facial nerve palsy, neuropathy, and psychiatric symptoms.

Other Extrathoracic Disease

Symptoms related to hepatic involvement are uncommon, and clinical evidence is usually limited to abnormalities in one or more hepatic enzymes. Parotid gland enlargement, lacrimal gland infiltration, bone lesions, splenomegaly, and myopathy due to granulomas within muscle tissue may also be seen.

Hypercalcemia occurs in fewer than 10% of patients and is thought to be due to elevated levels of 1,25-dihydroxyvitamin D. Elevated levels of ACE occur in 40 to 90% of patients.

Diagnostic Evaluation

The diagnosis of sarcoidosis is confirmed by the finding of well-formed, non-caseating granulomas in one or more affected organ systems or tissues, with appropriate additional studies to exclude other causes of granulomas. Flexible bronchoscopy with transbronchial lung biopsy is particularly useful, with a yield of 60 to 95%. In patients with symmetrical bilateral hilar lymphadenopathy, either in association with erythema nodosum (Löfgren's syndrome) or in the absence of any symptoms, physical findings, or screening laboratory data that might indicate another cause, many clinicians believe that a clinical diagnosis of sarcoidosis can be made without needing histologic confirmation. A commonly used staging system considers the pattern of involvement seen on the chest radiograph (Table 6–14).

Treatment

For pulmonary disease, intrathoracic nodal involvement is not an indication for treatment, but parenchymal lung disease is a potential indication. Presentation with Löfgren's syndrome does not warrant therapy, except as needed for symptoms. Corticosteroids acutely suppress the manifestations of the disease but have never been demonstrated to alter natural history. Typically, prednisone is started at a dose of 0.5 mg/kg/day. Many clinicians taper to 10 to 30 mg every other day. Treatment durations of 6 to 12 months are typical.

For more information about this subject, see: *Cecil Textbook of Medicine,* 21st edition. Philadelphia, W.B. Saunders Company, 2000. Chapter 81, Sarcoidosis, pages 432 to 436.

Table 6–14 ■ RADIOGRAPHIC STAGING OF INTRATHORACIC SARCOIDOSIS

STAGE	HILAR ADENOPATHY	PARENCHYMAL DISEASE	PERCENT AT ONSET	PERCENT WITH RESOLUTION
0	No	No	<10	NA
1	Yes	No	50	65 (<10% progress to parenchymal disease)
2	Yes	Yes	30	20–50
3 or 4	No	Yes (with fibrosis in stage 4)	10–15	<20

NA = not applicable.

Table 6–15 ■ ROUTES OF BACTERIAL INOCULATION OF THE LUNGS

ROUTE	EXAMPLES
Microaspiration of oropharyngeal secretions	Most bacterial pneumonias, anaerobic pleuropulmonary infections
Inhalation of airborne organisms	*Mycobacterium tuberculosis, Legionella* sp.; many viruses, including influenza virus
Blood stream	Staphylococcal endocarditis, septic emboli
Direct extension	Amebic liver abscess

OVERVIEW OF PNEUMONIA

Pneumonia indicates inflammation of the terminal airways, alveolar spaces, and interstitium. Bacterial pneumonia results when host defense mechanisms fail to contain a bacterial challenge presented to the lungs (Table 6–15).

Signs and Symptoms

Previously healthy persons may complain of a brief prodromal upper respiratory illness followed by fever, chills, pleuritic chest pain, and a cough productive of purulent sputum. Physical examination may reveal signs of consolidation, but elderly patients may present with only deterioration in mental function, and physical examination may reveal only rhonchi without signs of consolidation. A thorough physical examination, posteroanterior and lateral chest radiographs, and blood leukocyte count with differential cell count should be performed. In most patients, the history, physical examination, radiographic studies (Table 6–16), and evaluation of

Table 6–16 ■ COMMON ETIOLOGIC AGENTS OF COMMUNITY-ACQUIRED PNEUMONIA IN APPROXIMATE ORDER OF FREQUENCY

OUTPATIENT MANAGEMENT (AGE <60 YR, NO UNDERLYING DISEASE)	HOSPITALIZED PATIENT	SEVERE PNEUMONIA, INTENSIVE CARE
Streptococcus pneumoniae	*S. pneumoniae*	*S. pneumoniae*
Mycoplasma pneumoniae	*Haemophilus influenzae*	*Legionella* sp.
Respiratory viruses	Aerobic gram-negative bacilli	Aerobic gram-negative bacilli
Chlamydia pneumoniae	*Legionella* sp.	*M. pneumoniae*
Miscellaneous, including *Legionella* sp.	Miscellaneous, including *M. pneumoniae,* viruses	Respiratory viruses

Adapted from American Thoracic Society: Guidelines for the initial management of adults with community-acquired pneumonia: Diagnosis, assessment of severity, and initial antimicrobial therapy. Am Rev Respir Dis 148:1418, 1993.

Table 6–17 ■ COMMON RADIOGRAPHIC PATTERNS OF PNEUMONIA AND ASSOCIATED PATHOGENS

PATTERN	PATHOGENS
Lobar or segmental consolidation	*Streptococcus pneumoniae, Klebsiella pneumoniae, Haemophilus influenzae,* other gram-negative bacilli
Inhomogeneous infiltrates (patchy or streaky opacities)	*Mycoplasma pneumoniae,* viruses, *Legionella* sp.
Diffuse interstitial infiltrates	*Legionella* sp., viruses, *Pneumocystis carinii*
Cavitary infiltrates	*Mycobacterium tuberculosis,* gram-negative bacilli, *Staphylococcus aureus* (multiple modules)
Pleural effusion plus infiltrate	*S. pneumoniae, S. aureus,* anaerobes, gram-negative bacilli, *Streptococcus pyogenes*

6

the sputum by Gram stain provide all the required data for microbiologic diagnosis (Table 6–17).

For more information about this subject, see: *Cecil Textbook of Medicine,* 21st edition. Philadelphia, W.B. Saunders Company, 2000. Chapter 82, Overview of Pneumonia, pages 436 to 439.

LUNG ABSCESS

Lung abscess, which is a cavity containing pus and necrotic debris, may be caused by many different microorganisms. A relatively insidious onset of infection is seen in many patients. Weeks to months of malaise and low-grade fever may be associated with cough, weight loss, and anemia. Following cavitation, putrid sputum is usually noted.

The classic radiographic appearance of lung abscess is a cavity with an air-fluid level, with or without surrounding infiltrate; in some patients, however, repeat chest radiographs or computed tomographic (CT) scanning may be needed to detect the cavity. A similar radiographic appearance can be seen with a variety of other conditions (Table 6–18). Bronchoscopy with a protected specimen brush or BAL can obtain specimens for microbiologic testing.

Treatment

Antimicrobial therapy for 1 to 3 months and drainage are the keystones of treatment. For anaerobic infections, clindamycin is the drug of choice, given initially at a dose of 600 mg every 6 hours intravenously and then (when the patient is afebrile and improved) at 300 mg orally every 6 hours (Table 6–19). When penicillin is used, it should be given in high doses (12 million U/day intravenously in average-sized adults with normal renal function) and in combination with clindamycin or metronidazole 2 g/day intravenously in four divided doses. Postural drainage is important. Surgical resection of necrotic lung may occasionally be needed.

Table 6–18 ■ ORGANISMS AND CONDITIONS WITH THE RADIOGRAPHIC APPEARANCE OF LUNG ABSCESS

Infectious

Bacterial aspiration/pneumonia
- Anaerobes: pigmented and non-pigmented *Prevotella, Fusobacterium, Peptostreptococcus, Bacteroides fragilis,* and *Clostridium perfringens*
- Aerobes: streptococci, *Staphylococcus aureus,* Enterobacteriaceae, *Pseudomonas aeruginosa, Klebsiella pneumoniae, Legionella* sp., *Nocardia asteroides, Haemophilus influenzae, Eikenella corrodens, Salmonella* sp., *Burkholderia pseudomallei, Burkholderia mallei, Rhodococcus equi*

Bacterial embolic
- *S. aureus, P. aeruginosa*

Mycobacteria (often multifocal)
- *M. tuberculosis, M. avium* complex, *M. kansasii,* other mycobacteria

Fungi
- *Aspergillus* sp., Mucoraceae, *Histoplasma capsulatum, Pneumocystis carinii, Coccidioides immitis, Blastomyces dermatitidis, Cryptococcus neoformans*

Parasites
- *Entamoeba histolytica, Paragonimus westermani, Strongyloides stercoralis* (post-obstructive)

Empyema (with air-fluid level)
Septic embolism (endocarditis)

Predisposing Conditions

Fluid-filled cysts or bullae
Infarction without infection
- Pulmonary embolism
- Vasculitis
  - Goodpasture's syndrome
  - Wegener's granulomatosis
  - Polyarteritis nodosa

Bronchiectasis
Post-obstructive pneumonia (neoplasm, foreign body)
Pulmonary sequestration
Pulmonary contusion
Neoplasm

For more information about this subject, see *Cecil Textbook of Medicine,* 21st edition. Philadelphia, W.B. Saunders Company, 2000. Chapter 83, Lung Abscess, pages 439 to 441.

PULMONARY EMBOLISM

Although thrombus from the deep veins of the lower extremities is the most common material to embolize to the lungs, other substances such as neoplastic cells, air bubbles, carbon dioxide, intravenous catheters, fat droplets, and even talc in intravenous drug abusers are potential sources of emboli. Deep venous thrombosis and pulmonary embolism represent a continuum of one disease entity (venous thromboembolism).

The incidence of venous thromboembolism is especially high in hospitalized patients, particularly in the postoperative setting. More

Table 6–19 ■ DRUGS OF CHOICE FOR ANAEROBES INVOLVED IN LUNG ABSCESS*

Principal Pathogens

Prevotella: metronidazole, clindamycin, β-lactam/β-lactamase inhibitor combinations, carbapenems
Fusobacterium: as for *Prevotella*
Peptostreptococcus: β-lactam/β-lactamase inhibitor combinations, carbapenems, penicillin (high dosage)
Streptococcus (anaerobic, microaerophilic strains): penicillin (high dosage), β-lactam/β-lactamase inhibitor combinations, carbapenems

Less Common Pathogens

Bacteroides: metronidazole, β-lactam/β-lactamase inhibitor combinations, carbapenems
Clostridium: metronidazole, β-lactam/β-lactamase inhibitor combinations, carbapenems, penicillin
Actinomyces: penicillin (high dosage), clindamycin
Eikenella corrodens (microaerophilic): penicillin, β-lactam/β-lactamase inhibitor combinations, carbapenems

Unknown Bacteriology

Metronidazole plus penicillin, β-lactam/β-lactamase inhibitor combinations, carbapenems

*Drugs listed for each group of organisms are roughly comparable in activity and are the drugs that are most active. Other drugs (e.g., cefoxitin or clindamycin, alone or with penicillin) may be useful in patients with abscess of unknown bacteriologic origin who are only mildly to moderately ill.

than 95% of pulmonary emboli arise from the proximal deep veins in the lower extremities.

The predominant factor explaining hypoxemia in acute pulmonary embolism is the mismatch between pulmonary blood flow and regional alveolar ventilation. More than 50% obstruction of the pulmonary arterial bed is usually required before substantial elevation of the mean pulmonary artery pressure is seen. The dual pulmonary circulation, which includes both the pulmonary and bronchial arteries, prevents most emboli from causing pulmonary infarction. However, pulmonary infarction may be evident in areas of the peripheral lung supplied by smaller vessels and is more common in patients with preexisting heart failure.

Clinical Manifestations

The history and physical examination are notoriously nonsensitive and nonspecific (Table 6–20). The differential diagnosis depends on the clinical presentation and the presence of concomitant disease (Table 6–21; Fig. 6–5). Hypoxemia is common, but young patients without underlying lung disease may have normal PaO_2. When the D-dimer level is 500 μg/L or greater, the sensitivity for pulmonary embolism may be as high as 96 to 98%, but the specificity is much lower. Only one third of patients with massive or submassive emboli have manifestations of acute cor pulmonale, such as the $S_1Q_3T_3$ pattern, right bundle branch block, P wave pulmonale, or right axis deviation.

Common radiographic findings include pleural effusion, atelectasis, pulmonary infiltrates, and mild elevation of a hemidiaphragm.

Table 6–20 ■ SYMPTOMS AND SIGNS IN 117 PATIENTS WITH ACUTE PULMONARY EMBOLISM WITHOUT PRE-EXISTING CARDIAC OR PULMONARY DISEASE

SYMPTOMS	PERCENT OF PATIENTS	SIGNS	PERCENT OF PATIENTS
Dyspnea	73	Tachypnea (≥20/min)	70
Pleuritic pain	66	Rales (crackles)	51
Cough	37	Tachycardia (>100/min)	30
Leg swelling	28	S_4	24
Leg pain	26	Increased pulmonary component of S_2	23
Hemoptysis	13		
Palpitations	10	Deep venous thrombosis	11
Wheezing	9	Diaphoresis	11
Angina-like pain	4	Temperature >38.5° C	7
		Wheezes	5
		Homans' sign	4
		Right ventricular lift	4
		Pleural friction rub	3
		S_3	3
		Cyanosis	1

Adapted from Stein PD, Terrin ML, Hales CA, et al: Clinical, laboratory, roentgenographic and electrocardiographic findings in patients with acute pulmonary embolism and no pre-existing cardiac or pulmonary disease. Chest 100:598, 1991.

A normal chest radiograph in the setting of severe dyspnea and hypoxemia without evidence of bronchospasm or anatomic cardiac shunt is strongly suggestive of pulmonary embolism.

The ventilation-perfusion scan remains the most common diagnostic test utilized when pulmonary embolism is suspected (Tables 6–22 and 6–23). Pulmonary arteriography, the gold standard technique for the diagnosis of acute pulmonary embolism, is indicated when the diagnosis of pulmonary embolism must be made urgently and prior tests have been non-diagnostic. Spiral CT scanning is now another option instead of angiography.

Table 6–21 ■ DIFFERENTIAL DIAGNOSIS OF ACUTE PULMONARY EMBOLISM

Myocardial infarction
Pericarditis
Congestive heart failure
Pneumonia
Asthma
Chronic obstructive pulmonary disease
Pneumothorax
Pleurodynia
Pleuritis from collagen-vascular disease
Thoracic herpes zoster ("shingles")
Rib fracture
Musculoskeletal pain
Primary or metastatic intrathoracic cancer
Infradiaphragmatic processes (e.g., acute cholecystitis, splenic infarction)
Hyperventilation syndrome

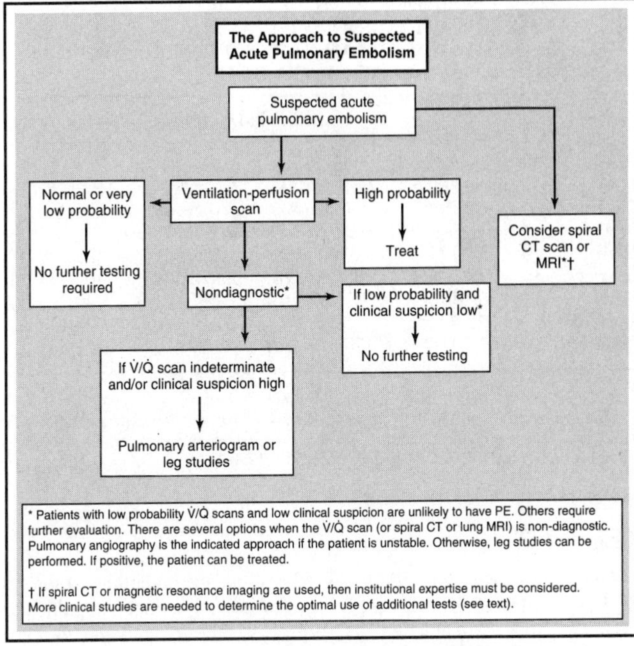

FIGURE 6–5 ■ An algorithm for the diagnostic approach to suspected acute pulmonary embolism. CT = computed tomography; MRI = magnetic resonance imaging; $\dot{V}/\dot{Q}$ = ventilation-perfusion; PE = pulmonary embolism.

6

Table 6–22 ■ INTERPRETATION OF VENTILATION-PERFUSION ($\dot{V}/\dot{Q}$) LUNG SCANS

CATEGORY	PATTERN
Normal	No perfusion defects
Low probability	Small $\dot{V}/\dot{Q}$ mismatches
	$\dot{V}/\dot{Q}$ matches without corresponding radiographic changes
	Perfusion defect substantially smaller than radiographic density
Intermediate probability	Marked, diffuse obstructive pulmonary disease with perfusion defects
	Perfusion defect of same size as radiographic change
	Single segmental mismatch*
High probability	Two or more segmental mismatches*
	Perfusion defect substantially larger than radiographic density

*Controversy exists regarding the importance of a single segmental mismatch, which has been considered either of high or intermediate probability. The more conservative interpretation, that is, intermediate probability, has been used in this table.

Adapted from Biello DR: Radiological (scintigraphic) evaluation of patients with suspected pulmonary thromboembolism. JAMA 257:3257, 1987.

Table 6–23 ■ PIOPED: POSITIVE PREDICTIVE VALUE OF PULMONARY EMBOLISM (PE) AT ANGIOGRAPHY BASED ON LUNG SCAN CATEGORY AND CLINICAL LIKELIHOOD OF PE

	CLINICAL PROBABILITY			
LUNG SCAN CATEGORY	80–100% No. of PE/No. of Pts. (%)	20–79% No. of PE/No. of Pts. (%)	0–19% No. of PE/No. of Pts. (%)	0–100% No. of PE/No. of Pts. (%)
High	28/29 (96)	70/80 (88)	5/9 (56)	103/118 (87)
Intermediate	27/41 (66)	66/236 (28)	11/68 (16)	104/345 (30)
Low	6/16 (40)	30/191 (16)	4/90 (4)	40/296 (14)
Very low	0/5 (0)	4/62 (6)	1/61 (2)	5/128 (4)
Total	61/90 (68)	170/569 (30)	21/228 (9)	252/887 (28)

PIOPED = Prospective Investigation of Pulmonary Embolism Diagnosis.

Adapted from PIOPED Investigators: Value of the ventilation/perfusion scan in acute pulmonary embolism. Results of the Prospective Investigation of Pulmonary Embolism Diagnosis (PIOPED). JAMA 263:2757, 1990.

Treatment

Heparin should be administered as an intravenous bolus of 80 U/kg followed by 18 U/kg/hour; further adjustment should also be weight-based (Table 6–24). Warfarin therapy may be initiated as soon as the activated partial thromboplastin time (aPTT) is in a therapeutic range. At least 5 days of intravenous heparin therapy is generally recommended. Low-molecular-weight heparin (LMWH) can be administered once or twice per day subcutaneously, even at therapeutic doses, and does not require monitoring of the aPTT. Selected patients may be treated as outpatients.

The primary indications for placement of an inferior vena cava (IVC) filter include contraindications to anticoagulation, recurrent embolism while receiving adequate therapy, and significant bleeding complications during anticoagulation. Thrombolytic therapy is often recommended in patients with massive pulmonary embolism,

Table 6–24 ■ WEIGHT-BASED NOMOGRAM FOR INITIAL INTRAVENOUS HEPARIN THERAPY

aPTT*	DOSE (IU/kg)
Initial dose	80 bolus, then 18/hr
<35 sec (<1.2×)	80 bolus, then 4/hr
35–45 sec (1.2–1.5×)	40 bolus, then 2/hr
46–70 sec (1.5–2.3×)	No change
71–90 sec (2.3–3.0×)	Decrease infusion rate by 2/hr
>90 sec (>3.0×)	Hold infusion 1 hr, then decrease infusion rate by 3/hr

aPTT = activated partial thromboplastin time.

*Figures in parentheses show comparison with control.

Adapted from Raschke RA, Reilly BM, Guidry JR, et al: The weight-based heparin dosing nomogram compared with a "standard care" nomogram. A randomized controlled trial. Ann Intern Med 119:874–881, 1993.

hemodynamic instability (hypotension), or severely compromised oxygenation (Fig. 6–6). Although a small percentage of patients with acute pulmonary embolism ultimately develop chronic dyspnea and hypoxemia due to chronic thromboembolic pulmonary hypertension, most patients who survive the acute episode have no long-term pulmonary sequelae.

Non-Thrombotic Pulmonary Emboli

Fat embolism commonly occurs in the setting of traumatic fracture of long bones. A characteristic syndrome of dyspnea, petechiae, and mental confusion often develops. Treatment is generally supportive, including oxygen and mechanical ventilation, and the prognosis is generally good. 6

Amniotic fluid embolism occurs during or after delivery when amniotic fluid gains access to uterine venous channels and then to the pulmonary and general circulations. The syndrome is heralded by the sudden onset of severe respiratory distress; hypotension and death frequently result. The differential diagnosis includes pulmonary thromboembolism, septic and hemorrhagic shock, venous air

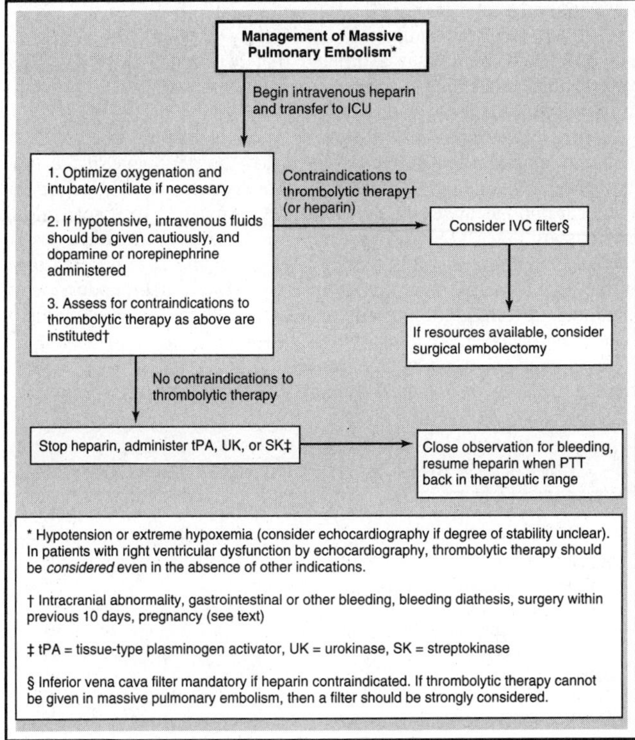

FIGURE 6–6 ■ An algorithm for the approach to the patient with massive acute pulmonary embolism. ICU = intensive care unit; IVC = inferior vena cava; PTT = partial thromboplastin time.

embolism, aspiration pneumonia, heart failure, abruptio placentae, and ruptured uterus. The primary treatment is supportive, with oxygen and mechanical ventilation.

The consequences of venous *air embolism* range from none to death. In the setting of a patient foramen ovale, embolization to the coronary or cerebral circulation is of most concern. Dyspnea, wheezing, chest pain, cough, agitation, confusion, tachycardia, and hypotension may be evident. The treatment of venous air embolism includes immediate placement of the patient in the Trendelenburg or left lateral decubitus position and administration of 100% oxygen. If a central venous catheter is in place near the right atrium, air aspiration should be attempted.

For more information about this subject, see *Cecil Textbook of Medicine,* 21st edition. Philadelphia, W.B. Saunders Company, 2000. Chapter 84, Pulmonary Embolism, pages 441 to 449, and Chapter 188, Antithrombotic Therapy, pages 1021 to 1028.

PULMONARY NEOPLASMS

Bronchogenic carcinoma can be divided into two subgroups: small cell lung cancer (SCLC) and non–small cell lung cancer (NSCLC), which includes the subtypes adenocarcinoma, squamous cell carcinoma, and large cell carcinoma (Table 6–25).

Tobacco smoking causes approximately 87% of cases in men and 85% in women. It is estimated that between 5000 and 15,000 excess lung cancer deaths, mostly in smokers, are caused annually in the United States by radon.

Adenocarcinoma is now the most frequent histologic type. Adenocarcinomas may be derived from either the periphery of the lung or the central airways. *Bronchoalveolar carcinoma,* subcategory of adenocarcinoma, arises in the periphery and tends to spread along pre-existing alveolar septa. *Squamous cell carcinoma* tends to originate in the central airways. *Large cell carcinoma* is undifferentiated at the light microscopic level but may exhibit neuroendocrine or glandular differentiation markers when studied by immunohistochemistry or electron microscopy. *Bronchial carcinoids* are well-differentiated neuroendocrine tumors. *Small cell lung cancer* is characterized by small, dark-staining cells with little cytoplasm.

Table 6–25 ■ MALIGNANT PULMONARY NEOPLASMS

	INCIDENCE (%)
Common	99
Non–small cell lung cancer	~75
Adenocarcinoma	~35
Squamous cell carcinoma	~30
Large cell carcinoma	~10
Small cell lung cancer	~20
Carcinoids	~5
Rare	<1
Lymphoma, carcinosarcoma, mucoepidermoid carcinoma, malignant fibrous histiocytoma, melanoma, sarcoma, blastoma	

Lung cancer is clinically silent for most of its course. Symptoms are caused by tumor growing locally or by metastatic disease. Paraneoplastic syndromes indicate late disease and poor prognosis.

Either a new cough or a change in the nature of a chronic cough is the most common presenting symptom. Hemoptysis, either gross or minor, commonly occurs when mucosal lesions ulcerate. Airway obstruction can result in wheezing, atelectasis, or postobstructive pneumonia. Local invasion can produce chest pain, dyspnea from pleural effusion, and symptoms referable to nerves, heart, and great vessels. The *superior vena cava syndrome* is characterized by facial suffusion and swelling due to blockage of the superior vena cava by either tumor or associated thrombosis. *Horner's syndrome* results from disruption of the cervical sympathetic nerves and is characterized by unilateral facial anhidrosis and miosis in its full-blown form. Hoarseness can occur from invasion of the recurrent laryngeal nerve. *Pancoast's syndrome,* caused by local invasion into the brachial plexus, results in shoulder and arm pain. Common sites of metastases of bronchogenic carcinomas include brain, bone, adrenal, and liver. Systemic manifestations are often nonspecific and can include weight loss, anorexia, and fever. The endocrine and neurologic manifestations of bronchogenic carcinoma are more specific (see Chapter 194 in *Cecil Textbook of Medicine*). Digital clubbing occurs most commonly in association with bronchogenic carcinoma. Hypertrophic pulmonary osteoarthropathy is often associated with clubbing and commonly presents with exquisite tenderness over the long bones.

Diagnosis and Staging

The chest radiograph is the most important radiologic study to diagnose lung cancer (see Fig. 6–2). CT scans reliably detect enlarged lymph nodes and can include the liver and adrenals to assess common sites of metastatic disease. Intrathoracic lymph nodes that exceed 1 cm in size have a high likelihood of harboring metastatic disease.

Sputum cytology is approximately 60 to 70% sensitive for central lesions but much less accurate for small peripheral lesions. Laboratory studies include a complete blood cell count, liver function tests, and serum calcium assay. More invasive diagnostic and staging studies include bronchoscopy, needle biopsy, video-assisted thoracoscopy, cervical mediastinoscopy, and thoracotomy. The staging systems for NSCLC and SCLC are different: in NSCLC a TNM (tumor-node-metastasis) staging system is used, whereas in SCLC, patients are divided into those with limited and extensive disease (Tables 6–26, 6–27, and 6–28).

Treatment

NON–SMALL CELL LUNG CANCER. Patients with stages I through IIIA NSCLC are routinely considered for surgery, with 5-

Table 6–26 ■ STAGING OF SMALL CELL LUNG CANCER

Limited	Tumor confined to chest plus supraclavicular nodes, but excluding cervical, axillary nodes
Extensive	Tumor outside of above confines

Table 6–27 ■ STAGING, DEFINITIONS FOR NON–SMALL CELL LUNG CANCER

Tumor	
T0	No tumor
TX	Primary tumor cannot be assessed; or positive cytology, no apparent tumor
Tis	Carcinoma in situ
T1	Tumor <3 cm diameter; no visceral pleural or main bronchial involvement
T2	Tumor >3 cm diameter, visceral pleural or main bronchial involvement >2 cm from carina; atelectasis extending to hilum but not involving whole lung
T3	Direct extension to chest wall, diaphragm, mediastinal pleura, parietal pericardium or <2 cm from carina, but not involving carina; atelectasis involving whole lung
T4	Invades heart, great vessels, esophagus, trachea, carina, vertebrae, malignant pleural or pericardial effusion, or satellite tumor nodules within the ipsilateral primary tumor lobe of lung
Nodes	
N0	No involvement
NX	Cannot assess regional lymph nodes
N1	Ipsilateral peribronchial or hilar nodal involvement and intrapulmonary nodes involved by direct extension
N2	Ipsilateral mediastinal or subcarinal nodal metastasis
N3	Contralateral mediastinal or hilar nodal metastasis; any supraclavicular or scalene nodal metastasis
Metastasis	
M0	None detected
M1	Any distant metastasis

From Mountain CF: Revisions in the International System for Staging Lung Cancer. Chest 111:1710, 1997.

Table 6–28 ■ STAGE GROUPING AND SURVIVAL FOR NON–SMALL CELL LUNG CANCER

		5-YR SURVIVAL (%)	
STAGE	DEFINITION	Clinical Staging	Pathologic Staging
0	Carcinoma in situ		
IA	T1N0M0	60	67
IB	T2N0M0	38	57
IIA	T1N1M0	34	55
IIB	T2N1M0, T3N0M0	22–24	38
IIIA	T3N1M0, T1N2M0 T2N2M0, T3N2M0	9–13	25
IIIB	T4, any N, M0 T1–3, N3, M0	3–7	
IV	Any T, any N, MI	1	

T = tumor; N = node; M = metastasis.

year survival rates ranging from 60 to 80% for patients with stage 1 disease to 15 to 25% for selected patients with stage IIIA disease. With the exception of peripheral solitary pulmonary nodules without hilar or mediastinal lymphadenopathy, a firm tissue diagnosis should almost always be obtained prior to surgical therapy. With the advent of lung-sparing operations, many patients who previously would not have been considered surgical candidates are now undergoing pulmonary resection. Patients with an FEV_1 of greater than 60% predicted or more than 2 L will likely tolerate a pneumonectomy. Radiation therapy is often used to palliate symptoms; distant metastases also are frequently treated primarily with radiation. Several trials treating stage IIIB patients with chemotherapy plus radiation have demonstrated a longer survival than with radiation alone.

SMALL CELL LUNG CANCER. Chemotherapy is the cornerstone of treatment for both limited- and extensive-stage SCLC. Surgery for patients with SCLC, with the exception of rare stage I disease, is not indicated.

Prognosis

The overall prognosis for patients with lung cancer remains grim, with a 5-year survival rate of 14%. Patients with stage I and II NSCLC treated by surgery have a 40 to 85% 5-year survival rate.

For more information about this subject, see *Cecil Textbook of Medicine,* 21st edition. Philadelphia, W.B. Saunders Company, 2000. Chapter 85, Pulmonary Neoplasms, pages 449 to 455.

DISEASES OF THE DIAPHRAGM, PLEURA, AND MEDIASTINUM

Diaphragm

Unilateral diaphragmatic paralysis is usually secondary to phrenic nerve involvement by a tumor, with bronchogenic carcinoma being the most frequent. Paralysis may also result from neurologic diseases such as myelitis, encephalitis, poliomyelitis, and herpes zoster; from trauma to the thorax or cervical spine; or from compression by benign processes such as a substernal thyroid, aortic aneurysm, and infectious collections.

Diaphragmatic hernias occur through congenitally weak or incompletely fused areas of the diaphragm, through the esophageal hiatus (>70% of all hernias), or because of traumatic rupture of the muscle. Symptom severity depends on the extension of abdominal contents into the thorax and the presence of strangulation. In the asymptomatic adult, observation is indicated, but surgery may be needed for diagnosis or to relieve strangulation.

Pleura

The parietal pleura and the visceral pleura are separated by a virtual cavity, which is lubricated by 5 to 10 mL of fluid with a low protein concentration (<2 g/dL) and a pH and glucose similar to that of blood.

Pleural Effusions

Pain, dyspnea, or cough, is neither sensitive nor specific for diagnosis. The physical examination shows decreased breath sounds and excursions in the affected hemithorax, with dullness and absent tactile fremitus over the area. Frequently there are E to A changes (egobronchophony) at the upper fluid border where the underlying lung parenchyma is compressed.

On radiologic examination, an effusion is suspected when there is blunting of the costophrenic angle. Up to 300 mL of fluid may fail to be seen in a posteroanterior chest radiograph, whereas as little as 150 mL may be seen in a lateral decubitus view.

A thoracentesis is diagnostic in approximately 75% of patients. As a rule, newly discovered effusions should be tapped. Relative contraindications to thoracentesis include a bleeding diathesis, anticoagulation, a small volume, mechanical ventilation, and low benefit-to-risk ratio.

Transudates (Table 6–29) are due to imbalances in hydrostatic and oncotic pressures. Heart failure is the most common cause; effusions are often bilateral, usually larger on the right, and associated with vascular congestion and cardiomegaly. Transudates occur in 5 to 10% of patients with liver cirrhosis and in up to 20% of patients with nephrotic syndrome.

Exudates (Table 6–30) are defined by the presence of at least one of the following criteria: (1) pleural fluid–serum protein ratio greater than 0.5; (2) pleural fluid–serum lactate dehydrogenase (LDH) ratio of more than 0.6; and (3) pleural fluid LDH greater than 200 IU/L. A fluid cholesterol level greater than 45 mg/dL may also be helpful. Biopsy, either percutaneous or via thoracoscopy, is indicated to evaluate patients with undiagnosed exudative effusion (particularly those with lymphocytic predominance) because the most frequently diagnosed disease is malignancy or tuberculosis. If the effusion is also purulent and has bacteria, immediate drainage is necessary and is best achieved with a chest tube. If drainage is not effective because of loculation, instilling intrapleural streptokinase may be effective. In some patients, thoracotomy with drainage and decortication may be life-saving.

Malignant effusions probably are the most common cause of exudate in patients older than age 60 years. The effusion may have abundant red blood cells (30,000–50,000/mL) and mononuclear cells (lymphocytes >50%). Cytology is positive in close to 60% of cases. The best method, short of pleurectomy or pleural abrasion,

Table 6–29 ■ CHARACTERISTICS OF PLEURAL FLUID TRANSUDATES

	ABSOLUTE VALUE	PLEURAL FLUID/ SERUM VALUE
Protein	<3 g/dL	<0.5
Lactate dehydrogenase	<200 IU/L	<0.6
Glucose	>60 mg/dL	1.0
White blood cell count	$<1000/mm^3$	—
Cholesterol	<45 mg/dL	

Table 6–30 ■ CORRELATION OF PLEURAL FLUID EXUDATE FINDINGS AND CAUSATIVE DISEASE

TESTS	DISEASE(S)
pH <7.2	Empyema, malignancy, esophageal rupture; rheumatoid, lupus, and tuberculous pleuritis
Glucose (<60 mg/dL)	Infection, rheumatoid pleurisy, tuberculous and lupus effusions, esophageal rupture
Amylase (>200 μ/dL)	Pancreatic disease, esophageal rupture, malignancy, ruptured ectopic pregnancy
Rheumatoid factor, antinuclear antibody, LE cells	Collagen-vascular diseases
Complement (decreased)	Lupus erythematosus, rheumatoid arthritis
Red blood cells (>5000/μL)	Trauma, malignancy, pulmonary embolus
Chylous effusion (triglycerides >110 mg/dL)	Violation of thoracic duct (trauma, malignancy)
Biopsy (+)	Malignancy, tuberculosis

to control recurrent malignant effusion is to instill tetracycline, talc, or medroxyprogesterone intrapleurally after chest tube drainage.

Frank blood in the pleural space (hematocrit >20%) is usually the result of trauma, hematologic disorders, pulmonary infarction, or pleural malignancies. Left-sided pneumothorax, particularly with a widened mediastinum, may indicate rupture of the aorta.

Leakage of the lymph (chyle) from the thoracic duct most commonly results from mediastinal malignancy (50%), especially lymphoma. Chylothorax, diagnosed by the presence of a triglyceride concentration greater than 110 mg/dL, may also result from thoracic surgery (20%) or trauma (5%).

Clinical pleurisy occurs in close to 5% of patients with rheumatoid arthritis. Pleuritic pain or effusion can be the presenting manifestation in 5% of patients with systemic lupus erythematosus and occurs at some point in the course in up to 50% of patients.

Meigs' syndrome is the triad of benign fibroma or other ovarian tumors with ascites and large pleural effusions (usually on the right side).

Malignant Mesothelioma

Asbestos exposure precedes 80 to 90% of malignant mesotheliomas. The effusion may be massive and is often bloody; in 70% of cases, the pH is less than 7.30. Median survival is 8 to 12 months after diagnosis.

Pneumothorax

Pneumothorax be caused by (1) perforation of the visceral pleura and entry of gas from the lung; (2) penetration of the chest wall, diaphragm, mediastinum, or esophagus; (3) gas generated by microorganisms in an empyema.

Simple spontaneous pneumothorax occurs most commonly in previously healthy men aged 20 to 40 and is due to spontaneous rupture of subpleural blebs at the apex of the lungs. Patients usually present with acute pain, dyspnea, and cough. Physical exami-

Table 6–31 ■ MOST FREQUENT CAUSES OF MEDIASTINAL MASSES

ANTERIOR	MIDDLE	POSTERIOR
Thymoma	Lymphoma	Neurogenic tumors
Lymphoma	Cancer	Enteric cysts
Teratogenic tumors	Cysts	Esophageal lesions
Thyroid	Aneurysms	Aneurysms
Parathyroid	Hernia (Morgagni's)	Diaphragmatic hernias (Bochdalek's)
Aneurysms		

nation shows decreased breath sounds and tactile fremitus with ipsilateral hyperresonance.

Tension pneumothorax can cause mediastinal shift and compromise circulation. For a small pneumothorax (<20% of the hemithorax) in an asymptomatic patient, observation may suffice. A chest tube, which can be connected to suction or placed under water seal, is required for a pneumothorax that occupies more than 50% of the hemithorax.

Secondary or *complicated pneumothorax* results from trauma or pulmonary disease. Patients should be hospitalized and a chest tube inserted because spontaneous expansion is rare. In patients on ventilatory support, a pneumothorax is always under tension and requires immediate insertion of a chest tube.

Mediastinum

Most patients with mediastinal masses are asymptomatic, and the finding is incidental on a chest radiograph. The most common symptoms are chest pain, cough, hoarseness, and dyspnea, whereas stridor, dysphagia, and Horner's syndrome are less frequent. Chest CT is the procedure of choice. The most common cause of a mediastinal mass in older patients is a metastatic carcinoma (Table 6–31).

For more information about this subject, see *Cecil Textbook of Medicine,* 21st edition. Philadelphia, W.B. Saunders Company, 2000. Chapter 86, Diseases of the Diaphragm, Chest Wall, Pleura, and Mediastinum, pages 455 to 462.

OBSTRUCTIVE SLEEP APNEA-HYPOPNEA SYNDROME

During *obstructive apnea,* respiratory efforts persist, but airflow is absent at the nose and mouth. *Central* or *non-obstructive apnea* occurs when both airflow and respiratory efforts are absent. Many adult patients exhibit *mixed apnea,* in which both central and obstructive patterns occur.

Hypoventilation (*hypopnea*) arises by mechanisms similar to those that produce apnea. Overall prevalence is approximately 2 to 4% with a male predominance of 2 to 4:1. The essential features of the obstructive sleep apnea-hypopnea syndrome include loud disruptive snoring, nocturnal choking or gasping, daytime fatigue, and impaired concentration (Table 6–32).

The definitive diagnostic test is the monitoring of the patient during sleep with continuous measurements of breathing and gas

Table 6–32 ■ DEFINITION OF OBSTRUCTIVE SLEEP APNEA-HYPOPNEA SYNDROME

Episodes of upper airway obstruction during sleep result in recurrent arousals associated with:
- Excessive daytime sleepiness, unexplained by other factors, and two or more of the following:
  - Loud disruptive snoring
  - Nocturnal choking/gasping/snorting
  - Recurrent nocturnal awakening
  - Unrefreshing sleep
  - Daytime fatigue
  - Impaired concentration

AND

- Overnight sleep monitoring documenting >5 episodes of hypopnea and apnea per hour

exchange. Treatment should be tailored to the individual patient (Table 6–33). Even a 5 to 10% decrease in body weight can be accompanied by clinical and objective remission.

For more information about this subject, see *Cecil Textbook of Medicine,* 21st edition. Philadelphia, W.B. Saunders Company, 2000. Chapter 87, Obstructive Sleep Apnea-Hypopnea Syndrome, pages 462 to 466.

Table 6–33 ■ THERAPY FOR OBSTRUCTIVE SLEEP APNEA-HYPOPNEA SYNDROME

Electromechanical: Nasal continuous positive airway pressure (CPAP), orthodontic devices, nasal splints, electrical stimulation

Surgical: Tracheostomy, uvulopalatopharyngoplasty, hyoplasty, linguoplasty, mandibular advancement; plastic remodeling of the uvula (laser-assisted or radiofrequency ablation)

Medical: Vasoconstrictive anti-inflammatory nasal sprays,* weight loss medications,* oxygen, and miscellaneous agents (e.g., progesterone, serotonin receptor blockade, acetazolamide, methylxanthines*)

*Not formally approved for obstructive sleep apnea-hypopnea syndrome.

CHAPTER 7

CRITICAL CARE MEDICINE

RESPIRATORY FAILURE

Hypoxic respiratory failure (Table 7–1) defines any condition that severely reduces arterial oxygen tension ($PaO_2 < 50$ mm Hg) and that cannot be corrected by increasing the inspired oxygen fraction to greater than 50% ($FIO_2 > 0.5$). *Hypercapnic-hypoxic respiratory failure* (Table 7–2) may be defined as a life-threatening condition with inadequate CO_2 excretion. During hypoventilation under ambient conditions, the PCO_2 and PO_2 levels change in opposite directions by nearly the same amount. The clinical presentation is dictated primarily by the condition causing the functional impairment, by the level of PaO_2, and by any resulting tissue hypoxia (Table 7–3).

The consensus definition of *adult respiratory distress syndrome* (ARDS) includes severe hypoxemia not responsive to supplemental oxygen ($PaO_2/FIO_2 < 200$) and widespread pulmonary infiltrates (involvement of three of six lung regions) not explained by cardiovascular disease or volume overload (Table 7–4). The crucial stimulus seems to be an inflammatory response to distant or local tissue injury. The spectrum of *acute lung injury* includes less severe cases, which frequently can be identified by PaO_2/FIO_2 less than 300. The differential diagnosis is primarily between cardiogenic pulmonary edema versus ARDS (Table 7–5). ARDS management requires aggressive attempts to maintain adequate oxygenation (Fig. 7–1) and to support the patient medically (Table 7–6).

Chronic obstructive pulmonary disease (COPD) and asthma represent the major causes of acute hypercapnic-hypoxic respiratory failure. The physician must closely follow blood gas measurements (Tables 7–7 and 7–8), transfer sick patients to an intensive care unit (ICU) (Table 7–9), and manage ventilation carefully (Tables 7–10 and 7–11; Fig. 7–2).

Table 7–1 ■ CAUSES OF HYPOXIC RESPIRATORY FAILURE

Adult respiratory distress syndrome
Pneumonia: lobar, multilobar
Pulmonary emboli (massive)
Atelectasis (acute lobar)
Cardiogenic pulmonary edema or shock
Lung contusion or hemorrhage: trauma, Goodpasture's disease, idiopathic pulmonary hemosiderosis, systemic lupus erythematosus

For more information about this subject, see *Cecil Textbook of Medicine,* 21st edition. Philadelphia, W.B. Saunders Company, 2000. Part IX: Critical Care Medicine, pages 483 to 525.

Table 7–2 ■ COMMON CAUSES OF HYPERCAPNIC-HYPOXIC RESPIRATORY FAILURE

1. Altered control
   a. Primary intracranial disease (tumor, hemorrhage)
   b. Trauma and raised intracranial pressure
   c. Drugs, poisons, and toxins
   d. Central hypoventilation
   e. Excess oxygen administration in hypercapnic patient
2. Neuromuscular disease
   a. Spinal cord lesions (trauma, tumor, vascular)
   b. Acute polyneuritis
   c. Myasthenia gravis
   d. Polymyositis, dermatomyositis
   e. Parkinson's disease
3. Metabolic derangements
   a. Severe acidosis
   b. Severe alkalosis
   c. Hypokalemia
   d. Hypophosphatemia
   e. Hypomagnesemia
4. Lungs and airway disease
   a. Upper airway disease (fixed, variable, or sleep-dependent)
   b. Lower airway disease (COPD, asthma)
5. Musculoskeletal alterations
   a. Kyphoscoliosis
   b. Ankylosing spondylitis
6. Obesity-hypoventilation syndrome

COPD = chronic obstructive pulmonary disease.

Table 7–3 ■ CLINICAL MANIFESTATIONS OF HYPOXIA AND HYPERCAPNIA

HYPOXEMIA*	HYPERCAPNIA*
Tachycardia	Somnolence
Tachypnea	Lethargy
Anxiety	Restlessness
Diaphoresis	Tremor
Altered mental status	Slurred speech
Confusion	Headache
Cyanosis	Asterixis
Hypertension	Papilledema
Hypotension	Coma
Bradycardia	
Seizures	
Lactic acidosis†	

*Listed in order of development with progressive alteration in PaO_2 or $PaCO_2$.

†Usually requires additional reduction in oxygen delivery due to inadequate cardiac output, severe anemia, or redistribution of blood flow.

Table 7–4 ■ DISORDERS ASSOCIATED WITH ADULT RESPIRATORY DISTRESS SYNDROME

Aspiration
Gastric contents
Fresh and salt water
Hydrocarbons
Central nervous system
Trauma
Anoxia
Seizures
Increased intracranial pressure
Drug overdose or reactions
Hematologic alterations
Disseminated intravascular coagulation
Massive blood transfusion
Leukoagglutination reactions
Infection
Sepsis (gram-positive or -negative)
Pneumonia: bacterial, viral, fungal
Inhalation of toxins
Oxygen
Smoke
Corrosive chemicals (NO_2, Cl_2, NH_3, phosgene)
Pancreatitis
Shock (rare in cardiogenic or embolic; uncommon in pure hemorrhagic)
Trauma
Fat emboli (long bones usually)
Lung contusion
Non-thoracic (severe)
Cardiopulmonary bypass

Positive pressure ventilation may cause barotrauma manifested as pneumothorax, subcutaneous and mediastineal emphysema, and systemic air embolism. Discontinuing assisted mechanical ventilation may be accomplished by connecting the endotracheal tube to a T piece for a few minutes each hour or a few hours each day; 2-hour trials have been used in most clinical studies. Synchronized intermittent mandatory ventilation can usually be discontinued if patients tolerate a ventilatory rate of less than 4/minute for 2 hours. In discontinuing pressure support ventilation, the pressure support ventilation level may be reduced in increments of 2 to 5 cm H_2O every 2 to 4 hours or so until patients tolerate a level of 5 cm H_2O for 2 hours. Mechanical ventilation can be discontinued more rapidly in patients using T piece trials and pressure support ventilation than with synchronized intermittent mandatory ventilation Positive end-expiratory pressure (PEEP) improves arterial oxygenation by recruiting alveoli for gas exchange (Table 7–12).

The specific recommendations for referral for transplant evaluation vary depending on the underlying disease (Table 7–13). Post-transplant survival rates are about 72% at 1 year and 45 to 50% at 5 years.

For more information about this subject, see *Cecil Textbook of Medicine,* 21st edition. Philadelphia, W.B. Saunders Company, 2000. Chapter 88, Respiratory Failure; Chapter 89, Surgical Ap-

Table 7–5 ■ FEATURES DIFFERENTIATING NON-CARDIOGENIC FROM CARDIOGENIC PULMONARY EDEMA

NON-CARDIOGENIC (ARDS)	CARDIOGENIC/VOLUME OVERLOAD
Prior History	
Younger	Older
No history of heart disease	Prior history of heart disease
Appropriate fluid balance (difficult to assess after resuscitation from shock, trauma, etc.)	Hypertension, chest pain, new-onset palpitations; positive fluid balance
Physical Examination	
Flat neck veins	Elevated neck veins
Hyperdynamic pulses	Left ventricular enlargement, lift, heave, dyskinesis
Physiologic gallop	S_3 and S_4; murmurs
Absence of edema	Edema: flank, sacrum, legs
Electrocardiogram	
Sinus tachycardia, non-specific ST–T wave changes	Evidence of prior or ongoing ischemia, supraventricular tachycardia; left ventricular hypertrophy
Chest Radiograph	
Normal heart size	Cardiomegaly
Peripheral distribution of infiltrates	Central or basilar infiltrates; peribronchial and vascular congestion
Air bronchogram common (80%)	Septal lines (Kerley lines), air bronchograms (25%); pleural effusion
Hemodynamic Measurements	
Pulmonary artery wedge pressure <15 mm Hg; cardiac index >3.5 L/min/m^2	Pulmonary capillary wedge pressure >18 mm Hg; cardiac index <3.5 L/min/m^2 with ischemia, may be >3.5 with volume overload

ARDS = adult respiratory distress syndrome.

proach to Lung Disease; and Chapter 90, Disorders of Ventilatory Control, pages 466 to 482.

SHOCK

It is valuable to classify different forms of shock according to etiology and cardiovascular physiology (Table 7–14). Many patients develop mixed shock. For example, septic shock patients often have a cardiogenic component due to myocardial depression.

One excellent physiologic and clinical measure of perfusion is arterial pressure, which is determined by cardiac output and vascular resistance and can be defined by the following equation:

$$MAP - CVP = CO \times SVR$$

where MAP = mean equation pressure, CVP = central venous

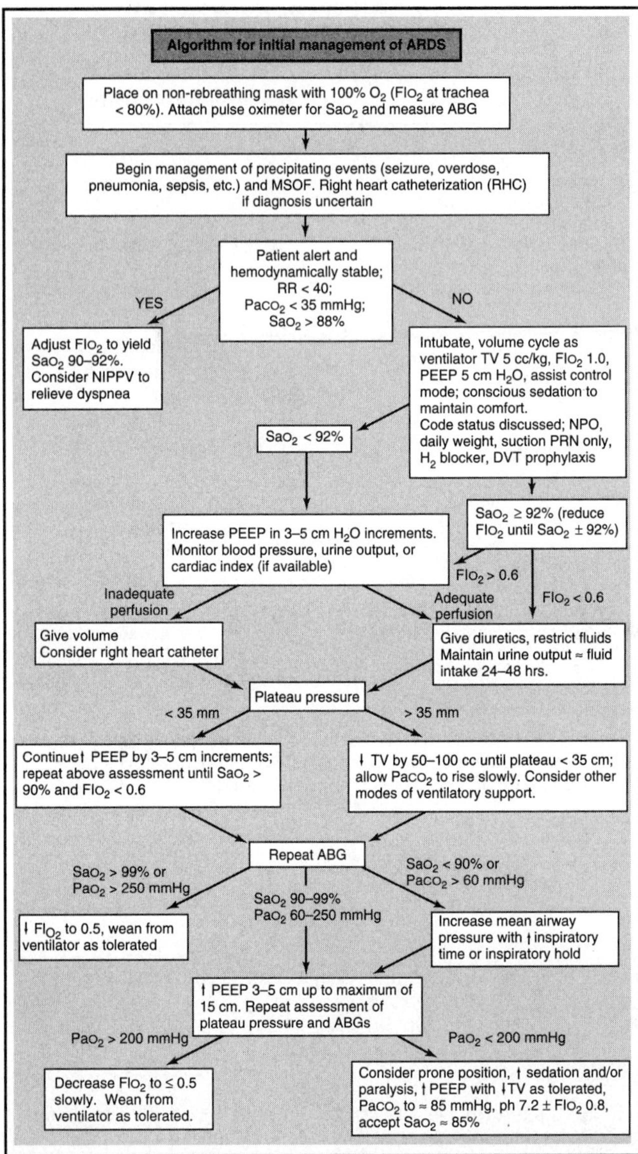
Algorithm for initial management of ARDS
Place on non-rebreathing mask with 100% O_2 (FIO_2 at trachea < 80%). Attach pulse oximeter for SaO_2 and measure ABG
Begin management of precipitating events (seizure, overdose, pneumonia, sepsis, etc.) and MSOF. Right heart catheterization (RHC) if diagnosis uncertain
Patient alert and hemodynamically stable; RR < 40; $PaCO_2$ < 35 mmHg; SaO_2 > 88%
YES
NO
Adjust FIO_2 to yield SaO_2 90–92%. Consider NIPPV to relieve dyspnea
Intubate, volume cycle as ventilator TV 5 cc/kg, FIO_2 1.0, PEEP 5 cm H_2O, assist control mode; conscious sedation to maintain comfort. Code status discussed; NPO, daily weight, suction PRN only, H_2 blocker, DVT prophylaxis
SaO_2 < 92%
SaO_2 ≥ 92% (reduce FIO_2 until SaO_2 ± 92%)
Increase PEEP in 3–5 cm H_2O increments. Monitor blood pressure, urine output, or cardiac index (if available)
FIO_2 > 0.6
FIO_2 < 0.6
Inadequate perfusion
Adequate perfusion
Give volume
Consider right heart catheter
Give diuretics, restrict fluids
Maintain urine output ≈ fluid intake 24–48 hrs.
Plateau pressure
< 35 mm
> 35 mm
Continue ↑ PEEP by 3–5 cm increments; repeat above assessment until SaO_2 > 90% and FIO_2 < 0.6
↓ TV by 50–100 cc until plateau < 35 cm; allow $PaCO_2$ to rise slowly. Consider other modes of ventilatory support.
Repeat ABG
SaO_2 > 99% or PaO_2 > 250 mmHg
SaO_2 90–99% PaO_2 60–250 mmHg
SaO_2 < 90% or $PaCO_2$ > 60 mmHg
↓ FIO_2 to 0.5, wean from ventilator as tolerated
Increase mean airway pressure with ↑ inspiratory time or inspiratory hold
↑ PEEP 3–5 cm up to maximum of 15 cm. Repeat assessment of plateau pressure and ABGs
PaO_2 > 200 mmHg
PaO_2 < 200 mmHg
Decrease FIO_2 to ≤ 0.5 slowly. Wean from ventilator as tolerated.
Consider prone position, ↑ sedation and/or paralysis, ↑ PEEP with ↓TV as tolerated, $PaCO_2$ to ≈ 85 mmHg, ph 7.2 ± FIO_2 0.8, accept SaO_2 ≈ 85%

FIGURE 7–1 ■ An algorithm for the initial management of adult respiratory distress syndrome (ARDS). ABG = arterial blood gas analysis; DVT = deep venous thrombosis; FIO_2 = inspired oxygen concentration; MSOF = multisystem organ failure; NIPPV = non-invasive intermittent positive pressure ventilation; $PaCO_2$ = arterial partial pressure of carbon dioxide; PaO_2 = arterial partial pressure of oxygen; PEEP = positive end-expiratory pressure; RR = respiratory rate; SaO_2 = arterial oxygen saturation; TV = tidal volume.

Table 7–6 ■ SUPPORTIVE MANAGEMENT OF ADULT RESPIRATORY DISTRESS SYNDROME

PRINCIPLE	GOAL	STRATEGY
Optimize fluid status	Lowest tolerated filling pressures; keep dry	Limit extraneous IV fluids, follow intake and output; diurese empirically; measure pulmonary capillary wedge pressure if fluid status unclear
Avoid gastrointestinal bleeding	Gastric pH >4; protect gastric lining	H_2-blockers, sucralfate, proton pump inhibitors
Prevent thromboembolism	Reduce clotting and venous stasis	Pneumatic and elastic compression stockings, subcutaneous heparin
Supply adequate nutrition	Replace resting energy expenditure	25–30 kcal/kg, 1.5 g/kg of protein; enteral feeding preferred, total parenteral nutrition if gut dysfunctional; some diets may improve outcome

7

pressure, CO = cardiac output, and SVR = systemic vascular resistance.

Blood flow to the heart and brain is carefully regulated and maintained over a wide range of blood pressure (from a mean arterial pressure of 50–150 mm Hg). With the onset of hemodynamic dysfunction in shock, homeostatic compensatory mechanisms attempt to maintain effective tissue perfusion, and many of the manifestations of shock represent the body's attempt to correct abnormalities. (Table 7–15). The clinical presentation of shock is quite variable and depends on the initiating cause and the response of multiple organs (Table 7–16).

Clinical Approach to Shock

Shock is a life-threatening emergency. The clinical approach must balance two important goals: the need to initiate therapy before shock causes irreversible damage to organs, and the need to

Table 7–7 ■ RECOMMENDED INITIAL FIO_2 BY VENTI-MASK OR NASAL O_2 BY CANNULA TO ACHIEVE PaO_2 > 60 mm Hg

INITIAL PaO_2 ON ROOM AIR (mm Hg)	VENTI-MASK FIO_2 (%)	NASAL CANNULA (L/min)
50	24	1
45–49	28	2
40–44	32	3
<40	35	4

Table 7–8 ■ SUGGESTED MODIFICATIONS OF TREATMENT (WITHOUT INTUBATION) BASED ON FOLLOW-UP ARTERIAL BLOOD GAS ANALYSES

FOLLOW-UP Pao_2 (mm Hg)	FOLLOW-UP $Paco_2$ (mm Hg)	FOLLOW-UP pH	THERAPEUTIC RECOMMENDATION
>60	<55	>7.30	No change in O_2; follow Sao_2 with pulse oximetry
>60	>55–<65	7.25	No change in O_2; repeat ABG in 3–4 hr
>60	>65–<80	<7.25–>7.20	No change O_2; repeat ABG in 1 hr
>60	>80	<7.20–>7.05	Add NIPPV; repeat ABG in 1 hr
<60	<55	Unchanged	Increase nasal O_2 flow 1 L/min
<60	>55	>7.25	Increase nasal O_2 flow until Sao_2 85%; check ABG in 1 hr

ABG = arterial blood gas analysis; NIPPV = non-invasive intermittent positive pressure ventilation.

perform a diagnostic evaluation to determine the cause of shock (Fig. 7–3). If the cause of shock remains undefined or the hemodynamic status requires repeated fluid challenges or vasopressors, a flow-directed pulmonary artery catheter should be placed and echocardiography should be performed.

Cardiogenic Shock

Cardiogenic shock is typically the result of an extensive myocardial infarction (MI) associated with damage to 40% or more of the left ventricular myocardium. Echocardiography can make the diagnosis of a mechanical complication, such as a ruptured papillary muscle or a ventricular septal defect, and can provide assessment of overall left ventricular function.

Text continues on page 187

Table 7–9 ■ INDICATIONS FOR INTENSIVE CARE UNIT ADMISSION OF PATIENTS WITH ACUTE COPD EXACERBATION

Severe dyspnea unresponsive to initial emergency therapy
Confusion, lethargy, or respiratory muscle fatigue (the last characterized by paradoxical chest wall motion)
Worsening hypoxemia despite supplemental oxygen or worsening respiratory acidosis (pH <7.30)
Assisted mechanical ventilation requiring endotracheal tube

COPD = chronic obstructive pulmonary disease.

Adapted from ATS Committee Statement. Inpatient management of COPD. Am J Respir Crit Care Med 152:S97–S106, 1995.

Table 7–10 ■ FEATURES OF HYPOXIC AND HYPERCAPNIC-HYPOXIC ACUTE RESPIRATORY FAILURE

	CONDITION	
FEATURE	**Hypoxic**	**Hypercapnic-Hypoxic**
Physiologic	Large right-to-left intrapulmonary shunt; hyperventilation usual	COPD: hypoventilation due to marked wasted (dead space) ventilation; minute ventilation normal to increased; $\dot{V}/\dot{Q}$ imbalance with increased A-a gradient. Neuromuscular and overdose: hypoventilation due to decreased minute ventilation, normal A-a gradient
Anatomic	Extensive edema; atelectasis or consolidation; hyaline membranes	Mucous gland hyperplasia (bronchitis); alveolar wall destruction (emphysema); hypertrophied bronchial muscle and mucous impaction (asthma); upper airway obstruction (fixed or variable)
Clinical Presentation		
Age	Any	Any; bronchitis and emphysema $>$55 yr
Medical history	Well; hypertension; heart disease	Chronic shortness of breath; weakness and wheezing
Present illness	Acute shortness of breath temporally related to some serious event (e.g., car accident, sepsis, worsening blood pressure, chest pain)	Recent upper respiratory tract infection; gradual worsening of shortness of breath, increased cough, sputum, and wheezing; drug overdose; new or increased muscle weakness
Physical examination	Evidence of acute illness, tachypnea ($>$35/min); tachycardia; hypotension; diffuse crackles; signs of consolidation	Tachypnea ($<$30/min); tachycardia; prolonged expiration; decreased breath sounds; wheezing; pedal edema; reduced strength; altered consciousness

Table continued on the following page

Table 7–10 ■ FEATURES OF HYPOXIC AND HYPERCAPNIC-HYPOXIC ACUTE RESPIRATORY FAILURE *Continued*

	CONDITION	
FEATURE	**Hypoxic**	**Hypercapnic-Hypoxic**
Laboratory Examination		
Chest radiograph	Small, white lungs; multiple patchy, diffuse infiltrates; lobar atelectasis or consolidation	Hyperinflation; large black lungs, bullae; wide interspaces; prominent bronchovascular marking with COPD or asthma; hypoinflation, small black lungs; with overdose or neuromuscular disease
Electrocardiogram	Sinus tachycardia; acute myocardial infarction; left ventricular hypertrophy	Right ventricular hypertrophy; "P" pulmonale; low voltage; clockwise rotation; normal
Laboratory	Nonspecific; hemoglobin low to normal; respiratory alkalosis; metabolic acidosis; raised BUN	Hemoglobin normal to high; respiratory acidosis; mixed metabolic and respiratory acidosis; low potassium

$\dot{V}/\dot{Q}$ = ventilation/perfusion; A-a = alveolar-arterial; BUN = blood urea nitrogen; COPD = chronic obstructive pulmonary disease.

Table 7–11 ■ MODES OF POSITIVE PRESSURE VENTILATION

MODE	DESCRIPTION	ADVANTAGES/DISADVANTAGES
Controlled mechanical ventilation (CMV)	Ventilator f, inspiratory time, and V_T (and thus $\dot{V}_E$) preset	May be used with sedation or paralysis; ventilator cannot respond to ventilatory needs
Assisted mechanical ventilation (AMV) or assist/control	Ventilator V_T and inspiratory time preset but patient can increase f (and thus $\dot{V}_E$)	Ventilator may respond to ventilatory needs; ventilator may under- or overtrigger, depending on sensitivity
Intermittent mandatory ventilation (IMV)	Ventilator delivers preset V_T, f, and inspiratory time, but patient also may breathe spontaneously	May decrease asynchronous breathing and sedation requirements; ventilator cannot respond to ventilatory needs
Synchronized intermittent mandatory ventilation (SIMV)	Same as IMV, but ventilator breaths delivered only after patient finishes inspiration	Same as IMV, and patient not overinflated by receiving spontaneous and ventilator breaths at same time
High-frequency ventilation (HFV)	Ventilator f is increased, and V_T may be smaller than V_D	May reduce peak airway pressure; may cause auto-PEEP
Pressure support ventilation (PSV)	Patient breathes at own f; V_T determined by inspiratory pressure and C_{RS}	Increased comfort and decreased work of breathing; ventilator cannot respond to ventilatory needs
Pressure control ventilation (PCV)	Ventilator peak pressure, f, and respiratory time preset	Peak inspiratory pressures may be decreased; hypoventilation may occur
Inverse ratio ventilation (IRV)	Inspiratory time exceeds expiratory time to facilitate inspiration	May improve gas exchange by increasing time spent in inspiration; may cause auto-PEEP
Airway pressure release ventilation (APRV)	Patient receives CPAP at high and low levels to simulate V_T	May improve oxygenation at lower airway pressure; hypoventilation may occur
Proportional assist ventilation (PAV)	Patient determines own f, V_T, pressures, and flows	May amplify spontaneous breathing; depends entirely on patient's respiratory drive.

f = respiratory rate; V_T = tidal volume; V_D = dead space; $\dot{V}_E$ = minute ventilation; PEEP = positive end-expiratory pressure; CPAP = continuous positive airway pressure; C_{RS} = respiratory system compliance.

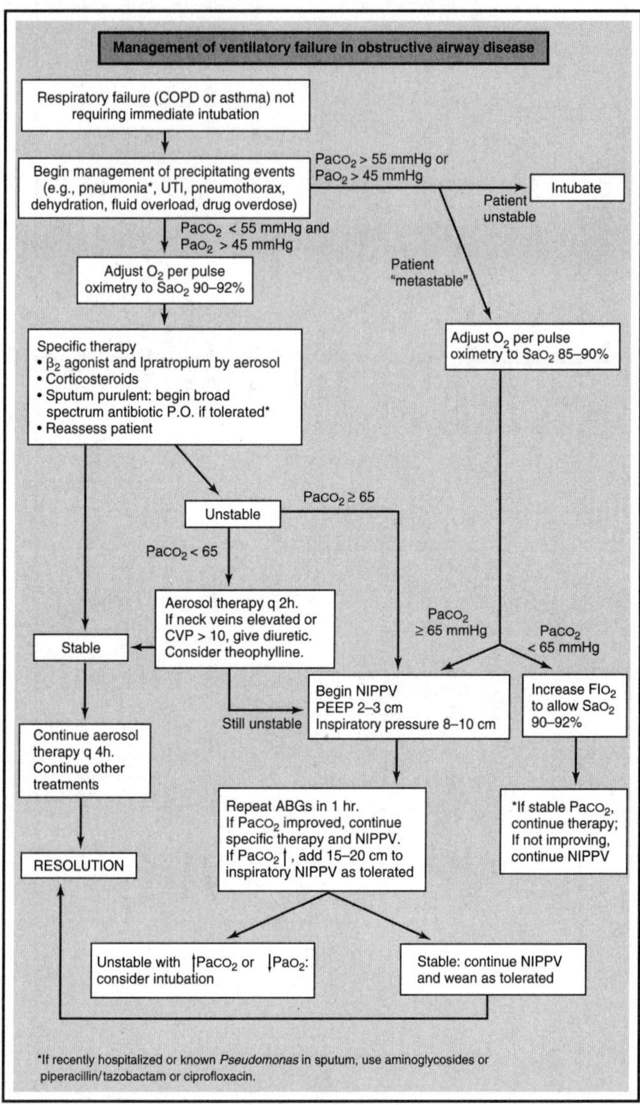

FIGURE 7–2 ■ An algorithm for the management of ventilatory failure in a patient with obstructive airway disease. COPD = chronic obstructive pulmonary disease; CVP = central venous pressure; HRF = hypoxic respiratory failure; UTI = urinary tract infection. (See Fig. 7–1 legend for key to other abbreviations.)

Table 7–12 ■ INDICATIONS FOR POSITIVE END-EXPIRATORY PRESSURE (PEEP)

To prevent or reverse atelectasis
To facilitate weaning from mechanical ventilation
To improve arterial oxygenation at a low inspired oxygen fraction
To reduce trigger-related work of breathing in patients with auto-PEEP

7

The prognosis of patients with cardiogenic shock remains grim. Vasopressor therapy to improve cardiac performance usually begins with dopamine 5 to 10 μg/kg/minute. Dobutamine 2 to 8 μg/kg/minute may be used in combination with dopamine to augment cardiac output further, but it does not usually increase arterial pressure further. In patients with resistant hypotension, norepinephrine 0.04 to 0.4 μg/kg/minute is usually used. Vasodilators such as intravenous (IV) nitroglycerin or nitroprusside are usually not used initially because they can aggravate hypotension; however, they may be used later or in combination with vasopressors and inotropic agents. At present, an aggressive approach appears to have the most potential to improve outcome (Fig. 7–4).

Shock Syndromes Related to Sepsis

Gram-negative and gram-positive organisms, as well as fungi, can cause sepsis and septic shock. The most recent definitions (Table 7–17) use the term *systemic inflammatory response syndrome* (SIRS) to emphasize that sepsis is one example of the body's inflammatory responses that can be triggered not only by infections but also by noninfectious disorders, such as trauma and pancreatitis. Organism-derived antigens and toxins stimulate the release of a large number of endogenous host-derived mediators from plasma protein precursors or cells (monocytes-macrophages, endothelial cells, neutrophils, and others) (Fig. 7–5).

Sepsis and septic shock produce three categories of clinical manifestations (Fig. 7–6). When the diagnosis is seriously entertained, blood cultures (usually three) and cultures of relevant body fluids and exudates should be obtained rapidly. Early, appropriate, broad-spectrum antimicrobial therapy (i.e., the pathogen has in vitro sensitivity to the chosen antibiotic regimen) improves patient survival. Once a specific pathogen is isolated, the antimicrobial spectrum can be narrowed. Corticosteroids and currently available inhibitors of endotoxin do not improve survival in human septic shock. Approximately 50% of patients who have hypotension secondary to sepsis and who are admitted to an ICU survive.

For more information about this subject, see *Cecil Textbook of Medicine,* 21st edition. Philadelphia, W.B. Saunders Company, 2000. Chapter 94, on Approach to the Patient with Shock; Chapter 95, Cardiogenic Shock; and Chapter 96, Shock Syndromes Related to Sepsis, pages 495 to 512.

Table 7–13 ■ GUIDELINES FOR LUNG TRANSPLANT REFERRAL

DISEASE	PULMONARY FUNCTION	ARTERIAL BLOOD GAS VALUES	NYHA CLASS	OTHER CONSIDERATIONS
Chronic obstructive lung disease	FEV_1 <25% predicted	PCO_2 >55 mm Hg		Pulmonary hypertension; progressive deterioration
Cystic fibrosis	FEV_1 <30% predicted or rapid decline	PCO_2 >50 mm Hg or PO_2 <55 mm Hg		Increasing admissions or rapid deterioration
Idiopathic pulmonary fibrosis	Vital capacity <60% predicted or DLCO <50% predicted	Exertional desaturation		Lack of response to therapy
Pulmonary hypertension			Functional Class III or IV despite vasodilator therapy	CI, <2 L/min/m^2; RAP, >15 mm Hg; mean PAP, >55 mm Hg
Eisenmenger's syndrome			Functional Class III or IV	

NYHA = New York Heart Association; FEV_1 = forced expiratory volume in 1 second; DLCO = diffusing capacity of carbon monoxide in the lungs; CI = cardiac index; RAP = right atrial pressure; PAP = pulmonary artery pressure.

Adapted from Joint Statement of American Society of Transplant Physicians/American Thoracic Society/International Society of Heart and Lung Transplantation: International guidelines for the selection of lung transplant candidates. Am J Respir Crit Care Med 158:335–339, 1998.

DISORDERS DUE TO HEAT AND COLD

Hyperthermic Syndromes

Heat exhaustion is due to severe dehydration and electrolyte loss. Patients frequently complain of cramps, headache, fatigue, nausea, and vomiting. They appear listless, with pallor of the skin and profuse sweating. Other clinical findings include orthostatic hypotension, core temperatures of 37.5 to 39° C (99.5 to 102.2° F), altered mental status, incoordination, and diffuse weakness. *Heatstroke* is manifested by central nervous system depression, hypohidrosis, core temperatures of 41° C or higher, and severe physiologic and biochemical abnormalities.

Neuroleptic malignant syndrome is a complex of extrpyramidal

Table 7–14 ■ CLASSIFICATION OF SHOCK

Hypovolemic

- Hemorrhagic
  - Trauma
  - Gastrointestinal
  - Retroperitoneal
- Fluid depletion (nonhemorrhagic)
  - External fluid loss
    - Dehydration
    - Vomiting
    - Diarrhea
    - Polyuria
  - Interstitial fluid redistribution
    - Thermal injury
    - Trauma
    - Anaphylaxis
- Increased vascular capacitance (venodilation)
  - Sepsis
  - Anaphylaxis
  - Toxins/drugs

Cardiogenic

- Myopathic
  - Myocardial infarction
    - Left ventricle
    - Right ventricle
  - Myocardial contusion (trauma)
  - Myocarditis
  - Cardiomyopathy
  - Post-ischemic myocardial stunning
  - Septic myocardial depression
  - Pharmacologic
    - Anthracycline cardiotoxicity
    - Calcium channel blockers
- Mechanical
  - Valvular failure (stenotic or regurgitant)
  - Hypertropic cardiomyopathy
  - Ventricular septal defect
- Arrhythmic
  - Bradycardia
  - Tachycardia

Table continued on following page

Table 7–14 ■ CLASSIFICATION OF SHOCK *Continued*

Extracardiac Obstructive

Impaired diastolic filling (decreased ventricular preload)
  Direct venous obstruction (vena cava)
    Intrathoracic obstructive tumors
  Increased intrathoracic pressure
    Tension pneumothorax
    Mechanical ventilation (with excessive pressure or volume depletion)
    Asthma
  Decreased cardiac compliance
    Constrictive pericarditis
    Cardiac tamponade
Impaired systolic contraction (increased ventricular afterload)
  Right ventricle
    Pulmonary embolus (massive)
    Acute pulmonary hypertension
  Left ventricle
    Aortic dissection

Distributive

Septic (bacterial, fungal, viral, rickettsial)
Toxic shock syndrome
Anaphylactic, anaphylactoid
Neurogenic (spinal shock)
Endocrinologic
  Adrenal crisis
  Thyroid storm
Toxic (e.g., nitroprusside, bretylium)

muscular rigidity and high core temperature occurring as an acute or subacute reaction to neuroleptic medications. *Malignant hyperthermia* is a hypermetabolic, myopathic syndrome that usually occurs when inducing anesthesia. Severe hyperthermia is also associated with ingestion of amphetamines, amphetamine congeners (MDMA, "ecstasy"), and cocaine.

Consequences of heat-induced cell damage are rhabdomyolysis, heart failure, cardiac arrhythmias, vasodilation, cytotoxic cerebral edema, hypotension, acute renal failure, ARDS, gastrointestinal hemorrhage, and acute hepatic failure. Laboratory abnormalities include hyperkalemia, hypercalcemia, hyperphosphatemia or hypophosphatemia, rising creatinine, consumptive coagulopathy, and lactic acidosis. PaO_2 values are incorrectly low and should be increased by 6% for each degree centigrade above 37° C; $PaCO_2$ is also lower and should be increased by 4.4% for each degree centigrade above 37° C; and pH is high and should be reduced by 0.015 unit for each degree centigrade above 37° C.

The primary goal of therapy is rapid cooling (Table 7–18).

Hypothermic Syndromes

Hypothermia is defined as a core body temperature lower than 35° C (95° F). An underlying illness or drug is often the predisposing factor.

PaO_2 values are incorrectly high and should be decreased by

Table 7–15 ■ CARDIOVASCULAR AND METABOLIC COMPENSATORY RESPONSES TO SHOCK

Maintain Mean Circulatory Pressure (Venous Pressure)

Volume
- Fluid redistribution to vascular space
  - From interstitium (Starling's effect)
  - From intracellular space (osmotic)
- Decrease renal losses
  - ↓ Glomerular filtration rate
  - ↑ Aldosterone
  - ↑ Vasopressin

Pressure
- Decrease venous capacitance
  - ↑ Sympathetic activity
  - ↑ Circulating (adrenal) epinephrine
  - ↑ Angiotensin
  - ↑ Vasopressin

Maximize Cardiac Performance

Increase contractility
- Sympathetic stimulation
- Adrenal stimulation

Redistribute Perfusion

Extrinsic regulation of systemic arterial tone
Dominant autoregulation of vital organs (heart, brain)

Optimize Oxygen Unloading

↑ RBC 2,3-DPG
Tissue acidosis
Pyrexia
↓ Tissue Po_2

↑ = increases; ↓ = decreases; RBC 2,3-DPG = red blood cell 2,3-diphosphoglycerate.

4.4% for each degree centigrade below 37° C; $Paco_2$ is also higher and should be decreased by 3.5% for each degree centigrade below 37° C; and pH is lower and should be increased by 0.015 unit for each degree centigrade below 37° C. When core temperature declines to 32° C, the classic Osborne (or J) wave appears on the downstroke of the R wave on the electrocardiogram (ECG).

The goals of management are to prevent further heat loss, increase core temperature, and anticipate and prevent complications (Table 7–19).

For more information about this subject, see *Cecil Textbook of Medicine,* 21st edition. Philadelphia, W.B. Saunders Company, 2000. Chapter 97, Disorders Due to Heat and Cold, pages 512 to 515.

ACUTE POISONING

The general approach to the poisoned patient may be divided into seven phases: (1) emergency management; (2) clinical evaluation; (3) elimination of poison from the gastrointestinal tract, skin, and eyes, or removal from the site of exposure in inhalation poi-

Table 7–16 ■ ORGAN SYSTEM DYSFUNCTION IN SHOCK

ORGAN SYSTEM	MANIFESTATIONS
Central nervous system	Encephalopathy (ischemic or septic)
	Cortical necrosis
Heart	Tachycardia, bradycardia
	Supraventricular tachycardia
	Ventricular ectopy
	Myocardial ischemia
	Myocardial depression
Pulmonary	Acute respiratory failure
	Adult respiratory distress syndrome
Kidney	Prerenal failure
	Acute tubular necrosis
Gastrointestinal	Ileus
	Erosive gastritis
	Pancreatitis
	Acalculous cholecystitis
	Colonic submucosal hemorrhage
	Transluminal translocation of bacteria/endotoxin
Liver	Ischemic hepatitis
	"Shock" liver
	Intrahepatic cholestasis
Hematologic	Disseminated intravascular coagulation
	Dilutional thrombocytopenia
Metabolic	Hyperglycemia
	Glycogenolysis
	Gluconeogenesis
	Hypoglycemia (late)
	Hypertriglyceridemia
Immune system	Gut barrier function depression
	Cellular immune depression
	Humoral immune depression

soning; (4) administration of an antidote; (5) elimination of any absorbed substance; (6) supportive therapy; and (7) observation and disposition. Resuscitation with airway establishment, adequate ventilation and perfusion, and restoration of all vital signs (including temperature) must be accomplished first.

A patient with acute poisoning often presents with coma, cardiac arrhythmia (Table 7–20), or seizures (Table 7–21). Naloxone 2 mg IV, thiamine 100 mg IV, and 50% glucose 50 mL IV (if the patient is hypoglycemic by Dextrostix) are given to all adult patients in coma after inserting an IV line and drawing appropriate blood samples. Activated charcoal, the single most important intervention, is considered safe and adequate treatment for all but a few overdoses (Table 7–22). For some poisoning, specific antidotes are indicated (Table 7–23). Specific methods are indicated to eliminate certain absorbed substances (Table 7–24).

Acetaminophen toxicity is likely to occur after a minimum acute ingestion of 140 mg/kg, or about 10 g in an adult. Acetaminophen poisoning clinically produces only nausea, vomiting, and anorexia 12 to 24 hours after ingestion, after irreversible hepatic necrosis

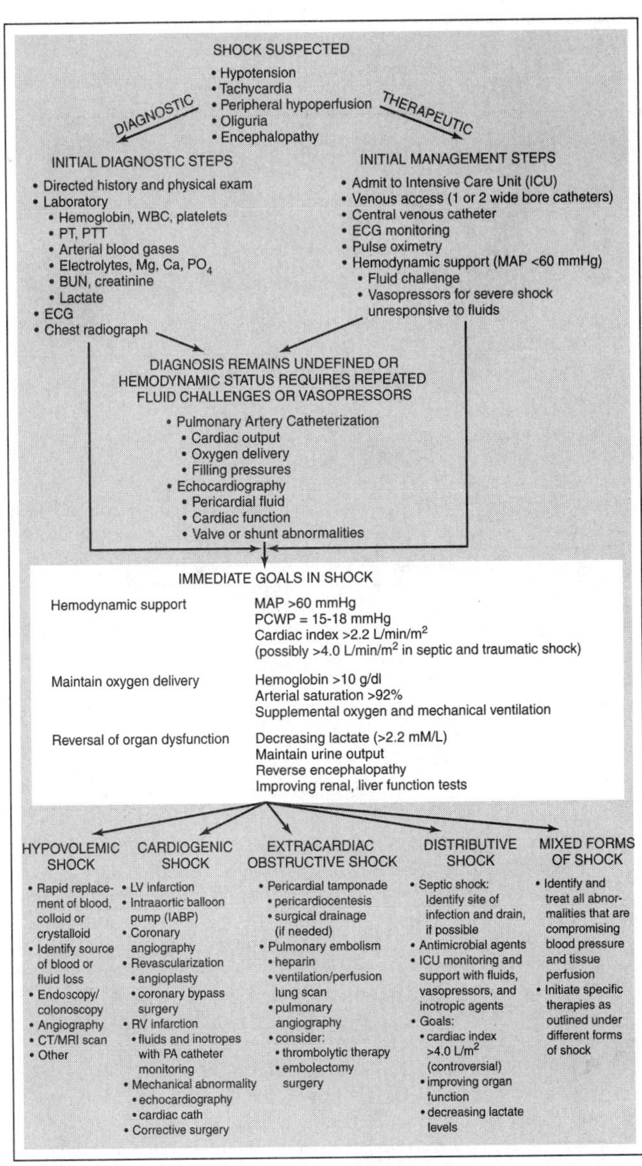

FIGURE 7–3 ■ An approach to the diagnosis and treatment of shock. MAP = mean arterial pressure, PCWP = pulmonary capillary wedge pressure; WBC = white blood cell count; PT = prothrombin time; PTT = partial thromboplastin time; BUN = blood urea nitrogen; CT = computed tomography; MRI = magnetic resonance imaging; LV = left ventricular; RV = right ventricular.

7

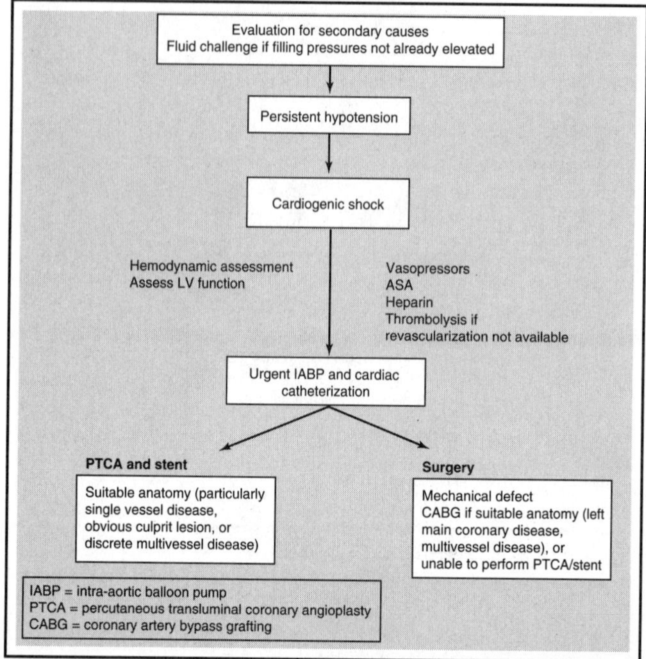

FIGURE 7–4 ■ Acute myocardial infarction with hypotension: an aggressive approach. LV = left ventricular; ASA = aspirin.

has already occurred. Acetylcysteine sodium (Mucomyst) given intravenously is the drug of choice.

A plasma *salicylate* level of more than 30 mg/dL indicates salicylate toxicity, and a level of 80 to 100 mg/dL indicates actual salicylate poisoning. The treatment of choice for salicylate poisoning is an alkaline diuresis with sodium bicarbonate. Hemodialysis is indicated if the salicylate level is higher than 80 to 100 mg/dL, if patients do not respond to a trial of bicarbonate therapy, or if the patient's condition is critical.

Although the *benzodiazepines* are common agents involved in overdose, they generally cause only coma and ataxia. Mortality is rare, and supportive care is all that is usually necessary.

For *calcium channel blockers,* persistent hypotension, bradycardia, pulmonary edema, or cardiac arrest may require whole-bowel irrigation with polyethylene glycol. A 10% calcium chloride 1-g bolus (over 5 minutes) IV may be life-saving, and 1 g IV every 15 minutes over the first hour may be necessary in critically ill patients, followed by 10% calcium chloride via continuous IV infusion.

A serum *iron* level higher than 500 μg/dL indicates serious intoxication. Management of iron poisoning includes gastric lavage with normal saline. Whole-bowel irrigation may be indicated after

Table 7–17 ■ DEFINITIONS OF SEPSIS

Infection: A microbial phenomenon characterized by an inflammatory response to the presence of microorganisms or the invasion of normally sterile host tissue by those organisms.

Bacteremia: The presence of viable bacteria in the blood.

Systemic inflammatory response syndrome: The systemic inflammatory response to a variety of severe clinical insults. The response is manifested by two or more of the following conditions:
- Temperature >38° C or <36° C
- Heart rate >90 beats/min
- Respiratory rate >20 breaths/min or Pa_{CO_2} <32 mm Hg (<4.3 kPa)
- White blood cell count >12,000 cells/mm^3, <4000 cells/mm^3, or >10% immature (band) forms

Sepsis: The systemic response to infection. This systemic response is manifested by two or more of the following conditions as a result of infection:
- Temperature >38° C or <36° C
- Heart rate >90 beats/min
- Respiratory rate >20 breaths/min or Pa_{CO_2} <32 mm Hg (<4.3 kPa)
- White blood cell count >12,000 cells/mm^3, 4000 cells/mm^3, or >10% immature (band) forms

Severe sepsis: Sepsis associated with organ dysfunction, hypoperfusion, or hypotension. Hypoperfusion and perfusion abnormalities that may include, but are not limited to, lactic acidosis, oliguria, or an acute alteration in mental status.

Septic shock: Sepsis with hypotension, despite adequate fluid resuscitation, along with the presence of perfusion abnormalities that may include, but are not limited to, lactic acidosis, oliguria, or an acute alteration in mental status. Patients who are on inotropic or vasopressor agents may not be hypotensive at the time that perfusion abnormalities are measured.

Hypotension: A systolic blood pressure <90 mm Hg or a reduction >40 mm Hg from baseline in the absence of other causes of hypotension.

Multiple organ system failure: Presence of altered organ function in an acutely ill patient such that homeostasis cannot be maintained without intervention.

Adapted from American College of Chest Physicians Society of Critical Care Medicine Consensus Conference: Definitions for sepsis and organ failure and guidelines for the use of innovative therapies in sepsis. Crit Care Med 20:864, 1992.

ingestion of sustained-release capsules. The treatment of choice is the antidote deferoxamine.

For *methanol,* or wood alcohol, treatment emphasizes IV ethanol, sodium bicarbonate, and hemodialysis. Hemodialysis is the treatment of choice for *ethylene glycol* poisoning. For *isopropyl alcohol,* treatment is generally conservative.

Even minute quantities of *organophosphates* cause abdominal pain, vomiting, headaches, and dizziness. The full-blown picture generally develops by 24 hours and includes coma, convulsions, confusion or psychosis, fasciculation, and weakness or paralysis. Atropine should be given as a physiologic antidote.

Tricyclic (or *cyclic*) *antidepressant* overdose causes cardiac arrhythmia and hypotension with ingestion of 1 g (10–20 mg/kg). A

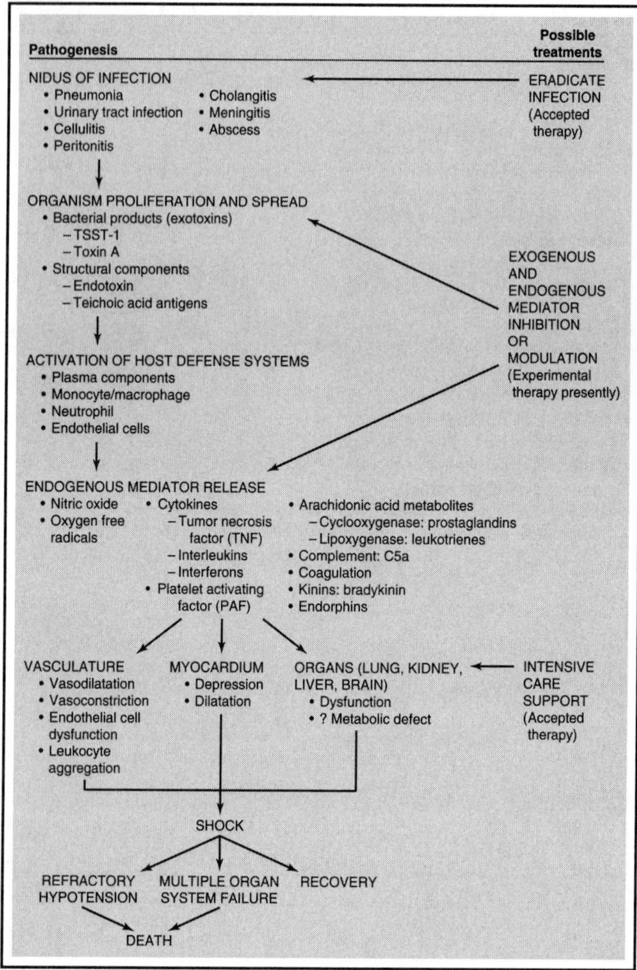

FIGURE 7–5 ■ Pathogenesis and possible treatment strategies in sepsis and septic shock. TSST-1 = toxic shock syndrome toxin-1.

QRS complex longer than 100 ms is a sign of severe toxicity and generally correlates with a plasma drug level higher than 1000 ng/mL. The treatment of choice for tricyclic antidepressant overdose is IV sodium bicarbonate via continuous infusion to maintain a blood pH of 7.5. Activated charcoal and supportive therapy are indicated. Phenytoin (Dilantin) has been reported to reverse QRS complex prolongation in tricyclic antidepressant overdose, but it is generally reserved for managing seizures. Physostigmine is no longer used in tricyclic antidepressant overdose.

For more information about this subject, see *Cecil Textbook of*

SUSPECTED SEPSIS

SYSTEMIC INFLAMMATORY RESPONSE SYNDROME (SIRS)
(presence of 2 of 4 findings)
- Fever or hypothermia
- Tachycardia
- Tachypnea
- Leukocytosis or leukopenia

SITE OF INFECTION
(physical exam, imaging or laboratory tests)
- Pneumonia, empyema
- Urinary tract infection
- Cellulitis
- Peritonitis
- Cholangitis
- Sinusitis
- Meningitis
- Abscess (peritoneum, skin, brain, paraspinal)
- No identifiable site (especially in neutropenic patients)

SEPSIS

INFECTED SITE

SURGICAL DRAINAGE

ANTIMICROBIAL AGENTS

ERADICATE INFECTION

REVERSAL OF SEPSIS

SURVIVAL

MULTIPLE ORGAN DYSFUNCTION SYNDROME (MODS)

– CARDIOVASCULAR: SEPTIC SHOCK
- Hypotension
- Tissue hypoperfusion (oliguria, lactic acidosis, cool extremities)

– RENAL
- Oliguria
- Acute renal insufficiency

– HEPATIC
- Hyperbilirubinemia

– CENTRAL NERVOUS SYSTEM
- Altered mental status

– PULMONARY
- Adult respiratory distress syndrome (ARDS)

CARDIOVASCULAR THERAPY
- ICU monitoring (cardiac rhythm, arterial and pulmonary artery catheters)
- Volume expansion
- Vasopressors
- Inotropic agents

PULMONARY THERAPY
- Supplemental oxygen
- Mechanical ventilation

CARDIOVASCULAR GOALS
- Mean arterial pressure ≥ 65 mmHg
- Pulmonary wedge pressure = 15-18 mmHg
- Hemoglobin level ≥ 10 g/dl
- Normal or decreasing blood lactate levels
- Cardiac index > 2.2 L/min/m^2 in non-septic shock and > 4.0 L/min/m^2 in septic shock

PULMONARY AND OTHER ORGAN SYSTEM GOALS
- O2 saturation > 92%
- Normal values or reversal of dysfunction in the following systems:
  - – pulmonary: arterial-alveolar oxygen gradient
  - – renal: blood urea nitrogen, creatinine, urine output
  - – hepatic: serum bilirubin
  - – brain: mental status

REVERSAL OF MODS

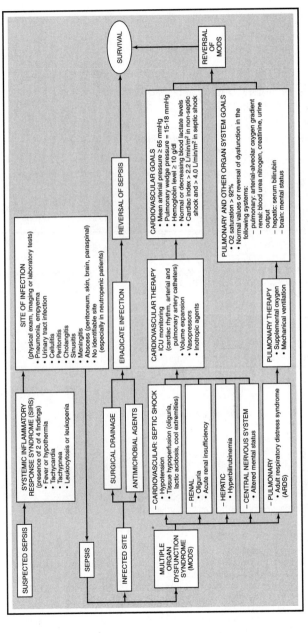

FIGURE 7–6 ■ Algorithm for diagnostic evaluation and management of sepsis and septic shock.

Table 7–18 ■ MANAGEMENT OF HYPERTHERMIA

1. Protect the airway
2. Insert at least two large-bore intravenous lines
3. Monitor core temperature
   a. Pulmonary artery
   b. Rectal probe
   c. Esophageal probe
4. Actively cool the skin until core temperature reaches 39° C
   a. Exposure to cool environment
   b. Wetting with water (avoid alcohol rubs)
   c. Continuous fanning
   d. Ice baths/immersion (22° C)
   e. Axillary/perineal ice packs
   f. Infusion of room-temperature saline
   g. Gastric/colonic iced saline lavage
   h. Peritoneal lavage with cool saline
5. If shivering occurs, administer chlorpromazine 10–25 mg intramuscularly
6. Monitor for seizures
7. Monitor electrocardiogram for dysrhythmia
8. Obtain serial diagnostic studies

Medicine, 21st edition. Philadelphia, W.B. Saunders Company, 2000. Chapter 98, Acute Poisoning, pages 515 to 522.

RHABDOMYOLYSIS

Rhabdomyolysis, a syndrome that results from destruction of skeletal muscle, is usually diagnosed by creatine kinase (CK) levels

Text continues on page 203

Table 7–19 ■ MANAGEMENT OF HYPOTHERMIA

Mild Hypothermia (34–36° C)

1. Remove from cold environment, replace wet clothing, cover with blankets or equivalent, use gentle passive rewarming techniques
2. Give warm oxygen through a mask or an endotracheal tube
3. Give warm dextrose/saline intravenous fluids
4. Warm the environment (thermostat, overhead lights)
5. Monitor electrocardiogram, respiratory status, core temperature
6. Obtain initial diagnostic studies

Moderate-to-Severe Hypothermia (≤33° C)

1. Admit to intensive care unit
2. Peripheral active rewarming: heating blankets, heating pads, hot-water bottles, warming lights, warm-water immersion
3. Actively warm central core; inhale heated, humidified oxygen, gastric lavage, colonic irrigation, and warmed intravenous fluids
4. Consider special beds, and protect against pressure necrosis
5. If core temperature is not rising 0.5–1.0° C/hr, consider warm fluid peritoneal dialysis, bladder lavage, hemodialysis, or bypass
6. Anticipate multiorgan dysfunction and secondary infection

Table 7–20 ■ COMMON TOXIC CAUSES OF CARDIAC ARRHYTHMIA

Tricyclic antidepressants*	Succinylcholine
Arsenic	Cyanide
β-Blockers	Digitalis
Calcium channel blockers	Phenothiazines
Carbon monoxide	Phosphorus
Chloral hydrate	Physostigmine
Clonidine	Quinine
Cocaine	

*Tricyclic antidepressants are listed first, as they remain the number one cause of prescription drug death; the list then follows alphabetically.

Table 7–21 ■ COMMON TOXIC CAUSES OF SEIZURES

Amoxapine	LSD
Anticholinergics	Oral hypoglycemics
Camphor	Parathion
Carbon monoxide	Phencyclidine
Cocaine	Phenothiazines
Ergotamine	Propoxyphene
Insulin	Propranolol
Isoniazid	Strychnine
Lead	Theophylline
Lindane	Tricyclic antidepressants
Lithium	

Table 7–22 ■ TOXINS NOT EFFECTIVELY ABSORBED BY CHARCOAL

Acids
Heavy metals
Alcohols
Hydrocarbons
Alkalis
Iron
Carbamates
Lithium
Cyanide
Organophosphates
Ethylene glycol

Table 7–23 ■ COMMON EMERGENCY ANTIDOTES

POISON	ANTIDOTE	ADULT DOSAGE*
Acetaminophen	*N*-acetylcysteine	140 mg/kg initial oral dose, followed by 70 mg/kg q 4 hr for 17 doses
Atropine	Physostigmine	Initial dose 0.5–2.0 mg IV; children: 0.02 mg/kg
Benzodiazepines	Flumazenil	0.2 mg (2 mL) IV over 15 sec; repeat 0.2 mg IV every minute as necessary; initial dose not to exceed 1 mg
β-Blockers	Glucagon	1 mg/mL ampule; 5–10 mg IV initially
Calcium channel blockers	Calcium	Calcium chloride 10%, 1 g (10 mL) IV over 5 min as initial dose; repeat as necessary in critical patients
Carbon monoxide	Oxygen	Hyperbaric oxygen in critical patients
Cyanide	Amyl nitrite	Pearls every 2 min
	Sodium thiosulfate	25% solution 50 mL IV over 10 min; 1.65 mL/kg for children
	Sodium nitrite	10 mL of 3% solution over 3 min IV; 0.33 mL (10 mg 3% solution)/kg initially for children
Digitalis	Digibind Fab antibodies (antigen-binding fragments)	IV dose of Digibind in critical patients with unknown ingestion: 800 mg (20 vials); dosage if serum digoxin and patient's weight (in kg) are known: the number of vials to administer = [concentration (in ng/mL) × 5.6 × kg]/600
Hydrofluoric acid	Calcium	Calcium gluconate gel or calcium carbonate paste; 10% calcium gluconate 10 mL in 40 mL D_5W via intra-arterial infusion over 4 hr may be indicated for significant digital hydrofluoric acid burns

Iron	Deferoxamine	Initial dose: 40–90 mg/kg IM not to exceed 1 g; 15 mg/kg/hr IV
Lead	Dimercaptosuccinic acid (succimer)	5-d course of 30 mg/kg/d in 3 divided doses; then 14-day course of 20 mg/kg/d divided in 2 doses
Mercury Arsenic Gold	Dimercaprol	5 mg/kg IM as soon as possible
Methyl alcohol Ethylene glycol	Ethyl alcohol	1 mL/kg of 100% ethanol initially in glucose solution; dilute ethanol to 10%; maintain blood level of 100 mg/dL; maintenance dose 0.15 mL/kg/hr (double during dialysis)
Nitrites	Methylene blue	0.2 mL/kg of 1% solution IV over 5 min
Opiates, propoxyphene, diphenoxylate-atropine	Naloxone	2.0 mg IV; 0.1 mg/kg IV for children; repeat as needed
Organophosphates	Pralidoxime (2-PAM) (Protopam Chloride)	Initial dose: 1 g IV; children: 25–50 mg/kg IV
	Atropine	Initial dose: 0.5–2.0 mg IV; 0.05 mg/kg IV initially for children
Tricyclic antidepressants	Sodium bicarbonate	Sodium bicarbonate 1–2 ampules IV; 1 mEq/kg IV bolus for initial dose; IV drip to maintain arterial pH of 7.5

*Dosages listed may require modification according to specific clinical conditions.

Updated and adapted from Haddad LM: Acute poisoning. *In* Bennett JC, Plum F (eds): Cecil Textbook of Medicine, 20th ed. Philadelphia, WB Saunders, 1996; and the American College of Emergency Physicians poster on poisoning, Dallas, Texas, 1980.

Table 7–24 ■ TREATMENT METHODS FOR ELIMINATION OF ABSORBED SUBSTANCE

- Alkaline diuresis
  - Phenobarbital
  - Salicylate
- Hemodialysis
  - Ethylene glycol
  - Lithium
  - Methanol
  - Salicylates
  - Theophylline
- Hemoperfusion
  - Barbiturates
  - Theophylline

Table 7–25 ■ PRECIPITATING FACTORS LEADING TO NON-HEREDITARY, NON-EXERTIONAL RHABDOMYOLYSIS

Alcoholism
Phosphate deficiency
Potassium deficiency
Various bacterial and viral infections
Drugs (e.g., cocaine, amphetamines, neuroleptics)
Toxins (e.g., tetanus, snake venom, toluene)
Direct injury (e.g., crush, electric shock, burns)
Ischemic injury (compression, sickle cell disease*)

*Listed as non-hereditary because the mechanism of injury is not related to a genetic defect in the synthesis of adenosine triphosphate.

Table 7–26 ■ TREATMENT OF RHABDOMYOLYSIS

1. Fluid replacement—be aggressive
2. Urine alkalinization—controversial. Benefit: increased solubility of uric acid, myoglobin. Harmful: HCO_3 could promote calcium deposition
3. Correct hyperkalemia
4. Management of hypocalcemia—avoid IV calcium unless tetany is present
5. Management of hypercalcemia—prevention is key. IV fluid, furosemide
6. Correction of hypoalbuminemia—usually not necessary
7. Disseminated intravascular coagulation—usually resolves spontaneously
8. Dialysis—if necessary
9. Hyperphosphatemia—oral binders, dialysis
10. Fasciotomy—relief of compartment syndromes

higher than 10,000 IU/L. A functionally useful approach is to classify patients into three broad categories: pure exertional rhabdomyolysis, exertional precipitation of rhabdomyolysis in the setting of a genetic defect in the synthesis of adenosine triphosphate (ATP), and a precipitating cause that may or may not be associated with exercise (Table 7–25).

Many patients who previously were thought to have "idiopathic" rhabdomyolysis instead have an inherited enzyme defect in ATP synthesis. The clinical suspicion for an enzymatic defect should be heightened if the patient has more than one episode of rhabdomyolysis or a positive family history of rhabdomyolysis.

If any of the classic metabolic findings (hypercalemia, hyperphosphatemia, hypocalcemia, hypermagnesemia, elevated uric acid level, elevated myoglobin level) of rhabdomyolysis are present, the patient should be admitted and treated aggressively (Table 7–26). Hypocalcemia is due to deposition of calcium phosphate in muscle and other soft tissues early in the course of rhabdomyolysis. The hypocalcemia often coexists with hyperphosphatemia that in part is due to phosphate leak from injured muscle. IV calcium generally should not be given to patients with rhabdomyolysis and hypocalcemia because it could worsen ectopic calcification. The only indications for IV calcium in patients with rhabdomyolysis are severe symptoms of hypocalcemia or severe hyperkalemia.

For more information about this subject, see *Cecil Textbook of Medicine,* 21st edition. Philadelphia, W.B. Saunders Company, 2000. Chapter 99, Rhabdomyolysis, pages 522 to 525.

CHAPTER 8

RENAL AND GENITOURINARY DISEASES

APPROACH TO THE PATIENT WITH RENAL DISEASE

For the kidney to maintain normal volume, electrolyte, and acid-base homeostasis, it is necessary that it receive normal amounts of substrate (normal blood flow) to form urine, has a normal glomerular filtration rate (GFR) and tubular function to form urine, and has a normal excretory path for urine. Thus, renal failure may be broadly classified as pre-renal (those conditions in which the kidney does not receive adequate blood flow), renal (those conditions in which components of the kidney per se do not function normally), and post-renal (those processes that impair normal excretion of urine after it has been formed). Renal failure is also classified according to the rate of progression of functional abnormality as being either *acute* or *chronic*.

Studies of Renal Function

GLOMERULAR FILTRATION RATE. Measuring GFR by collecting a 24-hour urine specimen is adequate in most circumstances and can give a good estimate by

$$C_{Cr} = \frac{U_{Cr} \cdot V}{P_{Cr}}$$

where C_{Cr} is a measure of creatinine clearance, U_{Cr} is urinary concentration of creatinine, V is urine volume for 24 hours, and P_{Cr} is plasma concentration of creatinine. Fractional excretion (FE) does not depend on accurate timed volume collections and is easy to calculate:

$$FE_x = \frac{U_x/P_x}{U_{Cr}/P_{Cr}} \cdot 100$$

where urinary (U) to plasma (P) concentrations of given electrolytes (X) are measured and divided by simultaneously measured urinary and plasma concentration of creatinine.

FE_{Na} generally has a value of less than 1% in pre-renal failure, whereas in syndrome of inappropriate antidiuretic hormone production (SIADH), acute tubular necrosis, or salt-losing nephropathy, the values are greater than 1% and tend to be greater than 3%.

For more information about this subject, see *Cecil Textbook of Medicine,* 21st edition. Philadelphia, W.B. Saunders Company, 2000. Part X: Renal and Genitourinary Diseases, pages 526 to 642.

Table 8–1 ■ INDICATIONS FOR RENAL BIOPSY

Nephrotic syndrome
Systemic disease
  Systemic lupus erythematosus
  Goodpasture's syndrome*
  Wegener's granulomatosis*
  Diabetes mellitus only if atypical course
Hematuria if persistent for >6 mo
Acute renal failure†
Transplanted kidney‡

* If the cause of the process cannot be determined with a renal biopsy.
† If unknown cause and not acute tubular necrosis.
‡ To help manage post-transplant state.

Radiologic Studies

Renal ultrasonography maybe performed to rule out hydronephrosis; to define the nature of renal cysts; to localize calculi; and to guide needles.

INTRAVENOUS PYELOGRAPHY (IVP). IVP is used predominantly to evaluate anatomic features of the renal excretory system.

RETROGRADE PYELOGRAPHY. If adequate definition of the urinary collecting system is not achieved by IVP, then the physician may consider a retrograde pyelogram.

RENAL ARTERIOGRAPHY. Renal arteriography is especially useful for defining the extent and type of fibromuscular dysplasia and is diagnostically helpful in differentiating other stenotic lesions such as arteriosclerosis, arterial dissections, emboli, thromboses, various types of vasculitides, and the effects of trauma.

COMPUTED TOMOGRAPHY (CT). Although CT scanning is not a primary modality to evaluate the kidney, it is especially useful in evaluating a non-functioning kidney; it is being used more and more frequently in the biopsy of renal masses, in which exact localization of small lesions is mandatory.

MAGNETIC RESONANCE IMAGING (MRI). The principal advantage of MRI at the present time is that it does not require radiocontrast material, nor does it expose the patient to radioactive compounds.

RADIONUCLIDE STUDIES. The principal use of radionuclide studies is to measure GFR and renal blood flow.

RENAL BIOPSY. See Table 8–1: for indication for renal biopsy.

For more information about this subject, see *Cecil Textbook of Medicine,* 21st edition. Philadelphia, W.B. Saunders Company, 2000. Chapter 100, Approach to the Patient with Renal Disease, pages 526 to 532.

FLUIDS AND ELECTROLYTES

Volume Disorders

In healthy adults, body water constitutes about 60% of body weight and exists in two compartments: the intracellular fluid (ICF)

Intracellular Water (2/3)		Extracellular Water (1/3)	
		Interstitial (2/3)	Blood (1/3)
±25	Na	140	
±150	K	4.5	
±15	Mg	1.2	
±0.01	Ca	2.4	
±2	Cl	100	
±6	HCO_3	25	
±50	Phos	1.2	

FIGURE 8–1 ■ Relative volumes of various body fluid compartments. In a normally built individual, the total body water content is roughly 60% of body weight. Because adipose tissue has a low concentration of water, the relative water-to-total body weight ratio is lower in obese individuals. The intracellular electrolyte concentrations are in millimoles per liter and are typical values obtained from muscle.

contains two thirds of body water, or 40% of body weight; the extracellular fluid (ECF) contains the remaining one third of total body water, and total blood volume; that is, plasma plus formed elements, constitutes one third of the total ECF volume. This "rule of thirds" for the body fluid compartments is useful in assessing most clinically encountered fluid and electrolyte disorders. Thus, in a healthy 70-kg man, total body water is about 40 L, of which 25 L is intracellular. The functional ECF volume is 15 L, 5 L of

Table 8–2 ■ **THE INTEGRATED VOLUME RESPONSE**

	SYSTEMIC HEMODYNAMIC CHANGES	EXTERNAL SALT AND WATER BALANCE
Response	Tachycardia ↑ Peripheral resistance ↓ Venous capacitance	Thirst Renal Na^+, water retention
Onset	Minutes	Hours
Major activators	Catecholamines ADH Angiotensin II Endothelin-1 Prostaglandin H_2 Thromboxane A_2	Catecholamines Aldosterone ADH
Major inactivators	Prostaglandin E_2 Atriopeptin Nitric acid	Prostaglandin E_2 Atriopeptin

ADH = antidiuretic hormone.

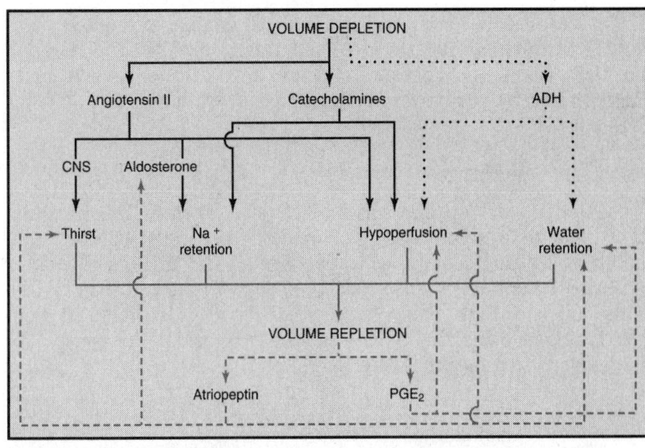

FIGURE 8–2 ■ The volume repletion reaction. The solid and dotted lines originating from "volume depletion" indicate positive mechanisms activated when volume depletion is either modest or severe, respectively. The dashed lines originating with "volume repletion" indicate negative feedback mechanisms. ADH = antidiuretic hormone; CNS = central nervous system; PGE_2 = prostaglandin E_2.

8

which is blood, and because the normal hematocrit is 40 to 45%, total plasma volume is 2.75 to 3.0 L (Fig. 8–1). Protection of the circulatory volume is the single most fundamental characteristic of body fluid homeostasis (Table 8–2; Fig. 8–2).

Volume-expanded states are characterized by an increase in total body water, which is usually accompanied by an increase in total body sodium. Total body salt and water may be increased while the ECF volume is decreased. In other words, certain volume-expanded states are characterized by dissociation between total body salt and water and the ECF volume (Table 8–3).

Table 8–3 ■ DISORDERS OF VOLUME EXCESS

Disturbed Starling Forces	Primary Hormone Excess
(Reduced effective circulating volume; edema formation)	(Increased effective circulating volume)
Systemic venous pressure increases	Primary aldosteronism
Right-sided heart failure	Cushing's syndrome
Constrictive pericarditis	SIADH
Local venous pressure increases	**Primary Renal Sodium Retention**
Left-sided heart failure	(Increased effective circulating volume)
Vena cava obstruction	Renal failure
Portal vein obstruction	
Reduced oncotic pressure	
Nephrotic syndrome	
Decreased albumin synthesis	
Combined disorders	
Cirrhosis	

SIADH = syndrome of inappropriate antidiuretic hormone production.

The recognition and management of volume-expanded states depend on proper identification and treatment of the underlying disorder. The cornerstones of therapy in volume-expanded states characterized by sodium excess include salt restriction and diuretics (Table 8–4).

Osmolality Disturbances

Osmoregulatory mechanisms are activated when ECF hypertonicity is due to a solute that is excluded from cells and therefore produces, at least acutely, cell shrinkage. If the ECF osmolality is increased by solutes, such as urea, which penetrate cell membranes, acute cell shrinkage does not occur to the degree predicted from freezing-point osmolality. The freezing-point osmolality can be approximated from the following formula:

$$\text{Osmolality} = 2[\text{Na}^+] + \frac{\text{glucose}}{18} + \frac{\text{BUN}}{2.8}$$

where the glucose and blood urea nitrogen (BUN) concentrations are expressed as milligrams per deciliter and the serum sodium concentration is expressed as milliequivalents per liter. In normal circumstances, glucose contributes 5.5 mOsm/kg H_2O to the serum osmolality. When hyperglycemia occurs, the effective ECF osmolality rises because glucose entry into cells is limited.

WATER BALANCE. The key elements regulating water balance are summarized in Figure 8–3.

Hypotonic Disorders

In a hypotonic disorder, the ratio of solutes to water in body fluids is reduced, and the serum osmolality and serum sodium are both reduced in parallel. True hypotonicity must be distinguished from apparent hypotonicity in which the *measured* serum sodium is low while the measured serum osmolality is either normal or increased (Table 8–5).

SIADH. In SIADH, hyponatremia occurs as a result of sustained endogenous production and release of antidiuretic hormone (ADH) or ADH-like substances; the ECF volume is normal or increased, and there are no other physiologic or pharmacologic stimuli to ADH release (Table 8–6).

Hypertonic Disorders

A hypertonic disorder is one in which the ratio of solutes to water in total body water is increased. All hypernatremic states are hypertonic. In some hypertonic disorders, such as uncontrollled hyperglycemia, the increase in effective ECF osmolaltiy is due to non-sodium solutes (Table 8–7).

Disturbances in Potassium Balance

Hypokalemia ($K^+ < 3.5$ mEq/L) (Table 8–8) and hyperkalemia ($K^+ > 5.5$ mEq/L) (Table 8–9) are common in the practice of medicine. Whereas the plasma potassium concentration is influenced by total body potassium stores, it should be recognized that factors influencing the distribution of potassium between extracellu-

Table 8–4 ■ CHARACTERISTICS OF COMMONLY USED DIURETICS

DIURETIC	PRIMARY EFFECT	SECONDARY EFFECT	COMPLICATIONS
Proximal Diuretics			
Acetazolamide	$\downarrow$ Na^+/H^+ exchange	$\uparrow$ K^+ loss, $\uparrow$ HCO_3^- loss	Hypokalemic, hyperchloremic acidosis
Metolazone	$\downarrow$ Na^+ absorption	$\uparrow$ K^+ loss, $\uparrow$ Cl^- loss	Hypokalemic alkalosis
Loop Diuretics			
Furosemide Bumetanide Ethacrynic acid	$\downarrow$ Na^+, K^+, $2Cl^-$ absorption	$\uparrow$ K^+ loss, $\uparrow$ H^+ secretion	Hypokalemic alkalosis Hearing deficits, hypomagnesemia
Early Distal Diuretics			
Thiazide Metolazone	$\downarrow$ NaCl absorption	$\uparrow$ K^+ loss, $\uparrow$ H^+ secretion	Hypokalemic alkalosis Hyperglycemia, hyperuricemia
Late Distal Diuretics			
Aldosterone antagonists Spironolactone Non-aldosterone antagonists Triamterene Amiloride	$\downarrow$ Na^+ absorption	$\downarrow$ K^+ loss, $\downarrow$ H^+ secretion	Hypokalemic acidosis

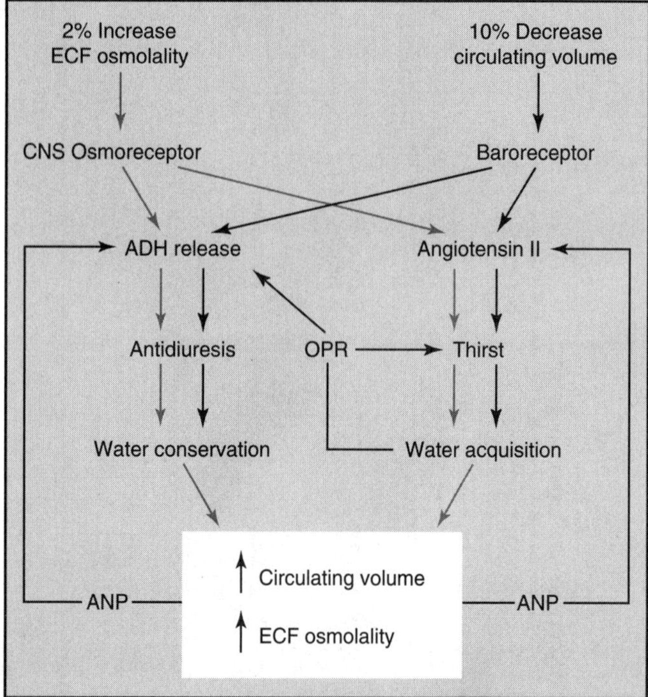

FIGURE 8–3 ■ The water repletion reaction. The white lines are positive water conservation processes activated by osmolality. The red lines are water conservation processes that are volume-activated. The black lines indicate negative feedback. ECF = extracellular fluid; CNS = central nervous system; ADH = antidiuretic hormone; ANP = atrial natriuretic peptide; OPR = oropharyngeal reflex. (From Reeves WB. Andreoli TE: The posterior pituitary and water metabolism. *In* Wilson JD. Foster DW [eds]: Williams Textbook of Endocrinology, 8th ed. Philadelphia, WB Saunders, 1992.)

lar and intracellular spaces are important determinants of plasma potassium concentration (Table 8–9). A rough rule of thumb is to recognize that serum potassium level rises by 0.6 mEq/L with metabolic decrease in plasma pH of 0.1 unit.

Disturbances in Acid-Base Balance

The relation between pH, bicarbonate, and carbonic acid concentrations in ECF may be expressed according to the familiar Henderson-Hasselbalch equation:

$$pH = pK + \log \frac{HCO_3^-}{H_2CO_3}$$

where pK is the carbonic acid dissociation constant, HCO_3 is the plasma bicarbonate concentration, and H_2CO_3 is the plasma carbonic acid concentration. The H_2CO_3 concentration is given by

Table 8–5 ■ DISTINCTION BETWEEN APPARENT AND REAL HYPOTONICITY

CONDITION	MEASURED SERUM (Na)	MEASURED SERUM OSMOLALITY
True hypotonicity	↓	↓
Increased non-sodium ECF solutes		
Hyperglycemia	↓	↑
Mannitol administration	↓	↑
Increased non-sodium ECF and ICF solutes		
Ethanol	Normal	↑
Ethylene glycol	Normal	↑
Methanol	Normal	↑
Isopropyl alcohol	Normal	↑
Laboratory artifact		
Hyperlipemia	↓	Normal
Hyperproteinemia	↓	Normal

ECF = extracellular fluid; ICF = intracellular fluid.

8

Table 8–6 ■ MAJOR CAUSES OF SYNDROME OF INAPPROPRIATE ANTIDIURETIC HORMONE PRODUCTION

Malignant Neoplasia

Carcinoma: bronchogenic, pancreatic, duodenal, ureteral, prostatic, bladder
Lymphoma and leukemia
Thymoma and mesothelioma

Central Nervous System Disorders

Trauma
Infection
Tumors
Porphyria

Pulmonary Disorders

Tuberculosis
Pneumonia
Fungal infections
Lung abscesses
Ventilators with positive pressure

Drug-Induced

Desmopressin
Oxytocin
Vincristine
Chlorpropamide
Nicotine
Cyclophosphamide
Morphine
Amitriptyline
Selective serotonin reuptake inhibitors

Table 8–7 ■ MAJOR CAUSES OF HYPERNATREMIA

IMPAIRED THIRST

Coma
Essential hypernatremia

SOLUTE DIURESIS

Osmotic diuresis: diabetic ketoacidosis, non-ketotic hyperosmolar coma, mannitol administration

EXCESSIVE WATER LOSSES

Renal
- Pituitary diabetes insipidus
- Nephrogenic diabetes insipidus

Extrarenal
- Sweating

COMBINED DISORDERS

Coma plus hypertonic nasogastric feeding

$\alpha PaCO_2$, where α is the CO_2 solubility constant and has a value of 0.0301 and $PaCO_2$ is the arterial carbon dioxide tension. Therefore the Henderson-Hasselbach equation becomes

$$pH = 6.1 + \log \frac{HCO_3^-}{0.03\ PCO_2}$$

The arterial pH is determined by the ratio of the bicarbonate–carbonic acid buffer system, as expressed in the Henderson-Hasselbalch equation (Fig. 8–4; Table 8–10).

Table 8–8 ■ MAJOR CAUSES OF HYPOKALEMIA

EXCESS RENAL LOSS

Mineralocorticoid excess
Bartter's syndrome
Diuresis
- Diuretics with a pre–late distal locus
- Osmotic diuresis

Chronic metabolic alkalosis
Antibiotics
- Carbenicillin
- Gentamicin
- Amphotericin B

Renal tubular acidosis
- Distal, gradient-limited
- Proximal

Liddle's syndrome
Gitelman's syndrome
Acute leukemia
Ureterosigmoidostomy

GASTROINTESTINAL LOSSES

Vomiting
Diarrhea, particularly secretory diarrheas

ECF → ICF SHIFTS

Acute alkalosis
Hypokalemic periodic paralysis
Barium ingestion
Insulin therapy
Vitamin B_{12} therapy
Thyrotoxicosis (rarely)

INADEQUATE INTAKE

EDF = extracellular fluid; ICF = intracellular fluid.

Table 8–9 ■ MAJOR CAUSES OF HYPERKALEMIA

Diminished Renal Excretion	Transcellular Shifts
Reduced glomerular filtration rate	Acidosis
Acute oliguric renal failure	β-Adrenergic blockade
Chronic renal failure	Cell destruction
Reduced tubular secretion	Trauma, burns
Addison's disease	Rhabdomyolysis
Hyporeninemic hypoaldosteronism	Hemolysis
Potassium-sparing diuretics	Tumor lysis
Voltage-dependent renal tubular acidosis	Hyperkalemic periodic paralysis
Trimethoprim-sulfamethoxazole	Diabetic hyperglycemia
Angiotensin-converting enzyme inhibitors	Insulin dependence plus aldosterone lack
	Depolarizing muscle paralysis
	Succinylcholine

8

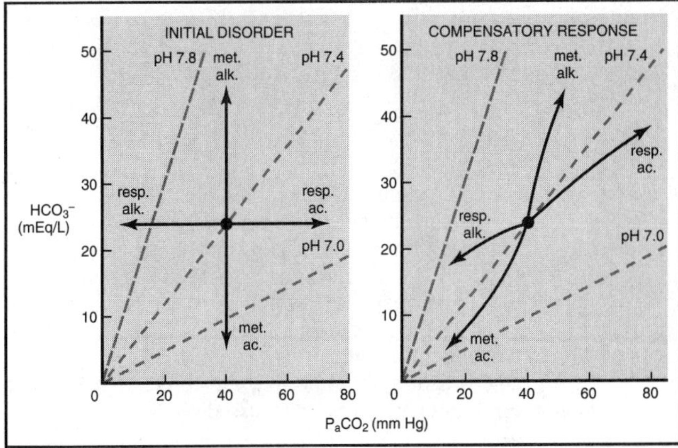

FIGURE 8–4 ■ Schematic frame of reference for considering acid-base disturbances. The dashed lines are the pH isobars for pH values of 7.8, 7.4, and 7.0 computed from the Henderson-Hasselbalch equation for given combinations of arterial bicarbonate (HCO_3^-) values (vertical axes) and arterial carbon dioxide ($Paco_2$) tensions (horizontal axes). The graph on the left shows the initial derangement in HCO_3^- concentrations in metabolic acidosis and metabolic alkalosis and the initial $Paco_2$ derangement in respiratory acidosis and respiratory alkalosis. Note that each of the four changes in either HCO_3^- or $Paco_2$ tends to displace the arterial pH from the pH 7.4 isobar. The graph on the right, labeled compensatory response, indicates the general trend of pH. HCO_3^- and $Paco_2$ changes were actually observed in the four primary acid-base disturbances: respiratory acidosis, respiratory alkalosis, metabolic acidosis, and metabolic alkalosis. Respiratory acidosis and alkalosis are accompanied by compensatory renal HCO_3^- retention and loss, respectively. Metabolic acidosis and alkalosis are accompanied by compensatory hyperventilation and hypoventilation, respectively. Note that the compensatory response in each of the four acid-base disorders tends to restore arterial pH values toward the pH 7.4 isobar.

Table 8–10 ■ RELATIONSHIPS BETWEEN HCO_3^- AND $P{CO_2}$ IN SIMPLE ACID-BASE DISORDERS

CONDITION	PRIMARY DISTURBANCE	PREDICTED RESPONSE
Metabolic acidosis	↓ HCO_3^-	$\Delta P{CO_2}$ (↓) = 1 − $1.4\Delta HCO_3^-$*
Metabolic alkalosis	↑ HCO_3^-	$\Delta P{CO_2}$ (↑) = 0.4 − $0.9\Delta HCO_3^-$*
Respiratory acidosis	↑ $P{CO_2}$	Acute: ΔHCO_3^- (↑) = $0.1\Delta P{CO_2}$ Chronic: ΔHCO_3^- (↑) = 0.25 − $0.55\Delta P{CO_2}$
Respiratory alkalosis	↓ $P{CO_2}$	Acute: ΔHCO_3^- (↓) = 0.2 − $0.25\Delta P{CO_2}$ Chronic: ΔHCO_3^- (↓) = 0.4 − $0.5\Delta P{CO_2}$

* After at least 12 to 24 hours.
From Hamm L: Mixed acid-base disorders. *In* Kokko JP, Tannen RL (eds): Fluids and Electrolytes, 3rd ed. Philadelphia, WB Saunders, 1996, p 344.

The *urinary anion gap,* defined as

$$\text{Urinary anion gap} = (Na^+ + K^+) - Cl^-$$

is useful in evaluating patients with hyperchloremic acidosis. The test provides an approximate index to urinary NH_4^+ excretion, as measured by a negative urinary anion gap, that is, urinary Na^+ + K^+ is less than urinary Cl^-. Thus, in hyperchloremic metabolic acidosis, a normal renal response would be a negative urinary anion gap, generally in the range of 30 to 50 mEq/L. In such an instance, the hyperchloremic acidosis is probably due to gastrointestinal losses rather than a renal lesion. In contrast, a positive urinary anion gap implies a renal tubular disorder.

Metabolic Acidosis

The major causes of metabolic acidosis are detailed in Table 8–11.

The major causes of increased plasma bicarbonate concentration are noted in Table 8–12.

For more information about this subject, see *Cecil Textbook of Medicine,* 21st edition. Philadelphia, W.B. Saunders Company, 2000. Chapter 102, Fluids and Electrolytes, pages 540 to 567.

ACUTE RENAL FAILURE

Many serious problems associated with acute kidney failure arise from the patient's limited capacity to achieve a balance between the intake and excretion of water and minerals and the accumulation of metabolic byproducts (chiefly from protein) that cause the symptoms of uremia. These two limitations may cause the serious complications of acute renal failure (ARF), including pulmonary edema, hyponatremia, hyperkalemia, acidosis, hyperphosphatemia,

Table 8–11 ■ MAJOR CAUSES OF METABOLIC ACIDOSIS

NORMAL ANION GAP	INCREASED ANION GAP
Renal Causes	**Endogenous Causes**
Bicarbonate loss	Uremic acidosis
Proximal RTA, type II	Lactic acidosis
Dilutional acidosis	Ketoacidosis
Carbonic anhydrase inhibitors	β-Hydroxybutyric acidosis
Primary hyperparathyroidism	**Exogenous Causes**
Failure of bicarbonate regeneration	Salicylates
Distral RTA, type I	Paraldehyde
Distal RTA, type IV	Methanol
Diuretics: amiloride, spironolactones, triamterene	Ethylene glycol
Gastrointestinal Causes	
Diarrheal states	
Small bowel drainage	
Ureterosigmoidostomy	
Acidifying Salts	
Ammonium chloride	
Lysine hydrochloride	
Arginine hydrochloride	
Parenteral hyperalimentation	

RTA = renal tubular acidosis.

anorexia, nausea, vomiting, and other uremic symptoms (Table 8–13). Evaluation of urine samples may point to a diagnosis of ARF (Table 8–14).

After initiation of ARF, four potential factors may depress renal function: vasoconstriction, decreased glomerular permeability, tubular obstruction, and backleak of filtrate. Clinical evidence of recovery may not be observed for days or weeks (average, 10 to 14 days) (Fig. 8–5; Table 8–15).

Treatment of ARF includes correction of reversible causes, prevention of additional injury, use of metabolic support during the maintenance and recovery phases of the syndrome, and attempts to convert oliguric to non-oliguric renal failure (Table 8–16). Maintaining fluid balance is crucial with daily measurements of weight. Peritoneal or hemodialysis should be performed if more conserva-

Table 8–12 ■ MAJOR CAUSES OF INCREASED PLASMA BICARBONATE CONCENTRATION

ECF volume contraction
Potassium depletion
Hypercapnia
Increased distal salt delivery
Mineralocorticoid excess

ECF = extracellular fluid.

Table 8–13 ■ CAUSES OF ACUTE RENAL FAILURE

PRIMARY DISORDER	CLINICAL EXAMPLES
	PRE-RENAL
Hypovolemia	Hemorrhage, skin losses (burns, sweating), gastrointestinal losses (diarrhea, vomiting), renal losses (diuretics, glycosuria), extravascular pooling (peritonitis, burns)
Ineffective arterial volume	Congestive heart failure, cardiac arrhythmias, sepsis, anaphylaxis, liver failure
Arterial occlusion	Bilateral arterial thromboembolism, thromboembolism of a solitary kidney, aortic or renal artery aneurysm
	POST-RENAL
Ureteral obstruction	Bilateral or in a solitary kidney (calculi, neoplasm, clot, retroperitoneal fibrosis, iatrogenic)
Urethral obstruction	Prostatitis, clot, calculus, neoplasm, foreign object
Venous occlusion	Bilateral or a solitary kidney (renal vein thrombosis, neoplasm, iatrogenic)
	INTRARENAL/INTRINSIC
Vascular	Vasculitis, microangiopathy, malignant hypertension, vasopressors, eclampsia, hyperviscosity states, hypercalcemia, iodinated radiocontrast agents
Glomerulus	Acute glomerulonephritis
Tubular injury	
Ischemia	Profound hypotension, post renal transplant, vasopressors, microvascular constriction, sepsis
Endogenous proteins	Hemoglobinuria, myoglobinuria, light-chain myeloma
Intratubular crystals	Uric acid, oxalate, sulfonamides, pyridium
Tubulointerstitial inflammation	Interstitial nephritis caused by drugs, infection, radiation
Nephrotoxins	Antibiotics (aminoglycosides, cephaloridine, amphotericin B); metals (mercury, bismuth, uranium, arsenic, silver, cadmium, iron, antimony); solvents (carbon tetrachloride, ethylene glycol, tetrachloroethylene); iodinated contrast agents; antineoplastic agents (bleomycin, cisplatin)

Table 8–14 ■ URINE INDICES IN ACUTE RENAL FAILURE

LABORATORY TEST	PRE-RENAL	ACUTE TUBULAR INJURY
Urine osmolality (mOsm/kg H_2O)	>500	<350
Urine sodium (mEq/L)	<20	>40
Urine/plasma creatinine ratio	>40	<20
Fractional sodium excretion*	<1	>1

$$* \frac{\text{Urine [Na]/serum [Na]}}{\text{Urine [creatinine]/serum [creatinine]}} \times 100.$$

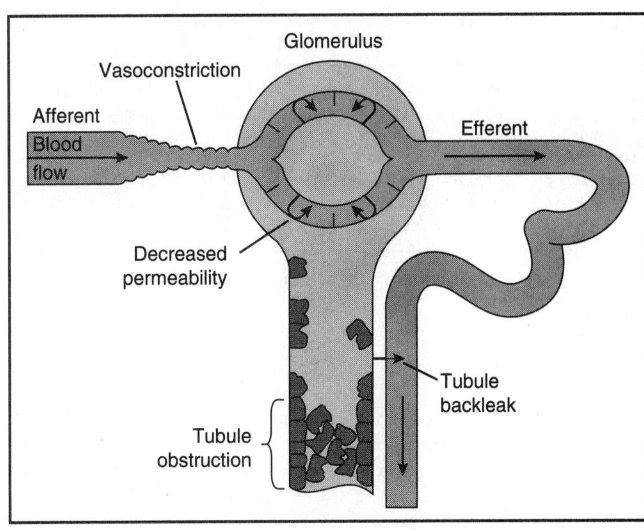

FIGURE 8–5 ■ Potential mechanisms causing oliguria in patients with acute renal failure.

8

Table 8–15 ■ DIAGNOSTIC CLUES TO THE CAUSE OF ACUTE RENAL FAILURE

PRIMARY DISORDER	URINALYSIS	CLINICAL FINDINGS
	PRE-RENAL	
Hypovolemia	Hyaline casts, no RBCs, or WBCs, low FE_{Na}	Rapid weight loss, postural hypotension
Ineffective arterial volume	Hyaline casts, no RBCs, or WBCs, low Fe_{Na}	Weight gain, edema, normal or low blood pressure
Arterial occlusion	Hyaline casts, rare to many RBCs	Occasional flank or low back pain
	POST-RENAL	
Ureteral obstruction	WBCs if infected, crystals or RBCs	Flank pain radiating into the groin
Urethral	WBCs and RBCs	Urethral pain
Venous occlusion	Proteinuria, hematuria	Occasional flank pain
	RENAL	
Vascular	Granular casts, proteinuria, RBCs and WBCs	Systemic illness suggesting vasculitis, hypertension
Glomerulus	RBC casts, granular casts, RBCs, WBCs, proteinuria	Systemic illness, hypertension
Tubular	Granular casts, tubular cells, RBCs, WBCs	Hypotension, sepsis

FE_{Na} = fractional sodium excretion; RBCs = red blood cell; WBCs = white blood cells.

Table 8–16 ■ GUIDELINES FOR TREATING ACUTE RENAL FAILURE

General	Avoid drugs that reduce renal blood flow (e.g., NSAIDs) and/or are nephrotoxic (e.g., radiocontrast agent)
Pre-renal	Restore blood pressure and vascular volume
Post-renal	Urologic evaluation
Intrinsic	Prevent hypotension and try to convert oliguria to non-oliguria; if edematous, try furosemide, 80–100 mg, but if non-edematous, try saline 500 mL intravenously

NSAIDs = non-steroidal anti-inflammatory drugs.

tive measures fail to prevent hyperkalemia, severe acidosis, volume overload, or uremia with urea nitrogen concentration greater than 100 mg/dL.

For more information about this subject, see *Cecil Textbook of Medicine,* 21st edition. Philadelphia, W.B. Saunders Company, 2000. Chapter 103, Acute Renal Failure, pages 567 to 571.

CHRONIC RENAL FAILURE

Chronic renal failure (CRF) is a progressive disease characterized by an increasing inability of the kidney to maintain normal levels of products of protein metabolism (such as urea), normal blood pressure and hematocrit, and sodium, water, potassium, and acid-base balance (Table 8–17). Once serum creatinine in an adult reaches about 3 mg/dL and no factors in the pathogenesis of the renal disease are reversible, the renal disease is highly likely to progress to end-stage renal disease (ESRD) over a very variable period (from a few years to as many as 20 to 25 years).

It is sometimes difficult to differentiate between acute and chronic renal failure when a patient with azotemia and an elevated

Table 8–17 ■ CAUSES OF CHRONIC RENAL FAILURE

- Diabetic glomerulosclerosis*
- Hypertensive nephrosclerosis*
- Glomerular disease
  - Glomerulonephritis
  - Amyloidosis, light-chain disease*
  - SLE, Wegener's granulomatosis
- Tubulointerstitial disease
  - Reflux nephropathy (chronic pyelonephritis)
  - Analgesic nephropathy (stones, BPH)
  - Myeloma kidney*
- Vascular disease
  - Scleroderma*
  - Vasculitis*
  - Renovascular renal failure (ischemic nephropathy)
  - Atheroembolic renal disease*
- Cystic diseases
  - Autosomal dominant polycystic kidney disease
  - Medullary cystic kidney disease

SLE = systemic lupus erythematosus; BPH = benign prostatic hypertrophy.
* Systemic disease involving the kidney.

serum creatinine concentration is recognized for the first time. (Table 8–18). Acute-on-chronic renal failure is a common circumstance, and reversible factors should always be sought when a diagnosis of CRF is made or when a patient with CRF shows unexpected rapid deterioration in renal function (Table 8–19).

For more information about this subject, see *Cecil Textbook of Medicine,* 21st edition. Philadelphia, W.B. Saunders Company, 2000. Chapter 104, Chronic Renal Failure, pages 571 to 578.

Dialysis can be performed on acute or chronic renal failure patients and is done either by employing an artificial membrane system using extracorporeal blood (hemodialysis) or by using peritoneal membrane (peritoneal dialysis). Hemodialysis uses blood pumps for ultrafiltration, whereas peritoneal dialysis uses the osmotic forces of high concentrations of glucose to remove water. Hemodialysis is considered more efficient, whereas peritoneal dialysis is considered somewhat simpler and less expensive. Patient selection for these two different forms of treatment is usually decided by special needs of the patient and the nephrologist's clinical judgment as to which treatment will be best tolerated.

Despite improved technologies, the annual mortality rates in the United States still average around 20% per year.

For more information about this subject, see *Cecil Textbook of Medicine,* 21st edition. Philadelphia, W.B. Saunders Company, 2000. Chapter 105, Treatment of Irreversible Renal Failure, pages 578–582.

GLOMERULAR DISORDERS

The mechanisms of glomerular injury are quite varied. Although certain common mechanisms may underlie the hematuria and proteinuria (e.g., loss of the glomerular charge barrier), the nature of the processes initiating this damage differs.

Several findings indicate the presence of a glomerular origin of any parenchymal renal disease. They include erythrocyte casts and/or dysmorphic erythrocytes in the urinary sediment and the presence of large amounts of albuminuria.

The Nephrotic Syndrome

The *nephrotic syndrome* is classically defined by albuminuria in amounts of more than 3.0 to 3.5 g/day accompanied by hypoalbuminemia, edema, and hyperlipidemia (Tables 8–20 and 8–21).

Glomerulonephritis

Rapidly progressive glomerulonephritis (RPGN) may progress to renal failure in a matter of weeks to months, with the presence of extensive extracapillary proliferation (i.e., crescent formation) (Table 8–22).

Anti-GBM disease (Table 8–23) is caused by circulating antibodies directed against the non-collagenous domain of type IV collagen that damages the GBM. This leads to an inflammatory response, breaks in the GBM, and the formation of a proliferative and often crescentic glomerulonephritis. If the anti-GBM antibodies cross-react with and damage the basement membrane of pulmonary capillaries, the patient develops pulmonary hemorrhage and hemo-

Table 8–18 ■ FEATURES OF CHRONIC RENAL FAILURE

Early

Hypertension
Proteinuria; elevated BUN or SCr
Nephrotic syndrome
Recurrent nephritic syndrome
Gross hematuria

Late (GFR < 15 mL/min, BUN > 60 mg/dL) ("Uremia")

Cardiac failure
Anemia
Serositis
Confusion, coma
Anorexia
Vomiting
Peripheral neuropathy
Hyperkalemia
Metabolic acidosis

BUN = blood urea nitrogen; SCr = serum creatinine; GFR = glomerular filtration rate.

Table 8–19 ■ POTENTIALLY REVERSIBLE FACTORS IN CHRONIC RENAL FAILURE

Pre-Renal Failure

ECF volume depletion
Cardiac failure
NSAIDs, ACE inhibitors

Post-Renal Failure

Obstructive uropathy

Intrinsic Renal Failure

Severe hypertension
Acute pyelonephritis
Drug nephrotoxicity (ATN, AIN, vasculitis)
Acute interstitial nephritis
Radiocontrast agents (ATN)
Hypercalcemia

Vascular

Renovascular
Renal vein thrombosis*
Atheroembolism

Miscellaneous

Hypoadrenalism
Hypothyroidism

* In nephrotic syndrome.

ECF = extracellular fluid; NSAIDs = non-steroidal anti-inflammatory drugs; ACE = angiotensin-converting enzyme; ATN = acute tubular necrosis. AIN = acute interstitial nephritis.

Table 8–20 ■ CAUSES OF THE NEPHROTIC SYNDROME

IDIOPATHIC OR PRIMARY NEPHROTIC SYNDROME	INCIDENCE (%)
Minimal change disease	10–15
Focal segmental glomerulosclerosis	20–25
Membranous nephropathy	25–30
Membranoproliferative glomerulonephritis	5
Other proliferative and sclerosing glomerulonephritides	15–30

ptysis. The association of anti-GBM antibody–mediated damage to the kidneys and lungs is called Goodpasture's syndrome.

8

Systemic Lupus Erythematosus

Renal involvement may greatly influence the course and therapy of systemic lupus erythematosus (SLE). The incidence of clinically detectable renal disease varies from 15 to 75% (Table 8–24).

For more information about this subject, see *Cecil Textbook of Medicine,* 21st edition. Philadelphia, W.B. Saunders Company, 2000. Chapter 106, Glomerular Disorders, pages 586 to 594.

TUBULOINTERSTITIAL DISEASES AND TOXIC NEPHROPATHIES

The tubules and interstitium of the kidney are separate structural and functional compartments that are intimately related, and any injury intially involving either of them will inevitably be associated with damage to the other, hence the term *tubulointerstitial diseases* (TIN).

As a rule, TIN is categorized as being *primary* or *secondary* in origin (Table 8–25). *Primary* TIN is defined as injury that affects the tubules and interstitium without significant involvement of the glomeruli or renal vasculature, at least in the early stages of the disease. *Secondary* TIN is defined as tubulointerstitial injury caused by diseases that initally affect the glomeruli or renal vasculature. Drugs have emerged as the most common cause of acute TIN (Table 8–26). Chronic TIN is the unifying features of an assorted group of diverse diseases (Table 8–27).

For more information about this subject, see *Cecil Textbook of Medicine,* 21st edition. Philadelphia, W.B. Saunders Company, 2000. Chapter 107, Tubulointerstitial Diseases and Toxic Nephropathies, pages 594 to 600.

OBSTRUCTIVE UROPATHY

"Obstructive uropathy" refers to the structural or functional changes in the urinary tract that impede the normal flow of urine. Deleterious effects of these obstructions are noted in Figure 8–6.

Clinical manifestations of obstructive uropathy depend on the location (upper or lower urinary tract), degree (complete or partial), and duration (acute or chronic) of the obstruction (Table 8–28).

The diagnostic approach to obstructive uropathy depends on the

Table 8–21 ■ NEPHROTIC SYNDROME ASSOCIATED WITH SPECIFIC CAUSES ("SECONDARY" NEPHROTIC SYNDROME)

Systemic Diseases

Diabetes mellitus
Systemic lupus erythematosus and other collagen diseases
Amyloidosis (amyloid AL-/ or AA-associated)
Vasculitic-immunologic diseases (mixed cryoglobulinemia, Wegener's granulomatosis, rapidly progressive glomerulonephritis, polyarteritis, Henoch-Schönlein purpura, sarcoidosis, Goodpasture's syndrome)

Infections

Bacterial (post-streptococcal, congenital and secondary syphilis, subacute bacterial endocarditis, shunt nephritis)
Viral (hepatitis B, hepatitis C, HIV infection, infectious mononucleosis, cytomegalovirus infection)
Parasitic (malaria, toxoplasmosis, schistosomiasis, filariasis)

Medication-Related

Gold, mercury, and the heavy metals
Penicillamine
Non-steroidal anti-inflammatory drugs
Lithium
Paramethadione, trimethadione
Captopril
"Street" heroin
Others—probenecid, chlorpropamide, rifampin, tolbutamide, phenindione

Allergens, Venoms, and Immunizations Associated with Neoplasms

Hodgkin's lymphoma and leukemia-lymphomas (with minimal change lesion)
Solid tumors (with membranous nephropathy)

Hereditary and Metabolic Disease

Alport's syndrome
Fabry's disease
Sickle cell disease
Congenital (Finnish type) nephrotic syndrome
Familial nephrotic syndrome
Nail-patella syndrome
Partial lipodystrophy

Other

Pregnancy-related (includes preeclampsia)
Transplant rejection
Serum sickness
Accelerated hypertensive nephrosclerosis
Unilateral renal artery stenosis
Massive obesity—sleep apnea
Reflux nephropathy

AL = primary amyloidosis; AA = secondary amyloidosis.

symptoms and the clinical findings of patients with asymptomatic renal insufficiency, renal colic, or ARF and anuria (Fig. 8–7).

For more information about this subject, see *Cecil Textbook of Medicine,* 21st edition. Philadelphia, W.B. Saunders Company, 2000. Chapter 108, Obstructive Uropathy, pages 600 to 605.

Table 8–22 ■ CLASSIFICATION OF RAPIDLY PROGRESSIVE ("CRESCENTIC") GLOMERULONEPHRITIS

Primary

Type I: Anti–glomerular basement membrane antibody disease (with pulmonary disease—Goodpasture's syndrome)
Type II: Immune complex–mediated
Type III: Pauci-immune (usually antineutrophil cytoplasmic antibody–positive)

Secondary

Membranoproliferative glomerulonephritis
IgA nephropathy—Henoch-Schönlein purpura
Post-streptococcal glomerulonephritis
Systemic lupus erythematosus
Polyarteritis nodosa, hypersensitivity angiitis

RENAL TUBULAR DISORDERS

Renal tubular disorders represent a group of conditions in which the renal tubular reabsorption of either ions or organic solutes is diminished, resulting in excessive amounts of either substance in the urine. The defect can be characterized by the nephron segment affected. Many of these disorders are inherited, although some are acquired and appear to involve the loss or formation of a defective transport carrier. The clinical syndromes associated with nephron defects are summarized in Table 8–29.

For more information about this subject, see *Cecil Textbook of Medicine,* 21st edition. Philadelphia, W.B. Saunders Company, 2000. Chapter 109, Specific Renal Tubular Disorders, pages 605 to 610.

Table 8–23 ■ COMMON RENAL DISEASES WITH ASSOCIATED PULMONARY DISEASES

DISEASE	MARKER
Goodpasture's syndrome	+ Anti–glomerular basement membrane antibodies
Wegener's granulomatosis, polyarteritis	+ Antineutrophil cytoplasmic antibodies
Systemic lupus erythematosus	+ Anti-DNA antibodies, low complement
Nephrotic syndrome, renal vein thrombosis, pulmonary embolus	+ Lung scan
Pneumonia with immune complex glomerulonephritis	− Low complement, circulating immune complexes
Uremic lung	− Elevated blood urea nitrogen and creatinine levels

Table 8–24 ■ WORLD HEALTH ORGANIZATION CLASSIFICATION OF LUPUS NEPHRITIS

CLASS	CLINICAL FEATURES
I. Normal glomeruli (LM, IF, EM)	No renal findings
II. (a) Mesangial disease normal by LM with mesangial deposits by IF and/or EM (b) Mesangial hypercellularity with mesangial deposits	Mild clinical renal disease; minimally active urinary sediment; mild to moderate proteinuria (never nephrotic) but may have active serology
III. Focal proliferative glomerulonephritis	More active sediment changes; often active serology; increased proteinuria (~25% nephrotic); hypertension may be present; some evolve into class IV pattern
IV. Diffuse proliferative glomerulonephritis	Most severe renal involvement with active sediment, hypertension, heavy proteinuria (frequent nephrotic syndrome), often reduced glomerular filtration rate; serology very active
V. Membraneous glomerulonephritis	Significant proteinuria (often nephrotic) with less active lupus serology

LM = light microscopy; IF = immunofluorescence; EM = electron microscopy.

DIABETIC NEPHROPATHY

Diabetes is the leading cause of CRF in the United States. About one third of patients who develop chronic renal failure in the United States do so because of diabetes. The natural course of the disease is depicted in Figure 8–8.

For more information about this subject, see *Cecil Textbook of Medicine,* 21st edition. Philadelphia, W.B. Saunders Company, 2000. Chapter 110, Diabetes and the Kidney, pages 610 to 613.

URINARY TRACT INFECTIONS AND PYELONEPHRITIS

Urinary tract infection (UTI) is a broad term that encompasses both asymptomatic microbial colonization of the urine and symptomatic infection with microbial invasion and inflammation of urinary tract structures. Common manifestations of UTI are noted in Table 8–30. Acute uncomplicated episodes of symptomatic infection (bacterial cystitis or urethritis) are treated most effectively with a short course of oral therapy (Table 8–31). Three-day treatment is recommended because it is more effective than single-dose therapy and is as effective as 7 to 10 days of treatment.

For more information about this subject, see *Cecil Textbook of Medicine,* 21st edition. Philadelphia, W.B. Saunders Company, 2000. Chapter 111, Urinary Tract Infections and Pyelonephritis, pages 613 to 617.

Table 8–25 ■ MORPHOLOGIC FEATURES OF ACUTE AND CHRONIC TUBULOINTERSTITIAL NEPHRITIS

MORPHOLOGY	ATN	ATIN	CTIN
Gross Renal Features			
Size	Enlarged	Enlarged	Small
Surface	Normal	Normal	Scarred
Echogenicity	Normal	Normal	Increased
Microscopic Features			
Interstitium			
Edema	+→++	+→++++	±→++
Fibrosis	None	Unusual	Severe
Cell infiltrates	Few	Prominent	Modest
Tubules			
Cells	Necrotic	Injured	Atrophy/ hypertrophy
Basement membrane	±→++	+→+++	Thickened
Shape	Preserved	Preserved	Atrophy/ dilation
Glomeruli			
Capillaries	Normal	Normal → MCD	Sclerosis
Capsule	Normal	Normal	Thickened/ fibrosed
Vasculature			
Endothelium	Normal → swollen	Normal	Normal
Wall	Normal	Normal	Variable sclerosis

ATN = acute tubular necrosis; ATIN = acute tubulointerstitial nephritis; CTIN = chronic tubulointerstitial nephritis; MCD = minimal change disease; + indicates presence, and the greater the number of + symbols, the more severe the morphologic feature.

Table 8–26 ■ PRINCIPAL CONDITIONS ASSOCIATED WITH ACUTE TUBULOINTERSTITIAL DISEASE

DRUGS

Antibiotics (penicillins, cephalosporins, rifampin)
Sulfonamides (cotrimoxazole, sulfamethoxazole)
Non-steroidal anti-inflammatory drugs (propionic acid derivatives)
Miscellaneous (phenytoin, thiazides, allopurinol, cimetidine)

INFECTIONS

Invasion of renal parenchyma
Reaction to systemic infections (streptococcal, diphtheria, Hantavirus)

SYSTEMIC DISEASES

Immune-mediated (lupus, transplanted kidney, cryoglobulinemias)
Metabolic (urate, oxalate)
Neoplastic (lymphoproliferative diseases)

IDIOPATHIC

Table 8–27 ■ CONDITIONS ASSOCIATED WITH CHRONIC TUBULOINTERSTITIAL DISEASE

DRUGS

Analgesics, non-steroidal anti-inflammatory drugs, cisplatin, cyclosporine, lithium

HEAVY METALS

Lead, cadmium

VASCULAR DISEASES

Hypertension, vasculitis, embolic disorders, radiation nephritis

URINARY TRACT OBSTRUCTION

Vesicoureteral reflux, mechanical

METABOLIC DISORDERS

Urate, oxalate, cystinosis

IMMUNE DISEASES

Systemic lupus erythematosus, allograft rejection, Goodpasture's syndrome, amyloidosis

GRANULOMATOUS DISEASES

Sarcoidosis, Wegener's granulomatosis

INFECTIONS

Bacterial, mycobacterial, viral, fungal

HEMATOLOGIC DISEASES

Plasma cell dyscrasias, sickle hemoglobinopathies, lymphomas

ENDEMIC

Balkan nephropathy

HEREDITARY

Cystic diseases, Alport's syndrome

IDIOPATHIC

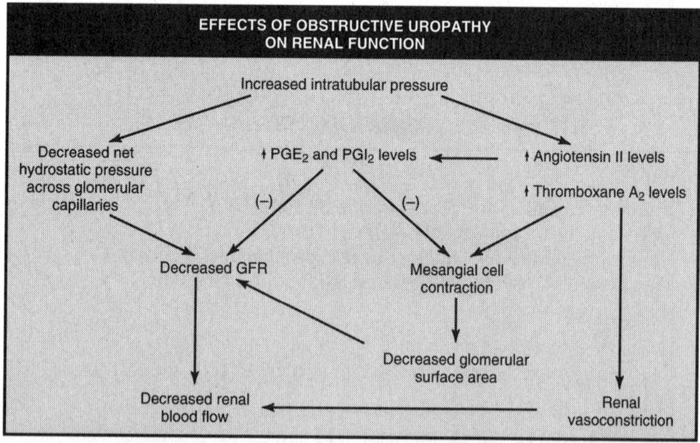

FIGURE 8–6 ■ Increased levels of prostaglandin E_2 (PGE_2) and prostacyclin (PGI_2) tend to antagonize (−) the effects of angiotensin II and thromboxane A_2 on mesangial cell contraction and renal vasoconstriction. Hence they tend to prevent the glomerular filtration rate (GFR) from decreasing further.

Table 8–28 ■ CLINICAL MANIFESTATIONS AND LABORATORY FINDINGS IN URINARY TRACT OBSTRUCTION

1. No symptoms (chronic hydronephrosis)
2. Intermittent pain (chronic hydronephrosis)
3. Elevated levels of BUN and serum creatinine with no other symptoms (chronic hydronephrosis)
4. Renal colic (usually due to utereral stones or papillary necrosis)
5. Changes in urinary output
   a. Anuria or oliguria (acute renal failure)
   b. Polyuria (incomplete or partial obstruction)
   c. Fluctuating urinary output
6. Hematuria
7. Palpable masses
   a. Flank (hydronephrotic kidney, usually in infants)
   b. Suprapubic (distended bladder)
8. Hypertension
   a. Flank (hydronephrotic kidney, usually in infants)
   b. Suprapubic (distended bladder)
9. Hypertension
   a. Volume-dependent (usually due to chronic bilateral obstruction)
   b. Renin-dependent (usually due to acute unilateral obstruction)
10. Repeated urinary tract infections or infection that is refractory to treatment
11. Hyperkalemic, hyperchloremic acidosis (usually due to defective tubular secretion of hydrogen and potassium)
12. Hypernatremia (seen in infants with partial obstruction and polyuria)
13. Polycythemia (increased renal production of erythropoietin)
14. Lower urinary tract symptoms: hesistancy, urgency, incontinence, post-void dribbling, decreased force and caliber of urinary stream, nocturia

BUN = blood urea nitrogen.

8

VASCULAR DISORDERS OF THE KIDNEY

The fact that the kidneys depend on systemic blood pressure to maintain normal renal blood flow, GFR, and tubular function underscores the vulnerability of the kidneys to diseases involving the renal vasculature.

Thrombosis of the renal arteries and segmental branches may arise as a result of intrinsic pathologic conditions of the renal arteries or as a complication of embolization of thrombi arising in distant vessels. A wide range of problems may cause renal artery thrombosis (Table 8–32).

For more information about this subject, see *Cecil Textbook of Medicine,* 21st edition. Philadelphia, W.B. Saunders Company, 2000. Chapter 112, Vascular Disorders of the Kidney, pages 617 to 620.

RENAL CALCULI (NEPHROLITHIASIS)

The development of kidney stones affects approximately 12% of the U.S. population, is two to three times more common in men than in women, and is uncommon in blacks and Asians.

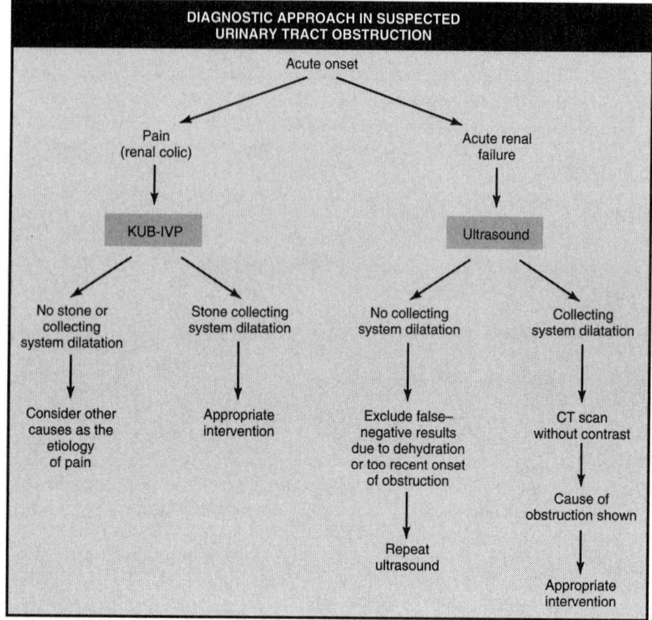

FIGURE 8–7 ■ Scheme of a diagnostic approach to urinary tract obstruction. KUB (kidney, ureter, bladder) = a flat film of the abdomen without contrast material; IVP = intravenous pyelography; CT = computed tomography.

The pain associated with passing a kidney stone is referred to as renal colic. Treatment should focus on two separate aspects: (1) work-up of etiology and associated preventive treatment, and (2) acute approach to relieving pain and urinary tract obstruction (Fig. 8–9). Avoidance of future bouts of stones is expected by determining the causes of urinary supersaturation that produce renal stone formation (Fig. 8–10). Effective therapy with drugs, dietary approaches, and increased fluid intake is fortunately available to treat most causes of nephrolithiasis.

For more information about this subject, see *Cecil Textbook of Medicine,* 21st edition. Philadelphia, W.B. Saunders Company, 2000. Chapter 114, Renal Calculi (Nephrolithiasis), pages 622 to 627.

CYSTIC DISEASES OF THE KIDNEY

Cystic diseases are among the few disorders that cause the kidneys to enlarge. The three major classifications of renal cystic disease are noted in Table 8–33.

Table 8–29 ■ CLINICAL SYNDROMES ASSOCIATED WITH NEPHRON TRANSPORT DEFECTS

PROXIMAL NEPHRON

I. *Selective Transport Defects*
   - A. Renal glycosurias
   - B. Renal aminoacidurias
   - C. Proximal renal tubular acidosis
   - D. Renal uric acid disorders (see Chapter 299)
   - E. Phosphate and calcium disorders (see Chapter 261)

II. *Non-selective Transport Defects: Fanconi's Syndrome*
   - A. Primary: idiopathic or genetic
   - B. Genetically transmitted systemic diseases
   - C. Dysproteinemic states
   - D. Secondary hyperparathyroidism with chronic hypocalcemia
   - E. Drugs and toxins
   - F. Heavy metals
   - G. Tubulointerstitial diseases
   - H. Other diseases

DISTAL NEPHRON

I. *Selective Transport Defects*
   - A. Classic distal renal tubular acidosis
   - B. Renal tubular acidosis of glomerular insufficiency
   - C. Hypermineralocorticoid and other potassium secretory disorders

II. *Non-selective Transport Defects: Generalized Distal Renal Tubular Acidosis, Hyperkalemia, and Renal Salt Wasting*
   - A. Primary mineralocorticoid deficiency
   - B. Hypoangiotensinemia
   - C. Hyporeninemic hypoaldosteronism
   - D. Mineralocorticoid-resistant hyperkalemia

LOOP OF HENLE

I. *Bartter's Syndrome*

II. *Drugs*
   - A. Furosemide
   - B. Bumetanide
   - C. Ethacrynic acid

LOOP AND MEDULLARY COLLECTING DUCTS

I. *Diabetes Insipidus* (see Chapter 238)

II. *Syndrome of Inappropriate Secretion of Antidiuretic Hormone* (see Chapter 102)

III. *Other Concentrating and Diluting Disorders*

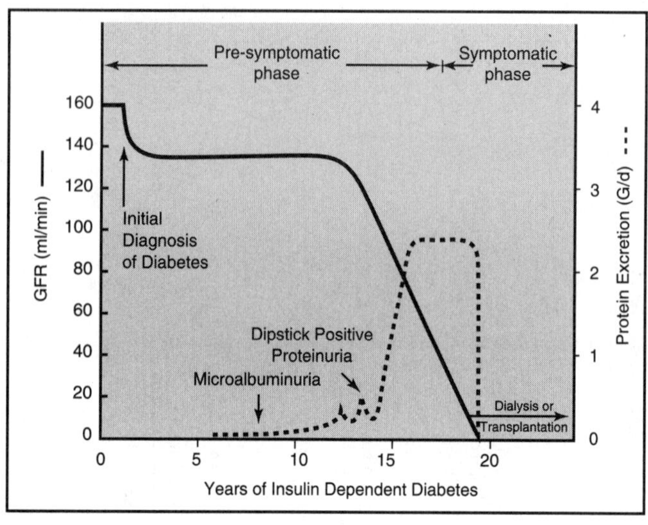

FIGURE 8–8 ■ Course of diabetic nephropathy.

For more information about this subject, see *Cecil Textbook of Medicine,* 21st edition. Philadelphia, W.B. Saunders Company, 2000. Chapter 115, Cystic Diseases of the Kidney, pages 627 to 630.

Table 8–30 ■ COMMON MANIFESTATIONS OF URINARY TRACT INFECTIONS

CLINICAL	LABORATORY
Urethritis or cystitis	Leukocyte esterase test positive
Frequent urination	Nitrite test may be positive
Burning on urination	Gram stain of uncentrifuged urine
Suprapubic discomfort	Leukocytes (≥5/hpf)
Lassitude	Gram-negative rods or gram-positive cocci (≥1/hpf)
Cloudy or blood-tinged urine	
Occasional low-grade fever	Urine culture (≥10^5 CFU/mL)
	Low-count bacteriuria (10^3–10^4 CFU/mL)
Acute pyelonephritis	Same findings as above *plus*
Sudden onset of fever	Leukocytosis
Shaking chills	Blood cultures positive (~20%)
Flank pain (may radiate)	Minimal effect on serum creatinine
Urinary symptoms may be absent	Decreased concentration ability

hpf = high-power field; CFU = colony-forming unit.

Table 8–31 ■ ORAL ANTIMICROBIAL DRUGS FOR UNCOMPLICATED URINARY TRACT INFECTIONS*

DRUG	DOSE	COMMENTS
Trimethoprim	100 mg q 12 hr†	About equally effective
Trimethoprim-sulfamethoxazole	80/400 mg q 12 hr†	
Nitrofurantoin	100 mg q 8 hr‡	Take with food
Cefixime	400 mg q day	Expensive
Cefuroxime axetil	250 mg q 12 hr	Expensive
Cefpodoxime	200 mg q 12 hr	Expensive
Norfloxacin	400 mg q 12 hr	Expensive§
Ciprofloxacin	100 mg q 12 hr	Expensive§
Ofloxacin	200 mg q 12 hr	Expensive§
Lomefloxacin	400 mg q daily	Expensive§
Enoxacin	200 mg q 12 hr	Expensive§
Carbenicillin indanyl	Two 382-mg tablets q/6 hr	For *Pseudomonas* spp.
Fosfomycin	3 g, single dose	Expensive

* Ampicillin, amoxicillin, cephalexin, or a tetracycline may be used if the bacteria are susceptible, but resistance to these drugs is common.

† Many clinicians prefer to use a double dose of these drugs.

‡ Contraindicated in patients with elevated serum creatinine levels. The monohydrate/macrocystal form is administered as 100 mg every 12 hours.

§ Bacteria rsistant to one quinolone are usually resistant to all others.

8

Table 8–32 ■ CAUSES OF RENAL ARTERY OCCLUSION

Thrombosis

Progressive atherosclerosis
Trauma, blunt
Aortic or renal artery aneurysm
Aortic or renal artery dissection
Aortic or renal artery angiography
Superimposed on inflammatory disorders
- Vasculitis
- Thromboangiitis obliterans
- Syphilis

Superimposed on structural lesions
- Fibromuscular dysplasia

Thromboembolism

Atrial fibrillation
Mitral stenosis
Mural thrombus
Atrial myxoma
Prosthetic valve
Septic or aseptic valvular vegetations
Paradoxical emboli
Tumor emboli
Fat emboli

Atheroemboli (Cholesterol Embolization)

Early patients with advanced atherosclerosis
Abdominal aortic surgery
Trauma, blunt
Angiographic catheters
Angioplasty or stent placement
Excessive anticoagulation

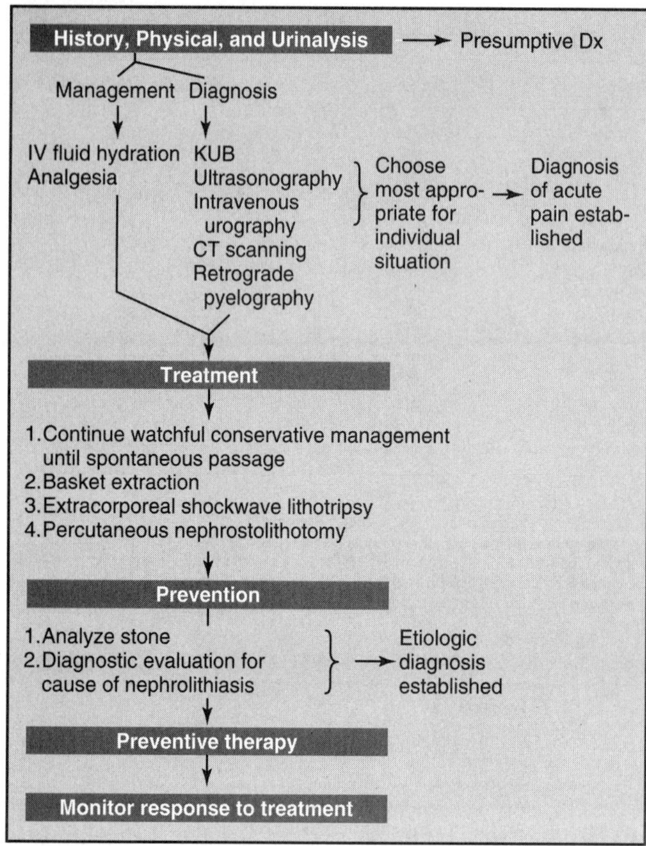

FIGURE 8–9 ■ Flow diagram for management of renal colic. See text for description of the approach to patients with acute stone episodes. KUB = kidney, ureter, bladder (film),

RENAL CELL CARCINOMA

Renal cell carcinoma is typically diagnosed during the sixth and seventh decades. The male-to-female ratio is 3:2. Approximately 29,900 new cancers are diagnosed annually. Renal cell carcinomas arise from the proximal renal tubular epithelium. Although most are solitary, some 7% are multicentric.

Hematuria is the most frequent presenting symptom, although pain and an abdominal mass are also common. The "classic triad" of hematuria, pain, and abdominal mass occurs in fewer than 10% of patients (Fig. 8–11).

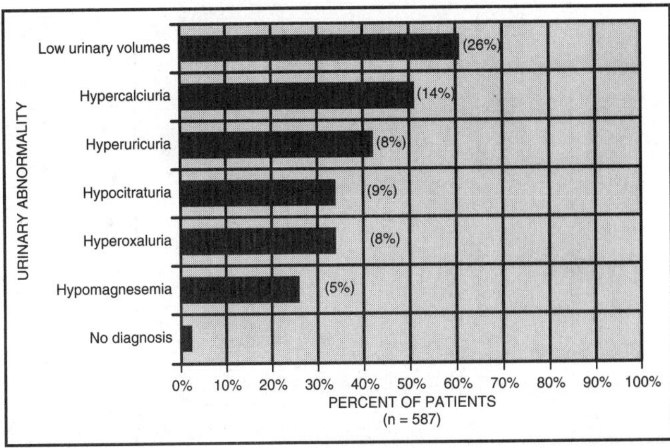

FIGURE 8–10 ■ Causes of urinary supersaturation in patients with nephrolithiasis: 587 consecutive patients seen in the stone center of St. Louis, Missouri, from 1987 to 1992 were evaluated with a standardized approach, described in the text section on preventing recurrent nephrolithiasis. Numbers in parentheses indicate sole occurrence of abnormality. (Data taken from Seltzer J, Winborn K. Hruska K [unpublished observation].)

Systemic symptoms such as fever, weight loss, anemia, polycythemia, hypercalcemia, and nonmetastatic hepatic dysfunction occur frequently and may represent the sole manifestation of renal cell carcinoma.

For more information about this subject, see *Cecil Textbook of Medicine,* 21st edition. Philadelphia, W.B. Saunders Company, 2000. Chapter 117, Tumors of the Kidney, Ureter, and Bladder, pages 631 to 635.

URINARY INCONTINENCE

Urinary incontinence is defined as involuntary loss of urine of sufficient severity to be a health or social problem, or both. A wide-ranging problem, prevalence and incidence are higher in women and increase with age. It can also be a sign of benign and malignant prostate enlargement in middle-aged and older men.

Persistent types of urinary incontinence can be categorized into four basic types (Table 8–34).

The most common method of managing urinary incontinence is adult diapers and pads. Where possible, reversible factors may be treated and a variety of behavioral therapies have been shown to be highly effective.

For more information about this subject, see *Cecil Textbook of Medicine,* 21st edition. Philadelphia, W.B. Saunders Company, 2000. Chapter 119, Urinary Incontinence, pages 640 to 642.

Table 8–33 ■ CHARACTERISTICS OF RENAL CYSTIC DISORDERS

	POLYCYSTIC		CYSTIC		MEDULLARY	
CHARACTERISTIC	**Dominant**	**Recessive**	**Simple**	**Acquired**	**Sponge Kidney**	**Cystic**
Prevalence	1:500–1:1000	1:16,000	Common	End-stage renal diseases	1:1000–1:5000	Rare
Symptoms	Common	Common	Rare	Occasional	Occasional	Common
Inherited	Yes	Yes	No	No	Unknown	Yes
Kidney size	Large	Large	Normal	Small to large	Normal	Small
Hypertension	Common	Common	Rare	Common	Rare	Rare
Hematuria	Common	Common	Occasional	Occasional	Unusual	Rare
Azotemia	Common	Common	No	Always	Rare	Common
Liver disease	40–60%	100%	No	No	No	No
Cranial aneurysm	5–20%	No	No	No	No	No
Differential diagnosis	ARPKD Tuberous sclerosis Multiple simple cysts	ADPKD Medullary sponge kidney	Tumor Diverticula of the renal pelvis	ADPKD Simple cysts Hippel-Lindau disease	Medullary cystic kidney Renal tubular acidosis Idiopathic nephrocalcinosis	End-stage renal disease Medullary sponge kidney

ARPDK = autosomal recessive polycystic kidney disease; ADPKD = autosomal dominant polycystic kidney disease.

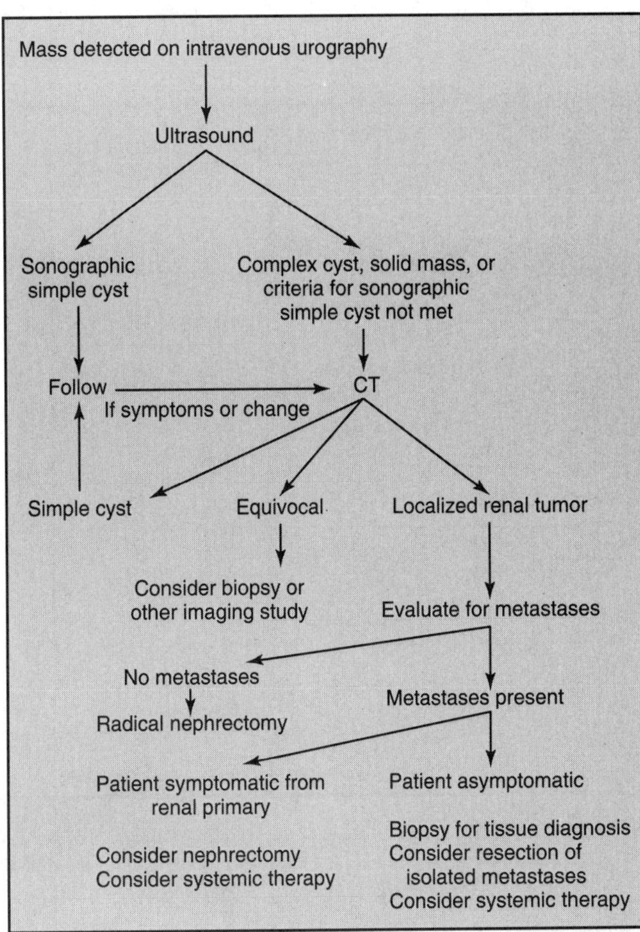

FIGURE 8–11 ■ Algorithm for work-up of incidental renal mass.

Table 8–34 ■ BASIC TYPES AND CAUSES OF PERSISTENT URINARY INCONTIENCE

TYPE	CLINICAL MANIFESTATIONS	COMMON CAUSES	PRIMARY TREATMENTS
Stress	Involuntary loss of urine (usually small amounts) with increases in intra-abdominal pressure (e.g., cough, laugh, exercise)	Weakness of pelvic floor musculature and urethral hypermobility Bladder outlet or urethral sphincter weakness	Pelvic muscle exercises and other behavioral interventions. β-Adrenergic agonists (phenylpropanolamine 75 mg bid) Periurethral injections Surgical bladder neck suspension or sling
Urge	Leakage of urine (variable but often larger volumes) because of inability to delay voiding after sensation of bladder fullness is perceived	Detrusor overactivity, isolated or associated with one or more of the following: Local genitourinary condition such as tumors, stones, diverticuli, or outflow obstruction CNS disorders such as stroke, dementia, parkinsonism, spinal cord injury	Bladder training and other behavioral interventions Bladder relaxants (tolterodine 2 mg bid; other anticholinergics)
Overflow	Leakage of urine (usually small amounts without warning) resulting from mechanical forces on an overdistended bladder or from other effects of urinary retention on bladder and sphincter function	Anatomic obstruction by prostate, stricture, cystocele Acontractile bladder associated with diabetes mellitus or spinal cord injury Neurogenic (detrusor-sphincter dyssynergy), associated with multiple sclerosis and other suprasacral spinal cord lesions	Surgical removal of obstruction Intermittent or chronic catheterization
Functional	Urinary accidents associated with inability to toilet because of impairment of cognitive and/or physical functioning, psychological unwillingness, or environmental barriers	Severe dementia and other neurologic disorders Psychological factors such as depression and hostility	Prompted voiding and other behavioral intervention Absorbent padding Drug treatment for bladder overactivity (selected patients)

From Kane RL, Ouslander JG, Abrass IB: Essentials of Clinical Geriatrics, 4th ed. New York, McGraw-Hill, 1998. Copyright © by McGraw-Hill, Inc. Used by permission of McGraw-Hill Book Company.

CHAPTER 9

GASTROINTESTINAL DISEASES

APPROACH TO THE PATIENT WITH GASTROINTESTINAL DISEASE

The diagnosis of gastrointestinal diseases derives predominantly from history and, to a lesser extent, from the physician's physical examination.

Nausea and Vomiting

Both hunger and appetite refer to the desire to eat. The determinants of *hunger* are usually physiologic mechanisms. *Appetite* is closely related to hunger, but it is thought to be influenced predominantly by environmental and psychological processes. *Satiety* refers to the gratification of hunger and appetite. *Anorexia* is a clinical symptom characterized by the absence of hunger or appetite.

9

Satiety and anorexia must be differentiated from *nausea,* which is the unpleasant feeling that one is about to vomit, and *vomiting* (or *emesis*), which is the forceful ejection of contents of the upper gut through the mouth. In contrast, *retching* involves coordinated, voluntary muscle activity of the abdomen and thorax. *Regurgitation* is the effortless return of gastric or esophageal contents into the mouth without nausea.

Medications are among the most common causes of nausea and vomiting. Opiates, digitalis, levodopa, bromocriptine, and anticancer drugs act on the chemoreceptor trigger zone. Drugs that frequently cause nausea through other mechanisms include nonsteroidal anti-inflammatory drugs (NSAIDs), erythromycin, cardiac antiarrhythmic medications, antihypertensive drugs, diuretics, oral antidiabetic agents, oral contraceptives, and gastrointestinal medications such as sulfasalazine. *Gastrointestinal* and *systemic infections,* both viral and bacterial, are probably the second most common cause of nausea and vomiting. Obstruction of the gastrointestinal tract or organs, labyrinthine disorders, severe psychogenic stress, uremia, diabetic ketoacidosis, hypercalcemia, hypoxemia, hyperthyroidism, Addison's disease, and radiation therapy are other common causes. The first trimester of pregnancy causes vomiting in approximately 70% of pregnant women. Postoperative nausea and vomiting complicate up to 40% of surgical operations.

Effective drugs for nausea and vomiting include phenothiazines, metoclopramide, domperidone, cisplatin, scopolamine, diphenhydramine, and cyclizine. The most effective of the antinausea drugs for chemotherapy-induced vomiting are the 5-HT_3 (serotonin) receptor antagonists such as ondansetron.

For more information about this subject, see *Cecil Textbook of Medicine,* 21st edition. Philadelphia, W.B. Saunders Company, 2000. Part XI: Gastrointestinal Diseases, pages 643 to 766.

Abdominal Pain

Abdominal pain is either acute or chronic; when chronic, it may be intermittent (e.g., recurrent biliary colic), unrelenting (e.g., chronic pancreatitis or pancreatic cancer), or intractable but of unclear cause (e.g., the functional abdominal pain syndromes). Pain from the esophagus, stomach, proximal duodenum, liver, biliary tree, and pancreas is perceived between the xiphoid and the umbilicus. Pain from the small intestine, appendix, and ascending and proximal two thirds of the transverse colon is perceived as periumbilical. Pain from the distal one third of the transverse colon, the descending colon, and the rectosigmoid is perceived between the umbilicus and the pubis. Referred pain is a helpful phenomenon; gallbladder pain may be perceived in the right shoulder or scapula, and pain from retroperitoneal processes such as pancreatitis is referred to the back.

The character of the pain (burning, steady, or colic), its duration, its time to reach peak intensity, and its relieving and aggravating factors (such as eating or passing gas or stool) are also helpful. Esophagitis is classically described as substernal burning pain relieved by antacids and aggravated by lying down. Peptic ulcer pain occurs when the stomach is empty (often around 4 A.M.), and it is relieved by eating or taking antacids. Gallbladder colic is perceived either in the midline or right upper quadrant, reaches a peak intensity within minutes to an hour, and usually persists for 1 to 4 hours. In contrast, the pain of cholecystitis and pancreatitis reaches its peak more slowly, becomes sustained, and lasts for days. Intestinal obstruction causes colicky pain that waxes and wanes over the course of minutes and is usually periumbilical.

Chronic intermittent abdominal pain may be due to obstructed viscera; to metabolic or genetic diseases, such as acute intermittent porphyria or familial Mediterranean fever; to neurologic diseases, such as diabetic radiculopathy, abdominal migraine, or vertebral nerve root compression; or to conditions such as Crohn's disease, endometriosis, lead poisoning, or mesenteric ischemia. Functional abdominal pain, which is common but of less clear pathophysiology, includes three major types: (1) irritable bowel syndrome, in which recurrent abdominal pain is accompanied by changes in gastrointestinal function (constipation, diarrhea, or alternating constipation and diarrhea); (2) non-ulcer dyspepsia, which is defined as ulcer-like symptoms in the absence of endoscopically definable anatomic or histologic evidence of inflammation; and (3) chronic, intractable abdominal pain, which is not accompanied by other symptoms of organ dysfunction.

Physical Examination

Distention, particularly if tympanic, suggests bowel obstruction, but simple obesity and ascites are more likely causes of distention without tympany. The character of bowel sounds (absent in peritonitis, high-pitched tinkles in intestinal obstruction) can be important. Palpation gives clues to the presence of severe peritoneal inflammation, as manifested by involuntary guarding, abdominal rigidity, or rebound tenderness. When these symptoms are accompanied by absent bowel sounds, perforation and peritonitis must be suspected.

The abdominal examination might reveal epigastric, right upper quadrant, right lower quadrant, or left lower quadrant tenderness to complement a compatible history for peptic ulcer disease, cholecystitis, Crohn's disease, or diverticulitis, respectively. An epigastric mass might suggest a pancreatic neoplasm or pseudocyst, whereas right lower quadrant and left lower quadrant masses suggest abscess due to inflammatory bowel disease and diverticulitis, respectively, or colonic cancer. Examination of the liver should focus primarily on its breadth and consistency.

A digital rectal examination is important to search for anorectal carcinoma and masses in the pouch of Douglas and also to determine the size and consistency of the prostate. Tenderness and masses laterally can occur in appendicitis, inflammatory bowel disease, diverticulitis, or abdominal cancers. The character and color of the stool and the presence of fecal occult blood should be assessed.

Diagnostic Procedures

In the jaundiced patient, ultrasonography (US) allows quick differentiation of obstruction of the intrahepatic and extrahepatic bile ducts from other causes of jaundice, such as hepatitis. US detects fatty liver as well as textural changes of cirrhosis, and it has a sensitivity between 80% and 90% for detection of hepatic neoplasm.

Computed tomography (CT) is an essential tool for evaluating and staging abdominal mass lesions; for diagnosis of hepatic, pancreatic, and splenic abscesses; and for detecting abscesses associated with disorders of the bowel such as appendicitis, diverticulitis, or Crohn's disease. In patients with biliary obstruction, CT is very useful for determining the cause of obstruction, including carcinoma of the pancreatic head or the ampulla, particularly when US evaluation remains inconclusive. Another important use of CT is to guide abdominal interventions such as percutaneous needle aspiration of mass lesions or abnormal fluid collections, placement of needles and probes for percutaneous tumor ablation, and drainage of abdominal abscesses.

Magnetic resonance imaging (MRI) is often used when US or CT is inconclusive. MRI can differentiate cavernous hemangiomas from other liver lesions, but technetium-99m (^{99m}Tc)–labeled red blood cell studies represent a more economic, alternative, noninvasive method to diagnose a cavernous hemangioma.

Biopsy and Drainage

Percutaneous US- or CT-guided biopsy of hepatic, pancreatic, or other abdominal mass lesions has become standard practice. The sensitivity of fine-needle biopsy of abdominal neoplasms is more than 90%, with a complication rate that is less than 1%.

Percutaneous drainage of abscesses and other abnormal fluid collections under US or CT guidance also has become a standard radiologic procedure. More than 90% of simple abdominal abscesses can be drained by percutaneous catheter drainage.

For more information about this subject, see *Cecil Textbook of Medicine,* 21st edition. Philadelphia, W.B. Saunders Company, 2000. Chapter 120, Approach to the Patient with Gastrointestinal

Disease, and Chapter 121, Diagnostic Imaging Procedures in Gastroenterology, pages 643 to 649.

GASTROINTESTINAL ENDOSCOPY

Endoscopy after appropriate preparation (Table 9–1) is the procedure of choice in most cases in which mucosal lesions or growths are suspected.

Upper Gastrointestinal Endoscopy

In patients with *gastroesophageal reflux disease* (GERD), the presence of dysphagia or odynophagia, weight loss, gastrointestinal bleeding, or frequent vomiting should lead to an early endoscopy. However, the overall sensitivity of endoscopy in GERD is only about 70%. When dyspepsia is recurrent and fails to respond to empiric therapy, endoscopy is commonly indicated.

In *dysphagia,* upper gastrointestinal (UGI) endoscopy is usually

Table 9–1 ■ ENDOSCOPIC COMPLICATIONS, PREPARATION, PRECAUTIONS, AND PROPHYLAXIS

Complications of Endoscopy

- General complications
  - Complications related primarily to sedation (cardiovascular and respiratory depression, aspiration)
  - Perforation
  - Bleeding
- Complications associated with specialized procedures
  - Pancreatitis (ERCP)
  - Cholangitis (ERCP)
  - Wound infections (PEG)

Preparation

- Upper endoscopy: nothing orally (solids: 6 hrs; liquids: 4 hrs)
- Colonoscopy: bowel purge the day before; optional enemas before the procedure
- Sigmoidoscopy: 1–2 enemas before the procedure

Precautions and Prophylaxis

- Hemodynamic and respiratory stabilization
- Prophylactic antibiotics
- Prevention of endocarditis, if indicated (patients with artificial valves, pulmonary-systemic shunts, previous history of endocarditis)
- Prevention of cholangitis (patients with biliary obstruction)
- Prevention of wound infection (PEG)
- Prevention of pancreatic infection (patients undergoing therapeutic pancreatic procedures)
- Patients on anticoagulants
  - Diagnostic procedure only: no adjustment required
  - High-risk procedure: discontinue anticoagulants 3–5 d before endoscopy and resume after the procedure; in patients at high risk for thromboembolism, heparin may be considered while the INR is subtherapeutic (discontinue heparin for 4–6 hr before the procedure)

ERCP = endoscopic retrograde cholangiopancreatography; PEG = percutaneous endoscopic gastrostomy; INR = international normalized ratio.

a second-line procedure. Dysphagia can often be categorized as oropharyngeal based on the clinical features of nasal regurgitation, laryngeal aspiration, or difficulty in moving the bolus out of the mouth. Conversely, the most common causes of esophageal dysphagia include malignant lesions, benign processes, and motility disturbances. Barium radiography can guide an endoscopy, suggest an underlying disturbance in motility, or occasionally detect subtle stenoses that are not appreciated on endoscopy.

When *dyspepsia* is recurrent and fails to respond to empiric therapy, endoscopy is commonly indicated. Endoscopy is mandatory in essentially all patients with *UGl bleeding*. It can detect and localize the site of the bleeding in 95% of cases and is clearly superior to contrast radiography. Patients with slower or inactive bleeding may be evaluated by endoscopy in a "semielective" manner (usually within 12 to 20 hours), but a case can be made for performing endoscopy very early, even in these stable patients.

Variceal bleeding is also effectively managed endoscopically, with a similar success rate to that with bleeding ulcers. Hemostasis is achieved using either band ligation, sclerotherapy, or a combination of both.

Colonoscopy and Sigmoidoscopy

In contrast to UGI bleeding, there is no single best test for acute *lower gastrointestinal bleeding* (Fig. 9–1). Colonoscopy is the most accurate test for detecting mass lesions of the large bowel that are suspected on clinical or radiologic grounds.

Pancreatobiliary Endoscopy

Endoscopic retrograde cholangiopancreatography (ERCP), involves a special side-viewing-endoscope (the duodenoscope) that is used to gain access to the second part of the duodenum. A small catheter is then introduced into the bile or pancreatic duct, and radiographic contrast medium is injected under fluoroscopic monitoring. Successful cannulation and imaging can be achieved in up to 95% of cases. Endoscopic stone removal is successful in 90% or more of cases and usually requires a sphincterotomy.

Endoscopic therapy has also revolutionized the palliative approach to malignant biliary obstruction. The technique, which requires the placement of indwelling stents, is superior to both radiologic and surgical techniques.

ERCP is also useful in patients with pancreatic diseases that do not present with obstructive jaundice, such as pancreatic cancer and, less commonly, chronic pancreatitis. It is also indicated in patients with acute or recurrent pancreatitis without any obvious risk factors on history or routine laboratory evaluation.

ERCP also has a role in some patients with *acute* pancreatitis that is likely caused by obstructing biliary stones. Patients presenting with severe biliary pancreatitis may benefit from an urgent ERCP early in their course, with the intention of detecting and removing stones from the common bile duct.

For more information about this subject, see *Cecil Textbook of Medicine,* 21st edition. Philadelphia, W.B. Saunders Company, 2000. Chapter 122, Gastrointestinal Endoscopy, pages 649 to 653.

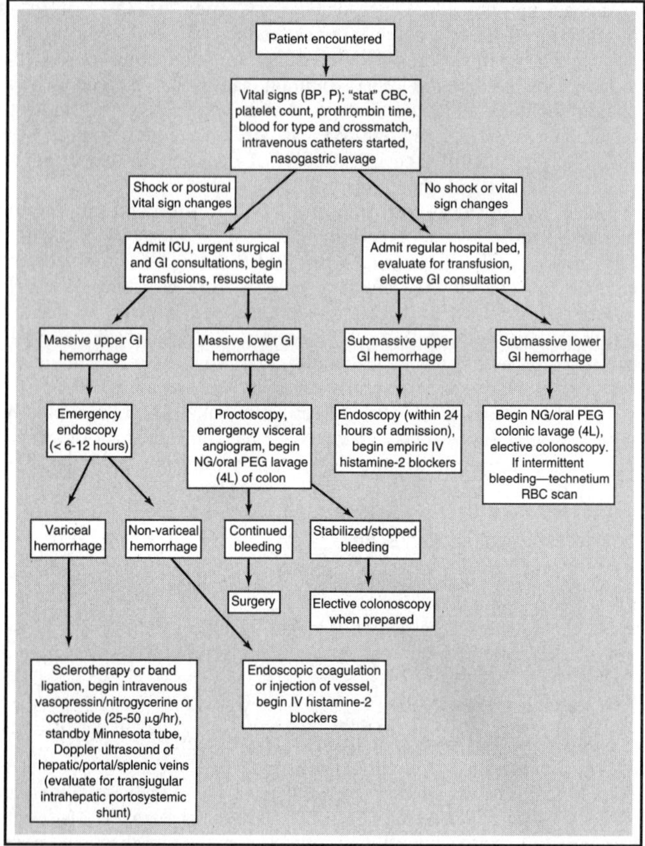

FIGURE 9–1 ■ Approach to the patient with gastrointestinal hemorrhage. BP = blood pressure; P = pulse; CBC = complete blood count; ICU = intensive care unit; GI = gastrointestinal; NG = nasogastric; PEG = percutaneous endoscopic gastrostomy; RBC = red blood cell.

GASTROINTESTINAL HEMORRHAGE AND OCCULT GASTROINTESTINAL BLEEDING

Gastrointestinal tract hemorrhage usually produces dramatic clinical signs and symptoms and brings patients promptly to the attention of physicians. *Hematemesis,* which is vomiting of gross blood, most frequently follows bleeding from the esophagus, stomach, or duodenum. *Melenemesis,* or "coffee grounds" vomiting, occurs when blood is in contact with gastric acid for at least 1 hour. *Melena,* usually noted by patients with bleeding from the proximal gastrointestinal tract, is characterized by dark-black, liquid, tarry, metallic-smelling stools. Melenic stools usually indicate UGI tract bleeding. *Hematochezia,* the passage of bright-red stools, is usually a sign of distal small bowel or brisk colonic hemorrhage. However, up to 10% of patients with hemodynamically significant hematochezia are actively bleeding from an upper, not lower, gastrointestinal tract lesion.

The most accurate non-invasive indicator of the severity of acute blood loss is the presence of shock or postural changes in vital signs. Shock indicates an acute blood volume loss of at least 15 to 20%. Postural vital sign changes (e.g., upright tachycardia, widening of the pulse pressure, and/or upright systolic hypotension) indicate acute intravascular volume loss of at least 10 to 15%.

Nasogastric lavage is helpful but highly inaccurate in estimating the severity of UGI bleeding. With acute hemorrhage, the hematocrit and hemoglobin levels are not reliable indicators of the severity of bleeding. For the hematocrit to fall, the blood plasma must have equilibrated with extracellular fluid or with administered intravenous (IV) fluids, and this equilibration may require 24 to 48 hours to occur.

Regardless of the site or cause of hemorrhage, all patients with significant active blood loss from the gastrointestinal tract should be evaluated in a similar manner (see Fig. 9–1). A rectal examination is essential to document stool color as well as to palpate for gross anorectal mass lesions such as polyps, cancers, or large hemorrhoids.

Upper Gastrointestinal Tract Bleeding

Ulcer disease, the most common cause of UGI tract bleeding, is responsible for 50% of moderately severe and 35% of severe bleeding episodes (Table 9–2). Hemorrhage from esophageal or gastric varices (responsible for nearly one third of the episodes of massive UGI hemorrhage) is usually associated with known or suspected

Table 9–2 ■ ETIOLOGY OF UPPER GASTROINTESTINAL TRACT HEMORRHAGE

- Esophagus
  - Esophagitis
  - Ulcer
  - Mallory-Weiss tear
  - Esophageal varices
- Stomach
  - Gastric ulcer
  - Prepyloric ulcer
  - Pyloric channel ulcer
  - Gastric erosions
  - Gastritis
  - Varices
  - Portal-hypertensive gastropathy
  - Gastric cancer
  - Polyp
  - Dieulafoy lesion
- Duodenum
  - Ulcer
  - Duodenitis
  - Diverticulum
- Aortoenteric fistula
- Pancreatic pseudocyst
- Postsphincterotomy

chronic liver disease. Mallory-Weiss tears of the gastroesophageal junction (causing 5% of minor and 20% of severe UGI hemorrhage) are usually associated with antecedent, forceful retching, but they may occur after forceful sneezing, coughing, or singultus. Esophagitis, particularly in the patient with long-standing reflux or regurgitation, is suggested by substernal burning pain occasionally relieved by ingestion of food or antacids. Gastrointestinal tract malignancies, such as esophageal and gastric cancer or carcinoma of the ampulla of Vater, rarely cause hemodynamically significant UGI bleeding. Rare causes include aortoduodenal fistulas in patients with atherosclerotic aneurysms of the abdominal aorta, acquired vascular ectasias, and ectasias associated with other systemic conditions, such as hereditary hemorrhagic telangiectasias (Osler-Weber-Rendu syndrome). Ectatic superficial arteries (Dieulafoy lesions), duodenal diverticula, and certain conditions related to the acquired immunodeficiency syndrome (AIDS) (cytomegalovirus [CMV] infection-related ulcers, Kaposi's sarcoma, and lymphoma) are also unusual.

Endoscopy, performed after adequate resuscitation and clinical assessment, is the diagnostic procedure of choice and can document the site of brisk hemorrhage in at least 95% of patients. Relative contraindications include acute myocardial infarction, severe chronic lung disease ($So_2 \leq 90\%$), hemodynamic instability, and patient agitation, but emergency endoscopy is commonly performed in these situations when diagnosis is critical and/or therapeutic interventions guided by the endoscopy are needed.

Endoscopy also offers definitive therapy for most active bleeding. Acute variceal bleeding, for example, can be controlled with endoscopic sclerotherapy or varix band ligation in nearly 90% of patients.

Barium contrast radiography is an acceptable alternative for diagnosing UGI lesions in patients who have not bled excessively, who have no stigmata of chronic liver disease, and who are not in need of endoscopic hemostasis. In those infrequent instances when the site of UGI bleeding is missed on endoscopy, angiography may localize the bleeding. In addition, selective infusion with vasopressin or coil embolization of actively bleeding arteries may control bleeding. For patients with less active blood loss, technetium red blood cell nuclear scintigraphy ("red cell scan") also can localize the site of bleeding.

Lower Gastrointestinal Bleeding

Colonic diverticula are responsible for nearly one fourth of all episodes of hemodynamically significant bleeding from the lower gastrointestinal tract (Table 9–3). Up to 10% of cases of hemodynamically significant hematochezia are caused by bleeding from UGI sites, particularly from duodenal ulcers. Other uncommon causes of lower gastrointestinal blood loss include aortoenteric fistulas, Meckel's diverticulum of the ileum, and mesenteric varices.

Proctoscopy with careful evaluation of the anorectal junction is the initial diagnostic step for all patients with hematochezia. If blood loss is modest (as evidenced by a normal hematocrit and vital signs), sigmoidoscopy may be followed by double-contrast barium radiography, which is highly accurate in detecting small

Table 9–3 ■ ETIOLOGY OF HEMATOCHEZIA IN 72 HOSPITALIZED PATIENTS*

SOURCE OF HEMORRHAGE	PERCENTAGE
Colonic cancer	7
Colonic polyps	11
Diverticula	23
Colitis	11
Vascular ectasia	1
Large hemorrhoids only	12
Ulcer tear (rectum)	10
Upper gastrointestinal or small bowel source	10
No site identified	15
	100

* Patients underwent colonoscopy (and endoscopy if colonoscopy was negative) at San Francisco General Hospital.

polyps and superficial mucosal abnormalities such as colitis. If signs and symptoms indicate lower gastrointestinal tract hemorrhage together with anemia, colonoscopy should be performed.

When bleeding is brisk, however, colonoscopy is usually not possible. Technetium red blood cell scintigraphy can detect active bleeding at a rate of at least 3 to 10 mL/hour. If bleeding continues at a rate exceeding 30 to 50 mL/hour, angiography can be extremely helpful in localizing the site of hemorrhage. An upper limit should be set on the number of units of blood transfused (perhaps as little as 6 to 8U) and the number of sessions of therapeutic endoscopy (realistically no more than two) before surgery is undertaken, particularly for patients with peptic ulcers, colonic neoplasms, or diverticular hemorrhage.

Occult Gastrointestinal Tract Hemorrhage

Occult gastrointestinal tract hemorrhage can be classified into three general categories: (1) patients with overt signs of UGI tract hemorrhage (i.e., hematemesis or melenemesis but a negative upper endoscopy), (2) patients with overt signs of apparent lower intestinal tract hemorrhage (i.e., hematochezia but a negative colonoscopy), and (3) patients presenting with positive fecal occult blood testing with or without iron deficiency anemia and negative routine upper *and* lower endoscopies (Table 9–4). Iron deficiency anemia with occult blood loss can be caused by colonic polyps or neoplasms, but a substantial minority have non-neoplastic lesions of the upper and/or lower gastrointestinal tract (Table 9–5).

For more information about this subject, see *Cecil Textbook of Medicine,* 21st edition. Philadelphia, W.B. Saunders Company, 2000. Chapter 123, Gastrointestinal Hemorrhage and Occult Gastrointestinal Bleeding, pages 653 to 658.

DISEASES OF THE ESOPHAGUS

The sensation of food bolus arrest during swallowing is *dysphagia:* even if transient, it indicates esophageal dysfunction. The sensation of a substernal lump (globus) about one half-hour after

Table 9–4 ■ SOURCES OF OCCULT GASTROINTESTINAL HEMORRHAGE

Occult Bleeding with Signs of Upper Gastrointestinal Hemorrhage

Epistaxis
Hemoptysis
Gingival/glossal/pharyngeal bleeding
Ingestion of blood—human or animal
Gastric cardia varices
Antral/duodenal varices
Dieulafoy lesions
Pancreaticobiliary bleeding
  Pancreatic pseudoaneurysm
  Hepatic neoplasms/trauma
Aortoduodenal fistula
Duodenal diverticulum
Vascular ectasias

Occult Bleeding with Signs of Lower Gastrointestinal Hemorrhage

Briskly bleeding duodenal ulcers
Small bowel Dieulafoy lesions
Vascular ectasias of colon
Meckel's diverticulum—distal ileum
Aortocolonic or arteriocolonic fistula
Solitary colonic ulcers
Colorectal varices

Blood Loss without Signs/Symptoms of Either Upper or Lower Bleeding

Small bowel neoplasms
  Adenocarcinoma
  Sarcoma
  Lymphoma
  Metastases—breast, lung, melanoma
Vascular ectasias
Crohn's disease of small bowel
Dieulafoy lesions
Small bowel varices

eating is not dysphagia. Dysphagia for a liquid bolus usually indicates an esophageal motor disorder. Dysphagia for solids can occur either with an organic obstruction (stricture or cancer) or with esophageal motor disorders. Pain on swallowing, *odynophagia,* can be seen after involvement of the mucosa by reflux, radiation, or viral or fungal infections and can be an uncommon manifestation of carcinoma.

Heartburn, which may occur in up to 20% of the population, is often worse after recumbency or lifting and may follow overeating or alcoholic indiscretion. Regurgitation of fluid contents into the mouth often accompanies heartburn. Regurgitation at night may lead to stridor or to wheezing, a hoarse voice, and other respiratory symptoms from unrecognized reflux. Abnormal contractile activity or spasm of the esophageal muscle can cause severe chest pain that is clinically indistinguishable from angina pectoris.

Gastroesophageal Reflux Disease

Gastroesophageal reflux disease refers to the varied clinical manifestations of reflux of stomach and duodenal contents into the

Table 9–5 ■ GASTROINTESTINAL LESIONS FOUND IN 100 PATIENTS WITH IRON DEFICIENCY ANEMIA*

SOURCE OF HEMORRHAGE	PERCENTAGE
Colon	
Cancer	11
Polyp	5
Vascular ectasia	5
Colitis	2
Cecal ulcer	2
Parasites	1
Total	26
Upper Gastrointestinal Tract	
Duodenal ulcer	11
Esophagitis	6
Gastritis	6
Gastric ulcer	5
Vascular ectasia	3
Anastomotic ulcer	3
Gastric cancer	1
Portal hypertensive gastropathy	1
Adenomatous polyp	1
Total	37

* Patients evaluated by colonoscopy followed by upper endoscopy under the same conscious sedation.

esophagus and is preferable to the term "reflux esophagitis." Two abnormalities of the lower esophageal sphincter (LES) may be associated with reflux: an LES with very low tone, as measured by LES pressure, or inappropriate relaxation of a normally competent LES.

Heartburn can vary from an occasional mild burning after overeating to severe discomfort that limits a patient's lifestyle. It may be accompanied by regurgitation of gastric contents, either into the mouth or into the respiratory tree. The latter group of patients may complain of nocturnal wheezing, coughing, hoarseness, a need to clear the throat repeatedly, or a sensation of deep pressure at the base of the neck.

Dysphagia is often present in patients with significant GERD. Blood loss may result from esophageal erosions and shallow ulcers.

DIAGNOSTIC APPROACH (Fig. 9–2). Monitoring esophageal pH for 24 hours can detect the relationship between symptoms (heartburn, chest pain, wheezing) and episodes of acid reflux. If pain, rather than heartburn, is the predominant symptom, a Bernstein test may be performed using the same catheter as is used for esophageal manometry. Reproduction of symptoms during acid infusion, followed by rapid symptom disappearance after returning to a saline infusion, suggests an esophageal cause of the discomfort. In approximately one half of patients with moderate to severe symptoms of GERD, the mucosa appears absolutely normal on endoscopy, but a biopsy may demonstrate the histologic changes of reflux.

COMPLICATIONS. Esophageal ulcers or strictures may complicate severe GERD. In some patients with chronic reflux esophagi-

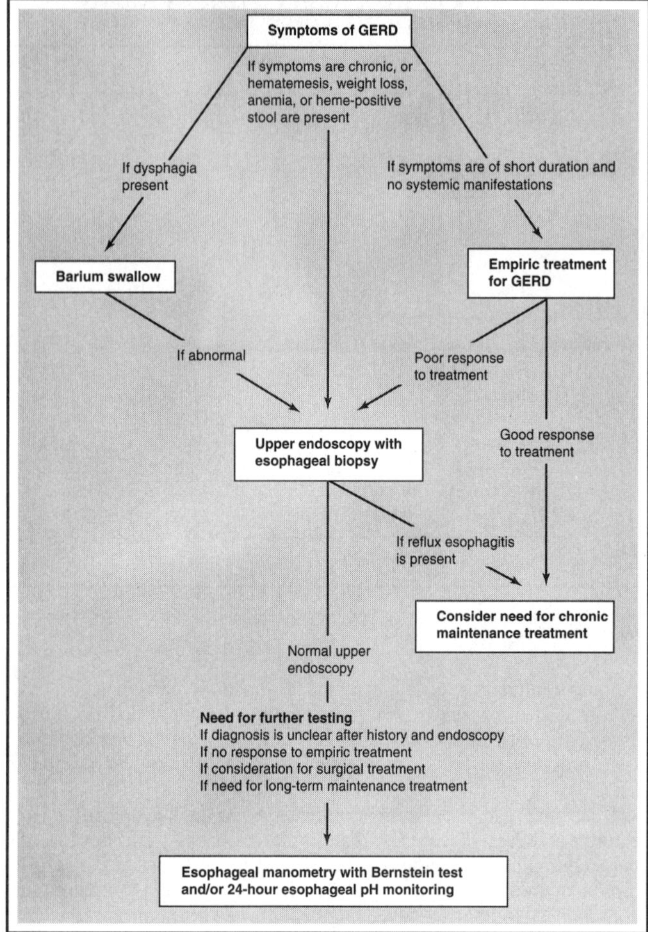

FIGURE 9–2 ■ Diagnosis and evaluation of patients with possible gastroesophageal reflux disease (GERD).

tis, the healing epithelium may be replaced not with squamous epithelium but with a specialized columnar (Barrett's) epithelium with intestinal metaplasia. Barrett's epithelium is not only a marker for severe reflux but also a precursor to adenocarcinoma of the esophagus.

If material refluxes above the upper esophageal sphincter, it may easily spill into the larynx and tracheobronchial tree. None of the clinical features of pulmonary aspiration, such as wheezing, hoarseness, or coughing, is pathognomonic, but together they may point toward reflux and aspiration as a possible cause.

TREATMENT (Table 9–6). Once healing of esophagitis has been achieved with either an H_2-antagonist or a proton pump inhibitor,

Table 9–6 ■ TREATMENT OF GASTROESOPHAGEAL REFLUX DISEASE (GERD)

Step 1. Simple measures (lifestyle changes and nonsystemic treatment)
- a. Elevate head of bed
- b. Avoid food and fluid intake before bedtime
- c. Avoid cigarettes, coffee, alcohol
- d. Avoid chocolate, peppermint
- e. Avoid tight clothing around the waist
- f. Take antacids 1 hr after meals, at bedtime, and as needed
- g. Reduce fat in diet
- h. Lose weight

Step 2. Measures for resistant cases (systemic treatment)

Step 2a. H_2-receptor antagonists
- a. Cimetidine 300 mg qid*
- b. Ranitidine 150 mg bid*
- c. Famotidine 20 mg bid*
- d. Nizatidine 150 mg bid*

Step 2b. Prokinetic agents
- a. Metoclopramide 10 mg qid*
- b. Bethanechol 10 mg qid*

Step 3. Measures for patients with GERD resistant to H_2-receptor antagonists
- a. Proton pump inhibitor: omeprazole 20 mg/d, or lansoprazole 30 mg/d*

Step 4. Measures for patients with GERD resistant to steps 1, 2, and 3 or patients who need long-term maintenance treatment
- a. Surgical fundoplication

* Higher doses or more frequent administration of an H_2-antagonist, proton pump inhibitor, or prokinetic agent may be required in some cases.

recurrence rates exceed 80% if no maintenance therapy is used. Maintenance therapy for esophagitis generally requires full dosage of an H_2-receptor antagonist or a proton pump inhibitor. Laparoscopic surgery is an alternative to long-term medical therapy and is recommended if there is good objective evidence of reflux and an adequate trial of medical management has not brought good results in a 6-month period.

Mildly symptomatic esophageal strictures can be handled by medical therapy, primarily proton pump inhibitors. Short, simple strictures can be dilated. Patients who do not tolerate dilation or require vigorous dilation every 3 to 4 weeks need a definitive antireflux operation, following which the stricture may regress.

Barrett's (columnar) epithelium may be premalignant and can be removed only by esophageal mucosal resection. Adequate antireflux therapy with high-dose H_2-antagonists or with a proton pump inhibitor causes regression of columnar epithelium in some patients. Patients with Barrett's epithelium should be followed with periodic endoscopic biopsies every 1 to 3 years to look for dysplasia and early changes of adenocarcinoma. The persistence of confirmed high-grade dysplasia is an indication for esophagectomy.

Treatment of the pulmonary complications of reflux in adults relies on improved night posture, gastric acid suppressants, and prokinetic agents. Caution is advised before recommending esophageal surgery in patients with reflux and predominantly pulmonary problems, because the cause-and-effect relationship may be uncertain in the individual patient.

Motor Disorders of the Esophagus

The motor disorders of the body of the esophagus have historically been classified as achalasia or diffuse spasm (Table 9–7). Weakness of the oropharyngeal musculature may cause transfer dysphagia. Solids are usually more trouble than liquids. If the LES fails to relax on deglutition (as occurs in achalasia), dysphagia occurs, and the contents are retained in the body of the esophagus. If primary muscle failure of the sphincter occurs, as in scleroderma, massive reflux and the consequences of GERD follow. Chest pain is the other major clinical presentation.

DIAGNOSIS. If the difficulty is thought to be in the oropharynx and upper esophageal sphincter (UES), a videoesophagram may reveal incoordination of tongue and palate, unilateral pharyngeal weakness, or aspiration of small amounts of barium into the trachea with swallowing. Manometric examination of the hypopharynx and UES can also aid in diagnosis.

Radiology of the esophageal body offers the best chance of diagnosis when motor disorders are associated with relatively static changes. When the motor abnormality is more intermittent, simultaneous contractions can be occasionally detected fluoroscopically. Prolonged esophageal pH and motility monitoring may help correlate symptoms of dysphagia or chest pain to reflux episodes or motility abnormalities.

TREATMENT. For achalasia, dilation with a pneumatic bag under radiographic control is the preferable initial therapy for almost all patients. Surgery is reserved for patients in whom bag dilation fails. Botulinum toxin, which reduces acetylcholine release and LES pressure, can be injected into the LES from an endoscopic approach to improve symptoms for several months. Patients with diffuse spasm can be given nitroglycerin, anticholinergics, or calcium channel antagonists. The treatment of scleroderma and other conditions marked by aperistalsis revolves mostly around the associated reflux.

Table 9–7 ■ MANOMETRIC CLASSIFICATION OF ESOPHAGEAL MOTOR DISORDERS

Achalasia
Diffuse esophageal spasm
Scleroderma
Isolated lower esophageal sphincter dysfunction
High pressure with normal relaxation
Normal pressure with impaired relaxation
Nonspecific esophageal motor disorder
High-amplitude peristaltic esophageal contractions ("nutcracker esophagus")
Repetitive esophageal contractions
Non-transmitted esophageal contractions
Low-amplitude esophageal contractions

Esophageal Tumors

Carcinoma of the esophageal epithelium, both squamous cell and adenocarcinoma, is by far the most common and important tumor of the esophagus. It is associated with both alcohol intake and tobacco smoking. Adenocarcinoma of the esophagus also arises in columnar (Barrett's) epithelium and appears to represent malignant degeneration in the metaplastic columnar tissue that develops in response to chronic inflammation from GERD. Benign neoplasms (leiomyoma, papilloma, and fibrovascular polyps) are rarer.

The most common clinical symptom of carcinoma is progressive dysphagia over a period of several months until only liquids can be taken. More advanced lesions manifest themselves with halitosis and weight loss.

DIAGNOSIS. The clinical suspicion of cancer of the esophagus should lead immediately to an esophagram. In the presence of suspicious symptoms and normal barium swallow results, endoscopy with biopsy and brushing of any suspicious lesion is indicated.

TREATMENT. Surgical resection of squamous cell carcinoma and adenocarcinoma of the lower third of the esophagus is preferred in most centers if the patient does not have widespread metastases. Perhaps only one fourth of all patients have a resectable tumor; of these patients, 10 to 20% do not survive the operative period, and 5-year survival is only 5 to 20% even with extensive resection.

Radiation therapy alone or in combination with surgery or chemotherapy has been a mainstay for squamous cell carcinoma, but adenocarcinomas are relatively radioinsensitive. Preliminary evidence suggests that multimodality treatment with radiation therapy plus chemotherapy with cisplatin and fluorouracil is superior to radiation therapy alone.

Other Conditions

Schatzki's ring, a common abnormality, is located in the terminal esophagus, has a symmetrical opening, and is usually at the junction between squamous and normal transitional or columnar epithelium of the stomach. All webs or rings can cause dysphagia for solids, and the impacted bolus usually has to be regurgitated. Symptomatic webs require mechanical disruption with either a dilator or an endoscope.

Zenker's diverticulum of the pharynx is not actually anatomically an esophageal diverticulum, as its neck is above the UES muscle. Zenker's diverticulum, if large, may require diverticulectomy. Scleroderma is occasionally associated with numerous wide-mouthed diverticula. If a patient with dysphagia is found to have a diverticulum, it is often difficult to determine whether the diverticulum or the associated motor disorder is the cause.

Infections afflicting the esophagus are usually fungal (*Candida*) or viral (CMV, herpes simplex virus [HSV]). Although both are most common in immunocompromised hosts, such as those receiving corticosteroids, undergoing cancer chemotherapy, or afflicted with AIDS, either or both can infect apparently healthy hosts. For mild, noninvasive candidal disease, topical therapy with nystatin

250,000 U every 2 hours or clotrimazole (dissolved in the mouth 5 times per day) suffices. For more serious infections, systemic treatment with oral fluconazole or occasionally ketoconazole is used. Fluconazole 100 mg/day given orally (PO) for 10 to 14 days is generally preferred over topical treatment in patients with AIDS. Low-dose IV amphotericin may be needed for patients who do not respond to oral treatment and those unable to swallow medications. Herpesvirus infection is treated with parenteral acyclovir. Ganciclovir or foscarnet can be tried for CMV infection.

For burns with solid lye or other solid agents, prednisone has been recommended at an initial dose of 80 mg/day, tapering to 20 mg/day until the esophagus heals. Tetracycline, doxycycline, potassium tablets, ascorbic acid, quinidine, and non-steroidal anti-inflammatory agents are the principal medications that cause pill-induced esophagitis. The esophagus can be involved either by blunt trauma or by penetrating missiles (e.g., gunshots or knife wounds).

Vomiting can cause esophageal injury, either mucosal (Mallory-Weiss) or through-and-through rupture (Boerhaave's syndrome). One fourth of patients shown to have a Mallory-Weiss tear have no prior history of vomiting. Diagnosis is almost always made at endoscopy.

For more information about this subject, see *Cecil Textbook of Medicine,* 21st edition. Philadelphia, W.B. Saunders Company, 2000. Chapter 124, Diseases of the Esophagus, pages 658 to 668.

GASTRITIS

Gastritis can be most readily classified by cause (Table 9–8). The most common cause of this inflammatory condition is infection with *Helicobacter pylori.*

With acute *H. pylori* infection, superficial gastritis develops in association with epigastric pain, nausea, and vomiting. With time and increasing severity of pangastritis, fundic gland atrophy can occur and cause a decrease in maximal acid secretion with age. Dysplastic epithelial changes can develop and progress to gastric cancer.

H. pylori can be detected using "non-invasive" modalities: serology with an enzyme-linked immunosorbent assay (ELISA) for IgG or IgA antibodies and ^{13}C- or ^{14}C-urea breath tests after an oral urea load. Invasive testing includes biopsy for histologic examination, urease test on antral biopsies, or culture.

Individuals with gastritis are usually asymptomatic. Non-ulcer dyspepsia is frequently due to functional disorders that are independent of *H. pylori.*

H. pylori–associated pangastritis can progress to fundic and antral gland atrophy, but the bacterium is frequently absent when hyposecretion of acid disrupts its unique ecologic niche in the acidic stomach and allows overgrowth of other bacteria.

Characteristic subepithelial hemorrhages are commonly found in individuals who abuse alcohol. Usually the bleeding is mild.

The immune gastritis of pernicious anemia predominantly involves the fundic gland mucosa. About 90% of patients with pernicious anemia have antibodies against parietal cells. Diagnosis re-

Table 9–8 ■ CLASSIFICATION OF GASTRITIS AND GASTROPATHY

Helicobacter pylori–induced gastritis (superficial, forms a spectrum from antral predominant, type B gastritis to pangastritis, type AB)
Atrophic gastritis
- Pernicious anemia (fundal gland predominant, type A, autoimmune markers)
- Atrophic pangastritis (involving antrum and fundal gland region, probably end-stage form of *H. pylori* gastritis)

Erosive hemorrhagic gastropathy
- Non-steroidal anti-inflammatory drug (NSAID) gastroenteropathy
- Stress-related mucosal disease
- Alcohol gastropathy

Unusual or specific forms of gastritis
- Phlegmonous gastritis
- Infections, usually in immunocompromised hosts
  - Viral (cytomegalovirus, herpes)
  - Fungal (*Candida, Histoplasma*)
  - Tuberculosis, syphilis
- Chronic erosive (diffuse varioliform) gastritis
- Postoperative alkaline reflux gastropathy
- Gastric ischemia
- Radiation-induced gastritis
- Ingestion of corrosive substances
- Ménétrier's disease (giant hypertrophic gastritis)
- Eosinophilic gastritis
- Granulomatous gastritis
- Vascular ectasia: watermelon stomach (antral vascular ectasia)
- Portal congestive gastropathy
- Lymphocytic gastritis

9

quires multiple biopsies because the histopathology may be patchy. Other than replacing vitamin B_{12}, no specific therapy exists for pernicious anemia. Gastric adenocarcinomas have been reported with increased frequency with pernicious anemia, but the assessment of increased risk is variable, ranging from none to threefold in different series. Only patients with dysplasia warrant close follow-up and/or surgical intervention.

Ménétrier's disease is defined by four features: (1) giant folds in the gastric fundus and body, (2) diminished acid secretory capacity, (3) hypoalbuminemia secondary to protein-losing gastropathy, and (4) histologic features of hyperplasia and a marked increase in mucosal thickness combined with gland atrophy and cystic dilation. Symptoms may include abdominal pain, nausea, vomiting, weight loss, and edema. The differential diagnosis includes gastrinoma syndrome, infiltrating carcinoma, lymphoma, and amyloidosis. HP infection should be treated, but the impact on gastric protein loss has not been established.

For more information about this subject, see *Cecil Textbook of Medicine,* 21st edition. Philadelphia, W.B. Saunders Company, 2000. Chapter 125, Gastritis and *Helicobacter pylori,* pages 668 to 670.

PEPTIC ULCER DISEASE

Epidemiology

Each year in the United States there are approximately 500,000 new cases and 4 million recurrences of peptic ulcer disease. The overall lifetime prevalence (combined gastric and duodenal ulcer) is estimated at approximately 12% in males and about 9% in females (Table 9–9). The daily use of NSAIDs significantly increases the risk of ulcer disease (relative risk = 10- to 20-fold). *H. pylori* increases the risk of developing duodenal ulcer disease by fivefold to sevenfold, yet only a small percentage (10 to 20%) of infected subjects develop peptic ulcer during a lifetime of infection. Curing HP infection reduces the risk of endoscopic ulcers during subsequent NSAID therapy.

It is important to distinguish between three types of NSAID-induced lesions; (1) superficial injury, which includes erosions and petechiae (punctate intramucosal hemorrhage); (2) "endoscopic ulcers," which are found in 10 to 25% of subjects taking NSAIDs; and (3) "clinical ulcers," which present as bleeding, perforation, or obstruction at a rate of 1 to 2% per patient-year of NSAID.

Mucosal prostaglandin production is decreased with doses as low as a "baby" aspirin tablet (82 mg) daily, and the ulcer risk is probably somewhat increased even with this low dose. A thorough evaluation is appropriate in any patient who bleeds while on NSAID therapy because the probability of finding lesions other

Table 9–9 ■ CAUSES AND ASSOCIATIONS OF PEPTIC ULCER

Common Forms of Peptic Ulcer

Helicobacter pylori–associated
NSAID-associated
Stress ulcer

Uncommon Specific Forms of Peptic Ulcer

Acid hypersecretion
- Gastrinoma: inherited—multiple endocrine neoplasia type I, sporadic
- Increased mast cells/basophils
  - Mastocytosis: inherited and sporadic
  - Basophilic leukemias
- Antral G cell hyperfunction/hyperplasia

Other infections
- Viral infection: herpes simplex virus type 1, cytomegalovirus
- ? Other infections

Duodenal obstruction/disruption (congenital bands, annular pancreas)
Vascular insufficiency: crack cocaine–associated perforations
Radiation-induced
Chemotherapy-induced (hepatic artery infusions)
? Rare genetic subtypes
- ? Amyloidosis type III (Van Allen–Iowa)
- ? Tremor-nystagmus-ulcer syndrome of Neuhauser

NSAID = non-steroidal anti-inflammatory drug.

Modified from Soll AH: Gastric, duodenal, and stress ulcer. *In* Sleisinger M, Fordtran J (eds): Gastrointestinal Disease, 5th ed. Philadelphia, WB Saunders, 1993, p 580.

than ulcers is at least as high as in subjects who are not taking NSAIDs.

Superficial mucosal damage (petechiae and erosions) is found in most patients hours after major operations or within 24 hours of the onset of major multisystem illness. Major bleeding in the setting of severe and prolonged physiologic stress occurs with discrete ulcers rather than from superficial mucosal lesions. Preventive therapy with H_2-receptor blockers is appropriate in high-risk patients or in patients with a history of peptic ulcer or gastrointestinal bleeding when exposed to severe, prolonged physiologic stress.

Clinical Manifestations

The majority of patients (approximately 70%) with epigastric distress ("dyspepsia") do not have evidence of active ulcer disease; conversely, up to 40% of patients with an active ulcer crater deny abdominal pain (Table 9–10). With the availability of endoscopy to confirm the presence or absence of a crater, antibiotics for curing *H. pylori* infection, and potent anti-ulcer therapies to heal virtually all ulcers, symptoms due to an active crater can be separated from symptoms due to other causes, thereby permitting appropriate clinical decisions. Physical examination is of limited value in patients with uncomplicated ulcer.

Diagnosis

Diagnostic confirmation requires either UGI endoscopy or barium contrast gastrointestinal radiography. Duodenal ulcers are almost never malignant. However, ulcerating lesions within the stomach may be due to gastric cancer, and approximately 4% of those that appear to be benign even by endoscopy are in fact malignant; therefore, under almost all circumstances it is imperative to obtain multiple biopsy specimens of gastric ulcers.

The American College of Physicians recommends that patients with uncomplicated dyspepsia be treated empirically with a short (4 to 8 weeks) course of anti-ulcer medication and observed to assess

Table 9–10 ■ DIAGNOSIS OF ULCER DISEASE BY SYMPTOMS ALONE IS IMPRECISE

	PREVALENCE (%)		
SYMPTOM	Duodenal Ulcer	Gastric Ulcer	Non-Ulcer Dyspepsia
Epigastric pain	~70	~70	~70
Nocturnal pain	50–80	30–45	25–35
Food causes pain relief	20–65	5–50	5–30
Episodic pain	50–60	10–20	30–40
Belching/bloating	30–65	30–70	40–80

Ulcers occur without symptoms (10–40%), and ulcer symptoms occur without ulcer (30–60%).

Modified from Isenberg JI, Walsh JH, Johnson LR: Peptic Ulcer Diseases. AGA Undergraduate Teaching Project—Unit 23. Timonium, MD, Milner-Fenwick, Inc, 1991.

their symptomatic response. Further evaluation is recommended only in patients who are unresponsive to this therapeutic trial or whose symptoms recurred after its discontinuation. By comparison, the American Gastroenterological Association recommends that patients with *uncomplicated* dyspepsia have routine *H. pylori* testing (Table 9–11) and that patients with positive results be treated to eradicate HP.

Determination of fasting and secretin-stimulated serum gastrin is indicated in patients who have intractable ulcer disease, those who will undergo elective duodenal ulcer surgery, and those in whom a diagnosis of Zollinger-Ellison (ZE; gastrinoma) syndrome is a consideration.

An important initial treatment alternative for patients with new-onset or previously undiagnosed dyspepsia is to perform serologic tests for *H. pylori.* The National Institutes of Health Consensus Conference concluded that only those ulcer patients (with duodenal and/or gastric ulcer) in whom *H. pylori* infection has been diagnosed by one of the sensitive and specific tests should be treated to eradicate the microorganism.

In general, most studies indicate that eradicating HP in patients with non-ulcer dyspepsia fails to alter dyspeptic symptoms significantly. However, there maybe a subgroup of patients with chronic dyspeptic symptoms related to *H. pylori* infection and chronic active gastritis. Therefore, in patients unresponsive to routine treatment for non-ulcer dyspepsia, testing for *H. pylori* is reasonable.

Ulcer Therapy

ANTISECRETORY DRUGS. The clinically equivalent doses of H_2-receptor antagonists are cimetidine, 800 mg, ranitidine or nizatidine, 300 mg, and famotidine, 20 mg. Proton pump inhibitors omeprazole (Prilosec) 20 to 40 mg/day and lansoprazole (Prevacid) 30 mg/day are the most effective antisecretory agents. Misoprostol is a relatively weak antisecretory drug whose primary role is to prevent ulcer and ulcer complications in NSAID users.

ANTIMICROBIAL THERAPY. A number of combination therapies are available that will reliably cure *H. pylori* infection (Table

Table 9–11 ■ DIAGNOSTIC TESTS FOR *HELICOBACTER PYLORI*

TEST	SENSITIVITY	SPECIFICITY	COMMENTS
Rapid urease test	80–98%	93–98%	Requires endoscopy
Histology	93–99%	95–99%	Requires endoscopy
Culture	77–92%	97–100%	Requires endoscopy
Serologic tests			
ELISA	88–99%	86–95%	Unsuitable for follow-up
Quick office test	94–96%	88–95%	Inexpensive, rapid
^{14}C- or ^{14}C-urea breath test	90–100%	89–100%	Good for diagnosis and follow-up

ELISA = enzyme-linked immunosorbent assay.

Modified from Walsh JH, Peterson WL: Treatment of *Helicobacter pylori* infection in the management of peptic ulcer disease. N Engl J Med 333:984–991, 1995.

9–12). Although few disagree that it is important to confirm the presence of infection before institution of antibiotic therapy, the role of post-therapy testing remains somewhat controversial. In general, failure to cure means that the organism was, or has become, resistant.

NSAID ULCERS. The best approach is to stop the NSAID and use antisecretory therapy to heal the ulcer. Patients who are NSAID users and who are also infected with *H. pylori* should also receive therapy for the infection.

Complications

Intractability, which is defined as failure of an ulcer to heal despite successful treatment of *H. pylori* infection and adequate antisecretory therapy, is rare and suggests a complicating factor such as the ZE syndrome; concomitant, and often covert, NSAID use; or another disease, such as Crohn's disease, masquerading as a peptic ulcer. Evaluation should include a determination of the serum gastrin and calcium levels and re-questioning about drug use, especially the use of over-the-counter medications that contain aspirin.

Peptic ulcer disease remains the most common cause of major *upper gastrointestinal bleeding;* between 15% and 20% of ulcer patients will experience hemorrhage during the course of their disease. Resuscitation takes precedence over diagnosis. Endoscopy provides rapid diagnosis, and endoscopically applied therapy has become the method of choice for initial management of UGI bleeding. Patients who have bled should be investigated for *H. pylori* status and for NSAID use. If NSAIDs are required, newer COX-2 inhibitors should be substituted after the ulcer has healed. Cotherapy with a proton pump inhibitor (e.g., omeprazole 20 mg/day, or lansoprazole 30 to 60 mg/day, in divided doses) or misoprostol 200 μg two to four times a day should be strongly considered. For cardiovascular indications, newer antiplatelet medication should be substituted for aspirin if possible.

The incidence of ulcer *perforation* is 7 to 10 per 100,000 population per year. The most common presentation is an abrupt onset of severe abdominal pain followed rapidly by signs of peritoneal inflammation. Initial management includes resuscitation by correction of fluid and electrolyte abnormalities, treatment of complications, continuous nasogastric suction, parenteral administration of broad-spectrum antibiotics (ampicillin-sulbactam and gentamicin) and, if a tension pneumoperitoneum is present, needle aspiration of the peritoneal cavity. Nasogastric suction is one of the mainstays of therapy. A randomized trial comparing non-operative treatment to emergency surgery showed that an initial period of non-operative observation yielded similar outcome, and the decision not to operate immediately could be based on the age and clinical condition of the patient.

Approximately 2% of ulcer patients develop *gastric outlet obstruction.* The mainstay of initial resuscitation and therapy is conservative medical management with decompression of the obstructed stomach; correction of fluid, electrolyte, and acid-base abnormalities; plus IV H_2-receptor antagonist therapy. Endoscopic

Table 9–12 ■ ANTIMICROBIAL THERAPIES SUCCESSFUL FOR TREATMENT OF *HELICOBACTER PYLORI* INFECTION

	H. PYLORI DRUGS				
THERAPY	**Drug 1**	**Drug 2**	**Drug 3**	**NOTES**	**SUCCESS**
Triple (3–4x/d)	Tetracycline 500 mg qid	Metronidazole 250 mg tid or qid or amoxicillin 750 mg tid, or clarithromycin 500 mg tid	Bismuth subsalicylate* 2 tablets qid	With meals for 14 d plus an H_2-blocker	~90%
Quadruple†	Tetracycline 500 mg qid	Metronidazole 500 mg tid, or clarithromycin 500 mg tid	Bismuth subsalicylate 2 tablets qid	With meals for 14 d plus a PPI‡ (bid)	~90%
Triple	Amoxicillin 500 mg qid	Clarithromycin 500 mg tid	Bismuth subsalicylate, 2 tablets qid	With meals for 14 d plus an H_2-blocker	~90%
MPpiC triple	Metronidazole 500 mg bid	PPI‡ bid	Clarithromycin 250–500 mg bid	With meals for 14 d	~90%
APpiC triple	Amoxicillin 1000 mg bid	PPI‡ bid	Clarithromycin 500 mg bid	With meals for 14 d	~90%
RBC triple	RBC 400 mg bid	Clarithromycin or metronidazole 500 mg bid	Tetracycline 500 mg bid	With meals for 14 d	~90%

RBC = ranitidine bismuth citrate.
* Bismuth subcitrate can be substituted.
† Possibly also effective with metronidazole-resistant *H. pylori*.
‡ PPI; lansoprazole and omeprazole can be used interchangeably.

Table 9–13 ■ INDICATIONS FOR EMERGENT/URGENT OPERATIONS IN PEPTIC ULCER DISEASE

Perforation
Bleeding
  Exsanguinating hemorrhage
  Bleeding >6 U of blood
  "Visible vessel," especially if bleeding
  Rebleeding on medical therapy or after endoscopic hemostasis
  Slow, persistent bleeding over days
  Age >65 yr
  Ulcer >2 cm
Gastric outlet obstruction unresponsive to medical therapy

balloon dilation and treatment of *H. pylori* infection have reduced the need for surgery to relieve obstruction.

Surgical Therapy

9

The overall role of surgery in ulcer therapy has declined over the past two decades (Table 9–13). A major recent advance in the surgical treatment of peptic ulcer disease is the use of laparoscopic techniques (Table 9–14).

Elective operation for duodenal ulcer is exceedingly rare. Normally, three conditions must obtain: (1) eradication of *H. pylori;* (2) ruling out of ZE syndrome; and (3) severe symptoms that interfere with the enjoyment of life or with work, despite well-supervised aggressive treatment.

Bleeding is a more serious complication in gastric ulcers than in duodenal ulcers. In a stable patient, the preferred procedure is distal gastrectomy that removes the ulcer and creates a gastroduodenal (Billroth I) anastomosis (Table 9–15).

H_2-receptor antagonists and proton pump inhibitors have been shown to be effective in treating most recurrent ulcers, particularly after previous vagotomy (Table 9–16). The incidence of ZE syndrome in patients with duodenal ulcer disease is only 1:1000 but rises to 1:50 in patients with postoperative recurrent ulcer.

Ulcer operations disrupt, to a greater or lesser degree, both the secretory functions and the motility of the stomach, sometimes

Table 9–14 ■ LAPAROSCOPIC SURGICAL PROCEDURES

PROCEDURE	COMMENTS
Laparoscopic closure of perforated peptic ulcer	Closure, omental patching, peritoneal toilet; gastric ulcers must be sampled in four quadrants
Laparoscopic suture ligation of bleeding peptic ulcer	Gastric ulcers must be sampled in four quadrants
Posterior truncal vagotomy and anterior highly selective vagotomy or seromyotomy (Taylor II)	Widely used, adequate results
Highly selective vagotomy	Best elective antiulcer procedure, 4–11% recurrence rate

Table 9–15 ■ SURGICAL OPTIONS FOR GASTRIC ULCERS

TYPE	LOCATION	INCIDENCE	TREATMENT OF CHOICE	COMMENTS
I	Body (lesser curve)	55–60%	Antrectomy Billroth I	Ulcer resected with specimen Mortality/recurrence rate of 2% Highly selective vagotomy and ulcer excision is a less than optimal approach
II	In association with duodenal ulcer	20–25%	Vagotomy and antrectomy	Acid reduction and ulcer excision accomplished
III	Prepyloric	20%	Vagotomy and antrectomy	Behaves like duodenal ulcer
IV	High-lying near gastroesophageal junction	<5%	Resection and esophagogastrojejunostomy (Csendes)	More common in South America

Table 9–16 ■ CAUSES OF POSTOPERATIVE ULCER RECURRENCE

Persistent *Helicobacter pylori* infection
Inappropriate primary operation
Highly selective vagotomy for gastric and prepyloric ulcer
Inadequate operation
Incomplete vagotomy
Inadequate drainage
Inadequate resection
Retained antrum
Hypersecretory states
Gastrinoma
Multiple endocrine neoplasia type I syndrome
G cell hyperplasia
Hypercalcemia
Ulcerogenic drugs
Non-steroidal anti-inflammatory drugs
Steroids
Reserpine

resulting in postgastrectomy syndromes, which include dumping, diarrhea, alkaline reflux gastritis, and maldigestion. All these complications are associated with truncal vagotomy and/or gastric resection. Highly selective vagotomy, which is the elective operation of choice, avoids these complications.

For more information about this subject, see *Cecil Textbook of Medicine,* 21st edition. Philadelphia, W.B. Saunders Company, 2000. Chapter 126, Peptic Ulcer Disease: Epidemiology, Pathophysiology, Clinical Manifestations and Diagnosis; Chapter 127, Peptic Ulcer Disease: Medical Therapy; Chapter 128, Complications of Peptic Ulcer; and Chapter 129, Peptic Ulcer Disease: Surgical Therapy, pages 671 to 684.

PANCREATIC ENDOCRINE TUMORS

The eight pancreatic endocrine tumors (Table 9–17) are classified as APUDomas (*a*mine *p*recursor *u*ptake and *d*ecarboxylation), sharing cytochemical features with carcinoid tumors, melanomas, and a number of other endocrine tumors (pheochromocytomas, medullary thyroid cancer). Except for insulinomas, each is frequently malignant.

Gastrinomas

The ZE syndrome is caused by a gastrin-releasing endocrine tumor that is usually located in the pancreas or duodenum and is characterized by clinical symptoms and signs due to gastric acid hypersecretion (ulcer disease, diarrhea, esophageal reflux disease). Twenty to 24 per cent of patients have ZE syndrome as part of the multiple endocrine neoplasia type I (MEN-I) syndrome, an autosomal dominantly inherited disease. These patients have hyperplasia or tumors of multiple endocrine glands, most commonly parathyroid hyperplasia (>90%), pituitary tumors (60%), and pancreatic endocrine tumors (80%).

Table 9–17 ■ PANCREATIC ENDOCRINE TUMORS

NAME OF TUMOR	NAME OF SYNDROME	MAIN SIGNS OR SYMPTOMS	LOCATION (%)	MALIGNANCY (%)	HORMONE CAUSING SYNDROME
Gastrinoma	Zollinger-Ellison syndrome	Abdominal pain Diarrhea Esophageal symptoms	Pancreas (30%) Duodenum (60%) Other (10%)	60–90	Gastrin
Insulinoma	Insulinoma	Hypoglycemic symptoms	Pancreas (100%)	5–15	Insulin
Glucagonoma	Glucagonoma	Dermatitis Diabetes/glucose intolerance Weight loss	Pancreas (100%)	60	Glucagon
VIPoma	Verner-Morrison Pancreatic cholera WDHA	Hypokalemia	Pancreas (90%) Other (10%) (neural, adrenal, periganglionic tissue)	80	Vasoactive intestinal peptide (VIP)
Somatostatinoma	Somatostatinoma	Diabetes mellitus Cholelithiasis Diarrhea	Pancreas (56%) Duodenum/jejunum (44%)	60	Somatostatin
GRFoma	GRFoma	Acromegaly	Pancreas (30%) Lung (54%) Jejunum (7%) Other (13%) (adrenal, foregut, retroperitoneum)	30	Growth hormone–releasing factor (GRF)
ACTHoma	ACTHoma	Cushing's syndrome	Pancreas (4–16% of all ectopic Cushing's)	>95	Adrenocorticotropic hormone (ACTH)
Nonfunctioning	PPoma Nonfunctional	Weight loss Abdominal mass Hepatomegaly	Pancreas (100%)	60–90	None (pancreatic polypeptide [PP] or chromogranin released but no known symptoms due to hypersecretion)

WDHA = *w*atery *d*iarrhea, *h*ypokalemia, and *a*chlorhydria.

The ZE syndrome may be suspected because of peptic ulcer disease that is recurrent, is non-healing despite treatment, is not associated with *H. pylori* infection, is complicated by bleeding, causes obstruction or esophageal stricture, is multiple or in unusual locations, or is associated with a pancreatic tumor or diarrhea. The initial measurement is a fasting serum gastrin level, which is elevated in 99 to 100% of patients.

Either omeprazole or lansoprazole starting at 60 mg/day is now the drug of choice. Long-term therapy appears safe. Selective vagotomy effectively reduces acid secretion, but many patients continue to require a low dose of drug. Parathyroidectomy should be performed in patients with hyperparathyroidism.

All patients should have imaging studies to localize the tumor, which can be identified in 95% of patients. Somatostatin receptor scintigraphy (SRS) using single-photon emission computed tomography (SPECT) after injection of ^{111}In-[DTPA-DPhe^{1}]octreotide is the localization method of choice. For pancreatic gastrinomas, endoscopic US is particularly sensitive. Surgical exploration for cure is now recommended in all patients without liver metastases, MEN-I, or complicating medical conditions limiting life expectancy. Surgical resection decreases the metastatic rate and results in a 5-year cure rate of 30%.

Glucagonomas

Glucagonomas are endocrine tumors of the pancreas that ectopically secrete glucagon, which causes a clinical syndrome whose cardinal features are a distinct dermatitis (necrolytic migratory erythema) (70 to 90%), diabetes mellitus or glucose intolerance (40 to 90%), weight loss (70 to 96%), anemia (30 to 85%), hypoaminoacidemia (80 to 90%), thromboembolism (10 to 25%), diarrhea (15 to 30%), and psychiatric disturbances (0 to 20%). The diagnosis is established by demonstrating elevation of plasma glucagon levels.

Subcutaneous (SC) administration of octreotide controls the rash in 80% of patients and improves weight loss, diarrhea, and hypoaminoacidemia, but usually does not improve the diabetes mellitus. Surgical resection is preferred, and even debulking the tumor may be of benefit. For residual disease, chemotherapy with dacarbazine or streptozotocin and doxorubicin, hepatic embolization, or chemoembolization may help control symptoms.

VIPomas

The VIPoma syndrome, also called the WDHA syndrome (for *w*atery *d*iarrhea, *h*ypokalemia, *a*chlorhydria) is due to an endocrine tumor, usually in the pancreas, that ectopically secretes vasoactive intestinal peptide (VIP). The cardinal clinical feature is severe, large-volume, watery diarrhea (>1 L/day) (100%) that occurs during fasting. Hypokalemia (80 to 100%) and dehydration (83%) commonly occur. The diagnosis is excluded when fasting stool volume is less than 700 mL/day. Elevated VIP levels are present in 90 to 100% of patients.

The symptoms can be controlled in more than 85% of patients by octreotide. Tumor localization studies with somatostatin receptor scintigraphy or surgical resection are preferred if possible; chemotherapy with streptozotocin and doxorubicin, hepatic chemoembolization, or hepatic embolization may benefit patients with unresectable or residual tumor.

Somatostatinomas

Somatostatinomas secrete somatostatin, which causes a distinct clinical syndrome of diabetes mellitus, gallbladder disease, diarrhea, steatorrhea, and weight loss. Duodenal somatostatinomas are frequently reported in patients with von Recklinghausen's disease and are usually asymptomatic. Sixty per cent of somatostatinomas occur in the pancreas and 40% occur in the duodenum or jejunum.

The diagnosis requires the demonstration of increased plasma and tumor concentrations of somatostatin-like immunoreactivity. Surgery, if possible, or chemotherapy, hepatic chemoembolization, or hepatic embolization may be of value.

For more information about this subject, see *Cecil Textbook of Medicine,* 21st edition. Philadelphia, W.B. Saunders Company, 2000. Chapter 130, Pancreatic Exocrine Tumors, pages 684 to 687.

FUNCTIONAL GASTROINTESTINAL DISORDERS: IRRITABLE BOWEL SYNDROME, NON-ULCER DYSPEPSIA, AND NON-CARDIAC CHEST PAIN

Based on clinical and epidemiologic studies, the functional gastrointestinal disorders have been classified according to the presumed anatomic site of the disorder (Table 9–18).

Irritable Bowel Syndrome

Symptoms consistent with irritable bowel syndrome are reported by one in six Americans. Only about one third of persons with irritable bowel syndrome consult a physician, but the condition still accounts for about 12% of primary care visits.

Accumulating evidence suggests that irritable bowel syndrome represents a true disorder of function. Basal colonic motility is normal in irritable bowel syndrome, but these patients tend to have an abnormally responsive colon to meals, drugs, gut hormones (e.g., cholecystokinin), and stress. Abnormal perception of gut sensation (visceral hypersensitivity) is another characteristic finding.

A high proportion of patients with a diagnosis of irritable bowel syndrome in tertiary referral centers (40 to 60%) have coexisting psychiatric disease. Approximately 20% of patients with irritable bowel syndrome identify a history of traveler's diarrhea or gastroenteritis (e.g., *Salmonella*) preceding the onset of symptoms. True food allergy appears to be very rare, but food intolerance may be more important.

Chronic or recurrent abdominal pain is always a feature. Classically, the pain is cramplike or aching and occurs in episodes. The pain of irritable bowel syndrome is relieved by defecation or is associated with a change in stool frequency or consistency.

An irregular disturbance of defecation (predominant constipation or diarrhea, or an alternating bowel pattern) is also a key feature of irritable bowel syndrome, and its absence excludes the diagnosis. Bloating is a common symptom, and symptoms of gastroesopha-

Table 9–18 ■ ROME CLASSIFICATION OF FUNCTIONAL GASTROINTESTINAL DISORDERS AND ESTIMATED PREVALENCE IN THE UNITED STATES

DISORDER	APPROXIMATE U.S. PREVALENCE (%)
Functional bowel disorders	
Irritable bowel syndrome	15
Abdominal pain or discomfort, relieved with defecation or associated with a change in the frequency or consistency of stools, *and*	
An irregular pattern of defecation (≥25% of the time) consisting of 3 or more of the following: altered stool frequency, altered stool form, mucus, bloating, or feeling of distention	
Functional abdominal bloating	30
Functional constipation	<5
Functional diarrhea	<5
Functional gastroduodenal disorders	
Functional (non-ulcer) dyspepsia	15*
Chronic or recurrent pain or discomfort centered in the upper abdomen (i.e., epigastrium)	
Endoscopy fails to identify a definite structural cause	
Aerophagia	20
Functional esophageal disorders	
Non-cardiac chest pain	15
Rumination syndrome	10
Globus	10
Functional abdominal pain	<5
Functional biliary pain (biliary dyskinesia)	<1
Functional anorectal disorders	
Functional incontinence	5
Functional anorectal pain	
Levator syndrome	5
Proctalgia fugax	10
Pelvic floor dyssynergia	10

* Assumes one third with dyspepsia have a structural explanation and are excluded.

geal reflux (heartburn or acid regurgitation) are reported by up to one third of patients with irritable bowel syndrome.

It is important to make a positive clinical diagnosis of irritable bowel syndrome by careful history and physical examination (Fig. 9–3). For patients with predominantly diarrhea, a small bowel radiograph is useful to rule out Crohn's disease. Bacterial overgrowth, detectable by a small bowel aspirate and quantitative culture, may occur in patients with small bowel diverticula or impaired small bowel motility.

TREATMENT. A change in medications may improve symptoms, and unnecessary drugs should be avoided. Increasing dietary fiber with unprocessed bran makes the stools bulkier, softer, and easier to pass and can relieve constipation.

Fad diets and high fat diets should be avoided. Cabbage, beans, legumes, and lentils may be worth avoiding because they are fer-

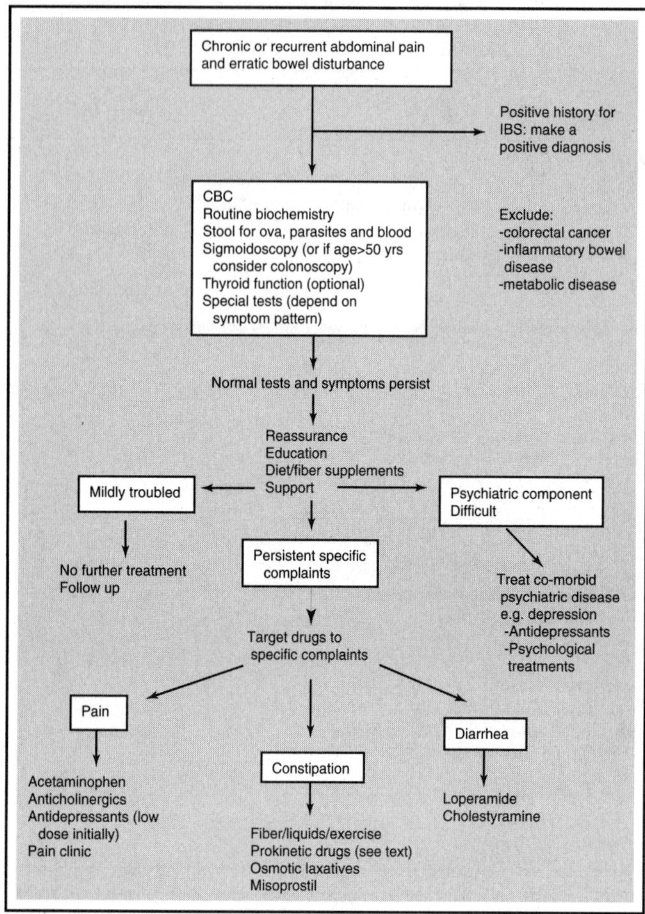

FIGURE 9–3 ■ Algorithm for the evaluation of suspected irritable bowel syndrome (IBS). CBC = complete blood count.

mented in the colon and may increase flatus. Avoidance of milk products may be helpful even in some patients without lactose intolerance.

The placebo response in irritable bowel syndrome is between 40% and 70%. In patients who complain of postprandial abdominal pain, antispasmodics are useful when administered 30 to 60 minutes before meals to reduce the gastrocolonic response. Alternatives include hyoscyamine (e.g., one to two timed-released capsules twice daily), belladonna 0.2 to 0.75 mL four times daily, dicyclomine 20 to 40 mg four times daily, and propantheline bromide 7.5 or 15 mg four times daily.

Patients who do not respond to dietary fiber for treatment of constipation may benefit from lactulose or milk of magnesia, the dose of which can be titrated depending on the clinical response. The pharmacologic agent of choice for predominant diarrhea is loperamide 2 to 4 mg three to four times per day. Simethicone is not helpful for bloating. Antidepressants are particularly useful in resistant patients.

Functional (Non-Ulcer) Dyspepsia

Symptoms in patients with functional dyspepsia are indistinguishable from the symptoms encountered in patients with peptic ulcer disease. Up to 50% of patients seen at tertiary referral centers with functional dyspepsia have delayed gastric emptying for solids, and a similar number have antral hypomotility after meals.

Patients with functional dyspepsia have a decreased pain threshold during balloon distention of the stomach. In general, patients who present for medical care with functional dyspepsia are more anxious and depressed than healthy controls and have higher neuroticism and somatization scores. Coffee may induce symptoms in approximately 50% of patients with functional dyspepsia.

The major organic causes to consider are chronic peptic ulcer disease, gastroesophageal reflux (with or without esophagitis), and, rarely but important, malignancy (Fig. 9–4).

Not all patients want or require medication for functional dyspepsia. Antacids are commonly used by patients with functional dyspepsia, but randomized controlled studies have all failed to show a significant benefit over placebo. The results of controlled trials testing full-dose H_2-receptor antagonists (cimetidine or ranitidine) have been conflicting. Reports have described promising improvement of ulcer-like dyspepsia during treatment with a proton pump inhibitor (omeprazole 20 mg/day, or lansoprazole, 30 mg/day) compared with placebo.

The dopaminergic receptor blockers metoclopramide and domperidone are widely used in functional dyspepsia, and convincing evidence from randomized controlled trials demonstrates that these prokinetics are superior to placebo. The prokinetic metoclopramide has an excellent safety profile.

Older patients (>45 years) with new, unexplained dyspepsia and those with alarming symptoms or on NSAIDs have an increased risk of organic disease and should undergo prompt upper endoscopic evaluation.

Non-Cardiac (Functional) Chest Pain

Clinical evaluation should be directed initially at excluding cardiac causes of chest pain (see Table 5–1). Ambulatory 24-hour esophageal pH monitoring, endoscopy, or acid perfusion (Bernstein) tests may be useful in diagnosing reflux. In the remaining patients, esophageal manometry may be considered, but the yield is low. An aggressive trial of acid suppression with proton pump inhibitors should be prescribed if there is any suspicion of reflux, with the dose doubled if there is no response after 1 to 2 weeks.

For more information about this subject, see *Cecil Textbook of*

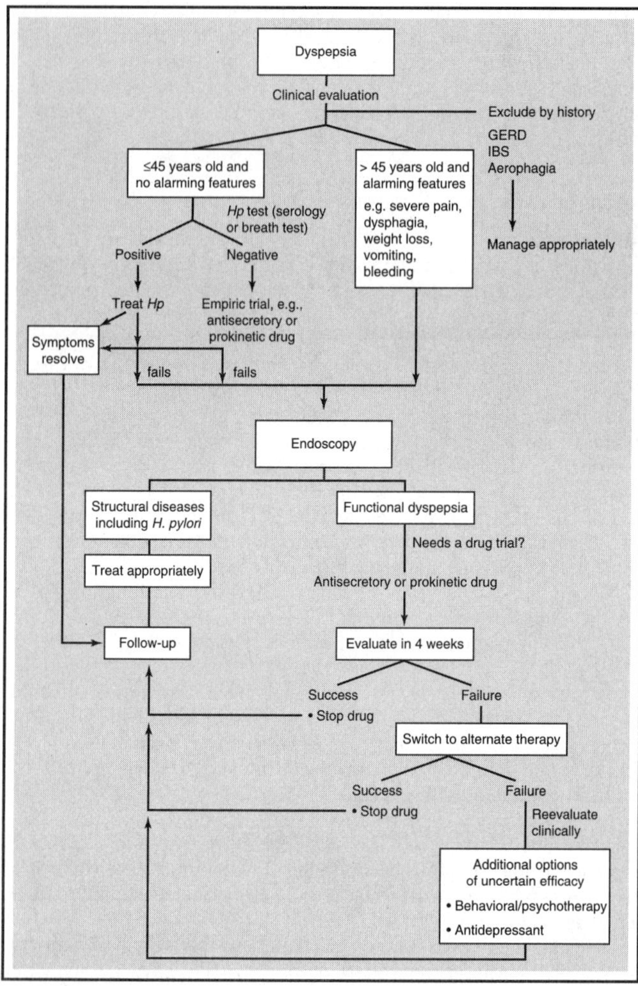

FIGURE 9–4 ■ Algorithm for the evaluation of dyspepsia. *Hp* = *Helicobacter pylori;* GERD = symptomatic gastroesophageal reflux disease; IBS = irritable bowel syndrome.

Medicine, 21st edition. Philadelphia, W.B. Saunders Company, 2000. Chapter 131, Functional Gastrointestinal Disorders: Irritable Bowel Syndrome, Non-Ulcer Dyspepsia, and Non-cardiac Chest Pain, pages 687 to 694.

DISORDERS OF GASTROINTESTINAL MOTILITY

Early satiety, nausea, and postprandial vomiting occur in patients with delayed transit through the stomach and upper small bowel.

Table 9–19 ■ MAJOR CAUSES OF VOMITING

Gastroenteritis
Gastritis/gastric ulcer
Motion sickness
Gastroparesis
Gastric outlet obstruction
Small bowel obstruction (usually above midjejunum)
Systemic illness (high fever/severe pain)
Peritonitis
Pregnancy (including hyperemesis gravidarum or acute fatty liver of pregnancy)
Drugs or toxins (including chemotherapy)
Increased intracranial pressure
Psychogenic vomiting/eating disorder

These symptoms can also result from organic non-motility disorders (Table 9–19).

Delayed Gastric Emptying

Delayed gastric emptying may be associated with other systemic diseases or may be due to a primary dysfunction of the stomach (Table 9–20). Acute gastroparesis, which is most frequently associated with an electrolyte disturbance, ketoacidosis, systemic infection, or an acute abdominal insult, is managed by treating the underlying disease, not the gastric motility disorder.

Metoclopramide improves the symptoms of gastric stasis in patients with diabetes mellitus both by increasing gastric emptying and decreasing the central nervous system recognition of nausea and distention. Bethanechol also stimulates an increase in gastric motility and improves symptoms in patients with diabetic gastric stasis. Erythromycin improves symptoms of gastroparesis by increasing antral contractions and fundal tone. Clonidine can improve gastric emptying and symptoms.

Disorders of Small Intestinal Motility

Small intestine motility may be hypoactive, hyperactive, or uncoordinated (Table 9–21). Diarrhea is generally the result of rapid intestinal transit. Patients with slow intestinal transit tend to complain of nausea, vomiting, abdominal distention, and periumbil-

Table 9–20 ■ GASTRIC MOTILITY DISORDERS

DELAYED GASTRIC EMPTYING	RAPID GASTRIC EMPTYING
Postvagotomy	Dumping syndrome
Diabetes mellitus	Pancreatic insufficiency
Viral infections	Celiac sprue
Reflux esophagitis	Zollinger-Ellison syndrome
Brain stem lesions	Duodenal ulcer
Anorexia nervosa	
Tachygastria	

Table 9–21 ■ SMALL INTESTINAL MOTILITY DISORDERS

Decreased Motility
Hollow visceral myopathy (primary intestinal pseudo-obstruction)
Progressive systemic sclerosis (late)
Amyloidosis
Muscular dystrophy
Duchenne's
Myotonic
Hypothyroidism
Jejunal diverticulosis
Jejunoileal bypass
Increased or Uncoordinated Motility
Primary visceral neuropathy
Carcinoma-associated visceral neuropathy
Progressive systemic sclerosis (early)
Irritable bowel syndrome
Diabetes mellitus
Infectious diarrhea
Mass lesion of brain stem
Amyloidosis
Hyperthyroidism
Carcinoid syndrome
Shy-Drager syndrome

ical abdominal cramps. Although constipation can occur with delayed intestinal transit, diarrhea is more common.

Hollow Visceral Myopathy (Primary Intestinal Pseudo-Obstruction)

Patients usually present with symptoms and signs of small intestinal stasis without evidence of an anatomic obstruction or of a secondary cause for pseudo-obstruction. Hollow visceral myopathy is familial, but random, non-familial cases are probably more common. With familial primary intestinal pseudo-obstruction, parts of the urinary system (bladder, renal pelvis) may also be dilated.

Approximately 40% of patients with progressive systemic sclerosis have defects in both neural and smooth muscle function of the intestine. Low doses of the somatostatin analogue octreotide stimulate phase 3 of the migrating motor complex and improve symptoms in systemic sclerosis.

Disorders of Colon Motility (Table 9–22)

The symptoms of painful colonic diverticular disease are similar to those of the irritable bowel syndrome but are more likely to be localized in the left lower quadrant. When diverticulitis occurs as a complication, the patient may have fever, left lower quadrant mass, leukocytosis, and occult blood in the stool. Painful diverticular disease of the colon is best treated by decreasing the intraluminal pressure, similar to therapy for the irritable bowel syndrome.

Hirschsprung's disease is the congenital absence of enteric neurons in the submucosal and myenteric plexuses. The severity of

Table 9–22 ■ PATHOGENESIS OF COLONIC MOTILITY DISORDERS

Slow Transit
Increased segmenting contraction
Primary constipation
Irritable bowel syndrome (spastic)
Diverticular disease
Anal outlet obstruction
Congenital-Hirschsprung's disease
Acquired
Decreased segmenting contractions
Irritable bowel syndrome (inertia)
Primary colonic pseudo-obstruction
Ogilvie's syndrome
Diabetes mellitus
Progressive systemic sclerosis
Spinal cord injury
Rapid Transit
Functional diarrhea
Bile salt diarrhea
Surreptitious abuse of laxatives

9

symptoms and the age at diagnosis are related to the length of the aganglionic segment. Patients may have chronic distention with a fecal impaction. Some patients have functional, painless diarrhea with fecal urgency but with no associated anatomic or histologic abnormality of the gastrointestinal tract. In treating functional diarrhea, antidiarrheal agents such as the opioid analogues, loperamide, and diphenoxylate decrease symptoms.

For more information about this subject, see *Cecil Textbook of Medicine,* 21st edition. Philadelphia, W.B. Saunders Company, 2000. Chapter 132, Disorders of Gastrointestinal Motility, pages 694 to 702.

DIARRHEA

Acute diarrheas are defined as those of less than 2 to 3 weeks', and rarely, 6 to 8 weeks' duration. The most common cause of acute diarrheas are infectious agents. *Chronic diarrheas* are those of at least 4 and, more usually, more than 6 to 8 weeks' duration. There are three categories of chronic diarrheas: osmotic (malabsorptive) diarrhea, secretory diarrhea, and inflammatory diarrhea.

Acute Diarrheas

Most infectious diarrheas are acquired through fecal-oral transmission from water, food, or person-to-person contact (Table 9–23). Patients with infectious diarrhea often complain of nausea, vomiting, and abdominal pain and have either watery, malabsorptive, or bloody diarrhea and fever (dysentery).

Diarrhea and the neurologic symptoms (tingling and burning around the mouth, facial flushing, sweating, headache, palpitations, and dizziness) of seafood poisoning may be caused by histamine release from the decaying flesh of a blood fish (dolphin, tuna,

Table 9–23 ■ EPIDEMIOLOGY OF ACUTE INFECTIOUS DIARRHEA AND INFECTIOUS FOOD-BORNE ILLNESS

VEHICLE	CLASSIC PATHOGEN
Water (including foods washed in such water)	*Vibro cholerae,* Norwalk agent, *Giardia,* and *Cryptosporidium*
Food	
Poultry	*Salmonella, Campylobacter,* and *Shigella* spp.
Beef, unpasteurized fruit juice	Enterohemorrhagic *Escherichia coli*
Pork	Tapeworm
Seafood and shellfish (including raw sushi and gefilte fish)	*V. cholerae, Vibrio parahaemolyticus,* and *Vibrio vulnificus; Salmonella* and *Shigella* spp; hepatitis A and B; tapeworm; and anisakiasis
Cheese, milk	*Listeria* spp.
Eggs	*Salmonella* spp.
Mayonnaise-containing foods and cream pies	Staphylococcal and clostridial food poisonings
Fried rice	*Bacillus cereus*
Fresh berries	*Cyclospora* spp.
Canned vegetables or fruits	*Clostridium* spp.
Animal-to-person (pets and livestock)	*Salmonella, Campylobacter, Cryptosporidium,* and *Giardia* spp.
Person-to-person (including sexual contact)	All enteric bacteria, viruses, and parasites
Day care center	*Shigella, Campylobacter, Cryptosporidium,* and *Giardia* spp; viruses, *Clostridium difficile*
Hospital, antibiotics or chemotherapy	*C. difficile*
Swimming pool	*Giardia* and *Cryptosporidium* spp.
Foreign travel	*E. coli* of various types; *Salmonella, Shigella, Campylobacter, Giardia,* and *Cryptosporidium* spp.; *Entamoeba histolytica*

Adapted from Powell DW: Approach to the patient with diarrhea. *In* Yamada T, Alpers DH, Owyang C, et al (eds.): Textbook of Gastroenterology, 3rd ed. Philadelphia, Lippincott–Raven, 1999.

marlin, or mackerel) after it is caught. This form of seafood poisoning is called *scomboid*. Plankton, algae, or dinoflagellates ingested by tropical and subtropical fish (amberjack, snapper, grouper, or barracuda) produce a toxin (ciguatoxin) that causes seafood poisoning known as *ciguatera*. The dinoflagellate toxins cause nausea, vomiting, abdominal pain, diarrhea, and neurologic symptoms such as weakness, pruritus, circumoral paresthesias, temperature reversal (hot drinks taste cold and vice versa) and even psychiatric abnormalities and memory loss. Shellfish poisonings are also due to algae or dinoflagellates ingested by bivalve mollusks; these different toxins may cause predominantly and occasionally severe neurologic symptoms (paralytic, neurotoxic or amnestic shellfish poisonings) or predominantly gastrointestinal symptoms (diarrheal shellfish poisoning). Puffer fish poisoning (tetrodotoxin) causes neurologic symptoms, respiratory paralysis, or even death.

The differential diagnosis of acute watery diarrhea includes food toxins, drugs, medications, and diseases (Fig. 9–5). Diarrhea may

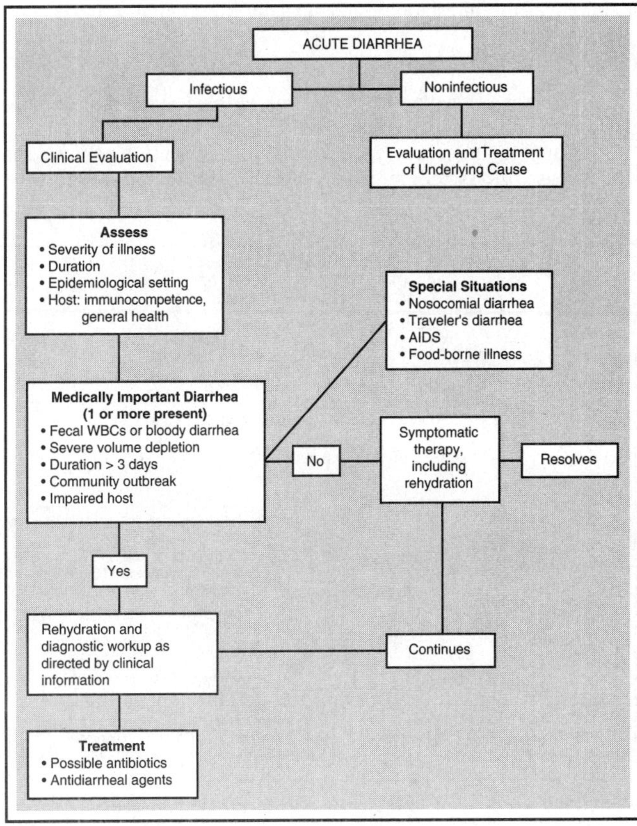

FIGURE 9–5 ■ Algorithm for the diagnostic approach to acute diarrhea. (Adapted from Parks SI, Giannella R: Approach to the patient with acute diarrhea. Gastroenterol Clin North Am 22:483, 1993.)

occur in up to 20% of patients receiving broad-spectrum antibiotics. Only half or fewer of these diarrheas are due to *Clostridium difficile* colitis (pseudomembranous colitis). Bacterial agents account for 85% of traveler's diarrhea.

Liquid formulations of any medication may cause diarrhea (elixir diarrhea) because of the high content of sorbitol used to sweeten the elixir. The incidence of acute, mild diarrhea with cancer chemotherapy or radiation therapy is quite high, approaching 100% with some agents such as amsacrine, azacitidine, cytarabine, dactinomycin, daunorubicin, doxorubicin, floxuridine, 5-fluorouracil (5-FU), 6-mercaptopurine (6-MP), methotrexate, and plicamycin.

Bismuth subsalicylate (Pepto-Bismol) is safe and efficacious in bacterial infectious diarrheas, whereas kaolin-pectin preparations are only minimally effective. Loperamide can be both useful and safe in acute or traveler's diarrhea, provided it is not given to patients with dysentery (high fever, with blood or pus in the stool) and especially when administered concomitantly with effective antibiotics. Certain infectious diarrheas should be treated with antibiotics: shigellosis, cholera, traveler's diarrhea, pseudomembranous enterocolitis, parasitic infestations, and sexually transmitted diseases.

Chronic Diarrhea

The goal in evaluating a patient with chronic diarrhea is to make a definitive diagnosis as quickly and inexpensively as possible (Fig. 9–6). Stool culture and examination may detect organisms that often cause protracted infectious diarrhea in adults: enteropatho-

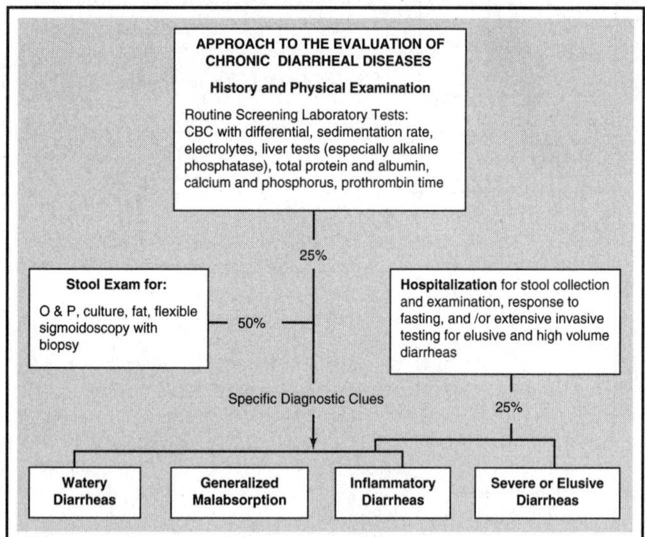

FIGURE 9–6 ■ Approach to the evaluation of malabsorption. CBC = complete blood count; O & P = ova and parasites. (Adapted from Powell DW: Approach to the patient with diarrhea. *In* Yamada T, Alpers DH, Owyang C, et al [eds]: Textbook of Gastroenterology, 3rd ed. Philadelphia, Lippincott–Raven, 1999.)

genic (enteroadherent) *Escherichia coli, Giardia, Entamoeba, Cryptosporidium, Aeromonas,* and *Yersinia enterocolitica.* If none of these organisms is found, a therapeutic trial of metronidazole or trimethoprim-sulfamethoxazole may be indicated. Up to 25% of patients will experience pain, bloating, urgency, a sense of incomplete evacuation, and loose stools for 6 months or longer after documented infectious diarrhea.

WATERY DIARRHEA. Chewing gum and elixir diarrhea can result from the chronic ingestion of dietetic foods, candy, chewing gum, or medication elixirs that are sweetened with unabsorbable carbohydrates such as sorbitol. Diets high in carbohydrate and low in fat may allow rapid gastric emptying and rapid small intestine motility, leading to carbohydrate malabsorption and osmotic diarrhea.

Bile acid–induced diarrhea can result from severe disease (e.g., Crohn's disease), resection, or bypass of the distal ileum, which allows dihydroxy bile salts to escape absorption. Bile acid diarrhea is also caused by measured increases in fecal bile acids in patients with postcholecystectomy diarrhea. Although many patients respond to cholestyramine, some do not.

True secretory diarrheas can be caused by metastatic carcinoid tumors of the gastrointestinal tract, gastrinomas, and non–beta cell pancreatic adenomas that secrete various peptide secretagogues, including VIP or calcitonin. Large (4 to 10 cm) adenomas of the rectum or rectosigmoid may cause a secretory form of diarrhea of 500 to 3000 mL/24 hours with hypokalemia. The diarrhea of systemic mastocytosis may be malabsorptive, secondary to mast cell infiltration of the mucosa with resulting villus atrophy, or intermittent and secretory.

Approximately 15% of patients referred for diarrhea to secondary or tertiary centers and 25% of patients with proven secretory diarrheas are found to be ingesting either laxatives or diuretics surreptitiously. Binge drinking of alcohol causes a brief diarrhea that usually lasts less than 1 day.

Up to 20% of young to middle-aged diabetics, particularly men between 20 and 40 years of age whose diabetes has been poorly controlled for more than 5 years, may have a profuse watery, urgent diarrhea, often occurring at night with incontinence. These patients usually have concomitant neuropathy, nephropathy, and retinopathy.

INFLAMMATORY DIARRHEAS. Patients with Crohn's disease or ulcerative colitis have diarrhea with stool volumes usually less than 1 L/24 hours. Infiltration of various layers of the gastrointestinal tract with eosinophils is a recognized clinical entity (eosinophilic gastroenteritis) that is accompanied by diarrhea in 30 to 60% of such patients. Peripheral eosinophilia is present in 75% of these patients. Intolerance to cow's milk and soy protein is a well-established cause of enterocolitis in infants. However, the role of food allergy in causing diarrhea in adults is less clear. Commonly suspected allergens include milk, eggs, seafood, nuts, artificial flavors, and food coloring.

Collagenous and microscopic colitis may be categorized as either inflammatory or secretory diarrheas. An epidemiologic relation to chronic NSAID use has been reported.

Severe protein loss through the gastrointestinal tract caused by ulceration, obstructed lymphatics, and immune-related vascular injury occurs in a variety of disease states: bacterial or parasitic infection, gastritis, gastric cancer, collagenous colitis, inflammatory bowel disease, congenital intestinal lymphangiectasia, sarcoidosis, lymphoma, mesenteric tuberculosis, Ménétrier's disease, sprue, eosinophilic gastroenteritis, systemic lupus erythematosus, or food allergies. The condition usually responds to corticosteroids or immunosuppressive therapy.

Patients receiving pelvic radiation for malignancies of the female urogenital tract or the male prostate may develop chronic radiation enterocolitis 6 to 12 months after total doses of radiation greater than 4 to 6 Gy. Chronic mesenteric vascular ischemia may present as watery diarrhea. Gastrointestinal tuberculosis and histoplasmosis present as diarrhea that may either be bloody or watery, as do certain immunologic diseases such as Behçet's syndrome or Churg-Strauss syndrome. *Fecal incontinence,* which may or may not be associated with diarrhea, has many causes (Table 9–24).

EVALUATION. A history of 10 to 20 bowel movements per day suggests secretory diarrhea. The important clinical manifestations of inflammatory diarrheas are the signs and symptoms of inflammation and/or the effects of severe chronic protein loss (Fig. 9–7). Qualitative tests on outpatient spot stool collections and quantitative tests (stool fat, electrolytes, and osmolality) or 48 to 72-hour stool collections can help define the causes of diarrhea, especially severe or elusive diarrheas.

Certain diseases may present radiographically as uniform thickening of the intestinal folds (e.g., amyloidosis, lymphoma, Whip-

Table 9–24 ■ CAUSES OF FECAL INCONTINENCE

- Normal sphincters and pelvic floor
  - Diarrhea
  - Fistula
- Abnormal function of sphincters and/or pelvic floor
  - Minor incontinence
    - Deficient internal sphincter
      - Trauma
      - Rectal prolapse
      - Third-degree hemorrhoids
    - Fecal impaction
      - Advanced age
      - Neurologic disorders
    - Minor external sphincter and pelvic floor denervation
  - Major incontinence
    - Congenital anomalies
    - Trauma
    - Complete rectal prolapse
    - Rectal carcinoma
    - Anorectal infection
    - Idiopathic
    - Drug intoxication
    - Neurologic
    - Upper motor neuron
      - Cerebral
      - Spinal
    - Lower motor neuron

Modified from Henry MM, Swash M (eds): Coloproctology and the Pelvic Floor: Pathophysiology and Management, Boston, Butterworths, 1985.

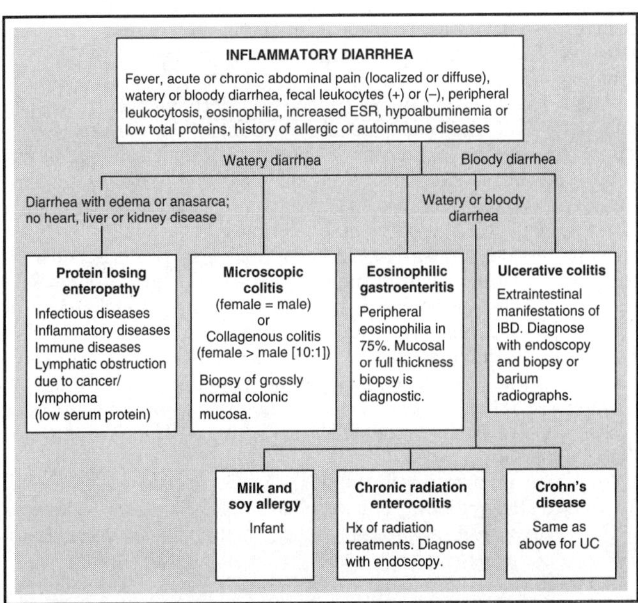

FIGURE 9–7 ■ Approach to the evaluation of inflammatory diarrheas. IBD = inflammatory bowel disease; UC = ulcerative colitis. (Adapted from Powell DW: Approach to the patient with diarrhea. *In* Yamada T, Alpers DH, Owyang C, et al [eds]. Textbook of Gastroenterology, 3rd ed. Philadelphia, Lippincott-Raven, 1999.)

9

ple's disease); others such as lymphoma or lymphangiectasia demonstrate uniform or patchy abnormalities. Routine contrast radiographs of the gastrointestinal tract are not usually helpful in the diagnosis of watery diarrheas. Upper endoscopy with distal duodenal biopsy should be undertaken if the presence of steatorrhea suggests small bowel mucosal malabsorption. Patients with severe watery or elusive diarrhea should have flexible sigmoidoscopy or, preferably, colonoscopy to exclude villous adenomas of the rectosigmoid, and biopsy to exclude microscopic or collagenous colitis, mastocytosis, or early inflammatory bowel disease.

For watery diarrhea, breath tests measure the respiratory excretion of labeled CO_2 after oral administration and metabolism of radioactive carbon-labeled substrates or of H_2 after administration of carbohydrates. These tests can assess fat, carbohydrate, and bile salt malabsorption or bacterial overgrowth. To test for lactase deficiency in patients in whom a therapeutic trial of carbohydrate-restricted free diet is inconclusive, breath hydrogen testing may be indicated.

The diagnosis of endocrine tumors such as carcinoids, gastrinoma, VIPoma, medullary carcinoma of the thyroid, glucagonoma, somatostatinoma, and systemic mastocytosis is made by demonstrating elevated blood levels of serotonin or urinary 5-hydroxyindole acetic acid and serum levels for gastrin, VIP calcitonin, glucagon, somatostatin, histamine, or prostaglandins, respectively.

Recently, somatostatin receptor scintigraphy has proven to be both sensitive and useful in the diagnosis and evaluation of ZE syndrome.

ANTIDIARRHEAL THERAPY. The bulk-forming agents (Kaopectate, psyllium, and methylcellulose) increase the consistency of stool and have no antisecretory activity. Bismuth salicylates, opiates, loperamide, clonidine, phenothiazine, and somatostatin have mild antisecretory activity but also cause dilation of the small intestine and colon and decrease peristalsis. Loperamide does not pass the blood-brain barrier and has a high first-pass metabolism in the liver. It has a high therapeutic-toxic ratio and is essentially devoid of addiction potential, so it is quite safe in adults, even in total doses of 24 mg/day. The usual dose is 2 to 4 mg two to four times daily. Octreotide has its major antisecretory effect in carcinoid syndrome and in neuroendocrine tumors because it inhibits hormone secretion by the tumor. Clonidine can be very useful in the diarrhea of opiate withdrawal and occasionally in patients with diabetic diarrhea.

For more information about this subject, see *Cecil Textbook of Medicine,* 21st edition. Philadelphia, W.B. Saunders Company, 2000. Chapter 133, Approach to the Patient with Diarrhea, pages 702 to 712.

MALABSORPTION SYNDROMES

Many diseases (Table 9–25) and drugs (Table 9–26) can cause malabsorption. Significant malabsorption of fat and carbohydrate usually causes chronic diarrhea, abdominal cramps, gas, bloating, and weight loss. Cheilosis and angular stomatitis can be due to riboflavin, iron, cobalamin, or folate deficiency. Manifestations of calcium, magnesium, or vitamin D malabsorption include paresthesias and tetany due to hypocalcemia or hypomagnesemia and bone pain due to osteomalacia or osteoporosis-related fractures. Paresthesias and ataxia are manifestations of cobalamin and vitamin E deficiency.

Diagnosis and Treatment

Chronic pancreatitis is the most common cause of pancreatic insufficiency. In the United States, chronic pancreatitis is most commonly due to alcohol abuse. Fat malabsorption due to chronic pancreatitis usually causes bulky, fat-laden stools, but fat-soluble vitamin absorption usually is preserved.

Malabsorption can occur in individuals with cholestatic liver disease or bile duct obstruction due to decreased bile salt synthesis and delivery. Osteoporosis is more common than osteomalacia.

Any condition that produces local stasis or recirculation of colonic luminal contents allows development of a predominantly "colonic" flora (coliforms and anaerobes such as *Bacteroides* and *Clostridum*) in the small intestine. Individuals with *bacterial overgrowth* can present with diarrhea, abdominal cramps, gas and bloating, weight loss, and signs and symptoms of vitamin B_{12} and fat-soluble vitamin deficiency. Acid-reducing agents should be stopped if possible. Treatment with antibiotics should be based on culture results when possible; otherwise, empiric treatment is given.

Table 9–25 ■ CAUSES OF MALABSORPTION

- Conditions that impair mixing
  - Partial gastrectomy with gastrojejunostomy
- Conditions that impair lipolysis
  - Chronic pancreatitis
  - Pancreatic cancer
  - Congenital pancreatic insufficiency
  - Congenital colipase deficiency
  - Gastrinoma
- Conditions that impair micelle formation
  - Severe chronic liver disease
  - Cholestatic liver disease
  - Bacterial overgrowth
  - Crohn's disease
  - Ileal resection
  - Gastrinoma
- Conditions that impair mucosal absorption
  - Congenital, primary, and secondary lactase deficiency
  - Congenital enterokinase deficiency
  - Abetalipoproteinemia
  - Giardiasis
  - Celiac disease
  - Tropical sprue
  - Agammaglobulinemia
  - Amyloidosis
  - AIDS-related (infections, enteropathy)
  - Radiation enteritis
  - Graft-versus-host disease
  - Whipple's disease
  - Eosinophilic gastroenteritis
  - Megaloblastic gut
  - Collagenous sprue
  - Ulcerative jejunitis
  - Lymphoma
  - Bacterial overgrowth
  - Short-bowel syndrome
  - Mastocytosis
- Conditions that impair nutrient delivery
  - Congenital intestinal lymphangiectasia
  - Lymphoma
  - Tuberculosis
  - Constrictive pericarditis
  - Severe congestive heart failure
- Conditions in which the mechanism of malabsorption is unknown
  - Hypoparathyroidism
  - Adrenal insufficiency
  - Hyperthyroidism
  - Carcinoid syndrome

Tetracycline 250 to 500 mg orally [PO] four times daily or a broad-spectrum antibiotic against aerobes and enteric anaerobes (ciprofloxacin 500 mg PO twice daily, amoxicillin/clavulanic acid 250 to 500 mg PO three times daily, cephalexin 250 mg PO four times daily with metronidazole 250 to 500 mg three times daily) should be given for 14 days. Motility disorders should be treated

Table 9–26 ■ DRUGS AND DIETARY PRODUCTS THAT IMPAIR NUTRIENT ABSORPTION

Cholestyramine
High fiber, phytates
Tetracycline
Antacids
Olestra
Orlistat
Metformin
Acarbose
Colchicine
Neomycin
Methotrexate
Phenytoin
Sulfasalazine

with prokinetic agents such as metoclopramide 10 mg PO four times daily, or erythromycin 250 to 500 mg PO four times daily. Octreotide 50 μg SC every day may improve motility in individuals with scleroderma.

With *ileal disease* or resection, the clinical consequences of bile salt malabsorption are directly related to the length of the diseased or resected terminal ileum. Fat absorption remains normal because of increased bile salt production, and micelle formation is preserved. Such patients can be treated with cholestyramine 2 to 4 g taken at breakfast, lunch, and dinner, an antimolity agent (loperamide or diphenoxylate hydrochloride), and a multiple vitamin and mineral supplement.

Acquired *lactase deficiency* is the most common cause of selective carbohydrate malabsorption. The diagnosis can be made by empiric treatment with a lactose-free diet, which results in resolution of symptoms, or by the hydrogen breath test after oral administration of lactose.

Celiac disease, also called celiac sprue, nontropical sprue, and gluten-sensitive enteropathy, is an inflammatory condition of the small intestine precipated by the ingestion of wheat, rye, and barley in individuals with certain genetic predispositions. The diagnosis of celiac disease is made by characteristic changes found on small intestinal biopsy. Antigliadin IgG and IgA antibodies are sensitive but not specific. Antiendomysial IgA antibodies (antibodies against the lining of smooth muscle bundles) are highly sensitive (90%) and specific (96 to 100%) for active celiac disease. Treatment consists of a lifelong gluten-free diet. Up to 90% of patients with celiac disease treated with a gluten-free diet experience symptomatic improvement within 2 weeks.

Tropical sprue is an inflammatory disease of the small intestine associated with the overgrowth of predominantly coliform bacteria. Treatment is a prolonged course of broad-spectrum antibiotics, oral folate, and vitamin B_{12} injections until symptoms resolve.

Giardia lamblia, the most common protozoal infection in the United States, can cause malabsorption in individuals infected with a large number of trophozoites, especially the immunocompromised or IgA-deficient host. Malabsorption occurs when a large number of organisms cover the epithelium. Stool for ova and parasites at

this stage of infection is often negative because of the attachment of organisms in the proximal small intestine. Diagnosis can be made by a stool and small intestinal biopsies.

AIDS-related diarrhea, malabsorption, and wasting are common findings in individuals with AIDS. Malabsorption is usually due to infection with cryptosporidia, *Mycobacterium avium-intracellulare* complex, *Isospora belli,* and microsporidia. *AIDS enteropathy,* a term used when no organism is identified, can also cause malabsorption.

Whipple's disease, a rare cause of malabsorption, manifests with gastrointestinal complaints in association with systemic symptoms such as fever, joint pain, or neurologic manifestations. Whipple's disease is caused by a gram-positive actinomycete, *Tropheryma whippelli.* Treatment is with a prolonged course of broad-spectrum antibiotics. Relapses are common.

Gastrointestinal dysfunction is common after *radiation* treatment to the pelvis or abdomen. Most individuals have an increased frequency of bowel movements for life.

Graft-versus-host disease (GVHD) causes diarrhea frequently after allogeneic bone marrow or stem cell transplantation. Immediately after transplant, diarrhea is due to the toxic effects of cytoreductive therapy on the intestinal epithelium. At 20 to 100 days after transplant, diarrhea is usually due to GVHD or infection.

9

For more information about this subject, see *Cecil Textbook of Medicine,* 21st edition. Philadelphia, W.B. Saunders Company, 2000. Chapter 134, Malabsorption Syndromes, pages 712 to 722.

INFLAMMATORY BOWEL DISEASE

In ulcerative colitis, inflammation begins in the rectum, extends proximally a certain distance, and then abruptly stops, with a clear demarcation between involved and uninvolved mucosa (Table 9–27). In Crohn's disease, the bowel wall is thickened and stiff. The mesentery, which is thickened, edematous, and contracted, fixes the intestine in one position. All layers of the intestine are thickened, and the lumen is narrowed. Skip lesions with two involved areas separated by a length of normal intestine suggest Crohn's disease. The earliest lesion of Crohn's disease is the aphthous ulcer, which typically occurs over Peyer patches in the small intestine and over lymphoid aggregates in the colon.

The dominant symptom in ulcerative colitis is diarrhea, which is usually associated with blood in the stool (Table 9–28). Systemic features, including fever, malaise, and weight loss, are more common if all or most of the colon is involved.

Crohn's disease presents with one of three major patterns: (1) disease in the ileum and cecum (40% of patients); (2) disease confined to the small intestine (30%); and (3) disease confined to the colon (25%). The predominant symptoms are diarrhea, abdominal pain, and weight loss. Fever and chills often accompany disease activity; a low-grade fever may be the patient's first warning sign of a flare. Aphthous ulcers of the lips, gingiva, or buccal mucosa are common.

The most common extraintestinal manifestation of inflammatory bowel disease (IBD) is arthritis, including colitic arthritis and ankylosing spondylitis. The hepatic complications of IBD include fatty

Table 9–27 ■ COMPARISON OF ULCERATIVE COLITIS AND CROHN'S DISEASE

	ULCERATIVE COLITIS	CROHN'S DISEASE
Pathology		
Rectal involvement	Always	Common
Skip lesions	Never	Common
Transmural involvement	Rare	Common
Granulomas	Occasional	Common
Perianal disease	Never	Common
"Cobblestone" mucosa	Rare	Common
Radiology		
"Collar button" ulcers	Common	Occasional
Small intestinal involvement	Never	Common
Discontinuous involvement	Never	Common
Fistulas	Never	Common
Strictures	Occasional	Common
Endoscopy		
Aphthous ulcers	Never	Common
Discontinuous involvement	Never	Common
Rectal sparing	Never	Common
Linear or serpiginous ulcers	Never	Common
Ulcers in terminal ileum	Never	Common

liver, pericholangitis, chronic active hepatitis, and cirrhosis. The biliary tract complications are sclerosing cholangitis (ulcerative colitis) and gallstones (Crohn's disease). The two common dermal complications of IBD are pyoderma gangrenosum and erythema nodosum. The ocular complications of IBD are uveitis and episcleritis.

Radiography and Endoscopy

In both ulcerative colitis and Crohn's disease, radiographic findings may not correlate well with disease activity. The patient's clinical response or endoscopic finding is more useful for this purpose.

The earliest endoscopic manifestations of ulcerative colitis are the development of diffuse erythema and loss of the fine vascular pattern seen in the normal rectal mucosa. The inflamed mucosa bleeds easily if touched with the endoscope; this easy bleeding is termed *friability*. In more severe disease, the mucosa bleeds sponta-

Table 9–28 ■ CRITERIA FOR SEVERITY IN INFLAMMATORY BOWEL DISEASE

Mild:	Fewer than 4 bowel movements per day with little or no blood, no fever, and sedimentation rate <20 mm/hr.
Moderate:	Between mild and severe.
Severe:	Six or more bowel movements per day with blood, fever, anemia, and sedimentation rate >30 mm/hr.

neously and small ulcerations appear. The earliest endoscopic manifestation of Crohn's disease is the apthous ulcer, a small discrete ulcer a few millimeters in diameter surrounded by a thin red halo of edematous tissue.

In ulcerative colitis, inflammation is seen in the rectum and extends proximally for some distance; in extensive disease, inflammation extends to the cecum. Although ulcerative colitis does not involve the small intestine, there may be a few centimeters of inflamed mucosa without ulceration in the terminal ileum. A major distinguishing mark in favor of Crohn's disease is the presence of transmural inflammatory changes.

Differential Diagnosis

Infections with *Shigella, Entamoeba, Giardia, E. coli* O157:H7 and *Campylobacter* organisms can present with bloody diarrhea, cramps, and an endoscopic picture identical to ulcerative colitis. An important distinction between these infectious diseases (except amebiasis) and IBD is that the diarrhea in the infectious diseases tends to be limited to a period of days to a few weeks.

Collagenous colitis is a chronic inflammatory disease marked histologically by the presence of a thick collagen deposition in the subepithelial layer of the colonic mucosa; biopsy with histology provides the diagnosis. Ischemic colitis is part of the differential diagnosis of the initial bout of IBD and should be considered in the elderly. Diverticulitis, which may be difficult to separate from acute Crohn's colitis, tends to be a more acute problem without chronic inflammation. Intestinal lymphoma can mimic the symptoms of Crohn's disease; in lymphoma, small bowel radiographs may show diffuse involvement with masses in the bowel wall.

Treatment

Antidiarrheal agents, usually loperamide or diphenoxylate, are useful in patients with mild IBD to reduce the number of bowel movements and to relieve rectal urgency. Anticholinergics (tincture of belladonna, clidinium, propantheline bromide, and dicyclomine hydrochloride) may reduce cramps, pain, and rectal urgency. Sulfasalazine has been used successfully as a single agent in mild to moderate acute attacks of ulcerative colitis and Crohn's colitis; it is the drug of choice in mild cases.

Oral corticosteroids are effective in mild to moderate ulcerative colitis and Crohn's disease. Parenteral therapy is reserved for moderate to severe disease. The typical initial dose of prednisone is 40 mg/day in moderate to severe disease. Maintenance therapy with corticosteroids is ineffective to prevent recurrences in ulcerative colitis or Crohn's disease in remission.

Azathioprine and 6-MP are effective in treating active Crohn's disease and in maintaining remission. Their roles in ulcerative colitis are less clear.

Except in cases of overt sepsis, there is little role for antibiotics in the management of ulcerative colitis. Antibiotics play a larger role in Crohn's disease; they are used in the management of the suppurative complications, especially abscess formation and perianal disease, although surgical drainage is the primary therapy for abscesses. Metronidazole 10 to 15 mg/kg/day is effective in perianal Crohn's disease and is as effective as sulfasalazine in Crohn's colitis.

MEDICAL MANAGEMENT OF ULCERATIVE COLITIS. The most common reason for hospitalization is intractable diarrhea, although blood loss is also a common problem. Patients with severe active ulcerative colitis should be evaluated for toxic megacolon. The mainstays of therapy for severe ulcerative colitis are bed rest, rehydration with IV fluids, and IV corticosteroids (hydrocortisone 300 mg/day; prednisolone, 60 to 80 mg/day, or methylprednisolone, 48 to 60 mg/day). Total parenteral nutrition may be necessary. Patients with peritoneal signs or symptoms of systemic infection should be treated with parenteral antibiotics. Patients who do not improve in 7 to 10 days should be considered for either colectomy or a trial of IV cyclosporine. Aminosalicylates reduce the incidence of recurrences in patients with ulcerative colitis; almost all patients should receive maintenance therapy. The efficacy of sulfasalazine at 3 to 4 g/day is greater than the efficacy of 2 g/day even though 2 g/day is the usual recommended maintenance dose. Corticosteroids are not effective as maintenance therapy and should not be used. Twenty to 25 per cent of patients with extensive ulcerative colitis eventually undergo colectomy. In ulcerative colitis, colectomy is a curative procedure.

MEDICAL MANAGEMENT OF CROHN'S DISEASE (Fig. 9–8). For patients who have been brought into clinical remission on corticosteroids, the rate at which the dose is tapered is arbitrary and not defined by controlled trials. The approach to severe Crohn's disease is similar to the approach to severe ulcerative colitis. The patient is hospitalized, given nothing by mouth, rehydrated with IV fluids, and given parenteral corticosteroids. Patients who respond to

TREATMENT ALGORITHM FOR CROHN'S DISEASE

CONDITION	TREATMENT
COLITIS OR ILEOCOLITIS	Oral 5-ASA drug or metronidazole —*Continued activity*→ Prednisone —*Continued activity or Steroid dependence*→ Immunomodulator —*Continued activity*→ Surgery
ILEITIS	Prednisone —*Continued activity*→ Immunomodulator —*Continued activity*→ Surgery
FISTULA	TPN or immunomodulator —*Failure to close*→ Surgery
ABSCESS	Antibiotics, drainage, and resection
OBSTRUCTION DUE TO INFLAMMATION	IV fluids, nasogastric suction, parenteral steroids —*Failure to respond*→ Surgery
OBSTRUCTION DUE TO SCARRING	IV fluids, nasogastric suction —*Failure to respond*→ Surgery
PERIANAL DISEASE	Antibiotics and surgical drainage
DISEASE IN REMISSION	Maintenance with oral 5-ASA drugs or immunomodulators

ASA=aminosalicylic acid
IV=intravenous
TPN=total parenteral nutrition

FIGURE 9–8 ■ Treatment algorithm for Crohn's disease.

parenteral corticosteroids are switched to high-dose oral corticosteroids (prednisone 40 mg/day), and the dose of prednisone is gradually reduced. Patients with severe Crohn's disease who do not respond to parenteral corticosteroids within a week should be considered for a course of treatment with the antitumor necrosis factor antibody, infliximab. Surgery can also be considered for those who do not respond to medical treatment. A course of total parenteral nutrition may be useful as adjunctive therapy.

Maintenance therapy with aminosalicylates is recommended for those brought into remission on corticosteroids or with surgery. Maintenance with 6-MP or azathioprine is recommended for patients brought into remission on those drugs or who were corticosteroid-dependent and then converted to those drugs. There is no role for cortricosteroids as maintenance therapy.

Within 10 years of diagnosis, approximately 60% of patients with Crohn's disease undergo surgery for their disease. Because surgical resection is not curative in Crohn's disease and recurrences are likely, the approach is more conservative in terms of the amount of tissue removed.

Complications

The most severe complication of ulcerative colitis is toxic megacolon, which is dilation of the colon to a diameter of greater than 6 cm associated with a worsening of the patient's clinical condition and the development of fever, tachycardia, and leukocytosis. Signs of improvement include a decrease in abdominal girth and the return of bowel sounds. Deterioration is marked by the development of rebound tenderness, increasing abdominal girth, and cardiovascular collapse. If the patient does not begin to show signs of clinical improvement during the first 24 to 48 hours of medical therapy, the risk of perforation increases markedly, and surgical intervention is indicated.

Abscesses and fistulas, which are common complications in Crohn's disease, are products of the extension of a mucosal fissure or ulcer through the intestinal wall and into extraintestinal tissue. The typical clinical presentation of intra-abdominal abscess is fever, abdominal pain, tenderness, and leukocytosis. Broad-spectrum antibiotic therapy, including anaerobic coverage, is indicated. The prevalence of fistulas is 20 to 40% in Crohn's disease. Total parenteral nutrition or immunomodulator therapy may induce fistula closure. Surgical therapy includes resection of the segment involved with active disease.

Small bowel obstruction in Crohn's disease may be caused by mucosal thickening from acute inflammation, by muscular hyperperplasia and scarring as a result of previous inflammation, or by adhesions. If the obstruction does not resolve with nasogastric suction and corticosteroids, surgery is necessary.

Perianal disease is an especially difficult complication of Crohn's disease. Limited disease can be approached with sitz baths and metronidazole, but in most cases adequate external drainage is also required.

Patients with extensive ulcerative colitis have a markedly increased risk for colon cancer, compared with the general population. Some practitioners perform surveillance colonoscopies with random biopsies in patients with long-standing ulcerative colitis beginning 8 to 10 years after the onset of disease and repeated every 1 to 2 years. The risk of colon cancer in Crohn's colitis is less than in ulcerative colitis but greater than in the general population.

For more information about this subject, see *Cecil Textbook of Medicine,* 21st edition. Philadelphia, W.B. Saunders Company, 2000. Chapter 135, Inflammatory Bowel Disease, pages 722 to 729.

MISCELLANEOUS INFLAMMATORY DISEASES OF THE INTESTINE

Appendicitis and Acute Abdomen

In *acute appendicitis,* abdominal pain is almost invariably the first manifestation. It is often poorly localized to the periumbilical area of the epigastrium. Pain is at first colicky, then steady, and increases in severity as the inflammatory process progresses. When the parietal peritoneum becomes inflamed, usually hours after the initial onset of symptoms, the pain becomes localized in the right iliac region; however, pelvic pain (pelvic appendix) or right upper quadrant pain may result. Anorexia is frequent, and the urge to eat argues against the diagnosis of appendicitis.

The most consistent physical finding is tenderness in the right iliac region at McBurney's point (one fingerbreadth from the anterosuperior iliac spine toward the umbilicus). With a retrocecal appendix, tenderness may be mild. Rectal examination may disclose tenderness anteriorly with a pelvic appendix or a bulge in the pelvic wall from an abscess. Rotating a flexed right hip when supine (obturator sign) or raising a straightened leg against resistance (psoas sign) may elicit pain.

A variety of disorders cause a subacute to acute right lower quadrant pain syndrome mimicking acute appendicitis (Table 9–29). For an acutely ill patient, early surgical consultation is mandatory.

In patients with an acute abdomen, the following studies should be performed: complete blood cell count with differential, serum electrolytes, blood urea nitrogen and creatinine, serum amylase, liver chemistry tests, urinalysis, and a pregnancy test in women of childbearing potential. An elevated polymorphonuclear (PMN) leukocyte count points to infection (appendicitis, cholecystitis), tissue necrosis (bowel infarction), or other inflammatory processes (pancreatitis).

Table 9–29 ■ CAUSES OF RIGHT LOWER QUADRANT PAIN SYNDROMES

INFLAMMATORY DISORDERS	NEOPLASMS	OTHER
Appendicitis	Carcinoid	Gynecologic disorders
Crohn's ileitis/colitis	Lymphoma	
Cecal diverticulitis	Cecal adenocarcinoma (perforated)	
Meckel's diverticulitis		
Yersinia ileocolitis		
Amebic colitis		
Tuberculous colitis		

Abdominal CT scanning has been invaluable in the evaluation of patients with an acute abdomen. Localized inflammatory processes of the right lower quadrant may suggest appendicitis or possibly Crohn's disease if the terminal ileum and/or right colon is thickened; however, overlap between these two entities may occur. CT also helps exclude diverticulitis, acute pancreatitis, biliary obstruction, luminal disorders such as small bowel or colonic infarction, and aortic dissection, as well as unsuspected processes of the liver and spleen.

When the diagnosis is in doubt, careful observation for 6 to 12 hours may be diagnostic. Surgical therapy is curative.

Diverticulitis of the Colon

Constant left lower quadrant pain and fever in the elderly are highly suggestive of acute diverticulitis. Leukocytosis is common, although non-specific.

Abdominal CT, which has become the test of choice, may demonstrate bowel wall thickening, abscess formation, and diverticula. Barium enema and CT are complementary because neither is 100% sensitive and specific.

Initial therapy includes broad-spectrum antibiotics such as a third-generation cephalosporin combined with anaerobic coverage (metronidazole). Early surgical consultation is important.

Radiation Enterocolitis

Radiation enterocolitis usually develops when the total dosage exceeds 50 Gy. During the early phases of radiation therapy, patients may report nausea, vomiting, and diarrhea, which may be bloody. Symptoms caused by the complications of high-dose radiation are not seen for months or even years following therapy (intestinal ulcerations with bleeding, obstruction from fibrosis and stricture, fistulas to other pelvic organs, abscesses, or chronic gastrointestinal bleeding and anemia from vascular ectasia). If a significant amount of small bowel is in the radiation field, malabsorption may be noted.

Intestinal and Colonic Ulceration

Isolated proximal small bowel ulcerations are most commonly caused by medications such as slow-release potassium pills or NSAIDs. Other disorders include infections, collagen-vascular diseases (Behçet's disease, systemic lupus erythematosus), and ulcerated neoplasms.

For more information about this subject, see *Cecil Textbook of Medicine,* 21st edition. Philadelphia, W.B. Saunders Company, 2000. Chapter 136, Miscellaneous Inflammatory Diseases of the Intestine, pages 729 to 732.

VASCULAR DISORDERS OF THE INTESTINE

Ischemic Disorders

The *celiac axis* and its branches supply the liver, biliary tract, spleen, stomach, duodenum, and pancreas; the *superior mesenteric artery* (SMA) gives off branches to the duodenum and pancreas and then supplies the entire small intestine as well as the ascending colon and a part of the tranverse colon; the *inferior mesenteric artery* anastomoses with the superior mesenteric artery to supply the transverse colon. The types of intestinal ischemia and their approximate incidences are colonic (60%), acute mesenteric (30%), focal segmental (5%) and chronic mesenteric (5%).

ACUTE MESENTERIC ISCHEMIA. Acute mesenteric ischemia is caused by superior mesenteric arterial embolus (50%), non-occlusive mesenteric ischemia (25%), superior mesenteric artery thrombosis (10%), focal segmental ischemia (5%), and acute mesenteric venous thrombosis (10%). SMA emboli usually originate from a left atrial or ventricular thrombus and lodge distal to the origin of a major branch.

Sudden severe abdominal pain developing in a patient with heart disease and arrhythmias, long-standing and poorly controlled heart failure, recent myocardial infarction, or hypotension should suggest the possibility of acute mesenteric ischemia. Increasing abdominal tenderness and muscle guarding indicate infarcted bowel. Right-sided abdominal pain associated with maroon or bright-red blood in the stool, although characteristic of colonic ischemia, also suggests acute mesenteric ischemia. Leukocytosis and metabolic acidemia are seen with advanced ischemic bowel injury. Early in the course of disease, plain films of the abdomen usually are normal. Later, formless loops of small intestine, ileus, or "thumbprinting" of the small bowel or right colon due to submucosal hemorrhage may develop.

Selective mesenteric angiography is the mainstay of diagnosis and initial treatment of both occlusive and non-occlusive acute mesenteric ischemia. The approach to diagnosing and managing acute mesenteric ischemia is based on several observations: (1) if the diagnosis is not made before intestinal infarction, the mortality rate is 70 to 90%; (2) both occlusive and non-occlusive forms can be diagnosed by angiography; (3) vasoconstriction may persist even after the initial cause of the ischemia is corrected; and (4) vasoconstriction can be relieved by vasodilators infused into the SMA.

Initial management of patients suspected of having acute mesenteric ischemia includes resuscitation, abdominal plain films, and selective angiography. Broad-spectrum antibiotics are begun immediately. Plain films of the abdomen are obtained, not to establish the diagnosis of acute mesenteric ischemia but to exclude other causes of abdominal pain. If no alternative diagnosis is made on the abdominal films, selective SMA angiography is performed.

Even when the decision to operate has been made based on clinical grounds, a preoperative angiogram should be obtained. Relief of mesenteric vasoconstriction is essential in treating emboli, thromboses, and "low flow" states and is accomplished by infusing papaverine at 30 to 60 mg/hour through the indwelling SMA angiography catheter.

Laparotomy is performed in acute mesenteric ischemia to restore arterial flow. Survival is in the range of 55%; 90% of patients with acute mesenteric ischemia diagnosed angiographically before the development of peritonitis survive.

MESENTERIC VENOUS THROMBOSIS. *Acute mesenteric venous thrombosis* resembles arterial forms of acute mesenteric ischemia. However, the tempo of illness is slower than that of arterial ischemia, and the mean duration of pain before hospital admission is 5 to 14 days. Underlying causes have been identified in more than 80% of patients and include antithrombin III, protein S and C deficiencies, and hypercoagulable states associated with polycythemia vera, myeloproliferative disorders, pregnancy, and neoplasms. As many as 60% of patients have a history of peripheral vein thromboses.

Characteristic findings on small bowel series include luminal narrowing from congestion and edema of the bowel wall, separation of loops due to mesenteric thickening, and thumbprinting. Selective mesenteric arteriography can differentiate venous thrombosis from arterial forms of ischemia, but US, CT, and MRI are more commonly used. Patients with suspected acute mesenteric ischemia have features suggesting mesenteric venous thrombosis; a contrast medium–enhanced CT scan is obtained before SMA angiography.

In the few patients with no physical finding of intestinal infarction in whom a diagnosis of mesenteric venous thrombosis is made by US, CT, or MRI, a trial of anticoagulant or thrombolytic therapy is worthwhile. All other patients should have prompt laparotomy, resection of non-viable bowel, and heparinization. The mortality of acute mesenteric ischemia is 20 to 50%.

9

FOCAL SEGMENTAL ISCHEMIA OF THE SMALL BOWEL. Focal segmental ischemia usually is caused by atheromatous emboli, strangulated hernias, vaculitis, blunt abdominal trauma, radiation, or oral contraceptives. Treatment is resection of the involved bowel.

COLON ISCHEMIA. Colon ischemia is the most common ischemic injury to the gastrointestinal tract. A spectrum of colon ischemic injury is recognized, including reversible colopathy (submucosal or intramural hemorrhage) (at least 30 to 40%); transient colitis (at least 15 to 20%); chronic ulcerating colitis (20 to 25%); stricture (10 to 15%); gangrene (15 to 20%); and fulminant universal colitis (<5%).

Five to 10 per cent of patients with colon ischemia have had a distal and potentially obstructing colonic or rectal lesion, including carcinoma, diverticulitis, stricture, or fecal impaction. Colon ischemia is a complication of elective aortic surgery in 1 to 7% of cases, but after surgery for ruptured abdominal aortic aneurysm it may be as high as 60%. Colon ischemia usually presents with sudden, crampy, mild, left lower abdominal pain, an urge to defecate, and passage of bright-red or maroon blood mixed with the stool within 24 hours.

Systemic low flow states usually involve the right colon; local nonocclusive ischemic injuries involve the "watershed" areas of the colon (i.e., the splenic flexure and rectosigmoid). Ligation of the inferior mesenteric artery produces changes in the sigmoid.

Colonoscopy or the combination of sigmoidoscopy and a gentle barium enema should be performed on the unprepared bowel within 48 hours of the onset of symptoms. Angiography may be indicated when the clinical presentation does not allow a clear distinction between colon ischemia and acute mesenteric ischemia.

In general, symptoms of colon ischemia subside within 24 to 48 hours, and healing is seen within 2 weeks. The prognosis of patients with colon ischemia complicating shock, heart failure, myocardial infarction, or severe dehydration is particularly poor, perhaps due to associated acute mesenteric ischemia.

If, as usual, colon ischemia completely resolves within 1 to 2 weeks, no further therapy is indicated. Recurrent fevers, leukocytosis, and septicemia in otherwise symptomatic patients with unhealed segmental colitis usually are caused by the diseased bowel, and elective resection is indicated.

CHRONIC MESENTERIC ISCHEMIA. Atherosclerosis is almost always the cause of chronic mesenteric ischemia or "abdominal angina." Abdominal pain probably results from a meal-induced increase in gastric blood flow that, in the presence of a fixed splanchnic arterial inflow, "steals" blood from the small bowel and makes it ischemic. Many patients have cardiac, cerebral, or peripheral vascular insufficiency.

The one consistent clinical feature of chronic mesenteric ischemia is abdominal discomfort or pain, which most commonly occurs 10 to 30 minutes after eating, gradually increases in severity, reaches a plateau, and then slowly abates over 1 to 3 hours.

Duplex US can detect a 70% stenosis of the celiac axis or SMA with a sensitivity of 97% and 87%, respectively. However, stenosis or occlusion of one or two or all of the major vessels by US or angiography does not by itself establish the diagnosis of chronic mesenteric ischemia, and patients with even three occluded vessels may be asymptomatic.

Vascular Lesions

Colonic vascular ectasia (angiodysplasia) is one of the most common causes of recurrent lower gastrointestinal bleeding in the elderly. It is almost always confined to the cecum or ascending colon. Patients may have bright-red blood, maroon-colored stools, and melena on separate occasions. Approximately 50% of patients with bleeding colonic vascular ectasias have evidence of cardiac disease, and up to 25% have been reported to have aortic stenosis.

Angiography was formerly the primary method to identify ectasias, but currently colonoscopy is preferable. Laser therapy, sclerosis, electrocoagulation, and the heater probe all have been used to ablate colonic vascular ectasias. None has been established as superior, but the heater probe and bipolar coagulation are most commonly used. Intra-arterial (SMA) vasopressin infusions stop hemorrhage in more than 80% of patients in whom extravasation is demonstrated. Right hemicolectomy should be performed only as a last resort.

Hereditary hemorrhagic telangiectasia (Osler-Weber-Rendu disease) is an autosomal dominant familial disorder characterized by telangiectases of the skin and mucous membranes and recurrent gastrointestinal bleeding. In most patients, bleeding presents as melena; hematochezia and hematemesis are less frequent. Lesions are usually present on the lips, oral and nasopharyngeal membranes, tongue, or periungual regions. Telangiectases occur in the colon but are more common in the stomach and small bowel. Similar vascular lesions are a prominent feature of progressive systemic sclerosis.

Dieulafoy's ulcer is an increasingly diagnosed cause of massive gastrointestinal hemorrhage. It is usually found in the stomach and sometimes in the small or large bowel. There is sudden onset of massive hematemesis or melena, usually followed by intermittent bleeding over several days. The bleeding site is usually 6 cm distal to the cardioesophageal junction.

Hemangiomas may be of cavernous, capillary, or mixed types. Bleeding from hemangiomas is usually slow, producing occult blood loss with anemia or melena. Diagnosis is best established by endoscopy.

Blue rubber bleb nevus syndrome describes a particular type of cutaneous vascular nevus associated with intestinal lesions and gastrointestinal bleeding. The lesions are distinctive: blue and raised, varying from 0.1 to 5.0 cm, and leaving a characteristic wrinkled sac when the contained blood is emptied by direct pressure.

Congenital arteriovenous malformations may be small and resemble ectasias or involve a long segment of bowel. Patients with significant bleeding should have resection of the involved segment.

For more information about this subject, see *Cecil Textbook of Medicine,* 21st edition. Philadelphia, W.B. Saunders Company, 2000. Chapter 137, Vascular Disorders of the Intestine, pages 732 to 738.

NEOPLASMS OF THE STOMACH

Gastric neoplasms are predominantly malignant, and nearly 90 to 95% of cases are adenocarcinomas. Less frequently observed malignancies include lymphomas, especially non-Hodgkin's lymphoma, as well as sarcomas, such as leiomyosarcoma. Benign gastric neoplasms include leiomyomas, carcinoid tumors, and lipomas.

Adenocarcinoma of the Stomach

Gastric adenocarcinoma was the most frequently observed malignancy in the world until the mid-1980s, and it remains extremely common in South America, some parts of the Caribbean, eastern Europe, and China. The intestinal type is typically in the distal stomach with ulcerations, is often preceded by premalignant lesions, and is declining in incidence in the United States. In contrast, the diffuse type involves widespread thickening of the stomach, especially in the cardia, and often affects younger patients; this form may present as linitis plastica, a nondistensible stomach with absence of folds and narrowed lumen due to infiltration of the stomach wall with tumor.

In its early stages, gastric carcinoma may often be asymptomatic or have only nonspecific symptoms, thereby making early diagnosis difficult. Later symptoms include bloating, dysphagia, epigastric pain, or early satiety. Gastric cancer often presents with gross or occult bleeding. Metastatic gastric cancer to the liver can lead to right upper quadrant pain, jaundice, and/or fever.

Paraneoplastic syndromes include Trousseau's syndrome, which is recurrent migratory superficial thrombophlebitis indicating a possible hypercoagulable state; acanthosis nigricans, which presents in flexor areas with skin lesions that are raised and hyperpigmented; neuromyopathy with involvement of the sensory and motor pathways; and central nervous system involvement with altered mental status and ataxia.

Laboratory studies may reveal iron deficiency anemia. Predisposing pernicious anemia can progress to megaloblastic disease.

The diagnostic accuracy of upper endoscopy with biopsy and cytology is far greater than for a UGI series, approaching 95 to 99% for both types of gastric cancer. Staging of gastric cancer, and at times diagnosis, has been greatly enhanced by the advent of endoscopic US.

The only chance for cure of gastric cancer remains surgical resection. However, complete resection is possible in only 25 to 30% of cases. Single-agent treatment with 5-FU, doxorubicin, mitomycin C, or cisplatin provides partial response rates of 20 to 30%. Radiation therapy is ineffective.

Approximately one third of patients who undergo a curative resection are alive after 5 years. In the aggregate, the overall 5-year survival rate of gastric cancer is less than 10%.

Lymphoma of the Stomach

Gastric lymphoma represents about 5% of all malignant gastric tumors and is increasing in incidence. The majority of gastric lymphomas are non-Hodgkin's lymphomas. Radiographically, gastric lymphoma usually presents as ulcers or as exophytic masses; upper endoscopy with biopsy and cytology is required for diagnosis and has an accuracy of nearly 90%. Treatment of large cell gastric lymphoma is usually subtotal gastrectomy followed by combination chemotherapy. For mucosa-associated lymphoid tissue (MALT) lesions, early data suggest that eradication of *H. pylori* infection with antibiotics induces regression of the tumor, but longer-term follow-up will be needed to be confident that such therapy is sufficient.

Other Tumors of the Stomach

Other gastric sarcomas include liposarcomas, fibrosarcomas, myosarcomas, and neurogenic sarcomas. Benign gastric tumors include leiomyoma, lipoma, neurofibroma, lymphangioma, ganglioneuroma, and hamartoma.

For more information about this subject, see *Cecil Textbook of Medicine,* 21st edition. Philadelphia, W.B. Saunders Company, 2000. Chapter 138, Neoplasms of the Stomach, pages 738 to 741.

NEOPLASMS OF THE LARGE AND SMALL INTESTINE

Neoplasms of the Large Intestine

POLYPS OF THE COLON. Polyps in the large intestine, whether noted at sigmoidoscopy, colonoscopy, or during barium enema, may be single or multiple, pedunculated or sessile, and sporadic or part of an inherited syndrome. Polyps become clinically significant because of bleeding or because of their potential for malignant transformation.

Hyperplastic polyps, which tend to be small and symptomatic, account for about one fifth of all polyps in the colon and for most of the polyps in the rectum and distal sigmoid colon. They are not considered neoplastic. Inflammatory polyps occur in chronic ulcerative colitis and also are not neoplastic.

Adenomatous polyps, also called colonic adenomas, increase with age in countries with a high or intermediate risk for colorectal cancer, occurring in 30 to 40% of individuals older than 60 years in the United States. The typical tubular adenoma is small and spherical and has a stalk. The villous adenoma may be large and sessile with a velvety surface. Tubulovillous lesions consist of a mixture of tubular and villous patterns. About 60% of adenomas are tubular, 20 to 30% are tubulovillous, and 10% are villous. All adenomas are dysplastic.

A period of approximately 5 years elapses between the diagnosis of adenoma and the development of carcinoma, but fewer than 5% of adenomas develop into carcinomas. The frequency of cancer in adenomas under 1 cm is 1 to 3%; in those between 1 to 2 cm, 10%; and in those over 2 cm, more than 40%. Invasive neoplasm has been found in 40% of the villous tumors, in fewer than 5% of the tubular adenomas, and in 23% of the tubulovillous variety.

Most adenomatous polyps are asymptomatic, but they may cause hematochezia. Because of the association of adenomas with the development of adenocarcinomas, colonic polyps should usually be removed or destroyed.

A follow-up colonoscopy is appropriate at 3 years to evaluate for the presence of any lesions missed at the previous procedure or to discover new lesions. If the colon is free of polyps at this examination, an interval of 3 years is appropriate before the next colonoscopy.

INHERITED POLYPOSIS SYNDROMES. The adenomatous polyposis syndromes include familial adenomatous polyposis and Gardner's syndrome. In both of these hereditary disorders, hundreds to thousands of colonic adenomas are present. Almost all patients with familial polyposis develop carcinoma of the colon by age 40 years if the colon has not been removed. The *Peutz-Jeghers syndrome* is characterized by melanotic spots on the lips, buccal mucosa, and skin, and by multiple hamartomatous polyps throughout the gastrointestinal tract from the stomach to the rectum.

HEREDITARY NONPOLYPOSIS COLORECTAL CANCER. Hereditary nonpolyposis colorectal cancer is inherited in a highly penetrant autosomal dominant fashion. The average age at diagnosis of cancer is the mid-40s, and it is characteristic to find multiple synchronous cancers with a majority of lesions proximal to the splenic flexure.

ADENOCARCINOMA OF THE LARGE BOWEL. The risk of colorectal cancer begins to increase at the age of 50 years and rises sharply at age 60 years. With each succeeding decade the risk doubles, reaching a peak by age 75 years. Approximately 2 to 4% of all patients with chronic ulcerative colitis develop colorectal carcinoma.

The adenomatous polyposis syndromes and hereditary nonpolyposis colorectal cancer together account for approximately 7% of colon cancers. As many as 50% or more of "sporadic" adenomas and cancers may exhibit a partially penetrant autosomal dominant inheritance.

Approximately 75% of colorectal cancers occur in the descending colon, rectosigmoid, and rectum. Approximately 50% are within the reach of the 60-cm fiberoptic sigmoidoscope. Carcinoma of the colon spreads by direct extension through the wall of the bowel into the pericolonic fat and mesentery, by invasion of surrounding organs, by way of the lymphatics to the regional lymph nodes, and via the portal vein to the liver.

Colorectal cancer must be suspected when patients present with rectal bleeding, a change in bowel habit, decrease in stool caliber, iron deficiency anemia, or unexplained abdominal pain. Metastases may be clinically apparent before or after resection of the primary colorectal cancer.

A digital rectal examination is essential to determining peritoneal or pelvic spread. In evaluating patients with symptoms or signs of colorectal cancer, colonoscopy is now the generally preferred approach. Endoscopic US is being used with increasing frequency to help in the staging of rectal cancers.

The modern approach to management is multidisciplinary. The most important goal of treatment for primary malignancies of the colon and rectum is complete removal, but surgery may be required for palliation as well as for cure. Preoperative radiation therapy is often combined with 5-FU and leucovorin in an effort to decrease local recurrence and distant spread. It may also be used to reduce tumor size and enable otherwise unresectable lesions to be resected. The postoperative administration of radiation (50 Gy) can decrease local recurrence and distant metastasis. For anal cancers the standard approach is to use a combination of radiation and chemotherapy, which usually shrinks or obliterates the cancer.

Patients with resected colonic cancer with lymph node spread have improved survival if treated with the combination of 5-FU and leucovorin for 6 months. The 10-year survival for patients with colorectal cancer after surgical resection is approximately 50% (Table 9–30), and survival correlates well with the stage of the disease: 80 to 90% 10-year survival for cancer confined to the mucosa; 70 to 80% 10-year survival for cancer extending through all areas of the bowel wall; and 30 to 55% 10-year survival for cancer involving the regional lymph nodes. Prior to surgical resection, the entire colon should be examined.

Colonoscopy should be repeated a year later and every 3 years

Table 9–30 ■ AMERICAN JOINT COMMITTEE ON CANCER: CLASSIFICATION OF COLON-RECTAL CANCER

Stage 0	Carcinoma in situ; the cancer does not extend beyond the smooth muscle that separates the mucosa from the submucosa (Tis, N0, M0)
Stage I	Cancer confined to the mucosa, submucosa, or external muscle; the cancer does not extend through the bowel wall (T1 or T2, N0, M0)
Stage II	Cancer that penetrates all layers of the bowel wall, with or without invasion of adjacent tissues (T3, N0, M0)
Stage III	Cancer involving regional lymph nodes or extending into nearby tissues or organs without spread to lymph nodes (any T, N1–N3, M0; or T4, N0, M0)
Stage IV	Cancer that has spread to distant sites, usually the liver or lungs (any T, any N, M1)

TNM = tumor, node, metastasis.

thereafter because new adenomas require 3 years or more to develop into large adenomas with malignant potential. After surgical resection, patients without known systemic metastases are evaluated for adjuvant therapy. Patients with colonic cancer and lymph node involvement should receive 5-FU and leucovorin, and those with rectal cancer and spread through the wall or with lymph node involvement should receive radiation plus chemotherapy.

Testing for fecal occult blood and flexible sigmoidoscopy are used for detecting early colorectal cancer in asymptomatic individuals. In three randomized controlled trials in the United States, Denmark, and the United Kingdom, colorectal mortality was significantly reduced (by 10 to 33%) by annual or biannual testing for fecal occult blood and appropriate colonoscopic follow-up. Case-control studies have demonstrated significant effectiveness of flexible sigmoidoscopy in reducing mortality (by 70%) from distal colorectal cancer. Current guidelines include several options. One is to test for fecal occult blood annually after age 50 years; patients with abnormal findings require careful diagnostic evaluation, including colonoscopy. Alternative screening approaches after age 50 years include flexible sigmoidoscopy every 5 years, double-contrast barium enema every 5 to 10 years, or colonoscopy every 10 years.

Neoplasms of the Small Bowel

The small bowel represents almost 90% of the mucosal surface of the gut, but small intestinal cancers account for only 1 to 2% of all gastrointestinal neoplasms. Adenocarcinomas, carcinoids, lymphomas, and leiomyosarcomas account for more than 90% of malignant small bowel tumors. More than half of all benign bowel tumors remain asymptomatic and may only be discovered incidentally at laparotomy or autopsy.

Carcinoids are the most frequently occurring small intestinal neoplasm, with more than half found incidentally either at autopsy or at operation for other diseases. Small carcinoid tumors may be asymptomatic, but larger carcinoid tumors can obstruct the lumen or bleed. Once metastasis occurs to the liver, features of the carcinoid syndrome become apparent.

The initial symptoms may be vague and poorly defined. Once bleeding occurs, causes such as peptic ulceration, Meckel's diverticulum, and vascular anomalies need to be considered. Intestinal obstruction may be due to adhesions, particularly in patients who have had prior abdominal operations, internal hernias, volvulus, or intussusception.

UGI tract barium radiographs and selective nasoenteric intubation (enteroclysis), which permits the introduction of barium and air into a relatively localized segment, may be useful in localizing tumors. Abdominal US and CT may determine the extent of hepatic involvement and assess intra-abdominal and retroperitoneal spread.

Treatment is primarily surgical; combination chemotherapy is used for extensive lymphoma.

For more information about this subject, see: *Cecil Textbook of Medicine,* 21st edition. Philadelphia, W.B. Saunders Company, 2000. Chapter 139, Neoplasms of the Large and Small Intestine, pages 741 to 750.

CARCINOMA OF THE PANCREAS

Ductal adenocarcinoma, which accounts for 90% of pancreatic cancers, is a relentlessly progressive and fatal disease. The remaining 10% of pancreatic cancers are endocrine tumors.

Currently, pancreatic cancer kills more Americans than any other neoplasm except breast, colorectal, lung, and prostate cancers. Pancreatic cancer occurs more frequently in men (1.5:1), and 80% occur between the ages of 60 and 80; the disease is unusual in people younger than 40 years. Pain occurs in 90% of patients. It may be vague and rather nonspecific and may occur up to 3 months before the onset of jaundice. Jaundice caused by obstruction of the common bile duct occurs early in the course of the disease in 60 to 70% of carcinomas of the head of the pancreas. Weight loss greater than 10% of ideal body weight is almost universal and is usually due to both malabsorption and decreased food intake. Glucose intolerance from increased plasma levels of islet amyloid polypeptide producing insulin resistance may be present in up to 80% of patients.

Hepatomegaly combined with jaundice is present in 80% and 30% of patients with carcinoma of the head and carcinoma of the body and tail, respectively. A palpable gallbladder (Courvoisier's sign) is present in 30% of patients. An abdominal mass or ascites is present in fewer than 20% of patients.

The preferred imaging test for diagnosing pancreatic cancer is a CT scan (Table 9–31). If a tumor is highly suspected but not found by CT scan, the most sensitive test is endoscopic US.

Surgical resection of pancreatic cancer offers the only chance of cure, and pancreaticoduodenectomy is the surgical procedure of choice. Unfortunately, only 10% of all pancreatic cancers are resectable, and the 5-year survival rate after resection is only 10%. Palliative procedures relieve symptoms of biliary obstruction, duodenal obstruction, or both. To decompress the biliary tree, endoscopic stenting is as successful as surgical decompression and may have lower morbidity.

Gemcitabine is the only single agent that may prolong survival. The combination of external beam radiation with 5-FU or with streptozotocin, mitomycin, and 5-FU improves survival when compared with radiation or chemotherapy alone.

For more information about this subject, see: *Cecil Textbook of*

Table 9–31 ■ DIAGNOSTIC ACCURACY (%) OF IMAGING MODALITIES IN DIAGNOSIS OF PANCREATIC CANCER

MODALITY	SENSITIVITY	SPECIFICITY	PREDICTIVE VALUE	
			Positive	Negative
Ultrasonography	74	84	78	79
Computed tomography	79	64	76	78
Endoscopic retrograde cholangiopancreatography	95	90	87	97

Medicine, 21st edition. Philadelphia, W.B. Saunders Company, 2000. Chapter 140, Carcinoma of the Pancreas, pages 750 to 752.

PANCREATITIS

Acute Pancreatitis

Acute pancreatitis is an acute inflammatory process with variable involvement of adjacent and remote organs. The risk of recurrent attacks is 20 to 50% unless the precipitating cause is removed. Local complications include acute fluid collections, pancreatic necrosis, and pancreatic abscess.

Among clinical causes known to precipitate acute pancreatitis (Table 9–32), choledocholithiasis and ethanol abuse account for 70 to 80% of all cases. Gallstones may cause pancreatitis by impacting in the ampulla of Vater. The stones usually pass spontaneously into the duodenum. The presence of lipemia, with serum triglyceride levels of more than 1000 mg/dL, represents a cause, not an effect, of pancreatitis.

9

CLINICAL PRESENTATION. Steady, dull, or boring midepigastric pain associated with nausea and vomiting is the classic presentation of acute pancreatitis. Pain radiates straight to the midline of the lower thoracic vertebral region in about 50% of patients. Initial physical examination reveals mild fever and tachycardia; hypotension is present in 30 to 40% of patients. There is marked tenderness to deep palpation of the upper abdomen, but signs of peritoneal irritation are absent. One to 2 weeks after the onset, large ecchymoses rarely appear in the flanks (Grey Turner sign) or the umbilical area (Cullen's sign).

DIAGNOSIS. The total serum amylase level rises 2 to 12 hours after onset of symptoms and remains elevated for 3 to 5 days in most cases. Values more than five times the upper limit of normal are highly specific for acute pancreatitis but are found in only 80 to 90% of cases. The magnitude of the rise in serum amylase does not correlate with the severity of the attack, nor does prolonged hyperamylasemia indicate developing complications. Serum lipase assays have similar specificity and sensitivity as serum amylase. Leukocytosis of up to 25,000/mm is present in 80% of patients; the hematocrit is frequently elevated due to hemoconcentration. Hypocalcemia occurs in up to 30% of patients. Transient, mild hyperglycemia is common. Elevated alanine aminotransferase (ALT) and alkaline phosphatase values suggest gallstone-associated pancreatitis.

Plain films of the abdomen should be obtained routinely. Changes caused by pancreatitis include localized ileus of a loop of jejunum ("sentinel loop"), generalized paralytic ileus, spasm of the transverse colon with absent colonic gas beyond ("colon cutoff sign"), and calcifications indicating the existence of underlying chronic pancreatitis.

US is the method of choice for detecting cholelithiasis and for determining the diameter of the extrahepatic and intrahepatic bile ducts. Dilation of these ducts suggests recent or persisting impaction of a stone in the distal common bile duct or the ampulla of Vater. CT scan is far superior to US for assessing the extent and local complications of pancreatitis.

Table 9–32 ■ FACTORS ASSOCIATED WITH ACUTE PANCREATITIS

Obstructive Causes

Choledocholithiasis
Ampullary obstruction by tumor or sphincter of Oddi hypertension
Choledochocele
Periampullary duodenal diverticulum
Pancreas divisum; annular pancreas
Primary or metastatic pancreatic tumor
Parasites in pancreatic duct: *Clonorchis, Ascaris*
Toxins
Ethanol
Methanol
Organophosphorus insecticides
Scorpion venom (*Tityus trinitatis*)
Drugs
Definite association: azathioprine; 6-mercaptopurine; valproic acid; estrogens; metronidazole; diuretics, including thiazides, furosemide, bumetanide; pentamidine; sulfonamides, including sulfasalazine; methyldopa; L-asparaginase; tetracyclines, cytarabine, dideoxyinosine
Probable association: chlorthalidone; mesalamine; ethacrynic acid; phenformin; angiotensin-converting enzyme inhibitors; nitrofurantoin; cocaine and amphetamine abuse; acetaminophen, cimetidine.

Metabolic Causes

Hypertriglyceridemia
Hypercalcemia

Trauma

Blunt abdominal trauma
Endoscopic retrograde cholangiopancreatographic procedures
Abdominal operations, cardiopulmonary bypass

Infections

Viral: mumps, coxsackie B, hepatitis A and B
Bacterial: Mycoplasma, Salmonella, Campylobacter jejuni

Vascular

Shock/hypoperfusion
Vasculitis
Cholesterol emboli

Miscellaneous

Penetrating duodenal ulcer
Organ transplantation
Crohn's disease of duodenum
Familial pancreatitis

Idiopathic

Several scoring systems predict the morbidity and mortality of acute pancreatitis attacks (Table 9–33). *Mild acute pancreatitis* is defined by the absence of systemic and local complications. About 80% of patients belonging to this category require less than 1 week of hospitalization.

TREATMENT. Volume restoration must be rapid and efficient. The patient should receive nothing by mouth. Nasogastric aspiration is indicated in the presence of vomiting or developing ileus; it

Table 9–33 ■ ADVERSE PROGNOSTIC FACTORS IN ACUTE PANCREATITIS

RANSON'S CRITERIA*—MAINLY ETHANOL-INDUCED	GLASGOW CRITERIA†—ALL CAUSES
On admission:	**Within 48 hrs:**
Age > 55 yr	Age > 55 yr
WBC > 16,000/mm³	WBC > 15,000/mm³
Glucose > 200 mg/dL‡	Glucose > 180 mg/dL‡
LDH > 350 IU/L	LDH > 600 IU/L
AST > 250 IU/L	BUN > 45 mg/dL
Within 48 hrs:	Albumin < 3.2 g/dL
Hematocrit decrease > 10%	Calcium > 8 mg/dL
BUN rise > 5 mg/dL	Arterial pO_2 < 60 mm Hg
Calcium < 8 mg/dL	
Arterial pO_2 < 60 mm Hg	
Base deficit > 4 mEq/L	
Fluid deficit > 6 L	

* Three or more positive criteria predict a complicated clinical course; mortality rises when ≥4 criteria are met. Data from Ranson JHC, Rifkind KM, Turner JW: Prognostic signs and nonoperative peritoneal lavage in acute pancreatitis. Surg Gynecol Obstet 143:209, 1976.

† Data from Blamey SL, Imrie CW, O'Neill WH, et al: Prognostic factors in acute pancreatitis. Gut 25:1340, 1984.

‡ No pre-existing hyperglycemia.

LDH = lactate dehydrogenase; AST = aspartate aminotransferase; BUN = blood urea nitrogen; WBC = white blood cell count.

need not be initiated routinely. The patient should receive sufficient analgesia.

Most systemic complications (Table 9–34) occur during the first week of illness. Ascending cholangitis and severe biliary pancreatitis present overlapping features and may coexist. Pancreatic necrosis is found by CT in approximately 80% of patients and resolves without incident in nearly 60% of patients.

Therapy and prognosis of the severely ill patient depend crucially on whether the necrotic tissue is infected; a Gram stain of

Table 9–34 ■ COMPLICATIONS OF ACUTE PANCREATITIS*

SYSTEMIC	LOCAL
Circulatory shock	*Impacted common bile duct stones*
Respiratory insufficiency	Pancreatic necrosis ± *infection*
Acute renal failure	Fluid collections ± *infection*
Sepsis	*Pancreatic abscess*
Coagulopathy (DIC)	*Colonic necrosis*
Hyperglycemia	*Bleeding*
Hypocalcemia	Splenic vein thrombosis
	Splenic necrosis

DIC = disseminated intravascular coagulation.

* Conditions in italics are life-threatening; they require prompt recognition and management.

the aspirate is more than 95% accurate in predicting the final results of bacterial cultures. Antibiotics with high penetration into pancreatic tissue include the fluoroquinolones, imipenem and cilastatin, and metronidazole. In patients with sterile pancreatic necrosis, prophylactic IV antibiotic therapy (e.g., ofloxacin 200 mg twice daily plus metronidazole 500 mg twice daily) appears to decrease the risk of conversion to infected pancreatic necrosis and, thus, of mortality.

Fluid collections occur within or around the pancreas in up to 50% of patients with severe pancreatitis. The majority resolve spontaneously. Pancreatic abscesses contain liquid pus and may be considered to represent infected fluid collections.

The search for the precipitating cause begins during the acute attack. After a second attack of idiopathic pancreatitis, ERCP with sphincter of Oddi manometry should be performed and will identify correctable obstructive causes of the pancreatitis attack in approximately one third of patients.

Chronic Pancreatitis

Chronic pancreatitis is marked by progressive fibrosis, leading to loss of exocrine and endocrine (islets of Langerhans) tissue and irregular dilation of pancreatic ductal structures (Table 9–35). Fully 70 to 80% of patients with chronic pancreatitis are chronic alcohol abusers. In approximately 40% of patients, chronic pancreatitis initially presents with episodes that are indistinguishable from acute pancreatitis; another 40% have pain of insidious onset. Spontaneous pain relief occurs in approximately 60% of patients within 6 to 12 years after the onset of symptoms. Pancreatic calcifications, diabetes mellitus, and malabsorption frequently appear when the pain begins to diminish. Malabsorption ultimately develops in about 40% of patients. Progressive loss of islets of Langerhans eventually leads to diabetes in 70% of patients, half of whom require insulin treatment.

Diagnosis depends on symptoms, tests of pancreatic function, and radiologic studies. The secretin test is the most sensitive test for chronic pancreatitis. Abdominal CT may detect small calcifica-

Table 9–35 ■ ETIOLOGIC ASSOCIATIONS WITH CHRONIC PANCREATITIS*

Etiologic Associations
Chronic Calcifying Pancreatitis
Chronic alcoholism
Tropical pancreatitis
Hereditary
Senile/pancreatic atrophy
Metabolic: hypercalcemia, hyperlipemia, post renal transplant
Idiopathic
Obstructive Chronic Pancreatitis
Tumors
Duct strictures
Pancreas divisum

* Hereditary isolated pancreatic enzyme deficiencies, congenital pancreatic insufficiency with neutropenia, and cystic fibrosis are separate nosologic entities.

tions missed on plain radiographs. The main value of ERCP is to identify potentially correctable lesions.

Control of abdominal pain is the most important and difficult task. Patients with intractable chronic or intermittent pain should be considered for a surgical procedure based on ERCP and CT evaluation of the duct system. For malabsorption, non–enteric-coated preparations of pancrelipase should be used, such as Viokase, Cotazyme, or Ilozyme, at doses of six tablets per meal. Concomitant suppression of gastric acid secretion with an H_2-recptor blocker is advisable.

One or more pseudocysts appear in up to 60% of patients with chronic pancreatitis. For large pseudocysts (>5 cm in diameter), internal drainage into the stomach, duodenum, or jejunum yields excellent results. The late incidence of adenocarcinoma of the pancreas is increased. The 10-year survival is 65% in alcoholics and 80% in patients with non-alcoholic chronic pancreatitis.

For more information about this subject, see *Cecil Textbook of Medicine,* 21st edition. Philadelphia, W.B. Saunders Company, 2000. Chapter 141, Pancreatitis, pages 752 to 759.

DISEASES OF THE PERITONEUM

Ascites

More than 90% of cases of ascites are due to portal hypertension, usually as a result of cirrhosis. Perhaps half of the remainder, or 5% of all cases of ascites, are due to peritoneal disease. The investigation of new-onset ascites, especially if unexplained by standard clinical examination and tests, should always include paracentesis (Table 9–36). Ascites associated with portal hypertension has a serum-ascites albumin gradient greater than 1.1 g/dL, whereas ascites caused by peritoneal inflammation or malignancy has a serum-ascites albumin gradient less than 1.1 g/dL. Whenever ascites is due to malignant infiltration of the peritoneum, either alone or accompanied by massive hepatic metastases, shedding of malignant cells into the ascites is almost invariable. In contrast, massive hepatic metastases without peritoneal studding or multilocular primary hepatocellular carcinoma arising in a cirrhotic liver rarely causes shedding of malignant cells into the ascitic fluid.

Medical management using diuretics and salt restriction is often effective in patients with portal hypertension. Conversely, ascites caused by peritoneal inflammation or malignancy alone does not respond to salt restriction and diuretics. Portal hypertensive ascites that fails to respond to salt restriction and diuretics is termed *refractory ascites.* Serial large-volume paracentesis is the simplest approach to management. Placement of a transjugular intrahepatic portosystemic shunt also improves ascitic control in cirrhotic patients with refractory ascites, albeit with the risks of encephalopathy and decompensation in hepatic function. The presence of ascites with positive neoplastic cytologic findings indicating peritoneal carcinomatosis signifies an expected survival of 6 months or less.

Chylous ascites is milky in appearance because of leakage of lymph into the peritoneal cavity; the triglyceride concentration is markedly elevated, always greater than 200 mg/dL. Chylous ascites is most often due to underlying malignancy, especially lymphoma.

Table 9–36 ■ DIAGNOSTIC TESTS IN ASCITES

FEATURE	DIAGNOSIS	ASCITIC WHITE BLOOD CELL COUNT (per mm^3)	ASCITIC RED BLOOD CELL COUNT	BIOCHEMICAL ANALYSIS	SERUM-ASCITES ALBUMIN GRADIENT (g/dL)
Portal hypertension	Cirrhosis	<250 PMN	Few or none	Protein usually <2.5 g/dL	>1.1
	SBP	>250 PMN	Few or none	Albumin <1 g/dL	>1.1
	Cardiac ascites	<250 PMN	Few or none	Protein >2.5 g/dL	>1.1
Malignancy	Peritoneal carcinomatosis	75% have >500	Few or none	Protein usually >2.5 g/dL	<1.1
	MHM	Usually <500	Few or none	Protein variable	>1.1
	Malignant chylous ascites	Often >300	Few or none	Triglycerides >200 mg/dL	Usually <1.1
	Hepatoma plus ascites	Often >500	Commonly increased		>1.1
Infection	Tuberculous peritonitis	80% >500, predominantly lymphocytes	Frequently present	Ascitic adenosine deaminase ≥32.3 U/L or LDH >90 U/L	50% have >1.1 (i.e., may have cirrhosis)
Miscellaneous	Pancreatic ascites	Frequently increased		Ascitic amylase greatly increased	Variable

PMN = polymorphonuclear leukocytes; SBP = spontaneous bacterial peritonitis; MHM = massive hepatic metastases; LDH = lactate dehydrogenase.

Acute Peritonitis

Secondary peritonitis results from any definable cause, such as perforation of a viscus owing to acute appendicitis or diverticulitis, perforation of an ulcer, and trauma, including iatrogenic intervention. Primary peritonitis, including spontaneous bacterial peritonitis, refers to peritonitis arising without a recognizable preceding cause. Tertiary peritonitis, which is persistent intra-abdominal sepsis without a discrete focus of infection, generally follows surgical treatment of prior severe peritonitis and occurs in severely ill patients in intensive care, especially patients who are immunosuppressed.

The classic features of acute peritonitis are abdominal pain, abdominal tenderness, and the absence of bowel sounds accompanied by fever, hypotension, tachycardia, and acidosis. However, peritonitis arising in patients with ascites is often very subtle in its manifestations. When suspected peritonitis is associated with ascites, paracentesis is mandatory.

Laparotomy is a cornerstone of therapy for secondary or tertiary acute peritonitis. Broad-spectrum systemic antibiotics are critical to cover bowel flora, including anaerobic species.

Spontaneous bacterial peritonitis (SBP) is a marker of severe hepatic failure and usually occurs in patients with low ascitic protein content and elevated serum bilirubin. The mechanism of SBP development is related to deficient opsonic activity in ascitic fluid. The offending organisms are almost always enteric gram-negative aerobes. SBP must be suspected not only whenever a cirrhotic patient has fever and abdominal pain more typical of acute peritonitis but also whenever a cirrhotic patient with ascites has a sudden deterioration in hepatic or renal function, worsening malaise, encephalopathy, or unexplained persistent leukocytosis. The key to establishing SBP is diagnostic paracentesis in which the ascitic fluid is found to have 250 or more PMN cells per cubic millimeter. A very elevated PMN cell count in ascites (e.g., $>5000/mm^3$) suggests an intra-abdominal abscess or a secondary cause of peritonitis. Three to 5 days of IV treatment with broad-spectrum antibiotics is usually adequate for SBP.

In *peritoneal tuberculosis,* ascites is almost invariable, whereas abdominal swelling and pain are common. Paracentesis reveals a lymphocytosis but rarely shows acid-fast bacilli on smear. Treatment of tuberculous peritonitis involves standard protocols using two or three drugs, usually for 9 months. All isolates must be tested for drug susceptibility.

Peritonitis in *continuous ambulatory peritoneal dialysis* patients is usually caused by gram-positive organisms. Treatment consists of infusing broad-spectrum antibiotics into the peritoneum through the abdominal wall catheter.

For more information about this subject, see *Cecil Textbook of Medicine,* 21st edition. Philadelphia, W.B. Saunders Company, 2000. Chapter 142, Diseases of the Peritoneum, Mesentery, and Omentum, pages 759 to 763.

CHAPTER 10

DISEASES OF THE LIVER, GALLBLADDER, AND BILE DUCTS

APPROACH TO THE PATIENT WITH LIVER DISEASE

The recognition of liver disease is not difficult when the patient presents with classic manifestations, such as overt jaundice, or with the classic stigmata of chronic liver disease, such as ascites, spider angiomas, liver palms, and asterixis. Jaundice may be the earliest manifestation of liver disease in some patients, and it is often noticed by the patient or his or her family members as scleral icterus. Pruritus may occur first in the course of obstructive jaundice (cholestasis) because retention of bile salts can occur before significant retention of bilirubin.

Liver diseases may present as symptoms related to other systems. For example, early hepatic encephalopathy may manifest as changes in sleep pattern or mild alterations in personality. Hepatitis C can present as glomerulonephritis or hemorrhagic skin lesions owing to the presence of cryoglobulinemia. Patients with hemochromatosis sometimes present with arthralgias, diabetes, or cardiac disease. Mild increases in aminotransferases in the asymptomatic patient may be the only manifestation of hepatitis C, whose ongoing inflammation silently destroys the liver.

Failure of homeostatic mechanisms in liver disease may produce hypoglycemia or glucose intolerance. Hypoglycemia may also occur in the absence of overt liver damage. For example, alcoholic hypoglycemia classically occurs in persons whose only important source of calories over a period of days is ethanol.

Fatty liver usually reflects excess accumulation of triglycerides. Alcoholic ketosis is attributed to an ethanol- or acetaldehyde-mediated impairment of the tricarboxylic acid cycle. The liver is the major site of chemical modification of a wide variety of exogenous drugs and toxins, as well as endogenous substances such as hormones.

Physical Examination

Spider angiomas occur on the upper trunk and face. Palmar erythema, except in the setting of pregnancy, may signal the presence of chronic liver disease. Scleral icterus may be detected before bilirubin levels of 3 to 4 are manifested by jaundice of the skin. Gynecomastia, the loss of hair, and reduction in the size or consist-

For more information about this subject, see in *Cecil Textbook of Medicine,* 21st edition. Philadelphia, W.B. Saunders Company, 2000. Part XII: Diseases of the Liver, Gallbladder, and Bile Ducts, pages 767 to 833.

ency of the testes are due to changes in estrogen metabolism. Chronic portal hypertension may lead to development of collateral circulation, which is manifested as caput medusa in the region of the umbilicus and epigastrium.

Ascites can be determined most easily by the demonstration of flank dullness. Shifting dullness and a fluid wave are more difficult to elicit and require more ascites.

The normal smooth liver with a sharp edge can be differentiated from the nodular liver of cirrhosis, the rock-hard liver of metastatic cancer, the tender liver of hepatitis or chronic passive congestion, and the pulsating liver of severe tricuspid insufficiency. In pancreatic carcinoma the palpable gallbladder is known as Courvoisier's sign. Splenomegaly is usually confirmation of portal hypertension. Evaluation for possible hepatic encephalopathy is crucial.

Laboratory Tests

Three patterns of liver injury are seen: necrosis, cholestasis, and infiltration (Table 10–1). In most liver diseases the ratio of aspartate aminotransferase (AST) to alanine aminotransferase (ALT) is typically 1 or less. However, ratios of 2 or greater are common in alcoholic hepatitis (Fig. 10–1). Serum alkaline phosphatase activity also may be increased in bone disorders (e.g., Paget's disease, osteomalacia, metastases to bone), the later stages of pregnancy, rapid bone growth, and chronic renal failure (Fig. 10–2). When the source of alkaline phosphatase is not apparent, levels of γ-glutamyl transpeptidase (GGT) or of 5′-nucleotidase, which tend to parallel levels of alkaline phosphatase in hepatobiliary disease but are not usually increased in bone disease, should be measured. Up to one third of patients with isolated elevations of serum hepatobiliary alkaline phosphatase activity have no demonstrable liver or biliary disease.

Higher plasma bilirubin levels are associated with a poorer prognosis. Chronic hemolysis cannot produce elevations of serum bilirubin above 5 mg/dL in the absence of liver disease. Levels greater than 30 mg/dL are uncommon in the absence of renal failure. During the recovery phase of prolonged hepatitis or cholestasis, normalization of serum bilirubin may require much longer than other liver tests. The level of serum ammonia is widely used to confirm the diagnosis of hepatic encephalopathy and to monitor the success of therapy, but the correlation of ammonia level with the degree of encephalopathy is only approximate.

Any acute or chronic liver disease may cause an abnormal prothrombin time by impairing the synthesis of essential clotting factors. Because the plasma half-life of these factors is typically less than 1 day, the prothrombin time responds rapidly to changes in hepatic synthetic function. This property makes the prothrombin time particularly useful for following the course of acute liver diseases; significant elevation often indicates an unfavorable prognosis.

Albumin, synthesized exclusively in the liver, has a long half-life in plasma (about 3 weeks in healthy adults). Low albumin levels are slow to develop and may persist for weeks after correction of the underlying problem. In cholestasis, the serum concentration of cholesterol increases.

Table 10–1 ■ TYPICAL LIVER TEST PATTERNS

	HEPATOCELLULAR NECROSIS			BILIARY OBSTRUCTION			
TEST	**Toxic or Ischemic**	**Viral**	**Alcohol**	**Chronic Complete**	**Chronic Partial**	**Acute Complete (First 24 hr)**	**INFILTRATION (CHRONIC)**
Aminotransferases	50–100x	5–50x	2–5x	1–5x	1–5x	1–50x	1–3x
Alkaline phosphatase	1–3x	1–3x	1–10x	2–20x	2–10x	May be normal	1–20x
Bilirubin	1–5x	1–30x	1–30x	1–30x	1–5x	Usually normal	1–5x
Prothrombin time	Prolonged in severe cases, unresponsive to vitamin K			May be prolonged, responsive to vitamin K	Usually normal	Usually normal	Usually normal
Albumin	Normal in acute illness, may be decreased in chronic disease			Usually normal, but may be decreased in biliary cirrhosis		Usually normal	Usually normal
Typical disorders	Acetaminophen toxicity, shock liver	Acute hepatitis A or B	Alcoholic hepatitis	Pancreatic carcinoma	Sclerosing cholangitis	Choledocholithiasis	Primary or metastatic carcinoma, *Mycobacterium avium-intracellulare* infection

Modified from Davern TJ, Scharschmidt B: Biochemical liver tests. *In* Feldman M, Scharschmidt BF, Sleisenger MH (eds): Sleisenger & Fordtran's Gastrointestinal and Liver Disease, 6th ed. Philadelphia, WB Saunders, 1998, pp 1112–1122.

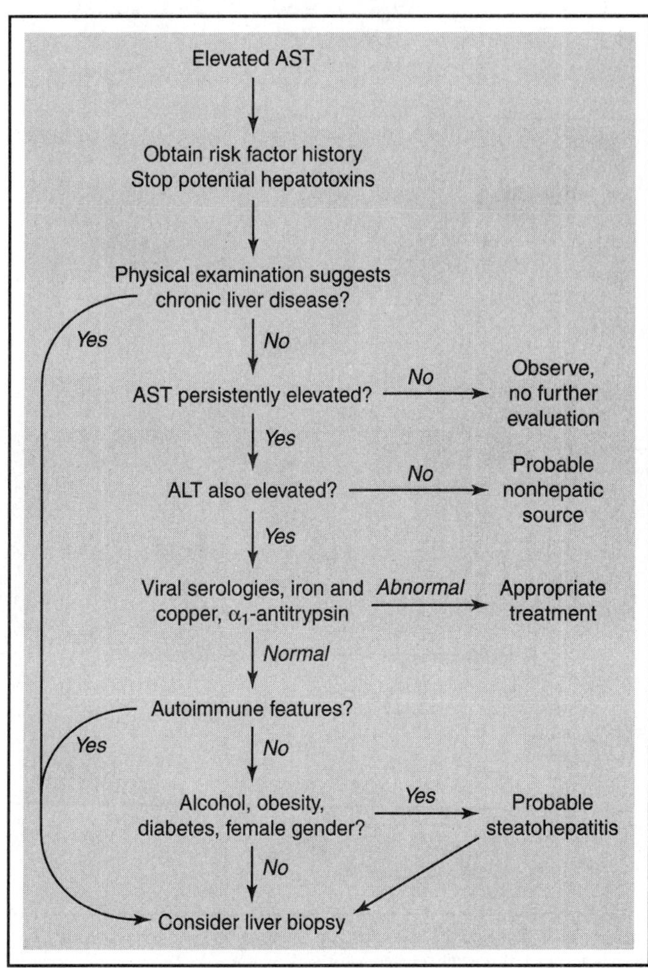

FIGURE 10–1 ■ Approach to the asymptomatic patient with isolated elevated levels of serum aspartate aminotransferase (AST). ALT = alanine aminotransferase.

In approximately 90% of patients with primary biliary cirrhosis, the serum contains antibodies against the inner mitochondrial membrane. Mitochondrial antibodies are also present in up to 25% of patients with histologically active chronic hepatitis and postnecrotic cirrhosis and in 7 to 8% of asymptomatic relatives of patients with primary biliary cirrhosis.

Approach to the Jaundiced Patient

Jaundice is a common feature of both acute and chronic generalized hepatic dysfunction (Table 10–2). The diagnostic approach to the jaundiced patient begins with a careful history, physical exami-

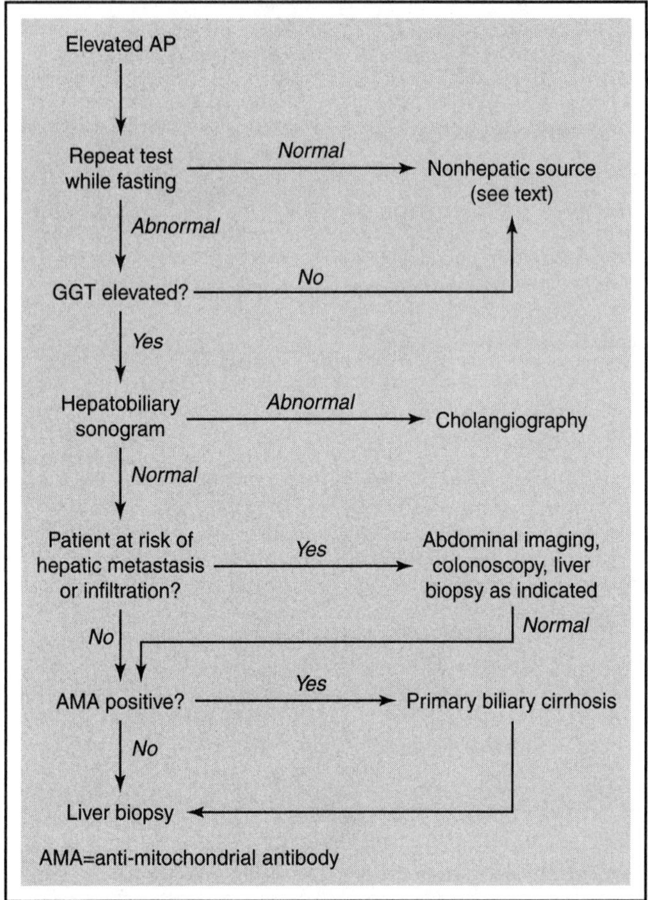

FIGURE 10–2 ■ Evaluation of isolated elevated levels of serum alkaline phosphatase (AP). GGT = γ-glutamyl transpeptidase.

nation, and screening laboratory studies (Fig. 10–3). The distinction between liver disease and extrahepatic obstruction is generally the most important aspect of the differential diagnosis (Table 10–3).

If the likelihood of obstruction is judged negligible, no imaging studies are necessary. Conversely, if the likelihood of obstruction is judged to be very high (e.g., fever and rigors in a patient with recent biliary tract surgery), direct cholangiography may be an appropriate initial choice. If obstruction is considered possible but not highly likely, non-invasive imaging with ultrasound (US) or computed tomography (CT) is a reasonable first study. The treatment of hyperbilirubinemia depends on the cause.

For more information about this subject, see *Cecil Textbook of Medicine,* 21st edition. Philadelphia, W.B. Saunders Company, 2000. Chapter 144, Approach to the Patient with Liver Diseases;

Table 10–2 ■ DIFFERENTIAL DIAGNOSIS OF JAUNDICE

Isolated Disorders of Bilirubin Metabolism

Unconjugated hyperbilirubinemia
- Increased bilirubin production
  - *Examples:* hemolysis, ineffective erythropoiesis, blood transfusion, resorption of hematomas
- Decreased hepatocellular uptake
  - *Examples:* drugs (e.g., rifampin)
- Decreased conjugation
  - *Examples:* Gilbert's syndrome, Crigler-Najjar syndrome, physiologic jaundice of the newborn

Conjugated or mixed hyperbilirubinemia
- Dubin-Johnson syndrome
- Rotor's syndrome

Liver Disease

Acute or Chronic Hepatocellular Dysfunction
- Acute or subacute hepatocellular injury
  - *Examples:* viral hepatitis, hepatotoxins (e.g., ethanol, acetaminophen, *Amanita*), drugs (e.g., isoniazid, methyldopa), ischemia (e.g., hypotension, vascular occlusion), metabolic disorders (e.g., Wilson's disease, Reye's syndrome), pregnancy-related (e.g., acute fatty liver of pregnancy, pre-eclampsia)
- Chronic hepatocellular disease
  - *Examples:* viral hepatitis, hepatotoxins (e.g., ethanol, vinyl chloride, vitamin A), autoimmune hepatitis, metabolic (Wilson's disease, hemochromatosis, α_1-antitrypsin deficiency)

Hepatic Disorders with Prominent Cholestasis

- Diffuse infiltrative disorders
  - *Examples:* granulomatous diseases (e.g., mycobacterial infections, sarcoidosis, lymphoma, drugs, Wegener's granulomatosis), amyloidosis, infiltrative malignancy
- Inflammation of intrahepatic bile ductules and/or portal tracts
  - *Examples:* primary biliary cirrhosis, graft-versus-host disease, drugs (e.g., chlorpromazine, erythromycin)
- Miscellaneous conditions
  - *Examples:* benign recurrent intrahepatic cholestasis, drugs, estrogens, anabolic steroids, total parenteral nutrition, bacterial infections, uncommon presentations of viral or alcoholic hepatitis, intrahepatic cholestasis of pregnancy, postoperative cholestasis

Obstruction of the Bile Ducts

Choledocholithiasis
- Cholesterol gallstones
- Pigment gallstones

Diseases of the bile ducts
- Inflammation/infection
  - *Examples:* primary sclerosing cholangitis, AIDS cholangiopathy, hepatic arterial chemotherapy, postsurgical strictures
- Neoplasms

Extrinsic compression of the biliary tree
- Neoplasms
  - *Examples:* pancreatic carcinoma, metastatic lymphadenopathy, hepatoma
- Pancreatitis
- Vascular enlargement (e.g., aneurysm, cavernous transformation of portal vein)

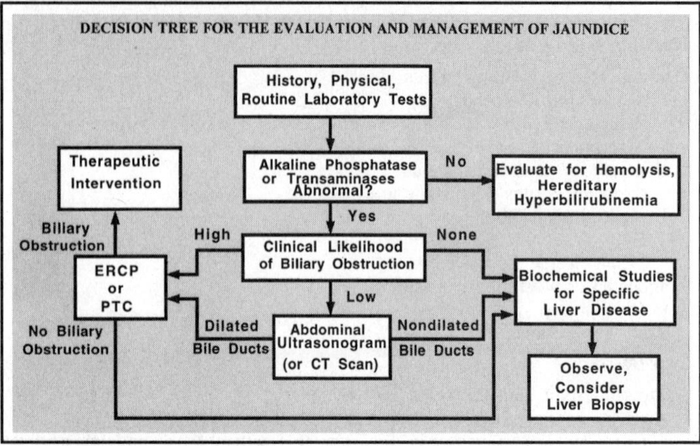

FIGURE 10–3 ■ Approach to the patient with jaundice. ERCP = endoscopic retrograde cholangiopancreatography: PTC = percutaneous transhepatic cholangiogram. (From Lidofsky SD, Scharschmidt BF: Jaundice. *In* Feldman M, Scharschmidt BF, Sleisenger MH [eds]: Gastrointestinal and Liver Disease, 6th ed. Philadelphia, WB Saunders, 1998, p 227.)

Table 10–3 ■ OBSTRUCTIVE JAUNDICE VERSUS CHOLESTATIC LIVER DISEASE

	SUGGESTS OBSTRUCTIVE JAUNDICE	SUGGESTS CHOLESTATIC LIVER DISEASE
History	Abdominal pain Fever, rigors Prior biliary surgery Older age	Anorexia, malaise, or myalgias suggestive of viral prodrome Known infectious exposure Receipt of blood products, use of intravenous drugs Exposure to known hepatotoxin Family history of jaundice
Physical examination	High fever Abdominal tenderness Palpable abdominal mass Abdominal scar	Ascites Stigmata of liver disease (e.g., prominent abdominal veins, gynecomastia, spider angiomas, Kayser-Fleischer rings) Asterixis, encephalopathy
Laboratory studies	Predominant elevation of serum bilirubin and alkaline phosphatase Prothrombin time that is normal or normalizes with vitamin K administration Elevated serum amylase	Predominant elevation of serum aminotransferase levels Prolonged prothrombin time that does not correct with vitamin K administration Blood tests indicative of specific liver disease

Chapter 145, Hepatic Metabolism in Liver Disease; Chapter 146, Bilirubin Metabolism, Hyperbilirubinemia, and Approach to the Jaundiced Patient; and Chapter 147, Laboratory Tests in Liver Disease, and Approach to the Patient with Abnormal Tests, pages 767 to 779.

TOXIC AND DRUG-INDUCED LIVER DISEASE

Drugs and toxins produce a variety of pathologic lesions in the liver (Table 10–4). Drug-induced liver disease is managed by discontinuing the implicated drug(s) and giving supportive care for acute hepatitis and hepatic failure as needed. In the case of severe, acute drug- or toxin-induced liver failure, urgent liver transplantation may be life-saving. Specific pharmacologic intervention is generally limited to the administration of *N*-acetylcysteine in acetaminophen overdosage.

In *acetaminophen* toxicity, patients develop nausea, vomiting, and diarrhea within a few hours of ingestion. Clinical and labora-

10

Table 10–4 ■ CLASSIFICATION OF DRUG-INDUCED LIVER DISEASE

CATEGORY	EXAMPLES
Zonal necrosis	Acetaminophen, carbon tetrachloride, simvastatin
Non-specific hepatitis	Aspirin, oxacillin
Viral hepatitis–like reaction	Halothane, isoniazid, phenytoin, diclofenac
Chronic hepatitis	
Autoimmune hepatitis–like	Methyldopa, dantrolene, diclofenac
Viral hepatitis–like	Isoniazid, halothane
Cholestasis	
Non-inflammatory	Estrogens, 17α-substituted steroids
Inflammatory	Amoxicillin-clavulanate, piroxicam
small duct injury (vanishing bile duct syndrome)	flucloxacillin, thiabendazole, haloperidol
Large duct injury (sclerosing cholangitis)	Fluorodeoxyuridine
Fatty liver	
Large droplet	Ethanol, corticosteroids
Small droplet	Tetracycline, valproic acid, didanosine
Phospholipidosis and steatohepatitis	Amiodarone, perhexiline maleate
Granulomas	Phenylbutazone, allopurinol
Fibrosis	Methotrexate, hypervitaminosis A
Tumors	
Adenoma	Estrogens
Angiosarcoma	Vinyl chloride
Vascular lesions	
Hepatic vein thrombosis	Estrogens
Veno-occlusive disease	Anticancer agents, azathioprine, *Senecio* alkaloids
Peliosis hepatis	Anabolic steroids, estrogens
Hepatic arteritis	Allopurinol, fluorodeoxyuridine
Nodular regenerative hyperplasia	Azathioprine, anticancer agents

tory signs of liver damage become evident 24 to 48 hours after ingestion. Serum aminotransferase levels of more than 5000 U/L are common. The plasma level of acetaminophen is the most reliable means of assessing prognosis. Levels in excess of 200 mg/L at 4 hours, 100 mg/L at 8 hours, or 50 mg/L at 12 hours after ingestion are predictive of severe liver damage and are indications for treatment with *N*-acetylcysteine. *N*-Acetylcysteine may afford some benefit after 10 hours, but its benefit after 24 hours is not established. The recommended oral dose is 140 mg/kg initially, followed by maintenance doses of 70 mg/kg every 4 hours for 72 hours. Survivors of acute acetaminophen toxicity usually recover completely without progressive or residual liver damage.

Halothane is a halogenated alkane anesthetic that rarely causes a viral hepatitis–like reaction. In severe cases, it may progress to fatal massive hepatic necrosis.

Isoniazid as single-drug chemoprophylaxis against tuberculosis is associated with a 10 to 20% incidence of subclinical liver injury. About 1% of patients receiving it develop significant liver injury. The onset usually occurs within 2 to 3 months after starting the drug, and initial symptoms are often non-specific, with malaise and anorexia preceding signs of liver disease.

For more information about this subject, see *Cecil Textbook of Medicine,* 21st edition. Philadelphia, W.B. Saunders Company, 2000. Chapter 148, Toxic and Drug-Induced Liver Disease, pages 779 to 783.

ACUTE VIRAL HEPATITIS

The five known causes of acute hepatitis are the hepatitis A (HAV), B (HBV), C (HCV), D or delta (HDV), and E (HEV) viruses: The *incubation period* varies from 2 to 20 weeks, largely on the basis of viral etiology and dose of exposure. The *pre-icteric phase* of illness is marked by the onset of fatigue, nausea, poor appetite, and vague right upper quadrant pain. The onset of dark urine marks the *icteric phase* of illness, during which jaundice appears and symptoms of fatigue and nausea worsen. Typically, acute viral hepatitis is rarely diagnosed correctly before the onset of jaundice, when the physical examination usually shows hepatic tenderness.

The duration of clinical illness is variable; it typically lasts 1 to 3 weeks. Recovery is first manifested by return of appetite and is accompanied by resolution of the serum bilirubin and aminotransferase elevations and clearance of virus. *Convalescence,* however, can be prolonged before full degrees of energy and stamina return.

Complications of acute viral hepatitis include chronic infection, fulminant hepatic failure, relapsing or cholestatic hepatitis, and extrahepatic syndromes. *Chronic hepatitis,* usually defined as at least 6 months of illness, eventuates in approximately 5% of adults with hepatitis B but in 75% of those with hepatitis C.

Acute liver failure or fulminant hepatitis occurs in 1 to 2% of patients with symptomatic acute hepatitis, most commonly with hepatitis B and D, and least commonly with hepatitis C. The most reliable prognostic factor in acute hepatic failure is the degree of prolongation of prothrombin time.

A proportion of patients with acute hepatitis develop a cholestatic pattern of illness, with prolonged and fluctuating jaundice and pruritus. Between 10 and 20% of patients develop a serum sickness–like syndrome during the pre-icteric phase of acute hepatitis, with variable combinations of rash, hives, arthralgias, and fever.

Hepatitis A

Hepatitis A is spread largely by the fecal-oral route (Fig. 10–4). Acute hepatitis A is invariably a self-limited infection; the virus can persist for months, but it does not lead to a chronic infection, chronic hepatitis, or cirrhosis. Severe and fulminant cases of hepatitis A can occur. The diagnosis of acute hepatitis A can be made based on the finding of IgM anti-HAV in the serum of a patient with the clinical and biochemical features of acute hepatitis. A safe and effective hepatitis A vaccine is available and is recommended for patients at high risk of acquiring hepatitis A.

Hepatitis B

Hepatitis B is spread predominantly by the parenteral route or by sexual contact (Fig. 10–5). The diagnosis of acute hepatitis B can be made on the basis of finding hepatitis B surface antigen (HBsAg) in the serum of a patient with the clinical and biochemical features of acute hepatitis. Testing for IgM anti–hepatitis B core (HBc) antigen is helpful, because this antibody arises early and is lost within 6 to 12 months of onset of illness. Loss of HBsAg and development of anti–hepatitis B surface (HBs) antigen denote recovery. Chronic hepatitis B develops in 2 to 7% of adults infected with HBV. Hepatitis B is also an important cause of fulminant hepatitis.

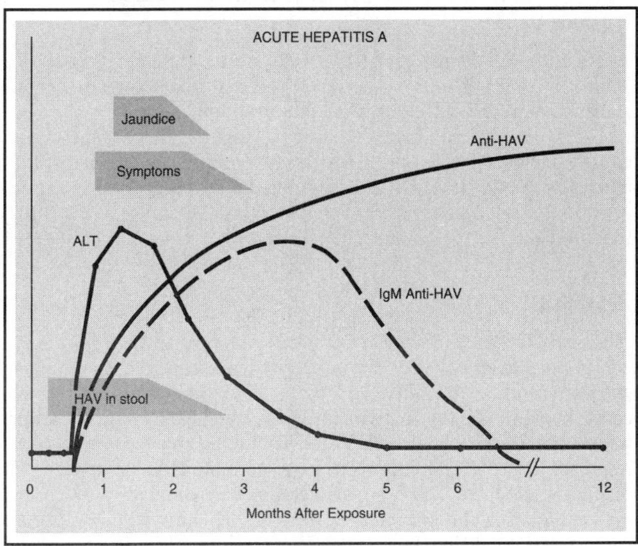

FIGURE 10–4 ■ The serologic course of acute hepatitis A. ALT = alanine aminotransferase; HAV = hepatitis A virus.

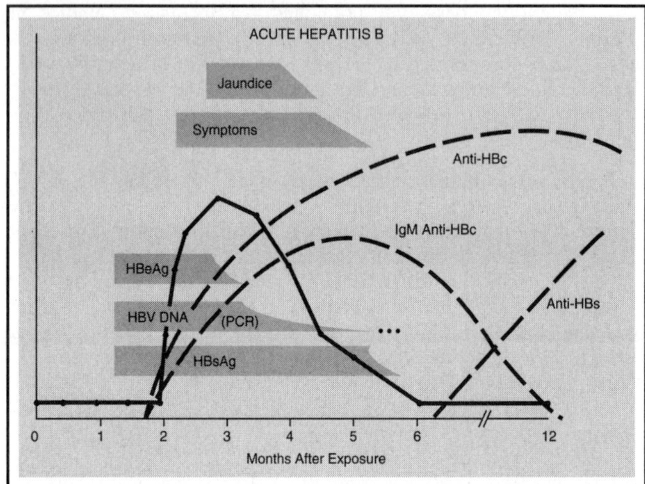

FIGURE 10–5 ■ The serologic course of acute hepatitis B. HBc = hepatitis B core; HBcAg = hepatitis B early antigen; HBs = hepatitis B surface; HBV = hepatitis B virus; PCR = polymerase chain reaction; HBsAg = hepatitis B surface antigen.

Vaccination against hepatitis B is now recommended for all newborns and children. Adults, especially in groups at high risk for acquiring hepatitis B, should also be vaccinated.

Hepatitis C

Hepatitis C is spread predominantly by the parenteral route (Fig. 10–6). Sexual transmission is rare. Maternal-infant spread occurs in approximately 5% of cases. The major complication of acute hepatitis C is the development of chronic hepatitis. Indeed, the clinical course depicted in Figure 10–6 is not typical, because hepatitis C does not resolve in 70% of cases, but rather progresses to chronic infection. The diagnosis of acute hepatitis C is generally made based on the finding of anti-HCV in serum.

Hepatitis D

Hepatitis D occurs in two clinical patterns, termed *co-infection* and *superinfection.* HDV co-infection represents the simultaneous occurrence of acute HDV and acute HBV infection. It resembles acute hepatitis B but may manifest a second elevation in aminotransferase levels. Acute HDV superinfection represents the occurrence of acute HDV infection in a chronic HBsAg carrier. The diagnosis of acute HDV superinfection can be made in a patient presenting with clinical features of acute hepatitis who had HBsAg and anti-HDV but no IgM anti-HBc in serum. Hepatitis D tends to be more severe than hepatitis B alone. There are no specific means of therapy for acute hepatitis D.

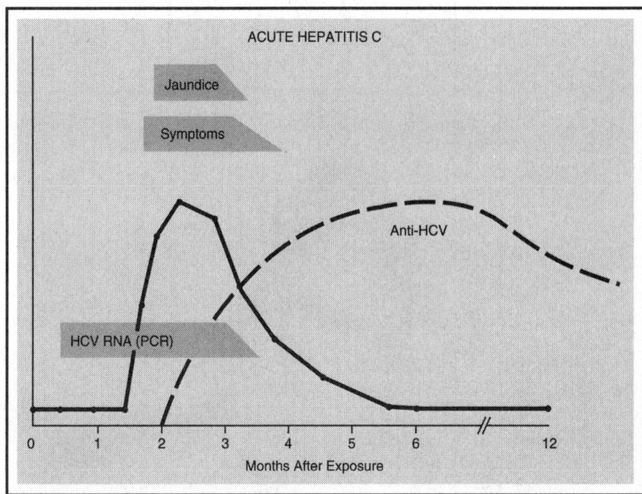

FIGURE 10–6 ■ The serologic course of acute hepatitis C. HCV = hepatitis C virus; PCR = polymerase chain reaction.

Hepatitis E

Hepatitis E is spread by the fecal-oral route. The clinical course of hepatitis E resembles that of other forms of hepatitis. Enzyme-linked immunoassays for IgM and IgG antibody to HEV (anti-HEV) have been developed and are reactive in at least 90% of patients at the onset of clinical illness. There are no known means of prevention or treatment of hepatitis E.

Hepatitis Non A . . . E

The syndrome of non-A . . . E hepatitis has been particularly associated with the complications of acute liver failure and aplastic anemia. Hepatitis non-A . . . E is a more common cause of fulminant hepatic failure than hepatitis A or B combined, often accounting for 30 to 40% of cases. Approximately one third of patients with non-A . . . E hepatitis develop chronic hepatitis, and a small percentage ultimately develop cirrhosis. Non-A . . . E hepatitis is a diagnosis of exclusion.

For more information about this subject, see *Cecil Textbook of Medicine,* 21st edition. Philadelphia, W.B. Saunders Company, 2000. Chapter 149, Acute Viral Hepatitis, pages 783 to 790.

CHRONIC HEPATITIS

Chronic hepatitis comprises several diseases that can lead insidiously to cirrhosis and end-stage liver disease (Table 10–5). The clinical symptoms of chronic hepatitis are typically non-specific, intermittent, and mild; a large proportion of patients have no symptoms of liver disease at all. The most common symptom is fatigue. In many cases, the diagnosis is made after liver test result abnormalities are identified when blood is drawn for a routine evalua-

Table 10–5 ■ DIFFERENTIAL DIAGNOSIS IN CHRONIC HEPATITIS

DIAGNOSIS	SCREENING TESTS	CONFIRMATORY TESTS	COMMENTS
Chronic hepatitis B	HBsAg	HBV DNA and HBeAg or HBcAg in liver	
Chronic hepatitis C	Anti-HCV	HCV RNA (using PCR)	Immunoblot for anti-HCV can be used to confirm antibody reactivity
Chronic hepatitis D	Anti-HDV	HDV RNA or HDV antigen in liver	
Autoimmune hepatitis	ANA (Anti-LKM1)	Exclusion of other causes and pattern of clinical disease	Suggested by raised IgG levels and by response to corticosteroid therapy
Drug-induced liver disease	History	Rechallenge if necessary	Medications most suspect include isoniazid, NSAIDs, methyldopa, nitrofurantoin
Wilson's disease	Ceruloplasmin	Urine and hepatic copper concentration	Suggested by hemolysis or severe chronic hepatitis in child or adolescent
Cryptogenic	Exclusion of other causes		Major differential is with autoimmune hepatitis and drug-induced liver disease

HBsAg = hepatitis B surface antigen; HCV = hepatitis C virus; HDV = hepatitis D virus; ANA = antinuclear antibody; LKM1 = liver-kidney microsomal 1 antibody; HBV = hepatitis B virus; HBeAg = hepatitis B e antigen; HBcAg = hepatitis B core antigen; IgG = immunoglobulin G; NSAIDs = non-steroidal anti-inflammatory drugs; PCR = polymerase chain reaction.

tion. Symptoms of advanced disease or an acute exacerbation include nausea, poor appetite, weight loss, muscle weakness, itching, dark urine, and jaundice.

Most typical are elevations in ALT and AST levels with little or no elevation in the alkaline phosphatase level. The elevations are usually in the range of one to five times the upper limit of normal. Hepatic histologic analysis is useful for grading the severity and for staging chronic hepatitis and is usually obtained to confirm the diagnosis.

Chronic Hepatitis B

Symptoms appear 30 to 150 days after exposure. The subsequent course is highly variable. Some patients continue to have active viral replication with high levels of HBV DNA and hepatitis B e antigen (HBeAg) in serum and progressive liver injury. In other patients, the disease is more indolent, leading insidiously in decades to cirrhosis. However, in a large proportion of patients, the disease eventually goes into remission with a fall in viral levels, loss of HbeAg, and transition to an "inactive" carrier state.

In the inactive carrier state, HBV DNA is not detectable in serum by using conventional hybridization assays sensitive to levels of 10^6 viral copies per milliliter. Testing for HBV DNA by polymerase chain reaction (PCR) usually demonstrates low levels of viral genome. Liver injury and pathogenesis of chronic hepatitis B are believed to be immunologically mediated, so the severity and course of disease do not correlate well with the level of virus in serum or antigen expression in liver.

The extrahepatic manifestations of chronic hepatitis B include mucocutaneous vasculitis, glomerulonephritis, and polyarteritis nodosa. Recommendations regarding indications and regimens as well as duration of antiviral therapy with interferon alfa, lamivudine, and perhaps other drugs will change as more effective combination antiviral therapies are developed.

Chronic Hepatitis D

On average, cirrhosis develops in 70% of patients with chronic hepatitis D. A prolonged course of rather high doses of interferon alfa (5 to 10 MU/day or thrice weekly) results in improvements in serum aminotransferase levels and liver histology in approximately one third of patients.

Chronic Hepatitis C

In the typical course, HCV RNA becomes detectable soon after exposure and remains present throughout the acute illness and thereafter. In 30 to 50% of infected individuals with chronic hepatitis by liver biopsy, serum aminotransferase levels fall and remain in the normal range despite persistence of HCV RNA.

A proportion of patients have severe and progressive disease, with cirrhosis and end-stage liver disease developing within a few years; other patients have a benign outcome. In patients followed from the time of acute infection, approximately 75 to 85% have chronic infection, but cirrhosis develops in only 10 to 20% within the first 20 years. However, when patients with established chronic hepatitis C are followed prospectively from the time of initial presentation, 30 to 50% develop cirrhosis.

The extrahepatic manifestations of chronic hepatitis C include cryoglobulinemia, glomerulonephritis, mucocutaneous vasculitis, non-Hodgkin's B cell lymphoma, porphyria cutanea tarda, lichen planus, and perhaps fibromyalgia.

The therapy of hepatitis C is rapidly evolving. The addition of ribavirin to interferon alfa therapy has increased the sustained response rate substantially. Even with combination therapy, the sustained response rate to interferon treatment in hepatitis C is less than 50%, and many patients find the therapy difficult to tolerate. For patients with decompensated liver disease due to hepatitis C, liver transplantation is indicated.

Autoimmune Hepatitis

Autoimmune hepatitis is characterized by the presence of autoantibodies, high levels of serum immunoglobulins, and frequent association with other autoimmune diseases. The pathogenesis is not known. The disease is more common in women and typically has its onset either in childhood or young adulthood or around the time of menopause.

Type 1 (classic) autoimmune hepatitis is characterized by the detection of antinuclear (ANAs), anti–smooth muscle (SMAs), antiactin, and anti-asialoglycoprotein receptor antibodies. Type 2 autoimmune hepatitis is characterized by the detection of anti–liver-kidney microsomal 1 antibodies (anti-LKM1) and anti–liver cytosol 1 antibodies, as well as the absence of ANA or SMA.

Most typical of autoimmune hepatitis is a rapid clinical response to corticosteroid therapy initiated in a dose of 20 to 30 mg/day. Corticosteroids or immunosuppressive therapy is usually continued indefinitely.

Cryptogenic Chronic Liver Disease

The term *cryptogenic chronic liver disease* is a diagnosis of exclusion and should be made only after hepatitis B, C, and D; autoimmune hepatitis; drug-induced liver disease; and inherited metabolic liver diseases such as Wilson's disease are excluded.

For more information about this subject, see *Cecil Textbook of Medicine,* 21st edition. Philadelphia, W.B. Saunders Company, 2000. Chapter 150, Chronic Hepatitis, pages 790 to 796.

PARASITIC, BACTERIAL, FUNGAL, GRANULOMATOUS, NEOPLASTIC, AND MISCELLANEOUS LIVER DISEASES

Bacterial Liver Abscess

A remarkable array of bacteria cause liver abscesses, with gram-negative enteric bacteria, especially *Escherichia coli, Klebsiella pneumoniae, Streptococcus faecalis,* and *Proteus vulgaris,* being the major contributors. The role of anaerobic organisms, especially *Bacteroides* and *Clostridium,* has been increasingly recognized.

A bacterial liver abscess may be suspected when a patient develops fever, leukocytosis, and right upper quadrant abdominal pain. Pyogenic liver abscess should be considered in any patient who has presumptive or definite evidence of septicemia in association with biochemical abnormalities of the liver. Most liver abscesses occur in the right lobe.

Directed aspiration of the abscess with culture and cytologic examination usually accurately identifies the causative organisms. The cornerstones of treating bacterial liver abscesses are effective drainage and antibiotics. Broad-spectrum antibiotics, including coverage for anaerobes, should begin immediately after aspiration, with later adjustments of treatment based on culture results. Antibiotics may be required for several weeks or even months.

Echinococcosis (Hydatid Disease)

Echinococcus-granulosa is a tapeworm living in dogs that acquire the infection from eating infected sheep viscera. Humans, like sheep, are intermediate hosts. The echinococcal cyst may remain asymptomatic or continue to expand. In some patients, cysts rupture into bile ducts or the peritoneal cavity, lungs, and other organs. Indirect hemagglutination and enzyme-linked immunosorbent assays are helpful for diagnosis. US, CT, and magnetic resonance imaging (MRI) are useful in diagnosing the presence of a cyst and may be highly suggestive of the echinococcal origin. Diagnostic aspiration is dangerous and may lead to dissemination of the infection. If feasible, surgical removal of the cyst is indicated.

Amebic Liver Abscess

The gradual onset of fever, malaise, and right upper quadrant abdominal pain is the usual presentation. Occasionally, the onset is abrupt, with fever and repeated rigors. Almost all patients have hepatic tenderness. Only a few patients have concomitant evidence of amebic colitis, and cysts are found in the stool in a minority of patients. The preferred site for abscess formation is superioanteriorly in the right lobe of the liver. Amebic abscesses should be considered in any patient who has resided in or traveled to an endemic area and in whom a hepatic filling defect is found on an imaging study. The indirect hemagglutination test indicates tissue invasion by amebae and is almost always indicative, although not diagnostic, of liver involvement. Metronidazole is the drug of choice.

Granulomatous Liver Disease

Major disorders in which hepatic granulomas are frequent include sarcoidosis, tuberculosis, histoplasmosis, and schistosomiasis. Coccidioidomycosis is a well-established cause of granulomas in the western United States. *Mycobacterium avium-intracellulare* is found in patients with AIDS. A variety of therapeutic drugs, including phenylbutazone, allopurinol, and carbamazepine, are well documented to cause granulomas. In addition, granulomas are characteristically found in the early stages of primary biliary cirrhosis.

Hepatic Tumors

Tumors of the liver are relatively uncommon but increasingly recognized, often incidentally, owing to the frequent use of abdominal radiologic imaging techniques (Table 10–6).

Table 10–6 ■ SELECTED FEATURES OF BENIGN AND MALIGNANT HEPATIC TUMORS

TUMOR	PATIENTS/RISK FACTORS	DIAGNOSIS	THERAPY
Benign			
Hemangioma	Healthy, incidental finding	Red blood cell–labeled scan	Observe; resect if symptoms
Adenoma	Young females on oral contraceptives	US/CT; sulfur-colloid scan: no uptake in lesion	Stop oral contraceptives; consider resection
Focal nodular hyperplasia	Middle-aged females, ±oral contraceptives	US/CT; sulfur-colloid scan: increased uptake in 60%	Stop oral contraceptives; observation
Focal fatty infiltration	Obesity, diabetes, corticosteroids, alcohol, weight changes, total parenteral nutrition	US/CT; sulfur-colloid scan: homogeneous uptake	Observation
Malignant			
Hepatocellular carcinoma	Cirrhosis, chronic viral hepatitis	US/three-phase CT, α-fetoprotein, biopsy	Resection, local ablation, liver transplantation
Fibrolamellar variant	Young, healthy, no risk factors	As above	As above
Cholangiocarcinoma	Sclerosing cholangitis, oriental cholangiopathies	US/CT/cholangiogram, carcinoembryonic antigen/CA 19-9	Resection, biliary drainage, chemotherapy/radiation
Metastatic	Extrahepatic malignancy (gastrointestinal, breast, lung)	US/CT, biopsy	Resection (colon cancer); treat underlying tumor
Angiosarcoma	Vinyl chloride, Thorotrast, arsenic exposure	US/CT/angiogram	Resection

US = ultrasonography; CT = computed tomography.

In most patients granulomas may be detected when a liver biopsy is being performed for some other reason, especially during evaluation of an increase in serum alkaline phosphatase. Treatment depends on the diagnosis established.

Liver Disease Unique to Pregnancy

Several liver diseases are related to pregnancy (Table 10–7). For the HELLP syndrome (*h*emolysis, *e*levated *l*iver *e*nzymes, and *l*ow *p*latelets), prompt delivery is the treatment of choice.

For more information about this subject, see *Cecil Textbook of Medicine,* 21st edition. Philadelphia, W.B. Saunders Company, 2000. Chapter 151, Parasitic, Bacterial, Fungal, and Granulomatous Liver Diseases; Chapter 152, Inherited, Infiltrative, and Metabolic Disorders Involving the Liver; and Chapter 156, Hepatic Tumors, pages 797 to 804, and 819 to 821.

ALCOHOLIC LIVER DISEASE, CIRRHOSIS, AND ITS MAJOR SEQUELAE

Cirrhosis represents the consequences of a sustained wound-healing response to chronic liver injury from a variety of causes (Table 10–8). Liver biopsy remains the gold standard for documenting cirrhosis.

Alcoholic Liver Disease

Although many patients who drink heavily develop hepatic enlargement and fatty accumulation, only a minority (~20%) of cases will progress to alcoholic hepatitis or cirrhosis. Risk factors for developing these more severe sequelae include duration and magnitude of alcohol ingestion, female sex, hepatitis B or C infection, genetic factors, and nutritional status.

Fatty liver is associated with moderate to marked hepatomegaly. Liver test results are generally normal or only modestly elevated.

Alcoholic hepatitis may lead to anorexia, fever, hepatomegaly, and jaundice. Liver tests characteristically reveal elevations of AST and ALT to less than 500 U/L, with AST values one to two times greater than ALT. In the hospitalized patient with acute alcoholic hepatitis, acute elevations of AST and ALT resolve over several days, followed by more persistent and sometimes marked elevation of bilirubin up to 20 times normal and alkaline phosphatase up to two to three times normal.

Fatty liver resolves completely within 4 to 6 weeks after alcohol ingestion is discontinued. In contrast, prognosis of alcoholic hepatitis is dependent on continued drinking, degree of inflammation, evidence of coagulopathy, ascites, hepatorenal syndrome, or encephalopathy.

Multivitamins (including thiamine, folate, vitamin K, and pyridoxine), fluids, and replacement of minerals (phosphate, magnesium) are usually warranted. In the patient with severe life-threatening alcoholic hepatitis, therapy with methylprednisolone 32 to 40 mg/day for 28 days will lessen short-term mortality. Corticosteroids are not appropriate in patients with mild hepatitis or with either gastrointestinal bleeding or concurrent bacterial infection.

Table 10–7 ■ LIVER DISEASES UNIQUE TO PREGNANCY

	TRIMESTER OF ONSET	SYMPTOMS	LABORATORY ABNORMALITIES	RECURRENCE WITH FUTURE PREGNANCIES
Hyperemesis gravidarum	1	Nausea, vomiting	Elevated AST/ALT (60–1000 U/L), occasionally hyperbilirubinemia	
Cholestasis	2, 3	Pruritus	Bile acids >8 μmol/L, elevated AST/ALT and bilirubin in more severe cases	Common
Acute fatty liver	3	Nausea, vomiting, abdominal pain	Elevated AST/ALT (100–1000 U/L), bilirubin >5 mg/dL, prolonged prothrombin time*	Rare
HELLP syndrome	2, 3, or post partum	Abdominal pain, nausea, vomiting	Elevated AST/ALT (60–1500 U/L), low platelets <100,000/mm^3, LDH >600 U/L, microangiopathic anemia	3–25%

AST = aspartate aminotransferase; ALT = alanine aminotransferase; HELLP syndrome = *h*emolysis, *e*levated *l*iver enzymes, *l*ow *p*latelets; LDH = lactate dehydrogenase.
* Useful diagnostic distinction from HELLP syndrome, in which prothrombin time and fibrinogen are usually normal.

Table 10–8 ■ CLASSIFICATION OF HEPATIC FIBROSIS AND CIRRHOSIS

I. Presinusoidal fibrosis
   A. Schistosomiasis
   B. Idiopathic portal fibrosis
II. Parenchymal (sinusoidal) fibrosis (true cirrhosis)
   A. Drugs and toxins
      Alcohol
      Methotrexate
      Isoniazid
      Vitamin A
      Amiodarone
   B. Infections
      Chronic hepatitis B or C
      Brucellosis
      Echinococcosis
      Congenital or tertiary syphilis
   C. Autoimmune
      Autoimmune chronic hepatitis—types 1, 2, and 3
   D. Vascular abnormalities
      Chronic, passive congestion due to right-sided heart failure, pericarditis
      Hereditary hemorrhagic telangiectasia (Osler-Weber-Rendu disease)
   E. Metabolic/genetic diseases
      Wilson's disease
      Hemochromatosis
      α_1-Antitrypsin deficiency
   F. Biliary obstruction
      Primary biliary cirrhosis
      Secondary ("mechanical") biliary obstruction
         Primary sclerosing cholangitis
         Neoplasm of bile ducts or pancreas
         Iatrogenic or inflammatory biliary stricture
      Cystic fibrosis
      Congenital biliary cysts
   G. Idiopathic/miscellaneous
      Non-alcoholic steatonecrosis (including jejunoileal bypass, obesity)
      Granulomatous liver disease
      Polycystic liver disease
III. Post-sinusoidal fibrosis
   A. Veno-occlusive disease

10

Primary Biliary Cirrhosis

The pathologic progression of primary biliary cirrhosis (PBC) is divided into four successive stages: florid duct lesion, ductular proliferation, fibrosis, and cirrhosis. The antigens against which antimitochondrial antibodies (AMAs) are directed are components of the E2 subunits of the 2-oxoacid dehydrogenase enzyme family (M2 antigen).

The disease typically occurs in middle-aged females, either as an incidental threefold to fourfold elevation of alkaline phosphatase or in evaluating complaints of fatigue and pruritus. Mild (twofold to threefold) elevation of aminotransferase levels is common. Identifying AMAs in serum usually leads to liver biopsy, which establishes the diagnosis. In addition to AMAs, characteristic laboratory abnormalities include increased serum IgM (95%), hypercholesterolemia, and other autoantibodies, including rheumatoid factor (70%), anti-SMAs (65%), and thyroid-specific or antinuclear antibodies.

PBC is a slowly progressive disease usually leading to liver failure over 5 to 10 years. A serum bilirubin value of more than 10 mg/dL by itself is a remarkably accurate indicator of impending liver failure.

Ursodeoxycholic acid (UDCA 8 to 10 mg/kg/day), a hydrophilic bile acid, has shown variable success in slowing the progression of PBC, possibly by reducing the concentration of toxic bile acids in the hepatic pool. Management should include correcting vitamin A, D, E, and K deficiencies and using antipruritics, including cholestyramine 16 to 32 g/day. Liver transplantation offers excellent quality of life in most patients with end-stage disease.

Secondary Biliary Cirrhosis

Secondary biliary cirrhosis occurs in response to chronic biliary obstruction from a variety of causes. *Primary sclerosing cholangitis* is the most common cause of intrahepatic cholestasis besides PBC. *Extrahepatic cholestasis* in adults most commonly results from structural or mechanical obstruction: choledocholithiasis, biliary or pancreatic cancer, iatrogenic stricture, or chronic pancreatitis. Disproportionately increased hepatic alkaline phosphatase (fourfold to fivefold increase) relative to other liver tests is typical of secondary biliary cirrhosis.

Recognizing and treating the underlying cause of cholestasis is the mainstay of therapy. Pruritus usually can be controlled with cholestyramine 16 to 32 g/day in two divided doses. Calcium and vitamin D supplementation may be required for bone disease.

Vascular Disorders Associated with Cirrhosis

Hepatic veno-occlusive disease occurs commonly as a complication of bone marrow transplantation and is characterized clinically by rapid onset of hepatomegaly, weight gain, and ascites. Hyperbilirubinemia and increased aminotransferases are typical. *Budd-Chiari syndrome,* like veno-occlusive disease, is not a true cirrhosis but rather an acute or subacute obstruction to hepatic venous outflow.

Miscellaneous Disorders Associated with Cirrhosis

Non-alcoholic steatonecrosis is a clinicopathologic syndrome remarkably similar to alcoholic liver disease, but it occurs in the absence of alcohol use. It is associated with diabetes mellitus, morbid obesity, and jejunoileal bypass surgery. Cirrhosis develops in at least one third of patients if the precipitant is not removed.

Major Sequelae of Cirrhosis

PORTAL HYPERTENSION. Portal hypertension should be suspected in any patient with ascites, splenomegaly, encephalopathy, or gastroesophageal varices (Table 10–9). Non-invasive abdominal imaging using US with Doppler probe can assess the hepatic parenchyma and the patency and flow characteristics of the portal and hepatic veins. If abdominal US with Doppler is not conclusive,

Table 10–9 ■ SEQUELAE OF CIRRHOSIS

1. Portal hypertension: bleeding from varices in esophagus/stomach (most common), duodenum, rectum, or surgical stomas; bleeding from congestive gastropathy; splenomegaly with hypersplenism
2. Ascites; spontaneous bacterial peritonitis; hepatic hydrothorax; abdominal hernia
3. Hepatorenal syndrome
4. Hepatic encephalopathy
5. Synthetic dysfunction/coagulopathy
6. Hepatopulmonary syndrome
7. Hepatocellular carcinoma
8. Feminization
9. Altered drug metabolism
10. Hepatic osteodystrophy

portal hemodynamics may be measured more directly by hepatic vein catheterization.

Hemorrhage from gastroesophageal varices is often the initial complication of portal hypertension, but 30 to 50% of bleeding episodes in patients with varices originate from non-variceal sources. Two endoscopic methods are equally effective in arresting active hemorrhage in more than 95% of patients: (1) direct or paravariceal injection with 1 to 2 mL of a sclerosant, and (2) band ligation. Pharmacologic control of acute hemorrhage may be achieved using either a combination of intravenous (IV) vasopressin 0.2 to 0.4 U/minute and nitroglycerin 5 μg/minute increased by 20 μg/minute to a maximum of 200 μg/minute, or octreotide 50 μg bolus, then 50 μg/hour, though not yet approved by the Food and Drug Administration (FDA) for this indication.

In patients who continue to bleed after endoscopic or pharmacologic therapy, a Minnesota or Sengstaken-Blakemore tube can be used for balloon tamponade. Emergent surgical portal decompression is an option in the rare patient in whom hemodynamic stabilization is not possible because of persistent hemorrhage. In a patient who is a potential candidate for liver transplantation, placing a transjugular intrahepatic portosystemic shunt (TIPS) is an attractive alternative to surgery. In the patient with moderate or large varices and well-preserved liver function, prophylactic use of β-blockers (propranolol or nadolol) to reduce the resting heart rate by 25% will lessen the risk of first variceal hemorrhage. In those in whom β-blockers fail or who are intolerant of β-blockers, obliterating varices by endoscopic sclerotherapy is equally effective. Elective portacaval shunt surgery is more effective at eliminating rebleeding than long-term sclerotherapy but is associated with higher initial transfusion requirement and cost.

ASCITES. Cirrhosis is the underlying cause in at least 80% of cases of ascites. All patients with new-onset ascites or those requiring hospitalization because of ascites should undergo diagnostic paracentesis (Table 10–10).

Most patients with cirrhotic ascites respond to dietary sodium restriction (40 to 60 mEq/day). Spironolactone should be started at 50 to 100 mg/day and can be advanced up to 400 mg to achieve a daily weight loss of 0.5 to 0.75 kg in patients without peripheral edema; more rapid weight loss is safe if peripheral edema is

Table 10–10 ■ DIAGNOSTIC EVALUATION OF ASCITES

Paracentesis

1. Fluid analysis: cell count, albumin, Gram stain
2. Calculate serum-ascites albumin gradient (SAAG):
   SAAG $\geq$ 1.1 g/dL: portal hypertension very likely
   SAAG $<$ 1.1 g/dL: suspect other causes
3. Direct bedside inoculation of ascites into blood culture broth
4. Optional: amylase, bilirubin, triglycerides, cytology, mycobacterial culture

Abdominal Ultrasonography with Doppler

1. Assess patency/flow in portal, hepatic, and splenic veins
2. Examine hepatic and splenic parenchyma
3. Exclude neoplasm or peritoneal disease
4. Assess biliary ductal size

present. Furosemide can be used instead of or in combination with spironolactone, beginning at a dose of 40 mg/day.

Ten per cent of patients with ascites fail to respond to standard therapy. In these patients, therapeutic paracentesis is safe and can remove 4 to 6 L or more per visit in those with peripheral edema. In non-edematous patients, safe paracentesis requires infusing 6 to 8 g of albumin per liter of ascites removed.

HEPATORENAL SYNDROME. Hepatorenal syndrome is renal failure associated with severe liver disease without an intrinsic abnormality of the kidney. The diagnosis is established in patients with cirrhosis by documenting very low urine sodium (<10 mEq/L) and oliguria in the absence of intravascular volume depletion. The most effective treatment is to correct the underlying liver disease, often by liver transplantation.

For more information about this subject, see *Cecil Textbook of Medicine,* 21st edition. Philadelphia, W.B. Saunders Company, 2000. Chapter 153, Alcoholic Liver Disease, Cirrhosis, and Its Major Sequelae, pages 804 to 812.

ACUTE AND CHRONIC LIVER FAILURE, HEPATIC ENCEPHALOPATHY, AND LIVER TRANSPLANTATION

Hepatic Encephalopathy

The impairment of the central nervous system in hepatic encephalopathy is probably multifactorial. The severity of neurologic dysfunction is variable and can be graded symptomatically (Table 10–11).

Acute encephalopathy is usually precipitated by identifiable factors, including gastrointestinal bleeding, excessive protein intake, hypokalemia, azotemia, infection, sedatives, hepatic insult (alcohol, drugs, viral hepatitis), or hepatocellular carcinoma. Hepatic encephalopathy is a diagnosis of exclusion. Concomitant problems such as intracranial lesions, infections, metabolic encephalopathies, alcohol intoxication or withdrawal, drug toxicity, postictal encephalopathy, and primary neuropsychiatric disorders must be excluded.

Lactulose, the mainstay of treatment, can be given orally, through a nasogastric tube, or rectally (less effective) in doses of

Table 10–11 ■ CLINICAL STAGING OF HEPATIC ENCEPHALOPATHY

STAGE	CONSCIOUSNESS	COGNITION	BEHAVIOR	MOTOR FUNCTION
1	Abnormal sleep	Decreased attention and calculation ability	Mood change, anxious, irritable, monotone voice	Dyscoordinated handwriting, tremor
2	Lethargy, ataxia, dysarthria	Memory decreased, disoriented to time	Dysinhibition, inappropriate	Asterixis, ataxia, dysarthria, yawning, sucking, blinking, expressionless
3	Confusion, delirium, semistupor, incontinence	Disoriented, incoherent, amnesia, rigidity	Bizarre, anger, paranoia, seizures	Abnormal reflexes, nystagmus, Babinski's reflex
4	Coma	None	Absent	Oculocephalic or oculovestibular response, decorticate or decerebrate posture, dilated pupils

30 to 120 mL/day. Neomycin (initially 1 to 2 g orally four times a day) can be used for short periods of time, and the dose should be decreased to 1 to 2 g/day after achievement of the desired clinical effect. Alternatively, metronidazole can be given at 250 mg orally three times a day alone or with neomycin. Ideally, the diet should contain at least 1.2 g/kg/day of protein, and higher total caloric intake may improve the tolerance to protein. However, restriction of protein to 70 g/day may be necessary.

Acute Liver Failure

In the United States, the most common causes of acute liver failure are HBV; non-A, non-B, non-C viral hepatitis; and exposure to certain drugs and toxins. Acetaminophen ingestion is responsible for 10% of acute liver failure cases in the United States. Massive liver cell necrosis from other drugs such as isoniazid, halogenated anesthetics, phenytoin, propylthiouracil, and sulfonamides accounts for another 10%. A well-recognized cause of acute liver failure is ingestion of poisonous mushrooms *(Amanita phalloides)*.

Clinical features of acute liver failure may result directly from the loss of functioning hepatocytes (jaundice, coagulopathy, hypoglycemia, metabolic acidosis) or from multiple systemic manifestations. Cerebral edema complicates stages 3 and 4 of hepatic encephalopathy in 50 to 85% of patients with acute liver failure.

Mannitol at a dose of 1 g/kg may decrease intracranial pressure (ICP) in selected patients with acute liver failure. In the absence of ICP monitoring, mannitol should be considered only in patients with progressive cerebral edema. Some authors advocate barbiturates (thiopentone 3 to 5 mg/kg IV infusion over 15 minutes). Prevention of hypoglycemia may require a continuous infusion of 5% or 10% glucose. Orthotopic liver transplantation offers a definitive treatment.

Chronic Liver Failure

The most common causes of end-stage liver disease include alcohol abuse, viral hepatitis (B, C, D), primary biliary cirrhosis, primary sclerosing cholangitis, hemochromatosis, α_1-antitrypsin deficiency, Wilson's disease, Budd-Chiari syndrome, schistosomiasis, drugs and toxins, steatohepatitis, and cryptogenic liver cirrhosis.

The Child-Pugh classification, which was developed to assess the severity of chronic liver failure, is based on five equally weighted clinical and laboratory parameters (encephalopathy, ascites, serum albumin, serum bilirubin, nutritional status) with a maximum score of 15 (Table 10–12). Patients with compensated chronic liver failure are Child-Pugh A (score 1 to 5), whereas those with advanced cirrhosis are Child-Pugh C (score 11 to 15).

Treatment includes identification and correction of potentially reversible factors such as sepsis, gastrointestinal bleeding, heavy loads of dietary protein, and unnecessary medications. Orthotopic liver transplantation should be considered.

Liver Transplantation

Early referral for transplantation is extremely important for patients with fulminant liver failure, including stage III or IV enceph-

Table 10–12 ■ CHILD-PUGH CLASSIFICATION OF LIVER CIRRHOSIS

PARAMETER/CLASS	A	B	C
Encephalopathy	Absent	Mild	Severe
Ascites	Absent	Moderate, easily treated	Severe, refractory to treatment
Serum albumin	>3.5	3.0–3.5	<3.0
Total bilirubin	<2.0	2.0–3.0	>3.0
Nutritional status	Good	Mild malnutrition	Severe malnutrition

alopathy developing less than 8 weeks after the onset of signs or symptoms without known pre-existing liver disease. Transplantation is performed for a wide variety of causes of chronic liver failure, with hepatitis C now the most common indication. Complications of liver transplantation are primarily vascular (e.g., thrombosis of the anastomosed hepatic artery or portal vein), biliary (relating to reconstruction of the biliary tract), infectious, or related to organ rejection. 10

For more information about this subject, see *Cecil Textbook of Medicine,* 21st edition. Philadelphia, W.B. Saunders Company, 2000. Chapter 154, Acute and Chronic Liver Failure and Hepatic Encephalopathy; and Chapter 155, Liver Transplantation, pages 813 to 819.

DISEASES OF THE GALLBLADDER AND BILE DUCTS

Disorders Associated with Cholestasis

INTRAHEPATIC CAUSES OF CHOLESTASIS. Small duct obliterative disorders, often collectively termed *vanishing bile duct syndromes,* include infiltrative neoplasms (discussed later); granulomatous disorders such as sarcoidosis; and the immune-mediated bile duct destruction of PBC, hepatic allograft rejection, and chronic graft-versus-host disease. Cholestasis of metabolic origin may be seen commonly in severely ill patients and is associated with trauma, surgery, sepsis, and parenteral hyperalimentation. Numerous drugs also can produce cholestasis.

DISEASES OF THE LARGE BILE DUCTS AND GALLBLADDER. Primary malignancies of the liver, bile ducts, gallbladder, ampulla of Vater, and pancreas typically present with jaundice caused by bile duct obstruction. Rare benign neoplasms that may obstruct the common bile duct distally include pancreatic cystadenoma and villous adenoma of the ampulla of Vater. Metastatic tumor from any source to lymph nodes in the porta hepatis can also cause extrinsic compression of the proximal common bile duct; this complication is a common cause of cholestasis in patients with cancers of the breast, lung, colon, or stomach. Extensive tumor metastases within the liver parenchyma may produce intrahepatic cholestasis by obstructing smaller intrahepatic ducts.

Cholangiocarcinoma arises from the intrahepatic or extrahepatic biliary epithelium. Cholangiocarcinomas tend to grow slowly and to infiltrate the wall of the duct and dissect along tissue planes.

The most useful imaging study is cholangiography, which typically demonstrates segmental narrowing or obstruction. Only one third of cholangiocarcinomas are resectable for cure at the time of presentation.

Gallbladder adenocarcinoma is an uncommon malignancy. There is a strong association of gallstones with carcinoma of the gallbladder (80 to 90% of carcinomatous gallbladders have stones). Gallbladder cancer is especially associated with very large gallstones (>3 cm in diameter) or calcification of the chronically inflamed gallbladder wall (porcelain gallbladder). However, because the incidence of adenocarcinoma of the gallbladder in patients with cholelithiasis is less than 1 per 1000 patient-years, the prevention of gallbladder cancer currently is not considered a sufficient indication for cholecystectomy in most patients with asymptomatic gallstones. Early symptoms of gallbladder cancer are non-specific and similar to those of cholelithiasis or cholecystitis; later, patients develop persistent pain and unremitting jaundice. New onset of cholestasis over days to weeks in any adult, especially older than age 50 years, is worrisome for cancer. US is generally the first imaging procedure in a cholestatic patient, but it may be preferable to go directly to CT or MRI if the clinical picture is strongly suggestive of cancer. When obstructing malignancy is not resectable for cure, relief of cholestasis by placement of internal stents without surgery is possible in most patients.

Choledochal cysts are congenital anatomic malformations of the bile duct. The triad of abdominal pain, jaundice, and a palpable mass is the classic presentation. The best method to establish diagnosis is endoscopic retrograde cholangiopancreatography (ERCP). Therapy is surgical.

Benign biliary strictures, which are fibrotic narrowings of the large bile ducts, occur as a result of trauma, inflammation, infection, or ischemia. *Chronic pancreatitis* commonly produces fibrotic narrowing of the common bile duct where it passes through the head of the pancreas.

Primary sclerosing cholangitis (PSC) is a disorder characterized by a patchy obliterative inflammatory fibrosis of the large bile ducts. Chronic inflammation leads to extensive bile duct strictures, cholestasis, and gradual progression to biliary cirrhosis. About 50% of cases occur in association with inflammatory bowel disease. Unlike other extraintestinal manifestations of ulcerative colitis, PSC shows little correlation with the severity of bowel inflammation and does not remit after colectomy. Patients with PSC typically present with insidious onset of chronic cholestasis, including jaundice, pruritus, fatigue, and malaise. There is no specific therapy, and PSC is a common indication for liver transplantation.

Cholangiopathy from AIDS describes a number of biliary tract abnormalities: cholecystitis, focal distal biliary stenosis at the ampulla of Vater, or multifocal stenosis of the biliary tree resembling PSC. AIDS cholangiopathy is strongly associated with colonization of bile with cryptosporidia or microsporidia. *Liver flukes* mature in the biliary tree, where they may cause ductal fibrosis and strictures.

Gallstones

Gallstone formation begins when bile becomes supersaturated with cholesterol or calcium. Black pigment gallstones are hard, dense, brittle concretions composed of calcium bilirubinate along with inorganic calcium salts of carbonate and phosphate. Brown pigment (earthy) gallstones have a soft, claylike consistency. In addition to calcium bilirubin, they contain a substantial proportion of calcium soaps of fatty acids.

Gallstone disease can be divided conceptually into four stages (Table 10–13). *Biliary colic* is thought to result from increased wall tension in the gallbladder and/or bile ducts due to impaction of a stone in the cystic duct or distal common bile duct. It is characterized by continuous severe pain in the epigastrium or right upper quadrant, sometimes radiating to the back or scapula, and typically lasting for more than 30 minutes. Biliary colic is frequently associated with nausea and vomiting. Transient elevation of bilirubin, alkaline phosphatase, AST, and ALT levels is sometimes noted. Attacks of *acute pancreatitis* may be triggered by passage of a gallstone through the ampulla of Vater.

Acute cholecystitis (inflammation of the gallbladder) typically presents as acute onset of constant, dull, right upper quadrant pain, fever, shaking chills, nausea, and vomiting. A characteristic physical finding is *Murphy's sign,* defined as tenderness of the gallbladder to palpation during examination of the abdomen. Patients with cholecystitis develop leukocytosis with a marked shift to the left, but bilirubin and alkaline phosphatase levels are usually not elevated. In most cases, the cholecystitis develops as a result of impaction of a stone in the neck of the gallbladder. In about 10% of cases, however, no gallstones are present; such *acalculous cholecystitis* may result from impaction of mucus or sludge, from ischemia in vasculitic disorders, or from direct infection of the gallbladder bile.

Some cases are sterile, but in the majority bacteria can be cultured from the gallbladder. The usual organisms present are *E. coli* and other enteric gram-negative bacteria. Antibiotic therapy will usually treat the infection and allow for elective surgery. However, acute cholecystitis should be considered a surgical disease requiring a surgical cure as promptly as it can be done safely.

Patients with long-standing gallstone disease frequently develop *chronic cholecystitis.* Other patients note vague, poorly defined,

Table 10–13 ■ STAGES OF GALLSTONE DISEASE

Lithogenic bile (stage 1)
↓
Asymptomatic gallstones (stage 2)
↓
Symptomatic gallstones (stage 3)
↓
Severe complications of gallstones (stage 4)

Acute:
- Acute cholecystitis (localized peritonitis, perforation, abscess, sepsis)
- Choledocholithiasis (obstructive jaundice, acute pancreatitis, ascending cholangitis)

Chronic:
- Chronic cholecystitis
- Choledochoduodenal fistula with gallstone ileus
- Gallbladder adenocarcinoma

non-specific intermittent epigastric discomfort, but many are asymptomatic.

Bacterial infection above an obstructing stone in the common bile duct is common and leads to *ascending cholangitis*. Patients with ascending cholangitis typically present with acute onset of high fever and signs of sepsis, right upper quadrant pain and tenderness, and jaundice. Leukocytosis with a shift to the left, conjugated hyperbilirubinemia, abnormally high alkaline phosphatase, and elevated aminotransferase levels are common. The usual pathogens observed in ascending cholangitis are enteric gram-negative bacteria, anaerobes, or occasionally enterococci. Antibiotics are indicated. Symptoms usually respond rapidly to biliary drainage through surgical, radiographic, or endoscopic means.

DIAGNOSTIC STUDIES IN GALLSTONE DISEASE. US is a sensitive, specific, non-invasive, and inexpensive test for diagnosis of gallstones. In general, US is the only diagnostic procedure needed to make the diagnosis of gallstones in the gallbladder, but it usually will not detect stones in the common bile duct.

Hepatobiliary radionuclide scans employ a variety of iminodiacetic acid (IDA) derivatives. Failure of these isotopes to enter the gallbladder or the intestine suggests obstruction of the cystic or common bile ducts, respectively.

Contrast material may be injected directly into the biliary tree through either a percutaneous, fluoroscopically guided approach (percutaneous transhepatic cholangiography, PTC) or a retrograde approach (ERCP). These tests represent the gold standard for examination of the biliary tree and generally will reveal stones or stenosis that are not detectable by other means.

THERAPY FOR GALLSTONES. No treatment is usually required for asymptomatic gallstones because of their low propensity to become symptomatic. Symptomatic gallstones are cured by cholecystectomy. Laparoscopic cholecystectomy is now preferred.

Gallstones in the common bile duct may be removed by the surgeon at the time of cholecystectomy. More recently, development of methods for direct choledochoscopy and stone extraction during surgery have reduced the need for common duct exploration. Alternatively, stones up to 1.5 cm in diameter can be extracted from the common bile duct by endoscopic methods after endoscopic sphincterotomy. Ascending cholangitis is treated aggressively with antibiotics and endoscopic sphincterotomy.

In addition to surgical therapy, cholesterol gallstones may be treated medically. Because oral dissolution therapy is slow and often not successful, it generally is reserved for patients with mildly symptomatic gallstones who are at very high risk for surgery.

For more information about this subject, see *Cecil Textbook of Medicine,* 21st edition. Philadelphia, W.B. Saunders Company, 2000. Chapter 157, Diseases of the Gallbladder and Bile Ducts, pages 821 to 833.

CHAPTER 11

HEMATOLOGIC DISEASES

APPROACH TO THE ANEMIAS

Impaired Production by the Bone Marrow

The bone marrow may produce inadequate erythrocytes because of erythropoietin deficiency, intrinsic bone marrow failure, or problems with erythrocyte development (Table 11–1).

Accelerated Destruction, Consumption, or Loss of Circulating Erythrocytes

In a patient with a normal bone marrow, accelerated loss of circulating erythrocytes always will be associated with increased erythropoiesis, which can be judged by the presence of an increased reticulocyte count. Anemia occurs only if the rate of production of erythrocytes by the bone marrow is unable to compensate completely for the loss or destruction of red blood cells (RBCs).

Abnormalities of RBC membrane proteins and lipids lead to deformed erythrocytes, which are prone to be removed prematurely from the circulation, primarily by the filtering functions of the spleen. Defects in enzymes in the hexose monophosphate shunt or those responsible for maintaining reduced glutathione to prevent oxidative injury to RBCs tend most frequently to be associated with episodic hemolysis during times of physiologic stresses, such as surgery, infections, or oxidants in foods or pharmacologic agents. More than 100 different structural variants of hemoglobin exhibit either reduced solubility or a higher susceptibility than normal to oxidation of amino acids within the globin chains.

In autoimmune hemolytic anemia, antibodies form against RBC membrane antigens. These antibody-coated erythrocytes are recognized by Fc or complement receptors on macrophages in the spleen (especially IgG) or liver (especially C3 complement). IgG-coated RBCs usually undergo repeated partial phagocytosis with progressive loss of their membrane until the cells that survive and re-enter the circulation are spherocytes, which have decreased deformability and eventually are sequestered and removed permanently from the circulation.

Although acute blood loss can result in anemia, it may be much more difficult to document slow, chronic blood loss, in which case the bone marrow almost always is able to compensate until the patient becomes iron-deficient.

The major factors that determine the specific response of the

For more information about this subject, see *Cecil Textbook of Medicine,* 21st edition. Philadelphia, W.B. Saunders Company, 2000. Part XIII: Hematologic Diseases, pages 834 to 1028.

Table 11–1 ■ PATHOPHYSIOLOGIC CLASSIFICATION OF ANEMIAS DUE TO IMPAIRED PRODUCTION OF ERYTHROCYTES BY THE BONE MARROW

Erythropoietin (EPO) deficiency (normocytic anemias)
- Renal insufficiency (worse after bilateral nephrectomy)
- Pure RBC aplasia due to anti-EPO antibodies (extremely rare)
- Anemia of chronic disease (inappropriately low EPO level is a partial contributing factor)

Quantitative deficiency of hematopoietic/erythroid progenitor cells (normocytic anemias)
- Idiopathic bone marrow aplasia/hypoplasia
- Secondary bone marrow aplasia/hypoplasia (drugs, toxins, infections, radiation, malnutrition)
- Myelofibrosis (primary or secondary)
- Bone marrow replacement by neoplastic cells (myelophthisis)
- Myelodysplasia (minority of myelodysplasia patients)
- PNH (10–15% of PNH patients)
- Pure RBC aplasia (antierythroid precursor cell antibodies, parvovirus B19 infection)

Impaired erythroid precursor cell division and DNA synthesis (macrocytic/megaloblastic anemias)
- Cobalamin (vitamin B_{12}) deficiency
- Folate deficiency
- Myelodysplasia
- Cancer chemotherapeutic drugs and some immunosuppressive and antimicrobial drugs

Impaired heme synthesis in differentiating erythroid cells (microcytic anemias)
- Iron deficiency
- Anemia of chronic disease/inflammation
- Sideroblastic anemias (particularly hereditary forms)

Impaired globin synthesis in differentiating erythroid cells (microcytic anemias)
- Thalassemias

RBC = red blood cell; PNH = paroxysmal nocturnal hemoglobinuria.

individual to anemia include the severity of anemia, rapidity of onset of anemia, age of the patient, his or her overall physical condition, and co-morbid events or disorders. Mild anemia often is associated with no clinical symptoms and may be discovered only when a complete blood cell count is done for another reason. The earliest clinical symptoms of mild to modest anemia tend to be fatigue, generalized weakness, and loss of stamina, followed by tachycardia and exertional dyspnea.

Weakness, fatigue, lethargy, decreased stamina, palpitations, dyspnea on exertion, and orthostatic lightheadedness are common symptoms in patients with chronic anemia. Co-morbid conditions, particularly with impaired blood supply or oxygenation of specific organs, may result in symptoms and signs resulting from organ-specific dysfunction. Splenomegaly raises the possibility of a chronic hemolytic anemia.

In a patient with acute severe hemolysis or blood loss, prominent early symptoms include resting or orthostatic hypotension due to a decrease in total blood volume, with subsequent lightheadedness or syncope; exertional, orthostatic, and/or resting tachycardia and palpitations; diaphoresis; anxiety; agitation; generalized severe weakness and lethargy; and possibly decreased mental function. Loss of 25 to 35% of the total blood volume in 12 to 24 hours cannot be ameliorated by the normal compensatory mechanisms, and loss of more than 40% of blood volume in 12 hours leads to profound symptoms due more to intravascular volume depletion than to anemia.

The initial diagnostic evaluation (Fig. 11–1) of anemia is based on readily available information, including a careful in-depth evaluation of the patient's past medical history and family history, physical examination (especially the presence or absence of splenomegaly), complete blood cell count, reticulocyte count, and microscopic evaluation of the peripheral blood smear (Table 11–2).

For more information about this subject, see *Cecil Textbook of Medicine,* 21st edition. Philadelphia, W.B. Saunders Company, 2000. Chapter 159, Approach to the Anemias, pages 840 to 847.

APLASTIC ANEMIA AND RELATED BONE MARROW FAILURE SYNDROMES

Aplastic anemia is a disease of the young, with a median age at onset of about 25 years (excluding aplasia secondary to cancer chemotherapy). The commonly accepted definition of severe disease is two of the following: (1) absolute neutrophil count (percentage of polymorphonuclear and band forms multiplied by the total white blood cell [WBC] count) of less than $500/mm^3$; (2) a platelet count less than $20{,}000/mm^3$; and (3) anemia with a reticulocyte count (corrected for hematocrit) less than 1% (or an absolute reticulocyte count $<40{,}000/mm^3$).

Most community-acquired aplastic anemia is caused by immune system attack on the bone marrow and resulting destruction of hematopoietic stem and progenitor cells (Table 11–3). *Pure RBC aplasia* without abnormalities of platelets or WBCs results from diverse causes (Table 11–4).

Bleeding is the most common early symptom of aplastic anemia. Patients commonly report days to weeks of easy bruising. In cases of more gradual onset, symptoms of anemia are described: usually lassitude, weakness, shortness of breath, and a pounding sensation in the ears. Petechiae and ecchymoses are frequently present, and there may be retinal hemorrhages. The diagnosis of aplastic anemia is usually straightforward, based on the combination of pancytopenia with fatty, empty bone marrow.

TREATMENT. Bone marrow transplantation offers the best therapy for a young patient with a fully histocompatible sibling donor. Early consideration of transplantation in a child or adolescent can avoid unnecessary transfusions. Transfusions increase the risk of graft rejection. Marrow transplantation is usually not recommended for patients who are older than 45 to 50 years.

Antithymocyte globulin (ATG) therapy leads to recovery of autologous bone marrow function in about 50% of patients. When therapy with ATG fails, about 50% of patients will respond to cyclosporine. The combination of ATG and cyclosporine, which is

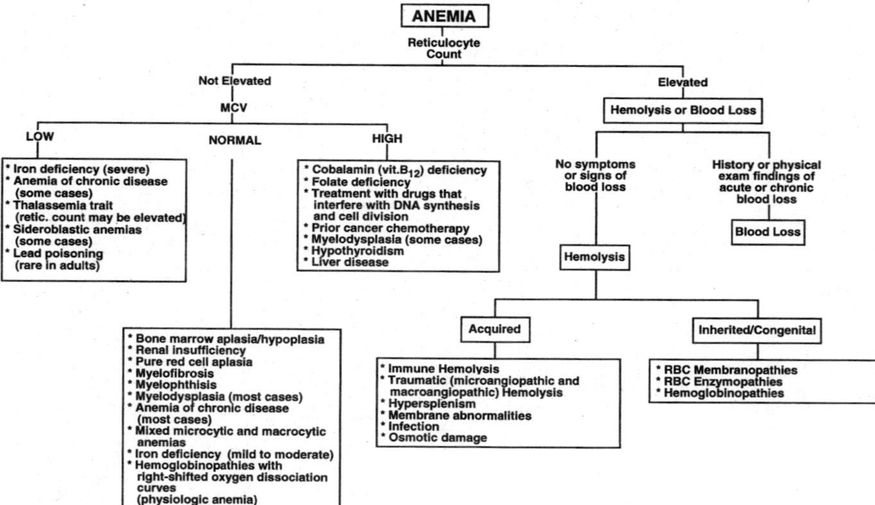

FIGURE 11–1 ■ Algorithm for diagnosis of anemias. MCV = mean corpuscular volume.

Table 11–2 ■ RED BLOOD CELL (RBC) MORPHOLOGIC ABNORMALITIES AS CLUES TO THE DIAGNOSIS OF ANEMIAS

RBC MORPHOLOGY	REPRESENTATIVE CAUSES OF ANEMIA
Microcytosis	Iron deficiency, anemia of chronic disease, thalassemia, and (rarely) lead poisoning, vitamin B_6 deficiency, or hereditary sideroblastic anemias
Macrocytosis	Polychromatophilia (reticulocytes), vitamin B_{12} (cobalamin) or folate deficiency, myelodysplasia, use of drugs that inhibit DNA synthesis
Basophilic stippling	Hemolysis, lead poisoning, thalassemia
Target cells	Thalassemia, hemoglobins C, D, E, and S, liver disease, abetalipoproteinemia
Microspherocytes	Autoimmune hemolytic anemia, alloimmune hemolysis, hereditary spherocytosis, some cases of Heinz body hemolytic anemias
Schistocytes and fragmented RBCs	Thrombotic thrombocytopenic purpura, disseminated intravascular coagulation, vasculitis, malignant hypertension, eclampsia, traumatic hemolysis due to prosthetic heart valve or damaged vascular graft, thermal injury (burns), postsplenectomy
Teardrop cells	Myelofibrosis, myelophthisis (bone marrow infiltration by neoplastic cells)
Sickle cells	Hemoglobin SS, SC, or S–β-thalassemia
Acanthocytes (spur cells)	Severe liver disease, malnutrition, McLeod blood group phenotype
Echinocytes (burr cells)	Renal failure, hemolysis due to malnutrition with hypomagnesemia and hypophosphatemia, pyruvate kinase deficiency, common in vitro artifact
Stomatocytes	Alcoholism, hereditary stomatocytosis
"Bite" cells or "blister" cells	Glucose-6-phosphate dehydrogenase deficiency, other oxidant-induced hemolysis, unstable hemoglobins
Howell-Jolly bodies	Postsplenectomy, hyposplenism
Intraerythrocytic parasitic or bacterial inclusions	Malaria (parasites), babesiosis (parasites), bartonellosis (gram-negative coccobacilli)
Agglutinated RBCs	Cold agglutinin disease, in vitro artifact
Rouleaux formation	Multiple myeloma, monoclonal gammopathy of undetermined significance

Table 11–3 ■ CLASSIFICATION OF APLASTIC ANEMIA AND SINGLE CYTOPENIAS

APLASTIC ANEMIA	CYTOPENIAS
Acquired	**Acquired**
Radiation	*Anemias*
Drugs and chemicals	Pure red blood cell aplasia (see Table 11–4)
Regular effects	Transient erythroblastopenia of childhood
Idiosyncratic reactions	*Neutropenias*
Viruses	Idiopathic
Epstein-Barr virus (infectious mononucleosis)	Drugs, toxins
Hepatitis (non-A, non-B, non-C hepatitis)	*Thrombocytopenias*
Human immunodeficiency virus (AIDS)	Drugs, toxins
Immune diseases	**Inherited**
Eosinophilic fasciitis	*Anemias*
Hypoimmunoglobulinemia	Congenital pure red blood cell aplasia
Thymoma and thymic carcinoma	*Neutropenias*
Graft-versus-host disease in immunodeficiency	Kostmann's syndrome
Paroxysmal nocturnal hemoglobinuria	Schwachman-Diamond syndrome
Pregnancy	Reticular dysgenesis
Idiopathic—the most frequent diagnosis	*Thombocytopenias*
Inherited	Thrombocytopenia with absence of radii
Fanconi's anemia	Idiopathic amegakaryocytic thrombocytopenia
Dyskeratosis congenita	
Schwachman-Diamond syndrome	
Reticular dysgenesis	
Amegakaryocytic thrombocytopenia	
Familial aplastic anemias	
Preleukemia (e.g., monosomy 7)	
Non-hematologic syndromes (Down, Dubovitz's, Seckel's)	

superior to ATG alone, produces hematologic responses in about 70% of cases.

Meticulous medical care is required so that the patient can survive to benefit from definitive therapy or, having experienced treatment failure, can maintain a reasonable quality of life in the presence of pancytopenia. Platelet and erythrocyte levels can be maintained by transfusion. Single-donor platelets from which leukocytes have been removed by filtration are the best product. RBCs should be transfused to allow a normal level of activity, usually to a hemoglobin value of 7.0 g/dL (9.0 g/dL if there is underlying cardiac or pulmonary disease).

For more information about this subject, see *Cecil Textbook of Medicine,* 21st edition. Philadelphia, W.B. Saunders Company, 2000. Chapter 160, Aplastic Anemia and Related Bone Marrow Failure Syndromes, pages 848 to 853.

Table 11–4 ■ CLASSIFICATION OF PURE RED BLOOD CELL APLASIA

Self-Limited
Transient erythroblastopenia of childhood
Transient aplastic crisis of hemolysis (parvovirus B19 infection)
Fetal Red Blood Cell Aplasia
Non-immune hydrops fetalis (in utero parvovirus infection)
Hereditary Pure Red Blood Cell Aplasia
Congenital pure red blood cell aplasia (Diamond-Blackfan syndrome)
Acquired Pure Red Blood Cell Aplasia
Thymoma and malignancy: thymoma, lymphoid malignancies (and more rarely other hematologic diseases), paraneoplastic to solid tumors
Connective tissue disorders with immunologic abnormalities: systemic lupus erythematosus, juvenile rheumatoid arthritis, rheumatoid arthritis, multiple endocrine gland insufficiency
Virus: especially persistent parvovirus B19; more rarely hepatitis, adult T-cell leukemia virus, Epstein-Barr virus
Pregnancy
Drugs: especially phenytoin, azathioprine, chloramphenicol, procainamide, isoniazid
Idiopathic

11

NORMOCHROMIC, NORMOCYTIC ANEMIAS

Under normal conditions, the marrow compensates for the 1.0 to 1.5% of the RBC mass that is lost each day. Anemia with small, or microcytic, RBCs (mean corpuscular volume [MCV] <80 fL) is most commonly due to iron deficiency or to thalassemia. Anemia with large, or macrocytic, cells (MCV >95 fL) is usually due to abnormalities in nucleic acid metabolism, with vitamin B_{12} or folate deficiency most commonly responsible. Anemias with RBCs of normocytic size (MCV 80 to 95 fL) have numerous causes, including faulty production and infiltrative marrow disorders. Low erythropoietin (EPO) states also result in normocytic anemias. The early stages of most anemias are also normochromic, normocytic because of the continued presence of the original, normal RBC population manufactured before the new pathologic lesion appeared.

Both acute blood loss and hemolytic anemia are normochromic, normocytic anemias with high reticulocyte counts and are accompanied by leukocytosis and thrombocytosis. These responses represent cytokine stimulation of all cell lines within the marrow in response to the anemia.

The anemia of *chronic renal failure* is due to progressive absence of adequate EPO production. Anemia usually supervenes once the creatinine clearance falls below 35 to 45 mL/minute. Treatment is initiated with EPO doses of 150 U/kg three times weekly and reduced to 50 to 100 U/kg per dose once the desired response has been obtained.

The *anemia of liver disease* is caused by progressive lipoprotein abnormalities that result in the sequential transformation of normochromic, normocytic RBCs into macrocytes, target cells, echinocytes, and, at the final and most severe stage, acanthocytes. Acanthocytes, or spur cells, are converted into spherocytes by the spleen.

An anemia, usually normocytic but sometimes macrocytic, accompanies *hypothyroidism* because of physiologic responses to decreased metabolic needs. *Deficiencies of stem cells,* as occurs with aplastic and hypoplastic anemias, cause a normochromic, normocytic (sometimes slightly macrocytic) anemia that is usually part of a pancytopenia. Most patients with the *anemia of chronic disease* have normochromic, normocytic RBC indices.

For more information about this subject, see *Cecil Textbook of Medicine,* 21st edition. Philadelphia, W.B. Saunders Company, 2000. Chapter 583, Normochromic, Normocytic Anemias, pages 853 to 855.

MICROCYTIC AND HYPOCHROMIC ANEMIAS

Iron Deficiency Anemia

Iron deficiency is the most common cause of anemia throughout the world and one of the most common medical problems that confronts general physicians. The prevalence is much higher in women than in men because of the toll of menstruation and pregnancy on iron stores.

Storage pools of iron in the form of ferritin and hemosiderin are present within the liver, spleen, and bone marrow. These reserves are approximately 1000 mg in males and 500 mg in females. Only a tiny fraction of iron (1 mg) is lost each day via the pathway of sweating and epidermal shedding from the gut and urinary tract.

In normal health, the body must guard itself against iron overload by absorbing only one tenth of the iron available in the diet. To maintain iron balance within the body, the adult male needs to absorb only 1.0 to 1.5 mg of iron each day, whereas an adult female needs to absorb a larger amount (2 to 3 mg) because of the iron losses from menstruation.

Because the iron-calorie ratio of the normal U.S. diet is 6 mg iron for every 1000 calories, males usually have no shortage of dietary iron; the restricted diets of some women may not provide a comparable surfeit. Diet-related iron deficiency may be aggravated by gastric achlorhydria.

The most common cause of iron deficiency anemia in both men and women is blood loss; this loss most frequently has its source in gastrointestinal bleeding in the former and menstrual bleeding in the latter. Even in the absence of occult blood in the stool or a history of melena, it is still imperative to examine the gastrointestinal tract because of its frequent involvement when iron deficiency is present. Less common causes of excessive iron loss include urinary tract bleeding and renal filtration of hemoglobin released from the breakdown of RBCs. Gastrojejunostomies and sprue may both result in iron deficiency as a result of loss of the necessary mucosal surface and/or increased intestinal transit time.

Iron deficiency anemia is characterized by a degree of fatigue that may be disproportionate to the apparent severity of the anemia, apparently because of depletion of essential tissue-based iron-containing enzymes. A sore tongue (glossitis), atrophy of the lingual papillae, and erosions at the corners of the mouth (angular stomatitis) are oral manifestations of iron deficiency. Dysphagia, attributable to an esophageal web, occurs most frequently in elderly women.

The laboratory findings in full-blown iron deficiency anemia include a reduction in all three RBC parameters (MCV, hemoglobin, hemoglobin concentration). In contrast, early iron deficiency anemia has normochromic, normocytic indices because the iron-deficient population of RBCs constitutes only a small percentage of the RBC mass. Only when the hematocrit falls below 31 to 32% do the RBC indices become microcytic.

Serum iron and transferrin (total iron-binding capacity) levels help confirm the diagnosis of iron deficiency, with a low serum iron and an elevated transferrin level resulting in a transferrin saturation of less than 10 to 15%. A low iron level is not in itself diagnostic of iron deficiency because many other systemic insults can alter the serum level of iron. Ferritin levels also permit recognition of iron deficiency, with a reduction to less than 10 ng/mL in uncomplicated iron deficiency. Bone marrow iron stores remain the final arbiter when any uncertainty exists regarding the presence of iron deficiency.

For treatment, the most commonly administered preparation is ferrous sulfate tablets, 300 mg/day. About 2 months of daily iron therapy are required for the hemoglobin level to return to normal. Return of ferritin levels to normal documents that iron stores have been restocked.

The Thalassemias

Abnormalities in globin chain synthesis, the thalassemias (pages 350 to 353), are a prominent consideration when microcytic and hypochromic anemia occurs in the appropriate ethnic groups.

Anemia of Chronic Disease

Anemia of chronic disease is the most common anemia in hospitalized patients. The anemia is moderate in degree, with the hematocrit usually in the range of 28 to 32%. The morphology is normochromic, normocytic in 60 to 70% of such patients, with the remainder having a mild hypochromic, microcytic anemia. The anemia is mild and well tolerated unless it is superimposed on other conditions.

Iron studies reveal low serum iron and transferrin levels. Anemia of chronic disease is a sideropenic anemia in the face of reticuloendothelial iron overload. Serum ferritin levels and bone marrow iron stores are both increased in anemia of chronic disease.

Confusion occurs with iron deficiency anemia because microcytic anemia occurs in 30 to 40% of cases and transferrin saturation may be reduced to levels seen in iron deficiency. Anemia of chronic disease is characterized by an elevation in ferritin levels, usually greater than 100 ng/mL. Bone marrow iron stores also distinguish the two because of the presence of marrow iron in anemia of chronic disease. EPO or transfusions can reverse the anemia but are rarely required because the anemia is mild.

Sideroblastic Anemias

A clue to the presence of sideroblastic anemias is the paradoxical finding of hyperferremia and nearly total transferrin saturation in a patient with a hypochromic anemia. The primary lesion results in a mismatch between iron delivery and its incorporation into heme. Consumption of large amounts of alcohol over a period of several weeks can induce a transient sideroblastic anemia that resolves upon abstinence from alcohol.

The morphologic evidence for the sideroblastic process is hypochromic RBCs. Transferrin levels are saturated, and ferritin levels are increased, although not usually to the same degree as in hemochromatosis.

Idiopathic refractory sideroblastic anemia develops in the elderly as a predominantly erythroid manifestation of a myelodysplastic syndrome. This form of sideroblastic anemia is characterized by macrocytic (rather than microcytic) indices. The lesion may evolve into leukemia. Treatment of the disorder remains experimental. The process may be very chronic, with no need for RBC transfusion until late in its course.

For more information about this subject, see *Cecil Textbook of Medicine,* 21st edition. Philadelphia, W.B. Saunders Company, 2000. Chapter 162, Microcytic and Hypochromic Anemias, pages 855 to 859.

MEGALOBLASTIC ANEMIAS

Etiologic categories of megaloblastic anemia are cobalamin deficiency, folate deficiency, drugs, and miscellaneous causes, including are enzyme deficiencies and unexplained disorders (Table 11–5). Chemically recognized pernicious anemia will develop in about 1.0% of people in the United States at some time during their lives.

All causes of megaloblastic anemia produce a common set of hematologic, laboratory, and other abnormalities (Table 11–6). The reticulocyte count is not elevated. Neutropenia and thrombocytopenia occur less commonly than anemia and are not usually severe. Megaloblastic anemia typically develops over many months and may not cause symptoms until the hematocrit falls below 20%.

Few, if any, patients with cobalamin or folate deficiency or other causes of megaloblastic anemia demonstrate all or even most of the classic hematologic or other abnormalities. Even anemia and increased MCV are frequently absent in patients with otherwise severe deficiencies of cobalamin or folate. Coexisting iron deficiency may also cause diagnostic problems inasmuch as all of the erythroid megaloblastic changes may be absent.

Cobalamin deficiency, unlike folate deficiency and other causes of megaloblastic anemia, produces a wide variety of neuropsychiatric abnormalities. *Combined systems disease* designates a spinal cord disorder marked by the insidious beginning and gradual progression of demyelination, initially of the dorsal (proprioceptive afferent) and later the lateral (corticospinal efferent) columns. Signs and symptoms are usually symmetrical and often include paresthesias in the extremities and impaired vibration and position sense. Cerebral and cranial nerve abnormalities and psychiatric abnormalities may be prominent. The severity of neuropsychiatric abnor-

Table 11–5 ■ ETIOLOGIC CLASSIFICATION OF THE MEGALOBLASTIC ANEMIAS

CATEGORY	ETIOLOGIC MECHANISMS
I. Cobalamin deficiency	
A. Decreased ingestion	
B. Impaired absorption	Intrinsic factor deficiency, chronic pancreatic disease, competitive parasites, intrinsic intestinal disease
C. Impaired utilization	Congenital enzyme deficiencies, lack of transcobalamin II, nitrous oxide administration
II. Folate deficiency	
A. Decreased ingestion	
B. Impaired absorption	Intestinal short circuits, tropical sprue, celiac disease, anticonvulsants, sulfasalazine, other drugs
C. Impaired utilization	Folic acid antagonists: methotrexate, triamterene, trimethoprim, pyrimethamine, ethanol
D. Increased requirement	Pregnancy, infancy, hyperthyroidism, chronic hemolytic disease, neoplastic disease, exfoliative skin disease
E. Increased loss	Hemodialysis
III. Drugs—metabolic inhibitors	Purine synthesis, pyrimidine synthesis, thymidylate synthesis, deoxyribonucleotide synthesis
IV. Miscellaneous	
A. Unexplained disorders	Myelodysplastic syndrome, acute myelogenous leukemia

11

malities actually bears a striking *inverse correlation* to the degree of anemia.

If drugs are excluded as a cause, the differential diagnosis of megaloblastic anemia in adults is usually limited to the important task of distinguishing between cobalamin deficiency and folate deficiency. In addition, patients should always be investigated for cobalamin deficiency in the presence of an unexplained neuropsychiatric abnormality.

The following distribution of serum cobalamin levels has been noted in clinically confirmed cobalamin-deficient patients: less than 100 pg/mL, approximately 50%; 100 to 200 pg/mL, approximately 40%; 200 to 350 pg/mL, approximately 10%; and higher than 350 pg/mL, approximately 0.1 to 1.0%. The distribution of serum folate levels in patients with clinically confirmed folate deficiency indicates that only about 75% of such patients have serum folate levels lower than 2.5 mg/mL, with almost all of the remaining 25% falling in the 2.5- to 5.0-ng/mL range.

The most useful follow-up tests for diagnosing and distinguishing between cobalamin and folate deficiency are serum levels of methylmalonic acid and homocysteine (Table 11–7). The only other conditions that also give rise to elevations in serum methyl-

Table 11–6 ■ HEMATOLOGIC AND OTHER ABNORMALITIES THAT MAY BE DUE TO ANY OF THE VARIOUS CAUSES OF MEGALOBLASTIC ANEMIA*

HEMATOLOGIC	OTHER
Anemia	Glossitis
Reticulocytopenia	Stomatitis
Macrocytosis (increased MCV)	Gastrointestinal symptoms
Neutropenia	Hyperpigmentation
Thrombocytopenia	Infertility
Peripheral blood smear	Orthostatic hypotension
Neutrophil hypersegmentation	Weight loss
Erythrocyte	
Variation in size	
Variation in shape	
Macro-ovalocytes	
Serum	
Elevated lactate dehydrogenase	
Elevated bilirubin	
Elevated iron	
Decreased haptoglobin	
Bone marrow	
Hypercellular	
Megaloblastic morphology	
Giant bands and metamyelocytes	

MCV = mean corpuscular volume.

*These abnormalities may be present in any number or combination in a given patient. Absence of any one or more of them occurs commonly in individual patients with all causes of megaloblastic anemia, including cobalamin deficiency and folate deficiency.

malonic acid or serum homocysteine are renal failure and intravascular volume depletion. With few exceptions, patients with serum cobalamin levels lower than 350 pg/mL or serum folate levels less than 5.0 ng/mL do not show objective hematologic or neuropsychiatric responses to cobalamin or folate therapy if their serum levels of methylmalonic acid and homocysteine are normal.

Oral cobalamin 1000 to 2000 μg/day is the treatment of choice for most patients with documented cobalamin deficiency. The abso-

Table 11–7 ■ TYPICAL SERUM FINDINGS IN MEGALOBLASTIC ANEMIA

		DEFICIENCY	
COMPONENT	NORMAL LEVELS	Cobalamin	Folate
Cobalamin	200–900 pg/mL	↓*	N
Folate	2.5–20 ng/mL	N	↓*
Methylmalonic acid	70–270 nmol	↑↑	N
Homocysteine	5–16 μmol	↑↑	↑↑

N = normal.

*A significant number of patients with cobalamin deficiency will have serum cobalamin levels in the lower portion of the normal range. The same is true with respect to folate deficiency and serum folate levels.

lute requirement of lifetime therapy must be well understood by the patient. For documented folate deficiency, the usual dose is 1 to 2 mg/day orally. By comparison, diagnostic trials of cobalamin or folate must be performed with physiologic levels of either vitamin (1 μg/day for cobalamin and 100 μg/day for folate) inasmuch as larger amounts can give hematologic responses even if the incorrect vitamin is administered.

For more information about this subject, see *Cecil Textbook of Medicine,* 21st edition. Philadelphia, W.B. Saunders Company, 2000. Chapter 163, Megaloblastic Anemias, pages 859 to 867.

HEMOLYTIC ANEMIAS: RED BLOOD CELL MEMBRANE AND METABOLIC DEFECTS

Membrane Defects

HEREDITARY SPHEROCYTOSIS. Molecular defects in spectrin, ankyrin, band 3, and protein 4.2 lead to spectrin deficiency as the "final common pathway" that characterizes all RBCs with hereditary spherocytosis. The clinical manifestations can vary from an insignificant hemolytic state that is fully compensated by increased marrow erythropoiesis to a life-threatening hemolytic state.

Common clinical complications of hereditary spherocytosis include splenomegaly, occasional aplastic crises, the formation of bilirubinate gallstones, and intermittent jaundice from hemolysis or biliary obstruction. Aplastic crisis is most often associated with parvovirus B19 infection. Megaloblastic crisis is caused by a relative lack of folic acid.

Laboratory features that are characteristic of hereditary spherocytosis include an elevated reticulocyte count and the presence of spherocytes on the blood smear. The differential diagnosis of spherocytosis includes autoimmune hemolytic anemia, which can be readily distinguished because it is associated with a positive direct antiglobulin (Coombs') test. The laboratory test most commonly used to confirm the presence of spherocytosis is the osmotic fragility test. Because hereditary spherocytic RBCs tend to be dehydrated, an elevated mean corpuscular hemoglobin concentration (MCHC) can be a helpful clue.

Splenectomy is highly effective in restoring a normal hematocrit and a near-normal reticulocyte count but should be reserved for patients with a degree of anemia that compromises oxygen delivery to vital organs, the development of extramedullary hematopoietic tumors, and the occurrence of bilirubinate gallstones. Splenectomy is generally deferred in patients with mild hereditary spherocytosis (hemoglobin >11 g/dL; reticulocyte count <8%). Failure of splenectomy to ameliorate the degree of hemolysis in hereditary spherocytosis, either immediately after the operation or many years later, is often due to the presence of an accessory spleen.

HEREDITARY ELLIPTOCYTOSIS. The great majority of individuals with mild hereditary elliptocytosis are heterozygous carriers. These patients have no anemia, little or no hemolysis (reticulocyte count, 1 to 3%), and no splenomegaly. Diagnosis is based on the presence of prominent elliptocytosis (often >40%) on the blood smear. Mild hereditary elliptocytosis requires no treatment. Spherocytic hereditary elliptocytosis should be treated like hereditary spherocytosis.

Red Blood Cell Metabolism Disorders

GLUCOSE-6-PHOSPHATE DEHYDROGENASE DEFICIENCY. The most common abnormal variants of the enzyme are called Gd^{A-}, found in about 10% of American blacks, and GD^{Med}, found in a smaller proportion of Mediterranean (Arabs, Greeks, Italians, Sephardic Jews, and others), Indian, and Southeast Asian populations. The inheritance pattern of G6PD deficiency is sex-linked.

Normal enzymes are slowly degraded over the lifetime of a normal RBC in vivo such that intracellular G6PD activity falls to half its original value in about 60 days. Even the oldest normal RBCs in the circulation retain sufficient G6PD activity to maintain intracellular reduced glutathione levels and to withstand nearly all oxidant stresses.

In the presence of severe oxidant stress, however, individuals with G6PD deficiency manifest hemolysis that can range from a chronic low-level hemolytic state, with a modest (3 to 4 g/dL) decrease in hemoglobin concentration and a modest increase in the reticulocyte count, to an acute episode of intravascular hemolysis characterized by anemia, hemoglobinemia, hemoglobinuria, hyperbilirubinemia, and jaundice. Changes in the blood smear include the appearance of Heinz bodies (visualized with supravital stains), bite cells (cells with small localized membrane invaginations, probably caused by splenic removal of Heinz bodies at the invagination sites), and blister cells (cells with a hemoglobin-free area adjacent to the membrane).

Hemolysis in the setting of G6PD deficiency is most often caused by acute infection, in which oxidant molecules are liberated in large amounts by granulocytes and mononuclear phagocytes. Oxidant drugs represent the other major category of oxidant stress that can lead to acute and/or chronic hemolysis. These include sulfonamides, sulfones, nitrofurans, chloramphenicol, antimalarials, anthelminthics, acetylsalicylic acid (aspirin; can give moderate doses), acetophenetidin (phenacetin), probenecid, vitamin K analogues, dimercaprol (BAL), methylene blue, and naphthalene. Ingestion of fava beans (broad beans) can also cause acute hemolysis in some patients with Gd^{Med}.

For more information about this subject, see *Cecil Textbook of Medicine,* 21st edition. Philadelphia, W.B. Saunders Company, 2000. Chapter 164, Hemolytic Anemias: Red Cell Membrane and Metabolic Effects, pages 867 to 876.

HEMOLYTIC ANEMIAS: AUTOIMMUNE

In general, two major classes of antierythrocyte antibodies produce hemolysis in humans: IgG and IgM. With antigens that are widely distributed on the erythrocyte surface, such as the antigens recognized by most antierythrocyte antibodies, many hundreds or thousands of IgG antibody molecules must be deposited on the erythrocyte membrane before two bind sufficiently close to one another to permit complement activation. IgG-sensitized erythrocytes are removed progressively from the circulation and sequestered predominately in the spleen.

By comparison, just a single molecule of IgM antibody bound to an erythrocyte membrane can bind C1 and activate the classic complement pathway. IgM-coated cells are cleared rapidly within the liver rather than the spleen.

IgG-induced immune hemolytic anemia can occur without an apparent underlying disease (idiopathic autoimmune hemolytic anemia); however, it can also occur with an underlying immunoproliferative disorder or systemic lupus erythematosus (Table 11–8). Some patients have immune thrombocytopenia in conjunction with IgG-induced autoimmune hemolytic anemia (Evans' syndrome), and some have immune granulocytopenia as well.

IgM-induced autoimmune hemolytic anemia is caused by an IgM antibody that reacts most efficiently with erythrocytes in the cold; thus this disorder has also been called "cold hemagglutinin disease." Chronic cold hemagglutinin disease is due to clonal expansion of lymphocytes in which a monoclonal antibody is produced. The symptom complex associated with multiple myeloma or Waldenström's macroglobulinemia does not develop in these patients.

Secondary cold hemagglutinin disease is most commonly associated with an underlying *Mycoplasma* infection. It may also occur with infectious mononucleosis, cytomegalovirus (CMV), and mumps. Cold hemagglutinin disease can also be seen in patients with an underlying immunoproliferative disorder and in patients with an underlying connective tissue disease, such as systemic lupus erythematosus.

Many of the symptoms of autoimmune hemolytic anemia are caused by the presence of anemia. If the hemolysis is significant,

Table 11–8 ■ DISEASES ASSOCIATED WITH AUTOIMMUNE HEMOLYTIC ANEMIA

Infections

Viral infections, especially respiratory infections
Infectious mononucleosis and cytomegalovirus infection
Mycoplasma, especially pneumonia
Tuberculosis

Non-Malignant Disorders

Systemic lupus erythematosus
Rheumatoid arthritis
Thyroid disorders
Ulcerative colitis
Chronic active hepatitis

Immunodeficiency Syndromes

Malignancies

Non-Hodgkin's lymphoma
Hodgkin's disease
Acute lymphocytic leukemia
Carcinoma
Thymoma
Ovarian cysts and tumors

mild jaundice may be noted. In addition, patients with an underlying disease often have symptoms associated with that disease. Massive splenomegaly suggests an underlying disorder such as lymphoma. The common initial symptoms are pallor, jaundice, dark urine, abdominal pain, and fever.

Laboratory data reveal the presence of anemia, reticulocytosis (if bone marrow function is adequate), and a positive result on the direct Coombs' test. The peripheral blood smear may show spherocytes, polychromasia, nucleated RBCs, and erythrophagocytosis.

Agglutination induced by anti-IgG (a γ-Coombs' test) indicates the presence of IgG on the surface of the RBCs, whereas agglutination with anti-C3 or anti-C4 (a non-γ-Coombs' test) is used to test for the presence of C3 and C4. In cold hemagglutinin disease, usually only a positive result in the non-γ-(C3) Coombs' test is observed. A cold agglutinin titer is also diagnostically helpful.

In many patients with IgG- or IgM-induced immune hemolytic anemia, no therapeutic intervention is necessary. Patients with IgG antibody–mediated autoimmune hemolytic anemia treated with glucocorticoids often respond within days of initiating therapy in dosages equivalent to 1 to 2 mg of prednisone per kilogram of body weight per day. By comparison, glucocorticoids are not usually effective in cold hemagglutinin disease.

Splenectomy should be considered in patients who are not responsive to steroids or require prednisone 10 to 20 mg/day or substantial dosages of steroid every other day for maintenance. Patients are selected for immunosuppressive therapy when a clinically unacceptable degree of hemolytic anemia persists following glucocorticoid therapy and splenectomy. Alternatively, patients may be corticosteroid resistant or intolerant and a poor surgical risk. The drugs most commonly used include the thiopurines (6-mercaptopurine, azathioprine, and thioguanine) and alkylating agents (cyclophosphamide and chlorambucil). Intravenous gamma globulin may be effective in patients with IgG-induced immune hemolytic anemia. Other measures that have been used effectively in some patients with IgG-induced immune hemolysis are vincristine, vinblastine infusions, and hormonal therapy.

Paroxysmal Nocturnal Hemoglobinuria

Paroxysmal nocturnal hemoglobinuria (PNH) is a primary bone marrow disorder that not only affects the RBC lineage but also affects the platelet, leukocyte, and pluripotent hematopoietic stem cell lines. Patients have a somatic mutation for a protein (phosphatidylinositol glycan class A) important in the pathway that controls formation of the phosphatidylinositol anchor of several membrane proteins.

Chronic intravascular hemolysis of varying severity is the most common finding. Patients commonly have iron deficiency anemia as well because of the large amount of iron lost in the urine during intravascular hemolysis via persistent hemoglobinuria and hemosiderinuria. Other frequent clinical complaints include abdominal, back, and musculoskeletal pain. Thrombosis of the hepatic veins (Budd-Chiari syndrome) and the portal, splenic, mesenteric, cerebral, and other veins may occur and is a common cause of death. Thrombotic episodes may require anticoagulant therapy.

Platelets and leukocytes also appear to have unusual susceptibility to lysis. Thrombocytopenia, granulocytopenia, or both are common and may be the initial manifestation(s) of the disease. PNH should be considered in everyone with aplastic anemia.

The diagnosis may be established by the sugar-water test, in which the patient's serum is mixed with D_5W and incubated with the patient's cells. In PNH, hemolysis ensues.

A prednisone dose of 15 to 40 mg every other day decreases the rate of hemolysis in some adult patients. Androgens may be effective. Bone marrow transplantation has been successful in some patients, but treatment of PNH generally has been unsatisfactory.

Drug-Induced Immune Hemolysis

Methyldopa and its derivatives (such as levodopa) produce a clinical syndrome virtually identical to IgG-induced immune hemolytic anemia. The hapten type of drug-induced immune hemolysis classically develops in patients exposed to high doses of penicillin. A portion of the penicillin molecule or its active metabolites combines with the erythrocyte surface, acts as a hapten, and induces an antibody response directed against the penicillin-coated erythrocyte membrane. The quinidine type of autoimmune hemolytic anemia usually occurs with quinidine, but it has been reported with quinine, stibophen, chlorpromazine, and sulfonamides. Commonly called an innocent bystander reaction, it is thought to be due to an antibody directed against quinidine and having a low affinity for the RBC surface.

For more information about this subject, see *Cecil Textbook of Medicine,* 21st edition. Philadelphia, W.B. Saunders Company, 2000. Chapter 165, Hemolytic Anemias: Autoimmune, pages 876 to 882.

HEMOLYTIC ANEMIAS: INTRAVASCULAR

Intravascular hemolysis is the result of a wide range of pathologic conditions including microangiopathic hemolytic anemia, valve hemolysis, exertional hemolysis, chemical agents, osmotic lysis, thermal injury, infections, PNH, cold agglutinin disease, and venoms.

Microangiopathic Hemolytic Anemias

The combination of small vessel damage and the appearance of fragmented RBCs in the peripheral blood defines microangiopathic hemolytic anemia (Table 11–9). Typical patients have anemia, reticulocytosis, and bizarre erythrocyte morphology—schistocytes, helmet cells, burr cells, and spherocytes. Because thrombotic thrombocytopenic purpura (TTP) often responds to plasmapheresis or plasma exchange, it is absolutely critical to review the peripheral blood film personally to identify fragmented RBCs in a patient with thrombocytopenia, particularly when the patient has neurologic or renal abnormalities.

A little-known consequence of exertion is a mild exertional hemolytic process marked by decreased serum haptoglobin and by hemoglobinuria in distance runners, marathoners, and triathletes. In

Table 11–9 ■ ERYTHROCYTE FRAGMENTATION SYNDROMES

Microangiopathic Hemolytic Anemia
Thrombotic thrombocytopenic purpura
Hemolytic-uremic syndrome
Disseminated intravascular coagulation
Disseminated carcinomatosis
Pregnancy-related
Preeclampsia/eclampsia
HELLP
Postpartum hemolytic-uremic syndrome
Glomerulonephritis
Malignant hypertension
Renal cortical necrosis
Allograft rejection
Vasculitis
Diabetic microangiopathy
Hemangiomas
Prosthetic Device and Large Vessel Disorders
Valve hemolysis
Septal patches
Vascular grafts
Arteriovenous fistulas
Circulatory assist devices

HELLP = *h*emolysis, *el*evated *l*iver enzymes, and *l*ow *p*latelet count.

diseases such as malaria, babesiosis, and bartonellosis, organisms infect RBCs and cause direct destruction. Infection with *Clostridium perfringens* also causes significant intravascular hemolysis.

Treatment is directed at the underlying disorder. Folate supplementation may be useful, and iron replacement may be necessary in a few individuals with valve hemolysis. Because thrombosis is a frequent complication of tumor-related microangiopathic hemolytic anemia, anticoagulation with heparin is sometimes recommended.

For more information about this subject, see *Cecil Textbook of Medicine,* 21st edition. Philadelphia, W.B. Saunders Company, 2000. Chapter 166, Hemolytic Anemias: Intravascular, pages 882 to 884.

HEMOGLOBINOPATHIES: THE THALASSEMIAS

The clinical syndromes associated with thalassemia arise from the combined effects of inadequate hemoglobin accumulation and unbalanced accumulation of globin subunits. The former causes hypochromia and microcytosis; the latter leads to ineffective erythropoiesis and hemolytic anemia. α-Thalassemia usually results from deletion of a single α-gene, while the β-thalassemias are rarely caused by major structural gene deletions. Reference laboratories can swiftly clone and directly sequence the α- or β-globin genes.

The α°-thalassemias result in completely abolished production of α-globin chains by the affected chromosome, whereas the α^{+}-thalassemias are defined by a variable amount of globin chain production resulting from the remaining α-globin genes on the chromosome (Fig. 11–2). Patients with α-thalassemia have a decrease in α-globin chain production relative to β-globin chain, with the formation of β_4 (hemoglobin H [Hb H]) inclusion bodies. RBCs bearing these inclusion bodies are rapidly removed from the circulation.

In contrast, patients with β-thalassemia have a decrease in β-globin chain production relative to α-globin chain production, which leads to an excess of α-globin chains. Unbound α-globin chains are extremely insoluble and precipitate in RBC precursors, leading to defective erythroid maturation. The few cells that do emerge into the peripheral circulation are rapidly removed in the spleen and liver.

The clinical spectrum of the α-thalassemia syndromes is directly related to the number of functioning α-globin genes. Accordingly, deletions of one or two α-globin genes are virtually asymptomatic. Hb H disease, which is caused by deletions of three genes (−−/-α), is manifested as a moderately severe anemia with splenomegaly and a hypochromic, microcytic blood film appearance. The hemolytic anemia in Hb H disease is partially compensated, with an average hemoglobin value of 8 to 10 g/dL. In its most severe form, in which all four genes are deleted, α-thalassemia is incompatible with life.

β-Thalassemia is ubiquitous, but especially common in Mediterranean, Asian, and African populations (and their American descendants). Whereas β-thalassemia trait is asymptomatic, disease occurs in homozygotes or compound heterozygotes such as β-thalassemia/Hb E (Table 11–10). In the presence of normal iron status, increased levels of Hb A_2 (to 4 to 6%) and/or increased Hb F (to 5 to 20%) by quantitative hemoglobin analysis supports the diagnosis.

α-Globin Gene	Genotype	Phenotype	# of Functional α-Genes
α α/α α	**Normal**	**Normal**	**4**
– α/α α	**α^+-thal heterozygote (mild)**	**Silent carrier α-thal trait**	**3**
– –/α α	**α^0-thal heterozygote (moderate)**	**Microcytosis α-thal trait**	**2**
– α/– α	**α^+-thal homozygote (moderate)**	**Microcytosis α-thal trait**	**2**
– –/– α	**α^0-thal x α^+-thal (severe)**	**Hb H disease**	**1**
– –/– –	**α^0-thal homozygote (lethal)**	**Hydrops fetalis with Hb Bart's**	**0**

FIGURE 11–2 ■ The genetic bases of the more common forms of α-thalassemia. (Adapted from Gelehrter TD, Collins FS: Principles of Medical Genetics. Baltimore, Williams & Wilkins, 1990.)

Table 11–10 ■ CLINICAL CLASSIFICATION OF THE THALASSEMIAS

CLASSIFICATION	GENOTYPE	CLINICAL SEVERITY*
	α-Thalassemia Syndromes	
α^+-carrier (silent)	$-\alpha/\alpha\alpha$†	Silent
α-Thalassemia trait	$-\alpha/-\alpha$; $--/\alpha\alpha$	Mild
Hb H disease	$-\alpha/--$	Mild–moderate, hemolytic anemia
Hydrops fetalis	$--/--$	Lethal
Hb Constant Spring genotypes	$\alpha\alpha^{cs}/\alpha\alpha$	Silent–mild
	β-Thalassemia Syndromes	
β-Thalassemia minor (trait)	β/β^+‡	Silent
β-Thalassemia intermedia	β/β^0; β^+/β^+; $\beta^+/\beta^0 = \beta^+$ HbE/β^0	Moderate–severe
β-Thalassemia major	$\beta^0/\beta^0 = \beta^0$	Severe
	Complex β-Thalassemia Syndromes	
Co-inherited β-thalassemia†	Various combinations of α- and β-thalassemia syndromes	
Hereditary persistence of fetal hemoglobin	Various point mutations or deletions in or around γ-globin gene	Mild–moderate
γ-Thalassemia	Deletion of 1 or more γ-genes	
δ-Thalassemia	Deletion of 1 or more δ-genes	
γ δ β-Thalassemia	Complex deletions of 1 or more γ-, δ-, β-genes in tandem	

*Silent = normal or minimally abnormal hematology values; mild = hemoglobin level normal or slightly reduced with disproportionate microcytic hypochromic indices; moderate = hemolytic anemia, icterus, splenomegaly, although no regular transfusion requirement; severe = profound anemia with transfusion dependency, extramedullary hematopoiesis, growth retardation, bone abnormalities, hemosiderosis; lethal = death in utero from anemic congestive heart failure.

†The α-thalassemia syndromes usually result from deletions in one or more α-genes, indicated by the minus sign, or from mutations in the coding sequence (e.g., α-Constant Spring, α^{cs}).

‡The β-thalassemia syndromes are typically the consequence of mutations that lead to a *decreased* level of normal β-chain production (β^+) or *absence* of β-chain production (β^0). Various combinations of these mutations give rise to syndromes of increasing severity.

Treatment

α-THALASSEMIA. Some deletions of one ($\alpha\alpha$/-α) or two (-α/-α, --/$\alpha\alpha$) α-globin genes are asymptomatic, and no therapy is indicated. For Hb H disease (three-gene deletion, --/-α), folic acid 1 mg orally, should be administered daily. Splenectomy may be indicated for progressive anemia and is often associated with a mean rise in hemoglobin of 2 to 3 g/dL.

β-THALASSEMIA. β-Thalassemia trait is asymptomatic and requires no treatment. For homozygotes or compound heterozygotes, dramatic improvement in life expectancy and morbidity has been observed over the last two decades, primarily because of aggressive transfusion support and the institution of effective iron chelation therapy in regularly transfused patients. Transfusion support is generally initiated once the hemoglobin level drops below 7 g/dL and remains there in the absence of infection or blood loss.

Although intensive transfusion programs have led to markedly improved survival, patients will die of iron overload unless chelation therapy is appropriately instituted and maintained. Many patients can be placed in iron balance by receiving a 12- to 24-hour infusion of deferoxamine 5 or 6 days a week. Allogeneic bone marrow transplantation is increasingly effective for patients with homozygous β-thalassemia.

11

For more information about this subject, see *Cecil Textbook of Medicine,* 21st edition. Philadelphia, W.B. Saunders Company, 2000. Chapter 167, Hemoglobinopathies: The Thalassemias, pages 884 to 889.

HEMOGLOBINOPATHIES: METHEMOGLOBINEMIAS, POLYCYTHEMIAS, AND UNSTABLE HEMOGLOBINS

Types of Methemoglobinemia

The most frequent type of methemoglobinemia is acquired or toxic. It can be induced by certain drugs and other chemicals (Table 11–11). Of the three types of hereditary methemoglobinemia, two are inherited as an autosomal recessive trait. In contrast to

Table 11–11 ■ MEDICATIONS AND CHEMICALS ASSOCIATED WITH METHEMOGLOBINEMIA

MEDICATIONS	CHEMICALS
Acetaminophen (nitrobenzene derivative)	Acetaniline
Dapsone	Aniline dyes
Flutamide	Nitric oxide
Metoclopramide	Nitrites
Nitroglycerin	Amyl nitrite
Paraquat/monolinuron	Isobutyl nitrite
Phenacetin	Sodium nitrite
Phenazopyridine (pyridium)	Nitrates (bacterial conversion to nitrites)
Primaquine	Nitrobenzenes/nitrobenzoates
Sulfamethoxazole	Nitroethane (nail polish remover)
	Nitrofurans
	4-Amino-biphenyl

the asymptomatic, chronically methemoglobinemic homozygotes, heterozygous individuals are at risk for developing acute, symptomatic methemoglobinemia after exposure to exogenous methemoglobin-inducing agents. To distinguish the hereditary forms of methemoglobinemia, biochemical analyses and interpretation of family pedigrees are required.

Methemoglobinemia may be clinically suspected by cyanosis, the slate-blue color of the skin, in the presence of a normal partial pressure of arterial oxygen. Other clinical symptoms of methemoglobinemia are generally seen only in acute toxic (acquired) methemoglobinemia and include headache, fatigue, dyspnea, and lethargy. Respiratory depression, altered consciousness, shock, seizures, and death may occur.

Offending agents should be discontinued if the patient is symptomatic. Methylene blue 1 to 2 mg/kg over 5 minutes should be used. For severe cases, hyperbaric oxygen and exchange transfusion have been anecdotally reported to be effective.

Hemoglobin Mutants Associated with Hemolytic Anemia: Unstable Hemoglobins

Approximately 100 different globin mutations have been reported to cause unstable hemoglobins. The diagnosis is suspected by demonstration of Heinz bodies in the RBCs.

For more information about this subject, see *Cecil Textbook of Medicine,* 21st edition. Philadelphia, W.B. Saunders Company, 2000. Chapter 168, Hemoglobinopathies: Methemoglobinemias, Polycythemias, and Unstable Hemoblobins, pages 889 to 893.

SICKLE CELL ANEMIA

The different sickle cell syndromes that result from distinct inheritance patterns of the sickle cell gene (β^S gene) are divided into sickle cell disease and sickle cell trait. The former is associated with chronic anemia and recurrent pain. The latter is largely asymptomatic. Common varieties of sickle cell disease are inherited as homozygosity for the β^S gene, called *sickle cell anemia* (Hb SS), or as compound heterozygosity of the β^S gene with another mutant β-globin gene—sickle cell-β^o thalassemia (HbS-β^o thal), sickle cell–Hb C disease (Hb SC disease), and sickle cell–β^+ thalassemia (HbS-β^+ thal).

Those cells that do not unsickle when reoxygenated, the "irreversibly sickled cells" (ISCs), are the least deformable sickle cells and have the shortest circulatory survival. Their number does not change with complications of disease (such as the acute painful episode), is generally constant in individual patients, and correlates mainly with the degree of anemia.

Sickle cells are destroyed randomly with a mean lifespan of 17 days. In addition, inappropriately low EPO levels contribute to the anemia. Clinical manifestations of sickle cell disease vary greatly between and among the disease genotypes. The current mean survival is 42 years for men and 48 years for women with sickle cell anemia.

EXACERBATIONS OF ANEMIA. The reasonably constant level of hemolytic anemia may be exacerbated by several different causes, most commonly aplastic crises. Aplastic crises are transient arrests of erythropoiesis characterized by abrupt falls in hemoglobin levels, reticulocyte number, and RBC precursors in the marrow. Parvovirus B19 specifically invades proliferating erythroid progenitors, accounting for its importance in sickle cell disease.

Acute splenic sequestration is characterized by acute exacerbation of anemia, persistent reticulocytosis, a tender enlarging spleen, and sometimes hypovolemia. Hyperhemolysis may occur with coexistent G6PD deficiency.

THE ACUTE PAINFUL EPISODE. Acute pain is often the first symptom of disease and is the most common reason why patients seek medical attention. Painful episodes are caused by vaso-occlusion and may be precipitated by cold, dehydration, infection, stress, menses, or alcohol consumption, but the cause of most episodes its indeterminate. Pain affects any area of the body, most commonly the back, chest, extremities, and abdomen. Half of painful episodes are associated with objective clinical signs—fever, swelling, tenderness, tachypnea, hypertension, nausea, and vomiting.

INFECTIONS. *Streptococcus pneumoniae* is the most common cause of bacteremia and *Haemophilus influenzae* is second. Urinary tract infections and bacteremia in older patients are more likely due to *Escherichia coli* and other gram-negative organisms. Bacterial pneumonia is one cause of the acute chest syndrome. *Mycoplasma pneumoniae* and *Chlamydia pneumoniae* account for approximately 20% of cases of acute chest syndrome. Osteomyelitis occurs more commonly in sickle cell disease, probably as a result of infection of infarcted bone.

NEUROLOGIC COMPLICATIONS. Neurologic complications occur in 25% of patients with sickle cell disease, and common events are transient ischemic attacks (TIAs), cerebral infarction, cerebral hemorrhage, seizures, and unexplained coma. Cerebral thrombosis accounts for 70 to 80% of cerebrovascular accidents (CVAs) and is due to large vessel obstruction rather than microvascular occlusion. Patients presenting with symptoms and signs suggestive of CVA should be evaluated immediately by computed tomographic (CT) scanning or magnetic resonance imaging (MRI).

PULMONARY COMPLICATIONS. The "acute chest syndrome" consists of dyspnea, chest pain, fever, tachypnea, leukocytosis, and pulmonary infiltrate. The usual causes are vaso-occlusion, infection, and pulmonary fat embolus from infarcted marrow.

HEPATOBILIARY COMPLICATIONS. Pigmented gallstones develop as a result of the chronic hemolysis of sickle cell disease and eventually will occur in at least 70% of patients. Chronic hepatomegaly and liver dysfunction are caused by trapping of sickle cells, transfusion-acquired infection, and iron overload.

RENAL COMPLICATIONS. Occlusion of the vasa recta compromises blood flow to the medulla, causing impaired urinary concentrating ability, papillary infarction, hematuria, incomplete renal tubular acidosis, and abnormal potassium clearance. Glomerular abnormalities result from vaso-occlusion, hyperperfusion, immune complex nephropathy, and parvovirus B19 infection. Hypertension, proteinuria, hyperkalemia, and worsening anemia may herald chronic renal insufficiency, the average age of onset of which is 23 years in sickle cell anemia and 50 years in Hb SC disease. Angiotensin-converting enzyme inhibitors diminish hyperperfusion and proteinuria but do not increase glomerular filtration.

Priapism, an unwanted painful erection, has been reported to affect from 6.4 to 42% of males with sickle cell disease. Recurrent priapism can be prevented by oral self-administration of the α-adrenergic agent etilefrine and by intracavernous injection for episodes lasting over an hour. Recurrences also may be prevented by the administration of diethylstilbestrol.

BONE COMPLICATIONS. Osteonecrosis may cause compression of vertebrae, shortening of cuboidal bones of the hands and feet, and acute "aseptic or avascular necrosis." Arthritic pain, swelling, and effusion may be the result of periarticular infarction or gouty arthritis.

DERMATOLOGIC COMPLICATIONS. Leg ulcers begin spontaneously or result from trauma, arise near the medial or lateral malleolus, and frequently occur bilaterally.

CARDIAC COMPLICATIONS. The chronic anemia of sickle cell disease is compensated by increased cardiac output, stroke and chamber volumes, and heart size.

Variant Sickle Cell Syndromes

In addition to homozygous sickle cell anemia, sickle cell syndromes result from simple heterozygous inheritance of the sickle cell gene (i.e., sickle cell trait) and from its compound heterozygous inheritance with other mutant β-globin genes (e.g., Hb SC disease, sickle cell–β-thalassemia).

SICKLE CELL TRAIT. The approximate prevalence of sickle cell trait is 9% among black Americans. Sickle forms are not seen on the peripheral blood smear. Few clinical complications are associated with sickle cell trait. Sickle cell trait is a common cause of hematuria among black Americans. The 30-fold greater frequency of unexplained sudden death in military recruits during basic training is the result of exercise-induced vaso-occlusion and rhabdomyolysis.

Hb SC DISEASE. As a result of a longer circulatory survival of Hb SC RBCs (i.e., 27 days compared with 17 days for Hb SS RBCs), the degree of anemia and reticulocytosis is frequently milder. Target cells predominate on the peripheral smear.

SICKLE CELL–β-THALASSEMIA. The frequency of β-thalassemia genes among black Americans is one tenth that of the β^S gene. Sickle cell–β-thalassemia RBCs are hypochromic and microcytic.

Diagnosis

Universal newborn screening of all ethnic backgrounds is recommended.

Therapy

Folic acid 1 mg/day orally, is administered. Non-invasive surveillance of cerebral blood flow using transcranial Doppler assessment is a useful predictor of CVA and should be performed regularly to identify those in whom chronic transfusion should be initiated to prevent this outcome. Immunization using conjugated vaccines for

S. pneumoniae and *H. influenzae* type b should be employed. Reimmunization for *S. pneumoniae* is recommended every 6 to 8 years.

INFECTIONS. Antibiotic therapy for the acute chest syndrome should provide coverage for *S. pneumoniae, H. influenzae* type b, *M. pneumoniae,* and *C. pneumoniae.* Cefuroxime and erythromycin combinations are recommended.

TRANSFUSION THERAPY. Patients with sickle cell disease have similar requirements for transfusion as do other patients. Preoperative transfusion is recommended for patients with sickle cell disease. Both simple transfusion to reduce Hb S to less than 60% and raise the hemoglobin level to 10 g/dL and aggressive partial exchange transfusion to reduce Hb S to less than 30% will reduce the incidence of perioperative acute chest syndrome. Deferoxamine chelation should be considered for those with elevated total body iron levels, that is, serum ferritin levels that exceed 2000 ng/mL.

PAIN MANAGEMENT. Neither RBC transfusion nor oxygen administration is indicated in treating the routine acute painful episode. Health care providers should be familiar with the pharmacology of characteristic analgesia and must overcome fears of narcotic addiction to treat pain. Intravenous morphine is recommended for prompt pain relief, and patient-controlled analgesia is an excellent means of subsequent pain control. The potent non-steroidal anti-inflammatory drug ketorolac can be given by injection or orally.

Hydroxyurea therapy results in significant reductions in sickle cell counts and increased levels of hemoglobin, hematocrit, MCV, Hb F, F cells, and F reticulocytes. Bone marrow transplantation has been used successfully for sickle cell anemia.

For more information about this subject, see *Cecil Textbook of Medicine,* 21st edition. Philadelphia, W.B. Saunders Company, 2000. Chapter 169, Sickle Cell Anemia and Associated Hemoglobinopathies, pages 893 to 905.

BLOOD TRANSFUSION

Whole blood is indicated when there are concomitant deficits of oxygen-carrying capacity, blood volume, and coagulation factors. *RBC transfusions* are used to alleviate signs and symptoms attributable to diminished oxygen-carrying capacity in patients unable to tolerate anemia pending the effect of iron, folic acid, vitamin B_{12}, exogenous EPO, or other specific therapeutic interventions to increase hemoglobin and hematocrit levels. Signs and symptoms attributable to anemia include fatigue, syncope, dyspnea on exertion, decreased exercise capacity, decreased mental acuity, tachycardia, angina, postural hypotension, or TIA (Fig. 11–3). With chronic anemia, symptomatic patients receive 2 to 3 U of blood at 2- to 3-week intervals. One unit of RBCs raises the hemoglobin by approximately 1 g/dL and the hematocrit by about 3%.

To date, there is no consensus about whether all patients or only certain patients, such as those receiving outpatient or perioperative transfusions, are most likely to benefit from leukocyte reduction transfusion. Washed RBCs are prepared by adding saline to blood cells. Washing removes plasma proteins, including IgA. Irradiated components are used to prevent graft-versus-host disease (GVHD)

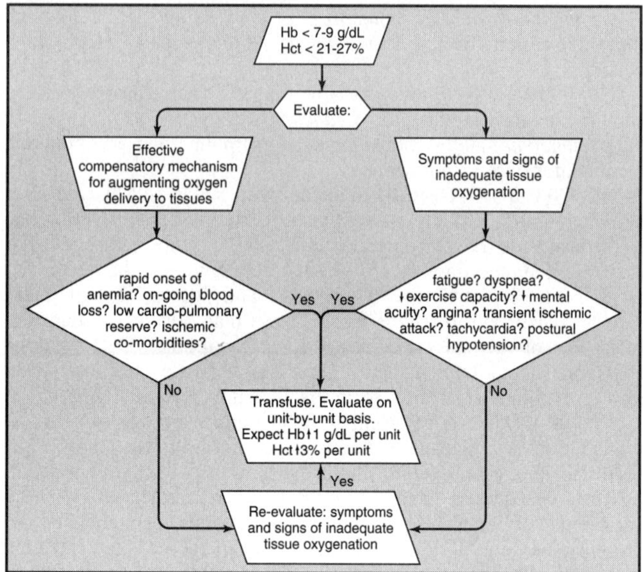

FIGURE 11–3 ■ An approach to deciding when to transfuse patients with anemia and/or blood loss. Hb = hemoglobin; Hct = hematocrit.

by eliminating the proliferative capacity of T lymphocytes. Autologous transfusion involves collection and reinfusion of a patient's own blood to reduce allogeneic blood exposure.

The majority of acute hemolytic reactions involve ABO incompatibility. Anaphylactic reactions develop in some IgA-deficient patients (approximately 1 in 500 to 1000 persons) who have IgE anti-IgA antibodies against IgA contained in donor plasma. If subsequent RBC transfusions are required, the components should be washed to remove IgA.

Adverse events associated with transfusion are listed in Table 11–12.

For more information about this subject, see *Cecil Textbook of Medicine,* 21st edition. Philadelphia, W.B. Saunders Company, 2000. Chapter 170, Blood Transfusion, pages 905 to 911.

DISORDERS OF PHAGOCYTE FUNCTION

Neutrophils may exhibit decreased adhesiveness and chemotaxis following exposure to a variety of drugs, the most common being corticosteroids and epinephrine (Table 11–13). The *hyperimmunoglobulin E syndrome* is characterized by reduced neutrophil motility accompanied by markedly elevated levels of serum IgE that lead to chronic dermatitis and recurrent sinopulmonary infections.

Familial Mediterranean fever is transmitted as an autosomal recessive trait. The disease is characterized by acute self-limited attacks of fever often accompanied by pleuritis, peritonitis, arthritis, pericarditis, inflammation of the tunica vaginalis of the testes, and

Table 11–12 ■ ADVERSE REACTIONS TO BLOOD TRANSFUSION

Acute
Hemolytic transfusion reactions
Fatal, hemolytic transfusion reactions
Febrile non-hemolytic transfusion reactions
Transfusion-related acute lung injury
Allergic reactions (urticaria)
Anaphylactic reactions
Hypervolemia
Bacterial transmission
Platelets
Red blood cells
Delayed
"Hemolytic" transfusion reactions
Serologic
Hemolytic
Graft-versus-host disease
Iron overload
Post-transfusion purpura
Transfusion-Transmitted Infections
Hepatitis
Retroviral infection
HIV-1 and -2
HTLV-I and -2
Cytomegalovirus

HIV = human immunodeficiency virus; HTLV = human T-cell lymphotropic virus.

erythematous skin lesions. The gene responsible for familial Mediterranean fever is located on chromosome 16. It encodes pyrin, which is expressed in neutrophils but not lymphocytes or monocytes. Acute attacks frequently last 24 to 48 hours and recur once or twice per month. Prophylactic colchicine 0.6 mg orally two or three times per day prevents or substantially reduces acute attacks of familial Mediterranean fever in 75 to 90% of patients.

Chédiak-Higashi syndrome is a rare autosomal recessive disease in which neutrophils, monocytes, and lymphocytes contain giant cytoplasmic granules. *Chronic granulomatous disease* is a genetic

Table 11–13 ■ ACQUIRED DISORDERS OF NEUTROPHIL DYSFUNCTION

Disorders of chemotaxis
Defects in the generation of chemotactic signals
Direct inhibition of neutrophil mobility
Drugs
Trauma, burns, pancreatitis
Immune complexes
Adhesion abnormalities
Trauma, burns, pancreatitis

Modified from Boxer LA: Neutrophil disorders: Qualitative abnormalities of the neutrophil. *In* Williams WJ, Beutler E, Erslev AJ, Lichtman MA (eds): Hematology, 5th ed. New York, McGraw Hill, 1994, p 828.

disorder affecting 4 to 5 per million humans. Neutrophils and monocytes from affected individuals ingest but do not kill catalase-positive microorganisms.

Deficiency of myeloperoxidase is the most common inherited disorder of neutrophil function. Lack of HOCl in the phagosome causes a delay in the microbicidal activity of neutrophils early after the ingestion of microorganisms. Eventually, however, effective killing of bacteria occurs. Clinically, myeloperoxidase deficiency is almost completely silent.

For more information about this subject, see *Cecil Textbook of Medicine,* 21st edition. Philadelphia, W.B. Saunders Company, 2000. Chapter 171, Disorders of Phagocyte Function, pages 911 to 919.

LEUKOPENIA AND LEUKOCYTOSIS

Neutropenia

When symptoms of neutropenia occur, they generally result from recurrent, often severe, bacterial infections. This risk of bacterial infection increases slightly as the peripheral neutrophil count falls below 1.0×10^9/L, but is substantially increased at levels below 0.5×10^9/L. Lungs, genitourinary system, gut, oropharynx, and skin are the most frequent sources of infection. The usual signs and symptoms of infection are often diminished or absent because the cell that mediates much of the inflammatory responses to infection is absent.

The patient with sepsis and severe neutropenia should be treated promptly with intravenous antibiotics after obtaining appropriate cultures but *without waiting for the results of those cultures.* Once these important initial questions are answered, the remainder of the diagnostic evaluation can proceed (Fig. 11–4).

TREATMENT. Immunosuppressive therapy, including glucocorticoids or azathioprine, almost always elicits a favorable response in patients with marrow failure mediated by cytotoxic T lymphocytes. Granulocyte-macrophage colony-stimulating factor (GM-CSF) and granulocyte colony-stimulating factor (G-CSF) are capable of increasing the neutrophil count in selected neutropenic patients. Patients with drug-induced neutropenia (e.g., after cancer chemotherapy) recover more rapidly if they receive either GM-CSF or G-CSF. Allogeneic transplantation should be reserved for patients with severe and symptomatic neutropenia caused by marrow failure.

Lymphocytopenia

The most common cause of reduced lymphocyte production throughout the world is protein-calorie malnutrition. Radiation and immunosuppressive agents, including alkylating agents and ATG, can induce lymphocytopenia. HIV does not frequently cause lymphocytopenia, but it infects the helper (CD4+) subset of T lymphocytes and destroys them, a process that results in a marked decline in the absolute numbers of helper (CD4+) T cells in the peripheral circulation. Losses of viable lymphocytes can also occur because of structural defects in sites of high-density lymphocyte traffic (i.e., through thoracic duct fistulas).

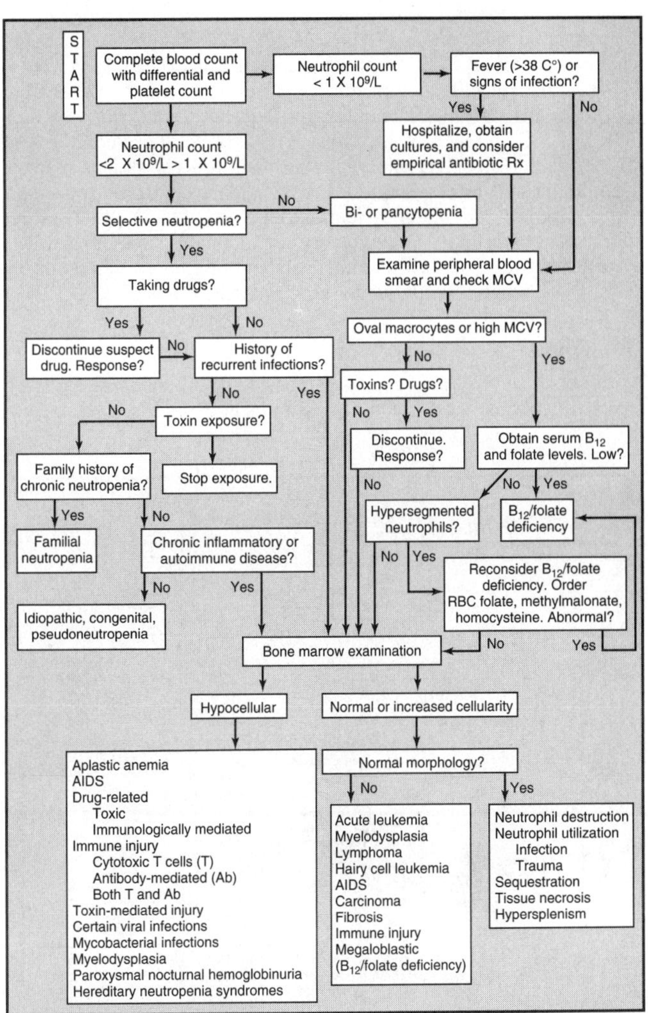

FIGURE 11–4 ■ A practical algorithm for the evaluation of patients with neutropenia. MCV = mean corpuscular volume; RBC = red blood cell.

There are no specific clinical manifestations of lymphocytopenia per se. Because lymphocytopenia ordinarily represents a response to an underlying disease, primary attention must be paid to establishing the nature of that disease and instituting therapy for it. Patients whose lymphocytopenia is accompanied by hypogammaglobulinemia may benefit significantly from administration of intravenous immunoglobulin.

Leukocytosis and Leukemoid Reactions

The terms *neutrophilia* (neutrophilic leukocytosis), *monocytosis, lymphocytosis, eosinophilia,* and *basophilia* suggest specific sets of diagnostic considerations. Leukocytosis is a common finding in acutely ill patients. When the leukocyte count exceeds 25 to 30 × 10^9/L, it is sometimes termed a *leukemoid reaction.* Leukemoid reactions are not synonymous with *leukoerythroblastosis,* which indicates the presence of immature WBCs and nucleated RBCs in the peripheral blood. Leukoerythroblastosis reflects serious marrow dysfunction and represents a clear indication to perform bone marrow aspiration and biopsy. Neutrophilia (Fig. 11–5) generally results from acute toxic, inflammatory, or traumatic stresses, and it is usually best to observe the course of neutrophilia to determine its degree of linkage with the underlying disease.

Monocytosis

Monocytosis is often seen in patients with tuberculosis, syphilis, fungal infections, ulcerative and granulomatous colitis, and sarcoid-

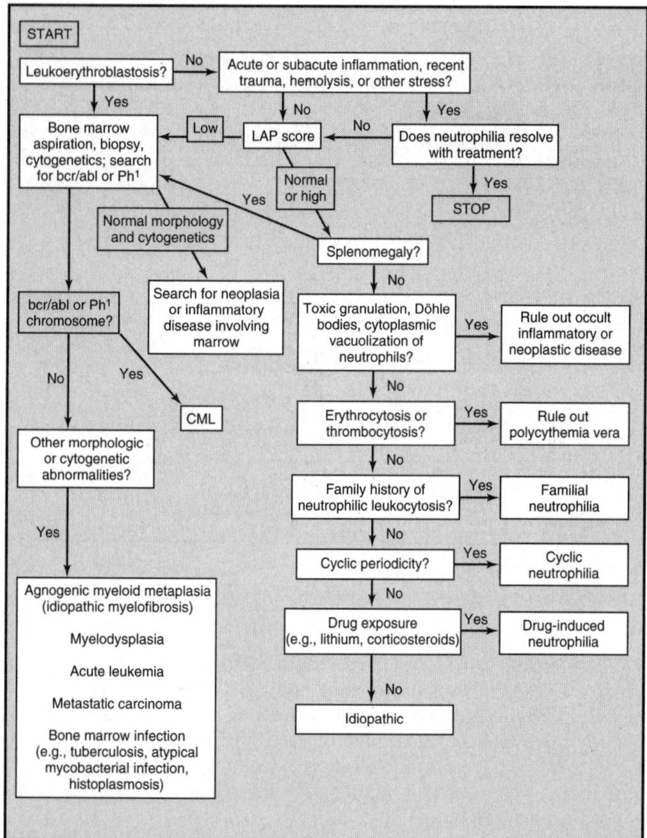

FIGURE 11–5 ■ Evaluation of patients with neutrophilic leukocytosis. LAP = leukocyte alkaline phosphatase; Ph[1] = Philadelphia chromosome; bcr/abl = the translocation of the c-*abl* gene from chromosome 9 to the *bcr* gene on chromosome 22q; CML = chronic myelogenous leukemia.

osis. Mild monocytosis is common in patients with Hodgkin's disease and a variety of cancers. High levels of monocytes in the blood are most often seen in patients with hematopoietic malignancies.

Lymphocytosis

Mild to moderate lymphocytosis is most commonly caused by viral infections, including infectious mononucleosis and infectious hepatitis. In infectious mononucleosis, many of the lymphocytes are large, with abundant cytoplasm. These are the characteristic "atypical" lymphocytes that exceed 20% of the total lymphocyte population.

Acute bacterial infections rarely cause lymphocytosis. One exception is pertussis, in which profound lymphocytosis is sometimes seen. Other causes include toxoplasmosis, brucellosis, tuberculosis, typhoid fever, carcinoma, Hodgkin's disease, acute lymphocytic leukemia (ALL) (early), chronic lymphocytic leukemia (CLL), Graves' disease, and drug reactions (e.g., tetracycline).

For more information about this subject, see *Cecil Textbook of Medicine,* 21st edition. Philadelphia, W.B. Saunders Company, 2000. Chapter 172, Leukopenia and Leukocytosis, pages 919 to 933.

EOSINOPHILIC SYNDROMES

Eosinophilia is not elicited by infections with single-celled protozoan parasites (with the exception of the intestinal coccidian parasite *Isospora belli*) but rather by the multicellular helminthic parasites. Even with severe helminthic diseases such as disseminated strongyloidiasis, superimposed bacterial infections can suppress eosinophilia. In evaluating a patient with unexplained eosinophilia, stool examinations for diagnostic ova and larvae should be performed (Table 11–14).

For more information about this subject, see *Cecil Textbook of Medicine,* 21st edition. Philadelphia, W.B. Saunders Company, 2000. Chapter 933, Eosinophilic Syndromes, pages 933 to 935.

MYELOPROLIFERATIVE DISEASES

Essential Thrombocythemia

If the clinical and laboratory evaluation is unrevealing for reactive thrombocytosis (Table 11–15), bone marrow examination is needed. Cytogenetic studies are recommended to distinguish essential thrombocythemia from the other chronic myeloid disorders. An increased RBC mass indicates polycythemia vera. The demonstration of t(9;22) or the *bcr-abl* rearrangement on DNA analysis is consistent with the diagnosis of chronic myelogenous leukemia (CML), even if the patient presents with isolated thrombocytosis.

Life expectancy in essential thrombocythemia is near normal, and the risk of leukemic conversion or post-thrombocythemic myelofibrosis is less than 5%. Vasomotor symptoms (headache, erythromelalgia, acroparesthesia, visual symptoms) may occur in more than one third of patients and are usually controlled by the use of

Table 11–14 ■ DISEASES ASSOCIATED WITH EOSINOPHILIA

"Allergic" diseases
- Atopic and related diseases
- Medication-related eosinophilias

Infectious diseases
- Parasitic infections, mostly with helminths
- Specific fungal infections: allergic bronchopulmonary aspergillosis, coccidioidomycosis (acute and sometimes disseminated)

Hematologic and neoplastic disorders
- Hypereosinophilic syndrome
- Leukemia
- Lymphomas, including nodular sclerosing Hodgkin's disease
- Tumor-associated
- Mastocytosis

Diseases with specific organ involvement
- Skin and subcutaneous diseases, including urticaria, bullous pemphigoid, eosinophilic cellulitis (Well's syndrome), episodic angioedema with eosinophilia
- Pulmonary diseases, including acute or chronic eosinophilic pneumonia, allergic bronchopulmonary aspergillosis
- Gastrointestinal diseases, including eosinophilic gastroenteritis
- Neurologic diseases (e.g., eosinophilic meningitis)
- Rheumatologic diseases, especially Churg-Strauss vasculitis; also eosinophilic fasciitis
- Cardiac diseases (e.g., endomyocardial fibrosis)
- Renal diseases, including drug-induced interstitial nephritis, eosinophilic cystitis, dialysis

Immunologic reactions
- Specific immunodeficiency diseases: hyper-IgE syndrome, Omenn's syndrome
- Transplant rejection: lung, kidney, liver

Endocrine
- Hypoadrenalism: Addison's disease, adrenal hemorrhage

Other
- Atheroembolic disease
- Irritation of serosal surfaces, including peritoneal dialysis
- Inherited

acetylsalicylic acid. Erythromelalgia refers to a burning pain and erythema of the extremities.

Compared with a control population, patients with essential thrombocythemia have a significantly increased risk for thrombosis (1% versus 7% per year). Bleeding complications, in the absence of antiplatelet therapy, are infrequent and usually non-consequential.

TREATMENT. Low-dose acetylsalicylic acid 81 mg/day is effective for controlling vasomotor symptoms. In high-risk patients (prior history of thrombosis or age >60 years), hydroxyurea significantly reduces thrombotic events compared with no treatment and is reasonable, starting at 500 mg orally twice a day. An alternative is anagrelide, which lowers platelet counts by interfering with the maturation of megakaryocytes. The starting dose is 0.5 mg orally three times a day. Interferon alfa controls thrombocytosis, splenomegaly, and disease-associated symptoms in approximately 80% of patients; it is currently considered a second-line therapeutic option.

Table 11–15 ■ CAUSES OF REACTIVE THROMBOCYTOSIS

Acute Conditions
Acute bleeding
Postsurgical period
Acute hemolysis
Infections
Tissue damage (acute pancreatitis, myocardial infarction, trauma, burns)
Coronary artery bypass grafting
Rebound recovery from chemotherapy or immune thrombocytopenia
Chronic Conditions
Iron deficiency anemia
Surgical or functional asplenia
Metastatic cancer, lymphoma
Inflammation (rheumatoid arthritis, vasculitis, allergies)
Renal failure, nephrotic syndrome

From Tefferi A, Silverstein MN: Chronic myeloproliferative disorders. *In* Wachter RM, Hollander H, Goldman L (eds): Hospital Medicine. Baltimore, Williams & Wilkins, 2000.

Polycythemia Vera

In view of the clonal nature of the disease, serum EPO levels are often suppressed in patients with polycythemia vera. The diagnosis is seriously considered when the low EPO level is associated with any one of the following: a hematocrit level of more than 60% (53% in women), splenomegaly, persistent leukocytosis, persistent thrombocytosis, microcytosis, unusual thrombotic history, post-bath pruritus, erythromelalgia, bone marrow panhyperplasia with atypical megakaryocytes, bone marrow reticulin fibrosis, clonal cytogenetic abnormalities, or in vitro formation of endogenous erythroid colonies.

A normal EPO level does not exclude the possibility of polycythemia vera. If a normal EPO level is associated with a hematocrit value of more than 60% (53% in women), then evaluation for secondary erythrocytosis is appropriate, followed, if negative, by bone marrow examination or in vitro testing for endogenous erythroid colony formation (Table 11–16).

At presentation, patients are either asymptomatic or manifest symptoms and signs related to hyperviscosity and tumor burden, including headaches, dizziness, visual symptoms, paresthesias, fatigue, abdominal discomfort, weight loss, and night sweats. Generalized pruritus (exacerbated by contact with water) is a poorly understood, frequent disease manifestation.

The primary morbid conditions associated with polycythemia vera are thrombosis and bleeding. In addition, patients may experience vasomotor disturbances (headache, dizziness, acral dysesthesia, erythromelalgia, visual symptoms). Furthermore, polycythemia vera is associated with a delayed risk of transformation into acute leukemia and myelofibrosis. Despite these complications, median survival in young patients exceeds 15 years.

TREATMENT. All patients should undergo phlebotomy, with the goal of keeping the hematocrit values less than 45% in men and

Table 11–16 ■ ACQUIRED CAUSES OF SECONDARY ERYTHROCYTOSIS

Appropriate erythropoietin response
Chronic lung disease
Arteriovenous or intracardiac shunts
High-altitude habitat
Chronic carbon monoxide exposure (smoking)
Pathologic erythropoietin production
Tumors (liver, kidney, cerebellum)
Uterine fibroids
Post renal transplant
Benign renal disorders (e.g., polycystic kidneys)

From Tefferi A, Silverstein MN: Chronic myeloproliferative disorders. *In* Wachter RM, Hollander H, Goldman L (eds): Hospital Medicine. Baltimore, Williams & Wilkins, 2000.

42% in women. Hydroxyurea appears to reduce early thrombosis without either compromising survival or significantly increasing the rates of acute leukemia or post-polycythemic myelofibrosis. Interferon alfa and anagrelide effectively lower platelet counts in patients with polycythemia vera. Radioactive phosphorus 2.3 mCi/m^2 may be considered if life expectancy is less than 10 years or compliance is an issue.

Agnogenic Myeloid Metaplasia and Myelofibrosis

Ineffective hematopoiesis, bone marrow fibrosis, and extramedullary hematopoiesis are associated with agnogenic myeloid metaplasia. The primary growth factor implicated in the pathogenesis of bone marrow fibrosis is transforming growth factor-β (TGF-β).

The peripheral blood smear provides the first clue to the diagnosis by revealing a leukoerythroblastic blood picture (the presence of nucleated RBCs, immature granulocytes, and teardrop-shaped RBCs). The diagnosis is confirmed by a bone marrow biopsy. Cytogenetic studies are strongly recommended before making the diagnosis.

Approximately one fifth of patients may present with asymptomatic splenomegaly. Of the remainder, about half present with mild to moderate anemia and the other half with severe anemia and marked splenomegaly.

Causes of death include heart failure, infection, and leukemic transformation, the last occurring in approximately 10% of patients. Most patients experience progressive anemia requiring frequent RBC transfusions and massive hepatosplenomegaly associated with the hypercatabolic symptoms of profound fatigue, weight loss, night sweats, and low-grade fever. In addition, some patients may develop extramedullary hematopoiesis.

TREATMENT. Except for allogeneic bone marrow transplantation, current therapy is not curative, does not prevent leukemic transformation, and may not prolong life. As initial treatment of anemia, a combination of an androgen preparation and a corticosteroid is used. In patients who do not respond to androgen therapy, a therapeutic trial of EPO may benefit the occasional patient. Splenectomy is considered for patients with symptomatic splenomegaly.

For more information about this subject, see *Cecil Textbook of Medicine,* 21st edition. Philadelphia, W.B. Saunders Company, 2000. Chapter 174, Myeloproliferative Diseases, pages 935 to 941.

MYELODYSPLASTIC SYNDROME

Myelodysplastic syndrome (MDS) refers to a heterogeneous group of acquired bone marrow disorders characterized by dysplastic growth of hematopoietic progenitors, a hypercellular bone marrow with peripheral cytopenia, and propensity to progress to acute myelogenous leukemia (AML). De novo MDS occurs only rarely in young patients, but therapy-related MDS is increasingly recognized as a potentially fatal complication of chemotherapy and/or radiation therapy for other malignancies. MDS is a clonal disorder with an acquired somatic mutation that affects an early hematopoietic progenitor and gives rise to clonally derived neutrophils, RBCs, and platelets.

The clinical presentation of MDS is frequently referable to cytopenia in one or more hematopoietic cell lineages. In the geriatric population, patients may present with symptoms related to comorbid illnesses. Any patient with a mild cytopenia in the setting of infection should have follow-up blood cell counts to determine if the cytopenia persists after the infection has resolved. The clinical course is characterized by inexorably progressive pancytopenia. 11

Granulocytes are poorly granulated and may be hyposegmented. RBCs are usually hypochromic with polychromasia. Mild macrocytosis is a hallmark of MDS, with MCV in the range of 100 to 110 fL.

The evaluation of a patient with unexplained cytopenia should always include exclusion of congenital disorders associated with cytopenia, exclusion of vitamin deficiencies, and, in particular, the possibility that drugs may be contributory. A careful physical examination for evidence of hypersplenism should be part of the evaluation. Alcoholic patients may resemble patients with MDS. Some physicians will incorporate testing for autoimmune diseases. When the initial physical examination, laboratory evaluation, and removal of potentially causative drugs fail to disclose a cause for a cytopenia, bone marrow aspiration and biopsy with cytogenetic analysis should be performed.

No treatment has been shown to prolong survival of MDS patients except for allogeneic bone marrow transplantation (BMT). Supportive care remains the mainstay of therapy. It may be reasonable to consider a trial of EPO.

For more information about this subject, see *Cecil Textbook of Medicine,* 21st edition. Philadelphia, W.B. Saunders Company, 2000. Chapter 175, Myelodysplastic Syndrome, pages 941 to 944.

THE CHRONIC LEUKEMIAS

Chronic Myelogenous Leukemia

CML is a disease characterized by overproduction of cells of the granulocytic, especially the neutrophilic, series and occasionally the monocytic series, leading to marked splenomegaly and very high WBC counts. The Philadelphia (Ph^1) chromosome is present in the bone marrow cells in more than 95% of cases. The fusion *bcr/abl* gene can be found in many cases of typical CML in which no cytogenetic abnormality occurs.

CML is increasingly being diagnosed in asymptomatic patients owing to the use of hematologic studies in routine physical examinations or in evaluations of other illnesses. The symptoms of CML, which usually are non-specific, are caused by anemia, large spleen size, or an increased basal metabolic rate, but most patients are asymptomatic or only mildly symptomatic. The serum uric acid level is commonly elevated. Neutrophil function is usually normal or only modestly impaired. Headaches, bone pain, arthralgias, pain from splenic infarction, and fever are uncommon in the early stages of CML but become more common as the disease progresses. Leukostatic symptoms, such as dyspnea, drowsiness, loss of coordination, or confusion, which are due to sludging in the pulmonary or cerebral vessels, are uncommon in the benign (chronic) phase of CML despite WBC counts that may exceed 400,000/μL. Splenomegaly occurs in more than 60% of cases.

All patients eventually develop a variety of changes in the disease. Most frequently there is a "blast crisis," a clinical picture resembling that of acute leukemia. This change can be abrupt, but more frequently it is preceded by a increasing splenomegaly, hepatomegaly, and infiltration of nodes, skin, bones, or other tissues; the appearance of blast cells; development of anemia and/or thrombocytopenia; or fever, malaise, and weight loss. These features, termed the *accelerated phase* of CML, demand re-evaluation of the bone marrow. Criteria for accelerated phase are an increase in blast cells (>15%) or basophils (>20%) in the blood or bone marrow, thrombocytopenia (<100,000/μL), serious anemia (hemoglobin <7 g/dL); documented extramedullary leukemia, or development of clonal evolution. Blast crisis is diagnosed when 30% or more blast cells are present in the bone marrow and/or peripheral blood.

All patients with untreated CML have an elevated WBC count, ranging from 10,000/μL to more than $1 \times 10^6/\mu$L. The predominant cells are of the neutrophil series; eosinophils and basophils are commonly increased. The bone marrow is hypercellular.

Leukocyte alkaline phosphatase (LAP) scores are markedly decreased in 90% or more of patients. Extremely high serum cobalamin values (e.g., vitamin B_{12} levels >10 times normal) are common.

The diagnosis is not difficult. The standard diagnostic test remains the cytogenetic analysis: the presence of the Ph^1 chromosome. The greatest diagnostic difficulty lies with patients who have splenomegaly and leukocytosis but who do not have the Ph^1 chromosome. When the Ph^1 chromosome is not found, molecular evidence for the presence of the hybrid *bcr/abl* gene should be sought. The Ph^1 chromosome is usually present in 100% of metaphases. CML must be differentiated from leukemoid reactions and from other myelodysplastic or myeloproliferative syndromes.

TREATMENT. Treatment is not necessary unless the WBC count exceeds 200,000/μL or there is evidence of leukostasis or unless painful splenomegaly suggests splenic infarction. Hyperuricemia should be treated with allopurinol.

Hydroxyurea is the preferred oral agent given at dosages of

1 to 4 g/day. Both human leukocyte interferon and recombinant interferon alfa (rIFN-A) can produce hematologic and cytogenetic remissions. BMT has been performed in patients with benign-phase CML. Long-term survival rates after BMT for accelerated and blast phases of CML are only 10 to 15%. Molecularly targeted therapy with a *bcr/abl* tyrosine kinase inhibitor is proving to be highly effective in ongoing trials.

Loss of control of CML with agents such as busulfan, hydroxyurea, or interferon is a feature of the development of the accelerated phase of CML. The blast crisis, or refractory accelerated phase of CML, is usually treated with regimens designed for the treatment of acute leukemia.

Hairy Cell Leukemia

Hairy cell leukemia (HCL) is uncommon (1 to 2% of all leukemias). The cell of origin of HCL is the B lymphocyte. Patients have fatigue due to anemia, fever, weight loss, and/or abdominal discomfort produced by splenomegaly. Sometimes the disease is diagnosed when patients have infection secondary to granulocytopenia or monocytopenia. The only consistent physical findings are slight to marked splenomegaly. More than two thirds of patients have anemia, neutropenia, thrombocytopenia, and monocytopenia. The cytopenias are due to a combination of bone marrow production failure caused by leukemic infiltration and of hypersplenism.

The peripheral blood film usually demonstrates relative or absolute lymphocytosis, composed of cells with cytoplasmic projections. Bone marrow biopsy demonstrates increased cellularity with a diffuse or occasionally patchy infiltrate with hairy cells.

TREATMENT. 2-Chlorodeoxyadenosine (2-CDA) produces complete remissions in more than 90% of HCL patients; this drug is becoming established as the first therapy of choice in HCL. Human leukocyte interferon (hIFN) or rIFN-A rapidly improves (1 to 3 months) granulocyte, platelet, and hemoglobin levels; reduces spleen size; and consistently decreases marrow infiltration. Pentostatin responses appear to be more durable than those seen in interferon-treated patients.

Chronic Lymphocytic Leukemia

CLL is a neoplasm characterized by accumulation of monoclonal lymphocytes, usually of B-cell immunophenotype (>95% of cases) and more rarely of T-cell immunophenotype. Most patients with CLL are older than 60 years of age. CLL is an accumulative rather than a proliferative disease. Most of the CLL cells in the blood and bone marrow are in the G_0 phase of the cell cycle. T-cell function is invariably abnormal.

Most patients with CLL are asymptomatic, and the disease is diagnosed when absolute lymphocytosis is noted in the peripheral blood. Symptoms such as fatigue, lethargy, loss of appetite, weight loss, or reduced exercise tolerance are non-specific. Many patients have enlarged lymph nodes. Fever, night sweats, and documented infections become more prominent as the disease progresses.

Lymphadenopathy with discrete, rubbery, mobile lymph nodes is present in two thirds of patients at diagnosis. Less commonly, and usually late in the disease, clinically significant infiltration of the skin, eyelids, heart, lungs, pleura, or gastrointestinal tract may occur. Later in the disease, massive adenopathy may develop.

CLL is characterized by absolute lymphocytosis in the peripheral blood—a minimal level of more than 5000/μL, but more usually in the range of 40,000 to 150,000/μL. Most physicians also document lymphocytosis in the bone marrow (>30% lymphocytes) and perform a bone marrow biopsy. Anemia (hemoglobin <11 g/dL) is present in 15 to 20% of patients at diagnosis and thrombocytopenia (platelet count <100,000/μL) in 10%. Autoimmune hemolytic anemia occurs in the course of 8 to 10% of cases, and hypogammaglobulinemia is common.

Patients with anemia and thrombocytopenia have a poor prognosis, while patients with lymphocytosis alone have an excellent prognosis. A high incidence of second malignant tumors (10 to 20% of patients) either precedes or follows the diagnosis of CLL.

Many diseases can cause lymphocytosis but their clinical pictures seldom are confused with that of B-cell CLL. The more difficult differential diagnosis is from other lymphoproliferative disorders, such as prolymphocytic leukemia (PLL), splenic lymphoma with villous lymphocytes (SLVL), HCL, the leukemic phase of mantle cell lymphoma, Waldenström's macroglobulinemia, and T-cell CLL. Small lymphocytic lymphoma (SLL) shares histopathologic and immunophenotypic features with CLL, differing only in lacking absolute monoclonal lymphocytosis in the peripheral blood. Occasionally, other lymphomas, such as follicular small cleaved cell lymphoma (FSCCL) and mantle cell lymphoma, manifest in a leukemic phase.

TREATMENT. It is traditional to delay treatment of early-stage CLL until the disease progresses. Development of anemia, thrombocytopenia, or neutropenia associated with infections is usually an indication for systemic antileukemic therapy unless an autoimmune cause is found; in these cases, corticosteroids should be tried before cytotoxic therapy.

Chlorambucil (less commonly, cyclophosphamide) is traditionally the first chemotherapeutic agent used. Corticosteroids are often used concurrently, but with no clearly demonstrated advantage in therapeutic response or survival. Fludarabine monophosphate and 2-CDS, both adenosine analogues, and pentostatin have exhibited striking therapeutic efficacy in CLL. Intravenous immunoglobulin significantly decreases the incidence of infections of minor to moderate severity in CLL patients with hypogammaglobulinemia.

The median survival of patients with CLL is 4 to 5 years after initiation of treatment. No current treatment strategy has demonstrated a survival advantage over conventional therapy with chlorambucil.

For more information about this subject, see *Cecil Textbook of Medicine,* 21st edition. Philadelphia, W.B. Saunders Company, 2000. Chapter 176, The Chronic Leukemias, pages 944 to 953.

THE ACUTE LEUKEMIAS

In acute leukemia, immature myeloid cells (in acute myelogenous leukemia [AML]) or lymphoid cells (in ALL), often called blasts, rapidly accumulate and progressively replace the bone marrow. Diminished production of normal RBCs, WBCs, and platelets ensues. This loss of normal marrow function in turn gives rise to anemia, infection, and bleeding. With time, the leukemic blasts pour out into the blood stream and eventually occupy the lymph nodes, spleen, and other vital organs.

The relative incidences for the four categories of leukemia are ALL, 11%; CLL, 29%; AML, 46%; and CML, 14%. ALL is the most common cancer and the second leading cause of death in children younger than 15 years. The incidence of AML gradually increases with age. The most important distinction is between AML and ALL (Table 11–17).

In most cases of acute leukemia, an abnormality in chromosome number or structure is found. These abnormalities are clonal. In AML, the most frequent changes are a gain of chromosome 8 or loss of part or all of chromosome 7 or 5. The most common cytogenetic abnormality seen in adults with ALL is the Philadelphia (Ph^1) chromosome, a translocation that results in fusion of the *bcr* gene on chromosome 22 to the *abl* tyrosine kinase gene on chromosome 9. The *bcr/abl* fusion is associated with both ALL and CML.

Anemia is present at diagnosis in most patients. Thrombocytopenia is usually present, and approximately one third of patients have clinically evident bleeding at diagnosis. Most patients with acute leukemia are significantly granulocytopenic at diagnosis. 11

In general, ALL tends to infiltrate normal organs more than AML. Enlargement of lymph nodes, liver, and spleen is common.

Table 11–17 ■ CLASSIFICATION OF ACUTE LEUKEMIAS

SUBTYPE	MORPHOLOGY
Acute Myelogenous Leukemias	
Acute undifferentiated leukemia	Uniform, very undifferentiated
Acute myeloid leukemia with minimal differentiation	Very undifferentiated, few azurophilic granules
Acute myeloid leukemia with differentiation	Granulated blasts predominate; Auer rods may be seen
Acute promyelocytic leukemia	Hypergranular promyelocytes
Acute myelomonocytic leukemia	Both monoblasts and myeloblasts are present
Acute monocytic leukemia, types a and b	Monoblasts predominate Type a, >80% monoblasts; type b, >20% promonocytes
Acute erythroleukemia	Erythroblasts and megaloblastic red blood cell precursors seen
Acute megakaryocytic leukemia	Undifferentiated blasts
Acute Lymphocytic Leukemias	
Acute lymphocytic leukemia, childhood variant	Small, uniform blasts, nucleoli indistinct
Acute lymphocytic leukemia, adult variant	Larger, more irregular nucleoli present
Burkitt-like acute lymphoid leukemia	Large with strongly basophilic cytoplasm and vacuoles

Leukemic cells sometimes infiltrate the skin and leptomeninges. In AML, leukemic blast cells, often referred to as chloromas or myeloblastomas, can occur in virtually any soft tissue.

Although most patients are granulocytopenic at diagnosis, the total peripheral WBC count is more variable; approximately 25% of patients have very high WBC counts (>50,000/μL), approximately 50% have WBC counts between 5000 and 50,000, and about 25% have a low WBC count (<5000/μL). In most cases, blasts are present in the peripheral blood. The diagnosis of acute leukemia is generally established by marrow aspiration and biopsy, which are generally hypercellular and contain 30 to 100% blast cells.

Evidence of tumor lysis syndrome may be noted at diagnosis, including hypocalcemia, hyperkalemia, hyperphosphatemia, hyperuricemia, and renal insufficiency. This syndrome, which is more commonly seen shortly after therapy is begun, can be rapidly fatal if untreated.

TREATMENT OF ALL. To prevent uric acid nephropathy, patients should be hydrated and given allopurinol 100 to 200 mg orally three times per day. If leukostasis occurs in the central nervous system (CNS), leukapheresis, immediate whole-brain irradiation, and hydroxyurea are indicated.

Initial therapy for ALL can be divided into three phases: remission induction, post-remission (consolidation) therapy, and CNS prophylaxis. A number of different chemotherapeutic combinations can be used to induce remission; all include vincristine and prednisone, and most add L-asparaginase and/or daunorubicin. Consolidation chemotherapy refers to short courses of further chemotherapy given at doses similar to those used for initial induction and thus requiring rehospitalization. Drugs include high-dose methotrexate, cyclophosphamide, and cytarabine. Effective regimens for CNS prophylaxis include intrathecal methotrexate alone, intrathecal methotrexate combined with 2400 cGy to the cranium, or 2400 cGy to the craniospinal axis.

About 25 to 45% of adults who initially achieve complete remission maintain complete remission for more than 5 years, and thus these patients are probably cured. The use of high-dose chemoradiotherapy followed by marrow transplantation from an HLA-identical sibling can cure 20 to 40% of patients with ALL who fail to achieve an initial remission or who have a relapse after an initial complete remission.

TREATMENT OF AML. A combination of an anthracycline (daunomycin or idarubicin) and cytarabine leads to complete remission in 60 to 80% of patients with AML. Intensive consolidation chemotherapy, with repeated courses of daunomycin and cytarabine at conventional doses, high-dose cytarabine, or other agents prolongs remission and improves disease-free survival.

Among patients in whom complete remission is achieved, 20 to 40% remain alive in continuous complete remission for more than 5 years, thus suggesting probable cure. Remissions of recurrent AML tend to be short-lived. Complete remissions can be induced in at least 80% of patients with acute promyelocytic leukemia (APL) by using all-*trans*-retinoic acid.

For patients with AML in whom an initial remission cannot be achieved or for patients who have a relapse after chemotherapy, marrow transplantation from an HLA-identical sibling offers the best chance for cure. Currently, transplantation is the treatment of choice for patients with AML who have suffered an initial relapse, and it should be strongly considered for most patients while in first remission. Autologous transplantation offers an alternative for patients without matched siblings.

For more information about this subject, see *Cecil Textbook of Medicine,* 21st edition. Philadelphia, W.B. Saunders Company, 2000. Chapter 177, The Acute Leukemias, pages 953 to 958.

APPROACH TO THE PATIENT WITH LYMPHADENOPATHY AND SPLENOMEGALY

Lymphadenopathy

The differential diagnosis of lymphadenopathy (Table 11–18) is vast. In patients actually seen with lymphadenopathy in practices in the United States, diagnoses will not be determined in a high proportion of patients. The occurrence of fever, sweats, or weight loss raises the possibility of a malignancy of the immune system. The particular sites of involvement can be important hints to the diagnosis inasmuch as infections and carcinomas are likely to cause lymphadenopathy in the lymphatic drainage of the site of the disorder. Lymph nodes that are tender are more likely to be due to an infectious process, whereas painless adenopathy raises the concern of malignancy. Typically, lymph nodes containing metastatic carcinoma are rock-hard, lymph nodes containing lymphoma are firm and rubbery, and lymph nodes enlarged in response to an infectious process are soft. The larger the lymph node, the more likely a serious underlying cause exists, and lymph nodes greater than 3 to 4 cm in diameter in an adult are of great concern.

Table 11–18 ■ CAUSES OF LYMPHADENOPATHY

Infection
- Bacterial (e.g., all pyogenic bacteria, cat-scratch disease, syphilis, tularemia)
- Mycobacterial (e.g., tuberculosis, leprosy)
- Fungal (e.g., histoplasmosis, coccidioidomycosis)
- Chlamydial (e.g., lymphogranuloma venereum)
- Parasitic (e.g., toxoplasmosis, trypanosomiasis, filariasis)
- Viral (e.g., Epstein-Barr virus, cytomegalovirus, rubella, hepatitis, HIV)

Benign disorders of the immune system (e.g., rheumatoid arthritis, systemic lupus erythematosus, serum sickness, drug reactions such as to phenytoin, Castleman's disease, sinus histiocytosis with massive lymphadenopathy, Langerhans' cell histiocytosis, Kawasaki syndrome, Kimura's disease)

Malignant disorders of the immune system (e.g., chronic and acute myeloid and lymphoid leukemia, non-Hodgkin's lymphoma, Hodgkin's disease, angioimmunoblastic-like T-cell lymphoma, Waldenström's macroglobulinemia, multiple myeloma with amyloidosis, malignant histiocytosis)

Other malignancies (e.g., breast carcinoma, lung carcinoma, melanoma, head and neck cancer, gastrointestinal malignancies, germ cell tumors, Kaposi's sarcoma)

Storage diseases (e.g., Gaucher's disease, Niemann-Pick disease)

Endocrinopathies (e.g., hyperthyroidism, adrenal insufficiency, thyroiditis)

Miscellaneous (e.g., sarcoidosis, amyloidosis, dermatopathic lymphadenitis)

CT provides an accurate assessment of lymph nodes. Lymph node aspiration or excisional biopsy is often necessary for an accurate diagnosis of the cause of the lymphadenopathy.

The approach to a patient complaining of newly discovered lymphadenopathy in the neck, axilla, or groin will depend on the size, consistency, and number of enlarged lymph nodes and the patient's general health. In general, very large or very firm lymph nodes in the presence of systemic symptoms such as unexplained fever, sweats, or weight loss should lead to a lymph node biopsy. For cervical lymph nodes in a patient with suspected head and neck cancer, excisional biopsy should be delayed until a full ear, nose, and throat examination has been performed (see pages 793 to 796).

For the most common situation, in which a lymph node is soft, not larger than 2 to 3 cm, and the patient has no obvious systemic illness, observation for a brief period is usually the best approach. Performance of a complete blood count and examination of a peripheral smear can be helpful in recognizing a systemic illness (e.g., infectious mononucleosis). These patients are often also given antibiotics. If the lymph node does not regress over the course of a few weeks or if it grows in size, a biopsy should be performed.

Splenomegaly

Conditions associated with splenomegaly are extremely numerous (Table 11–19). Splenic hyperfunction (i.e., a condition often referred to as hypersplenism) is associated with cytopenias.

Ultrasonography (US) can provide accurate determination of splenic size and is easy to repeat. CT will frequently give a better view of the consistency of the spleen and can identify splenic

Table 11–19 ■ CAUSES OF SPLENOMEGALY

Infection
- Bacterial (e.g., endocarditis, brucellosis, syphilis, typhoid, pyogenic abscess)
- Mycobacterial (e.g., tuberculosis)
- Fungal (e.g., histoplasmosis)
- Parasitic (e.g., malaria, toxoplasmosis, leishmaniasis)
- Rickettsial (e.g., Rocky Mountain spotted fever)
- Viral (e.g., Epstein-Barr virus, cytomegalovirus, HIV, hepatitis)

Benign disorders of the immune system (e.g., rheumatoid arthritis with Felty's syndrome, systemic lupus erythematosus, drug reactions such as to phenytoin, Langerhans' cell histiocytosis, serum sickness)

Malignant disorders of the immune system (e.g., acute or chronic myeloid or lymphoid leukemia, non-Hodgkin's lymphoma, Hodgkin's disease, Waldeström's macroglobulinemia, angioimmunoblastic-like T-cell lymphoma, malignant histiocytosis)

Other malignancies (e.g., melanoma, sarcoma)

Congestive splenomegaly (e.g., portal hypertension secondary to liver disease, splenic or portal vein thrombosis)

Hematologic disorders (e.g., autoimmune hemolytic anemia, hereditary spherocytosis, thalassemia major, hemoglobinopathies, elliptocytosis, megaloblastic anemia, extramedullary hematopoiesis)

Storage diseases (e.g., Gaucher's disease)

Endocrinopathies (e.g., hyperthyroidism)

Miscellaneous (e.g., sarcoidosis, amyloidosis, tropical splenomegaly, cysts)

Table 11–20 ■ AN APPROACH TO THE PATIENT WITH SPLENOMEGALY

1. Does the patient have a known illness that causes splenomegaly (e.g., infectious mononucleosis)? Treat and monitor for resolution.
2. Search for an occult infection (e.g., infectious endocarditis), hematologic disorder (e.g., hereditary spherocytosis), occult liver disease (e.g., cryptogenic cirrhosis), autoimmune disease (e.g., systemic lupus erythematosus), or storage disease (e.g., Gaucher's disease). If found, manage appropriately.
3. If systemic symptoms are present and suggest malignancy and/or focal replacement of the spleen is seen on imaging studies and no other site is available for biopsy, splenectomy is indicated.
4. If none of the above are true, monitor closely and repeat studies until the splenomegaly resolves or a diagnosis becomes apparent.

tumors or abscesses. In general, a splenic "biopsy" involves splenectomy. The approach to a patient with an enlarged spleen should focus initially on excluding a systemic illness that could explain the splenomegaly (Table 11–20).

For more information about this subject, see *Cecil Textbook of Medicine,* 21st edition. Philadelphia, W.B. Saunders Company, 2000. Chapter 178, Approach to the Patient with Lymphadenopathy and Splenomegaly, pages 958 to 962.

NON-HODGKIN'S LYMPHOMAS

The non-Hodgkin's lymphomas (NHLs) include over 20 discrete entities (Table 11–21).

B-Cell Chronic Lymphocytic Leukemia and Small Lymphocytic Lymphoma

Over 90% of B-cell chronic lymphocytic leukemias (B-CLLs) and small lymphocytic lymphomas (SLLs) are manifested as chronic lymphoid leukemias. Patients are typically older adults with bone marrow and peripheral blood involvement at diagnosis. Generalized lymphadenopathy, hepatosplenomegaly, and extranodal infiltrates may occur. Patients often have hypogammaglobulinemia, associated infectious complications, and autoimmune phenomena such as hemolytic anemia or thrombocytopenia.

Extranodal Marginal Zone B-Cell Lymphoma (Low-Grade B-Cell MALT Lymphoma)

The majority of low-grade gastric lymphomas and almost 50% of all gastric lymphoid neoplasms are MALT (mucosa-associated lymphoid tissue) lymphomas. Forty per cent of orbital lymphomas and the majority of indolent pulmonary, thyroid, and salivary gland B-cell malignancies are also MALT lymphomas. Recent studies suggest that therapy directed at the antigen (*Helicobacter pylori* in gastric lymphoma) may eliminate early lesions.

Follicular Lymphoma

Follicular lymphomas are composed of mixtures of small cleaved and large non-cleaved follicle center cells. Approximately 60% of

Table 11–21 ■ WORLD HEALTH ORGANIZATION CLASSIFICATION OF NEOPLASTIC DISEASES OF THE HEMATOPOIETIC AND LYMPHOID TISSUES: LYMPHOID NEOPLASMS

B-Cell Neoplasms

*Precursor B-cell lymphoblastic leukemia/lymphoma**
Mature B-cell neoplasms
- B-cell chronic lymphocytic leukemia/small lymphocytic lymphoma
- B-cell prolymphocytic leukemia
- Lymphoplasmacytic lymphoma
- Splenic marginal zone B-cell lymphoma
- Hairy cell leukemia
- Extranodal marginal zone B-cell lymphoma of the mucosa-associated lymphoid tissue type
- Mantle cell lymphoma
- Follicular lymphoma
- Nodal marginal zone lymphoma with or without monocytoid B cells
- Diffuse large B-cell lymphoma
- Burkitt's lymphoma
- Plasmacytoma
- Plasma cell myeloma

T-Cell Neoplasms

Precursor T-cell lymphoblastic lymphoma/leukemia
Mature T-cell and NK cell neoplasms
- T-cell prolymphocytic leukemia
- T-cell large granular lymphocytic leukemia
- NK cell leukemia
- Extranodal NK/T-cell lymphoma, nasal and nasal type
- Mycosis fungoides/Sézary syndrome
- Primary cutaneous anaplastic large cell lymphoma
- Subcutaneous panniculitis-like T-cell lymphoma
- Enteropathy-type intestinal T-cell lymphoma
- Hepatosplenic γ/δ T-cell lymphoma
- Angioimmunoblastic T-cell lymphoma
- Peripheral T-cell lymphoma (unspecified)
- Anaplastic large cell lymphoma, primary systemic type
- Adult T-cell lymphoma/leukemia (HTLV-1)

NK = natural killer; HTLV = human T-cell leukemia virus.
*The most common B- and T-cell malignancies are in italics.
Modified from Jaffe E, Bernard C, Harris N, et al: Proposed World Health Organization classification of neoplastic diseases of hematopoietic and lymphoid tissues. Am J Surg Pathol 21:114, 1997.

tumors are CD10+. Over 75 to 80% of indolent B-cell lymphomas are follicular lymphomas. These lymphomas are primarily diseases of older adults, who often have widespread nodal disease, as well as splenic and bone marrow involvement. Although the clinical course is usually indolent, follicular lymphomas are not curable with currently available standard therapy.

Mantle Cell Lymphoma

Most cases of mantle cell lymphoma are composed exclusively of small to medium-sized lymphoid cells with slightly irregular or "cleaved" nuclei. In contrast to follicular lymphoma, mantle cell lymphoma is usually CD10− and CD43+. Patients usually have widespread disease involving the lymph nodes, spleen, Waldeyer's ring, and extranodal sites, including bone marrow, blood, and the gastrointestinal tract.

Diffuse Large B-Cell Lymphoma

Diffuse large B-cell lymphomas are composed of large cells that resemble centroblasts or immunoblasts. The *bcl*-2 gene is rearranged in about 30% of diffuse large B-cell lymphomas. Over 30% of adult NHLs are diffuse large B-cell lymphomas. Patients often have single or multiple, rapidly enlarging symptomatic masses in nodal or extranodal sites. Primary diffuse large B-cell lymphomas are aggressive but potentially curable with intensive therapy.

Anaplastic Large Cell Lymphoma

Most anaplastic large cell lymphomas are manifested as systemic diseases involving the lymph nodes and/or extranodal disease sites. Whereas primary cutaneous anaplastic large cell lymphoma is very indolent, the systemic form behaves similarly to diffuse large B-cell lymphoma and may be cured with intensive therapy.

Precursor B-Cell Lymphoblastic Leukemia

Although the vast majority of cases of B-cell lymphoblastic leukemia and lymphoma are manifested as acute leukemias with bone marrow and peripheral blood involvement, a small proportion are solid tumors involving the skin, bone, and lymph nodes.

Burkitt's Lymphoma

Burkitt's lymphoma is most common in children. The majority of non-African Burkitt's lymphomas occur in the abdomen.

Peripheral T-Cell Lymphomas

Peripheral T-cell lymphomas represent fewer than 10% of all NHLs. Patients with peripheral T-cell lymphoma are usually initially seen with disseminated disease and occasional eosinophilia, pruritus, or hemophagocytic syndromes. Although the clinical course is usually aggressive, these diseases are potentially curable with combination chemotherapy.

The clinical entities of mycosis fungoides and Sézary syndrome are now recognized as different clinical manifestations of cutaneous T-cell lymphomas. The classic mycosis fungoides manifestation of cutaneous T-cell lymphoma begins with an erythematous macular eruption in sun-shielded areas; these lesions eventually become more palpable and subsequently develop into frank tumors.

Precursor T-Cell Lymphoblastic Lymphoma/Leukemia

Patients with T-cell lymphoblastic lymphoma/leukemia typically have mediastinal (thymic) masses and/or peripheral lymphadenopathy; CNS involvement is common. Patients with adult T-cell lymphoma leukemia are usually adults with detectable human T-cell lymphotropic virus, type 1 (HTLV-1) antibodies. Patients with "acute" adult T-cell lymphoma/leukemia have a high WBC count,

Table 11–22 ■ ANN ARBOR STAGING SYSTEM

Stage I	Involvement of a single lymph node region (I) or a single extralymphatic organ or site (IE)
Stage II	Involvement of two or more lymph node regions on the same side of the diaphragm (II) or localized involvement of an extralymphatic organ or site (IIE)
Stage III	Involvement of lymph node regions on both sides of the diaphragm (III) or localized involvement of an extra-lymphatic organ or site (IIIE), the spleen (IIIS), or both (IIISE)
Stage IV	Diffuse or disseminated involvement of one or more extra-lymphatic organs with or without associated lymph node involvement

Identification of the presence or absence of symptoms should be noted with each stage designation. A = asymptomatic; B = fever, sweats, weight loss greater than 10% of body weight.

hepatosplenomegaly, hypercalcemia, and lytic bone lesions; survival is often only a few months.

Staging Systems

Patients with NHL are currently staged with the Ann Arbor classification (Table 11–22). A widely accepted prognostic factor model for patients with aggressive NHLs uses the age, serum lactate dehydrogenase, performance status, stage, and number of extranodal disease sites (Table 11–23).

The initial history should include the duration and rate of lymph node enlargement; the presence or absence of fever, night sweats, and/or unexplained weight loss (B symptoms); and the presence or absence of symptoms that might indicate extranodal involvement. The size of the liver and spleen should be noted. Elevation of liver enzymes, bilirubin, and alkaline phosphatase may be signs of liver involvement.

In patients with abnormal chest radiographs, thoracic CT scans provide important additional information regarding the extent of disease. Abdominal-pelvic CT scans are recommended for evaluat-

Table 11–23 ■ THE INTERNATIONAL PROGNOSTIC INDEX FOR NON-HODGKIN'S LYMPHOMA

RISK GROUP (PATIENTS OF ALL AGES)	RISK FACTORS*	DISTRIBUTION OF CASES(%)	COMPLETE RESPONSE RATE (%)	5-YEAR SURVIVAL RATE (%)
Low	0.1	35	87	73
Low–intermediate	2	27	67	51
High–intermediate	3	22	55	43
High	4–5	16	44	26

*Age (≤60 versus >60 years); serum lactate dehydrogenase (normal versus >1× normal); performance status (0 or 1 versus 2 to 4); stage (I or II versus III or IV); and extranodal involvement (≤1 site versus >1 site).

Modified from Shipp M, Harrington DP, Anderson J, et al: International non-Hodgkin's lymphoma prognostic factors project: A predictive model for aggressive non-Hodgkin's lymphoma. N Engl J Med 329:987, 1993.

ing mesenteric and retroperitoneal disease. Gallium-67 scans are positive in nearly all aggressive lymphomas and in approximately 50% of indolent lymphomas at diagnosis. Unilateral bone marrow biopsies should be performed as part of the initial staging evaluation.

Treatment

B-CELL SMALL LYMPHOCYTIC LYMPHOMA AND CHRONIC LYMPHOCYTIC LEUKEMIA. Therapeutic approaches are discussed under The Chronic Leukemias (pages 367 to 370).

FOLLICULAR LYMPHOMA, GRADES 1 AND 2. Only 15% of patients with follicular lymphoma are initially seen with stage I or II disease. A number of studies have demonstrated the efficacy of directed radiation therapy in this setting. The optimal treatment strategy for advanced-stage (III–IV) patients remains to be determined. Patients can be treated conservatively with an approach that includes no initial treatment, followed by palliative single-agent (e.g., chlorambucil) or combination chemotherapy (e.g., cyclophosphamide, vincristine, and prednisone) or involved-field radiotherapy as needed. Alternatively, patients may be treated aggressively with initial combination chemotherapy (e.g., cyclophosphamide, doxorubicin [hydroxydaunomycin] vincristine [Oncovin], and prednisone [CHOP] or fludarabine-containing regimens) and/or radiation therapy. Rituximab, a chimeric monoclonal antibody targeting the CD20 antigen on B lymphocytes, is effective for relapsed, low-grade or follicular non–Hodgkin's lymphoma; it can also be used as initial systemic therapy for these patients.

FOLLICULAR LYMPHOMA, GRADE 3. The current approach to treatment of this disease is similar to that for diffuse large B-cell lymphoma. High-dose chemotherapy with or without total-body irradiation, followed by autologous bone marrow transplantation, has also been used as consolidation therapy for patients with recurrent follicular lymphoma and high-risk newly diagnosed follicular lymphoma.

MANTLE CELL LYMPHOMA. Mantle cell lymphoma has a pattern of continued relapse despite combination chemotherapy (e.g., cyclophosphamide, vincristine, and prednisone or CHOP).

DIFFUSE LARGE B-CELL, ANAPLASTIC, BURKITT'S, AND PERIPHERAL T-CELL LYMPHOMAS. Patients with localized disease are commonly treated with anthracycline-containing combination chemotherapy (e.g., CHOP). Salvage regimens typically incorporate drugs that were not used in the first-line induction therapy. Burkitt's and Burkitt's-like variant lymphomas are currently treated in the same way. Aggressive treatment with CHOP or other similar regimens may significantly improve survival in patients who have HIV-associated lymphoma.

For more information about this subject, see *Cecil Textbook of Medicine,* 21st edition. Philadelphia, W.B. Saunders Company, 2000. Chapter 179, Non-Hodgkin's Lymphomas, pages 962 to 969.

HODGKIN'S DISEASE

Hodgkin's disease has four histologic subtypes. The Reed-Sternberg cell is the diagnostic tumor cell. Nodular sclerosing Hodgkin's disease is the most common subtype and typically affects young females with early-stage supradiaphragmatic presentations. Mixed-cellularity Hodgkin's disease usually presents as generalized lymphadenopathy or as disease in extranodal sites, and produces associated systemic symptoms. Lymphocyte-predominant Hodgkin's disease is a rare form in which few Reed-Sternberg cells may be identified.

Lymphocyte-depletion Hodgkin's disease is a rare disorder. By the time of diagnosis, affected patients usually have advanced-stage disease, extranodal involvement, an aggressive clinical course, and poor prognosis.

Differential Diagnosis

More than 80% of patients present with lymphadenopathy above the diaphragm, often involving the anterior mediastinum; fewer than 10 to 20% present with lymphadenopathy limited to regions below the diaphragm. Unlike aggressive NHLs or other neoplasms, Hodgkin's disease rarely causes superior vena cava obstruction, phrenic nerve involvement with diaphragmatic paralysis, or laryngeal nerve compression and hoarseness. Cervical, supraclavicular, axillary, or, uncommonly, inguinal lymphadenopathy may be the initial complaint. Disseminated lymphadenopathy is infrequent. When present, it is usually associated with systemic symptoms. Isolated extranodal presentations (e.g., cutaneous nodules or gastric involvement) without nodal involvement usually denote an NHL.

In each anatomic stage (Table 11–24), the presence of B symptoms is an adverse prognostic indicator. *Unexplained fever* is defined as recurrent temperatures above 38° C during the previous month, night sweats are considered present if they are drenching and recurrent, and unexplained weight loss is significant only if at least 10% of body weight is lost within the preceding 6 months.

Table 11–24 ■ THE COTSWOLDS STAGING CLASSIFICATION FOR HODGKIN'S DISEASE

Stage I	Involvement of a single lymph node region or a lymphoid structure (e.g., spleen, thymus, Waldeyer's ring)
Stage II	Involvement of two or more lymph node regions on the same side of the diaphragm (i.e., the mediastinum is a single site, hilar lymph nodes are lateralized); the number of anatomic sites should be indicated by a subscript (e.g., II_2)
Stage III	Involvement of lymph node regions or structures on both sides of the diaphragm:
	III_1: With or without involvement of splenic, hilar, celiac, or portal nodes
	III_2: With involvement of para-aortic, iliac, or mesenteric nodes
Stage IV	Involvement of extranodal site(s) beyond that designated E

Designations applicable to any disease stage

A: No symptoms
B: Fever, drenching sweats, weight loss
X: Bulky disease:
  >⅓ the width of the mediastinum
  >10 cm maximal dimension of nodal mass
E: Involvement of a single extranodal site, contiguous or proximal to a known nodal site
CS: Clinical stage
PS: Pathologic stage

The initial laboratory studies should include a complete blood cell count with WBC differential and platelet count, an erythrocyte sedimentation rate (ESR), tests for liver and renal function, and assays for serum alkaline phosphatase and lactate dehydrogenase. Abnormalities of liver function studies should prompt further evaluation of that organ, with imaging and possible biopsy.

Radiologic studies should include a chest radiograph and CT scan of the chest, abdomen, and pelvis with intravenous contrast medium enhancement. Because chest CT scans may remain abnormal long after completion of therapy, a gallium scan assists in the evaluation of pretreatment involvement and response to therapy.

Unilateral iliac crest bone marrow biopsy should be part of the staging process. Laparotomy is not a routine staging procedure and should be considered only if the additional information may alter the choice of treatment.

Treatment

Radiation therapy and combination chemotherapy have resulted in the cure of more than 75% of all newly diagnosed patients with Hodgkin's disease. Radiation remains the gold standard for the management of most patients with early-stage disease, with a 15- to 20-year survival of nearly 90% and a relapse-free survival rate of 75 to 80%.

Early-stage patients with bulky mediastinal disease and significant B symptoms or clinically staged patients at high risk for subdiaphragmatic involvement attain better relapse-free survival rates with combined-modality therapy including chemotherapy with MOPP (mechlorethamine, vincristine [Oncovin], procarbazine, and prednisone) or ABVD (doxorubicin [Adriamycin], bleomycin, vinblastine, and dacarbazine). Six weeks to 3 months after mantle radiation therapy, approximately 15% of patients develop an electric shock sensation radiating down the backs of both legs when the head is flexed. Radiation pneumonitis and/or acute pericarditis may occur in fewer than 5% of patients. Later, mantle field radiation therapy can induce subclinical hypothyroidism. Thyroid replacement is recommended, even for asymptomatic patients. An increase in the risk of coronary artery disease has been reported for patients who have received mediastinal irradiation.

The mainstay of treatment in advanced Hodgkin's disease (stages IIIB and IV) is combination chemotherapy. ABVD is now considered the preferred drug combination in Hodgkin's disease treatment because it is at least equally effective and avoids exposure to the toxic drugs in MOPP. Results reveal a complete response rate of approximately 80%, a disease-free survival of complete responders of 50 to 60%, and an overall survival of 40 to 50%. Side effects include nausea and vomiting; pulmonary toxicity (bleomycin); vinblastine-associated peripheral autonomic neuropathy; and symptomatic phlebitis.

For patients who relapse after radiation therapy, combination chemotherapy such as ABVD is the treatment of choice. High-dose chemotherapy accompanied by autologous stem cell transplantation has become the preferred choice in patients who fail to attain a complete response with chemotherapy or who relapse early after completion of combination chemotherapy.

For more information about this subject, see *Cecil Textbook of Medicine,* 21st edition. Philadelphia, W.B. Saunders Company, 2000. Chapter 180, Hodgkin's Disease, pages 969 to 977.

PLASMA CELL DISORDERS

The plasma cell disorders (including monoclonal gammopathies, immunoglobulinopathies, paraproteinemias, and dysproteinemias) are a group of neoplastic or potentially neoplastic diseases associated with proliferation of a single clone of immunoglobulin-secreting plasma cells derived from the B-cell series of immunocytes. Each monoclonal protein (M protein, myeloma protein, or paraprotein) consists of two heavy (H) polypeptide chains of the same class and subclass and two light (L) polypeptide chains of the same type. The heavy polypeptide chains are designated by Greek letters: γ in immunoglobulin G (IgG), α in immunoglobulin A (IgA), μ in immunoglobulin M (IgM), δ in immunoglobulin D (IgD), and ϵ in immunoglobulin E (IgE). The light-chain types are kappa (κ) and lambda (λ). The presence of an M protein is most suggestive of monoclonal gammopathy of undetermined significance (MGUS), multiple myeloma, primary amyloidosis, Waldenström's macroglobulinemia, or other lymphoproliferative disease. Serum protein electrophoresis should be done when multiple myeloma or Waldenström's macroglobulinemia is suspected.

Monoclonal Gammopathy of Undetermined Significance

MGUS is characterized by a serum M-protein concentration of less than 3 g/dL; fewer than 5% plasma cells in the bone marrow; no or only small amounts of M protein in the urine; absence of lytic bone lesions, anemia, hypercalcemia, and renal insufficiency; and, most important, the stability of the amount of the M protein and the failure of other abnormalities to develop. The prevalence of MGUS is 1% of patients older than 50 years and 3% of those older than 70 years.

Approximately one fourth of patients develop multiple myeloma (18%), macroglobulinemia (3%), amyloidosis (3%), or related disorders (2%), with an actuarial rate of 16% at 10 years, 33% at 20 years, and 40% at 25 years. No technique reliably differentiates a patient with a benign monoclonal gammopathy from one who will subsequently have symptomatic multiple myeloma or other malignant disease. In general, the serum electrophoresis should be repeated at 3 to 6 months; if it is stable, it should be checked annually.

ASSOCIATION OF MONOCLONAL GAMMOPATHIES WITH OTHER DISEASES. An M protein is found in 3 to 4% of patients with a diffuse lymphoproliferative process but in fewer than 1% of those with a nodular lymphoma. Approximately 5% of patients with sensorimotor peripheral neuropathy of unknown cause have an associated monoclonal gammopathy. In half of those with an IgM monoclonal gammopathy and peripheral neuropathy, the M protein binds to myelin-associated glycoprotein. These patients have a slowly progressive sensorimotor neuropathy beginning in the distal extremities and extending proximally.

Multiple Myeloma

Multiple myeloma is characterized by the neoplastic proliferation of a single clone of plasma cells engaged in the production of a monoclonal immunoglobulin. This clone proliferates in the bone marrow and frequently invades the adjacent bone, producing extensive skeletal destruction that results in bone pain and fractures. Anemia, hypercalcemia, and renal insufficiency are other important features (Table 11–25). The median age at the time of diagnosis is about 65 years; only 2% of patients are younger than 40.

A normocytic, normochromic anemia is present initially in two thirds of patients but eventually occurs in nearly every patient. The serum protein electrophoretic pattern shows a peak or localized band in 80% of patients, hypogammaglobulinemia in almost 10%, and no apparent abnormality in the remainder. The urine reveals an M protein in approximately 75% of patients. In the bone marrow, plasma cells usually account for 10% or more of all nucleated cells. Conventional radiographs reveal abnormalities consisting of punched-out lytic lesions, osteoporosis, or fractures in 75% of patients.

Minimal criteria for the diagnosis are bone marrow containing more than 10% plasma cells or a plasmacytoma plus at least one of the following: (1) M protein in the serum (usually >3 g/dL), (2) M protein in the urine, and (3) lytic bone lesions. **11**

Myeloma kidney is characterized by the presence of large waxy laminated casts in the distal and collecting tubules. Hypercalcemia, which is present in 25% of patients, results from destruction of bone. Amyloidosis occurs in 10 to 15% of patients and may produce nephrotic syndrome or renal insufficiency or both. Radiculopathy, the single most frequent neurologic complication, is usually in the thoracic or lumbosacral area and results from compression of the nerve by the vertebral lesion or by the collapsed bone itself. Compression of the spinal cord occurs in up to 10% of patients. Propensity to infection results from impairment of antibody response, deficiency of normal immunoglobulins, and neutropenia. Bleeding may occur from coating of the platelets by the M protein.

TREATMENT. Patients with MGUS should not be treated. Indications for therapy include significant anemia, hypercalcemia, or

Table 11–25 ■ CLINICAL MANIFESTATIONS OF MULTIPLE MYELOMA

Skeletal involvement: pain, reduced height, pathologic fractures, hypercalcemia
Anemia: due mainly to decreased erythropoiesis; produces weakness and fatigue
Renal insufficiency: mainly due to "myeloma kidney" from light chains or hypercalcemia; rarely from amyloidosis
Recurrent infections: respiratory and urinary tract infections or septicemia due to gram-positive or gram-negative organisms
Bleeding diathesis: from thrombocytopenia or coating of platelets with M protein
Amyloidosis: develops in 10–15%
Extramedullary plasmacytomas: occur late in the disease
Cryoglobulinemia type I: rarely symptomatic

renal insufficiency; lytic bone lesions; and extramedullary plasmacytomas.

Chemotherapy is the preferred initial treatment for overt, symptomatic multiple myeloma in patients older than 70 years or in younger patients in whom transplantation is not feasible. The oral administration of melphalan and prednisone produces objective response in 50 to 60% of patients. Palliative radiation should be limited to a well-defined focal process that has not responded to chemotherapy.

If the patient is younger than 65 to 70 years, the physician should discuss the possibility of autologous peripheral blood stem cell transplantation, ideally as part of a prospective study. Autologous transplantation should not be performed if the patient has received long-term chemotherapy and has refractory multiple myeloma. Thalidomide can produce durable responses in patients who relapse after high-dose chemotherapy.

PROGNOSIS. Multiple myeloma has a progressive course, and almost all patients with multiple myeloma will eventually relapse. The median survival is approximately 3 years. Twenty to 30 per cent of patients survive 5 or more years, but fewer than 5% survive longer than 10 years.

Variant Forms of Multiple Myeloma

Patients with *plasma cell leukemia* have greater than 20% plasma cells in the peripheral blood and an absolute plasma cell count of at least 2000/μL. Treatment of plasma cell leukemia is unsatisfactory.

Patients with *non-secretory myeloma* have no M protein in either the serum or the urine and account for only 1% of those with myeloma. Response to therapy and survival are similar to those in patients with an M-protein-component.

Osteosclerotic myeloma (POEMS syndrome) is characterized by *p*olyneuropathy, *o*rganomegaly, *e*ndocrinopathy, *M* protein, and *s*kin changes (POEMS). The major clinical features are a chronic inflammatory-demyelinating polyneuropathy with predominantly motor disability and sclerotic skeletal lesions. Evidence of Castleman's disease may be found. Radiation therapy will produce substantial improvement of the neuropathy in more than half of the patients.

The diagnosis of *solitary plasmacytoma* of bone is based on histologic evidence of a tumor consisting of monoclonal plasma cells identical to those seen in multiple myeloma. Almost 50% of patients with solitary plasmacytoma are alive at 10 years.

Extramedullary plasmacytoma is a plasma cell tumor that arises outside the bone marrow. Treatment consists of tumoricidal irradiation.

Waldenström's Macroglobulinemia

Waldenström's macroglobulinemia is the result of an uncontrolled proliferation of lymphocytes and plasma cells in which a large IgM M protein is produced. The median age at the time of diagnosis is about 65 years.

Weakness, fatigue, and bleeding (especially oozing from the oronasal area) are common presenting symptoms. Blurred or impaired vision, dyspnea, loss of weight, neurologic symptoms, recurrent infections, and heart failure may occur. In contrast to multiple myeloma, lytic bone lesions, renal insufficiency, and amyloidosis are rare. Retinal hemorrhages, exudates, and venous congestion with vascular segmentation may occur. Sensorimotor peripheral neuropathy is common.

Almost all patients have moderate to severe normocytic, normochromic anemia. The bone marrow aspirate is often hypocellular, but the biopsy is hypercellular and extensively infiltrated with lymphoid cells and plasma cells. Rouleaux formation is prominent, and the ESR is markedly increased. About 10% of macroglobulins have cryoproperties.

The combination of typical symptoms and physical findings, the presence of a large IgM M protein (usually >3 g/dL), and lymphoid–plasma cell infiltration of the bone marrow provide the diagnosis.

Patients should not be treated unless they have anemia, constitutional symptoms, hyperviscosity, or significant hepatosplenomegaly or lymphadenopathy. Chlorambucil is usually given orally. Combinations of alkylating agents may be beneficial. Patients with symptomatic hyperviscosity should be treated with plasmapheresis.

Heavy-Chain Diseases

The heavy-chain diseases (HCDs) are characterized by the presence of an M protein consisting of a portion of the immunoglobulin heavy chain in the serum or urine or both. Patients with γ-HCD often present with a lymphoma-like illness, but the clinical findings are diverse and range from an aggressive lymphoproliferative process to an asymptomatic state. Treatment is indicated only for symptomatic patients.

α-HCD occurs in patients from the Mediterranean region or Middle East. Most commonly, the gastrointestinal tract is involved, resulting in severe malabsorption with diarrhea, steatorrhea, and loss of weight. It may respond to melphalan or to cyclophosphamide and prednisone. Antibiotics such as tetracycline may also produce a remission.

μ-HCD may present with chronic lymphocytic leukemia or lymphoma. Treatment with corticosteroids and alkylating agents has produced some benefit.

Cryoglobulinemia

Cryoglobulins precipitate when cooled and dissolve when heated. They are designated as idiopathic or essential when they are not associated with any recognizable disease.

Type I (monoclonal) cryoglobulinemia is most commonly of the IgM or IgG class associated with macroglobulinemia, multiple myeloma, or MGUS. Most patients are completely asymptomatic. Others with monoclonal cryoglobulins in the range of 1 to 2 g/dL may have pain, purpura, Raynaud's phenomenon, cyanosis, and even ulceration.

Type II (mixed) cryoglobulinemia typically consists of an IgM M protein and polyclonal IgG. Vasculitis, glomerulonephritis, lymphoproliferative disease, and chronic infectious processes are common. Purpura and polyarthralgias are frequently seen. Nephrotic syndrome may result. Hepatic dysfunction and serologic evidence of infection with hepatitis C virus are common.

Type III (polyclonal) cryoglobulins are also found in many patients with infections or inflammatory diseases. They are of no clinical significance.

Primary Amyloidosis

The median age at diagnosis of primary amyloidosis is 64 years, and only 1% of patients are younger than 40 years old (Table 11–26). Weakness or fatigue and loss of weight are the most frequent symptoms. Dyspnea, pedal edema, paresthesias, lightheadedness, and syncope are frequently seen. The liver is palpable in one fourth of patients, but splenomegaly occurs in only 5%. Macroglossia is present in 10%.

Proteinuria is present initially in 80% and renal insufficiency in almost 50% of patients. A localized band or spike in the serum protein electrophoretic pattern is found in about half of patients, but it is modest in size (median, 1.4 g/dL). An M protein is found in the serum or urine in almost 90% of patients at diagnosis. Less than one fifth of patients have more than 20% plasma cells in the marrow.

Early cardiac amyloidosis is characterized by abnormal relaxation, whereas advanced involvement is characterized by restrictive hemodynamics. Heart failure is present in approximately 20% of patients at diagnosis and develops during the course of the disease in an additional 10%. The electrocardiogram frequently shows either low voltage in the limb leads or features consistent with an anteroseptal infarction. Atrial fibrillation, atrial or junctional tachycardia, ventricular premature complexes, and heart block are common.

Sensorimotor peripheral neuropathy occurs in one sixth of patients. Autonomic dysfunction may be a prominent feature and is usually manifested by orthostatic hypotension, diarrhea, or impotence.

Table 11–26 ■ CLINICAL CLASSIFICATION OF AMYLOIDOSIS

AMYLOID TYPE	CLASSIFICATION	MAJOR PROTEIN COMPONENT
AL	Primary	κ or λ light chain
AA	Secondary	Protein A
AL	Localized	κ or λ light chain
ATTR	Familial	
	Neurologic	Transthyretin mutant (prealbumin)
	Cardiopathic	Transthyretin mutant (prealbumin)
	Nephropathic	
	Familial Mediterranean fever	Protein A
	Senile systemic amyloidosis	Normal transthyretin (prealbumin)
$A\beta_2M$	Long-term dialysis	β_2-Microglobulin

The initial diagnostic procedure should be abdominal fat aspiration, which is positive in 80% of patients. A bone marrow aspiration and biopsy are positive for amyloid in more than 50% of patients. If subcutaneous fat and bone marrow biopsies are negative, a rectal biopsy should be done, or tissue should be obtained from a suspected organ.

Melphalan- or prednisone-containing regimens are the treatment of choice. Median survival of patients with primary amyloidosis is 13 months.

For more information about this subject, see *Cecil Textbook of Medicine,* 21st edition. Philadelphia, W.B. Saunders Company, 2000. Chapter 181, Plasma Cell Disorders, pages 977 to 987.

STEM CELL TRANSPLANTATION

The two types of stem cell transplantation are (1) autologous, in which the patient is the cell donor, and (2) allogeneic, in which the stem cells are derived from a separate individual.

Allogeneic Transplantation

Initially, only sibling donors with an identical HLA genotype could safely be used. More recently, the development of international computer-linked panels consisting of millions of tissue-typed donors has made it possible to perform transplants between unrelated but phenotypically HLA-matched individuals. The morbidity of allogeneic stem cell transplantation largely results from alloreactivity, which causes graft-versus-host disease (GVHD).

Autologous Transplantation

One of the fundamental concepts of medical oncology is that intensification of therapy will increase the cure rate of chemosensitive and radiosensitive tumors. Dose intensification is limited by damage to normal organs, among the most sensitive of which is the bone marrow. One way of overcoming this limitation is to harvest and freeze hematopoietic stem cells. This material is then infused to produce hematologic rescue following doses of chemotherapy and/or radiotherapy that would otherwise be lethal from marrow ablation.

Sources of Hematopoietic Stem Cells

Peripheral blood stem cell (PBSC) harvest has become a preferred alternative to marrow harvesting for most autologous transplants and is increasing in popularity for allografts. Time to engraftment, particularly of platelets, is reduced (often by a week or more), probably because PBSCs contain greater numbers of more mature progenitor cells than marrow does.

Complications

Preparative chemoradiotherapy regimens before transplantation produce a number of potentially lethal adverse effects. The two most common severe problems are hepatic veno-occlusive disease and hemorrhagic cystitis. Veno-occlusive disease of the liver results from treatment-mediated damage to hepatic venous endothelium and is characterized by weight gain, hepatomegaly, and hyperbilirubinemia, often with ascites and refractory thrombocytopenia. Hemorrhagic cystitis occurs in 5 to 50% of patients following treatment with preparatory regimens containing high-dose cyclophosphamide. Gastrointestinal mucositis with painful oral ulceration, dysphagia, vomiting, and diarrhea occurs almost universally. Pneumonitis, acute carditis, capillary leak syndrome, and pulmonary alveolar hemorrhage can also occur.

Post-transplant immunodeficiency is associated with a high incidence of infection and considerable morbidity and mortality. Many post-transplant infections result from reactivation of latent herpesviruses, including CMV, Epstein-Barr virus (EBV), herpes simplex, and herpes zoster. Other viral infections, including respiratory syncytial virus, parainfluenza, and adenovirus, may cause significant morbidity and mortality after transplantation, particularly when they produce pneumonitis. Intravenous administration of the granulocyte growth factors G-CSF or GM-CSF may abbreviate the hospital stay, but it has been much harder to demonstrate that these agents substantially reduce morbidity or mortality.

Complications caused by alloreactivity are manifested as rejection (host dominant) or GVHD (donor dominant). The risk of rejection increases with increasing donor-recipient disparity. Rejection is also increased by graft manipulation intended to reduce the incidence of GVHD. GVHD occurs when the donor's CD4+ and CD8+ T lymphocytes recognize major or minor histocompatibility antigens on host tissue. The major targets for attack are the skin, gut, and liver. GVHD of the skin is manifested as erythema that initially affects the face, hands, and feet and then progresses to diffuse erythema with bullae and desquamation. In the gut, the complication is characterized by watery diarrhea that may progressively increase in volume and become bloody. In the liver, the disease is typically manifested by hyperbilirubinemia and an elevated alkaline phosphatase level. Fortunately, a number of recent advances in GVHD prophylaxis have helped reduce this toll. The combination of cyclosporine begun on day 1 with methotrexate after transplantation has proved very effective. Complete prevention of GVHD may not be of benefit. Destruction of host hematopoietic and immune system cells appears essential to ensure complete engraftment. This activity, termed the *graft-versus-leukemia effect,* has been especially well documented in myeloid leukemias.

The acute form of GVHD may be followed by chronic GVHD, although this complication may arise de novo after day 40. Chronic diffuse GVHD is often manifested as a systemic sclerosis-like syndrome affecting the skin, eyes, gut, liver, and lungs.

Most late effects of bone marrow transplantation are related either to chronic GVHD or to the toxicity of chemotherapy and radiotherapy conditioning regimens. Although recurrence of malignant disease is not strictly a complication of transplantation, it remains a major cause of treatment failure. Relapse is more common after autologous transplantation.

Outcome

Disease-free survival rates approaching or exceeding 90% can now be expected for patients with aplastic anemia, chronic myeloid leukemia in the first chronic phase, or thalassemia without liver damage. Conversely, survival rates for patients with advanced malignancy remain low; the combination of both severe regimen-related toxicities in these heavily pre-treated patients and a high relapse rate means that only 5 to 30% may survive 5 years.

For more information about this subject, see *Cecil Textbook of Medicine,* 21st edition. Philadelphia, W.B. Saunders Company, 2000. Chapter 182, Stem Cell Transplantation, pages 987 to 991.

APPROACH TO THE PATIENT WITH BLEEDING AND THROMBOSIS

There are three general clinical settings in which patients may be required to undergo evaluation for a possible bleeding disorder. First, patients may present with a history or physical signs of bleeding that provoke suspicion of a systemic coagulopathy. Second, asymptomatic patients may be incidentally discovered to have laboratory abnormalities that suggest a bleeding disorder. Third, patients may be asked to undergo routine testing for bleeding risk before surgery or an invasive procedure.

Not only should the patient be asked about spontaneous bleeding episodes in the past, but the response to specific hemostatic challenges should also be recorded. A history of prior bleeding suggests a coagulopathy, as does the finding of bleeding from multiple sites. The history must also include a survey of coexisting systemic diseases and drug ingestion that may affect hemostasis.

In general, patients with thrombocytopenia or qualitative platelet and vascular disorders present with bleeding from superficial sites in the skin and mucous membranes. In contrast, patients with inherited or acquired coagulation factor deficiencies, such as hemophilia or therapeutic anticoagulation, tend to bleed from deeper tissue sites and in a delayed manner after trauma.

Four simple, rapid screening tests are generally used in the initial evaluation of patients with a suspected coagulopathy: (1) platelet count, (2) bleeding time, (3) prothrombin time (PT), and (4) activated partial thromboplastin time (aPTT).

Thrombocytopenia, routinely reported by electronic particle counting, should be verified by examination of the peripheral smear. "Pseudothrombocytopenia," a laboratory artifact of ex vivo platelet clumping, may be caused by the ethylenediaminetetraacetic acid (EDTA) anticoagulant used in tubes for blood cell counts, other anticoagulants, or cold agglutinins acting at room temperature; it should be suspected whenever a very low platelet count is reported in a patient who does not exhibit any clinical bleeding. Pseudothrombocytopenia is indicated by the finding of platelet clumps on the peripheral smear.

The bleeding time measures the time to cessation of bleeding after a standardized incision over the volar aspect of the forearm. The bleeding time is prolonged in (1) thrombocytopenia, (2) qualitative platelet abnormalities, (3) defects in platelet–vessel wall interactions (e.g., von Willebrand's disease [vWD]), or (4) primary vascular disorders.

The PT measures the integrity of the extrinsic and common pathways of coagulation (Factors VII, X, V, prothrombin, and fibrinogen). The aPTT measures the integrity of the intrinsic and common pathways of coagulation (high-molecular-weight kininogen, prekallikrein, Factors XII, XI, IX, VIII, X, and V, prothrombin, and fibrinogen).

With a few exceptions, normal results for all four of the screening tests of hemostasis essentially exclude any clinically significant systemic coagulopathy. Patients with Factor XIII deficiency may have a serious bleeding diathesis but have normal screening tests. Patients with vWD sometimes have normal bleeding times and usually do not have sufficiently reduced levels of Factor VIII to affect the aPTT. Rare disorders of fibrinolysis may also be associated with normal screening tests.

A prolonged bleeding time in the absence of thrombocytopenia should initially be approached by determining if the patient is taking any drugs that might interfere with platelet function (e.g., aspirin, other non-steroidal anti-inflammatory drugs) or has coexisting diseases that might explain the finding (e.g., renal failure). If these conditions are not found, or if the bleeding fails to correct after discontinuing any potential offending drugs, further specialized testing may include platelet aggregation studies to identify specific qualitative abnormalities of platelet function and specific assays to exclude one of the types of vWD.

The finding of a prolonged PT and/or aPTT indicates that there is either a deficiency of one or more coagulation factors or an inhibitor, usually an antibody, directed at one or more components of the coagulation system. These two possibilities can be readily distinguished by performing an inhibitor screen, which involves a 1:1 mix of patient and normal plasma. If the 1:1 mix fails to correct the prolonged PT and/or aPTT, an inhibitor is likely to be present in the patient's plasma.

Patients with lupus anticoagulants typically have prolongations of the aPTT, and sometimes also the PT, yet they more often have thrombotic rather than bleeding complications. In patients with heparin-induced thrombocytopenia, a marked decrease in the platelet count is sometimes associated with arterial and venous thrombosis.

Increasing evidence from many studies now indicates that routine screening of all preoperative patients is not only uninformative but may even be counterproductive. Laboratory testing is indicated in patients whose bleeding histories are suspicious as well as in those who are to undergo procedures in which even minimal postoperative hemorrhage could be hazardous.

Evaluation of the Patient with a Possible Hypercoagulable State

Many, and possibly most, patients with venous thromboembolism have an inherited basis for hypercoagulability. The primary or hereditary hypercoagulable states result from specific mutations, mostly in genes encoding a plasma protein that serves as a physiologic anticoagulant. Evaluation for occult malignancy need not be exhaustive and can be limited to a thorough history, physical examination, a routine complete blood cell count and chemistries, test of fecal occult blood, urinalysis, mammogram (in women), and chest radiograph.

For more information about this subject, see *Cecil Textbook of Medicine,* 21st edition. Philadelphia, W.B. Saunders Company, 2000. Chapter 183, Approach to the Patient with Bleeding and Thrombosis, pages 991 to 995.

HEMORRHAGIC DISORDERS: ABNORMALITIES OF PLATELET AND VASCULAR FUNCTION

Platelets circulate for 9 to 10 days. Approximately one third reside in a splenic pool, which exchanges freely with the circulating pool. Low platelet counts (thrombocytopenia) (Table 11–27 and Fig. 11–6) can be caused by disturbances in production, distribution, or destruction. With a platelet count of 50,000 to 100,000/μL, patients may bleed longer than normal with severe trauma; with a platelet count of 20,000 to 50,000/μL, bleeding occurs with minor trauma, but spontaneous bleeding is unusual; with a platelet count less than 20,000/μL, patients may have spontaneous bleeding; and when the platelet count is less than 10,000/μL, patients are at high risk for severe bleeding. Decreased production of platelets may be due to abnormal maturation of megakaryocytes as seen in deficiency of either vitamin B_{12} or folate and in hematopoietic dysplasias.

Idiopathic Thrombocytopenic Purpura

Idiopathic thrombocytopenic purpura (ITP) is an autoimmune bleeding disorder characterized by the development of antibodies to one's own platelets, which are then destroyed by phagocytosis in the spleen and, to a lesser extent, the liver. Petechiae, ecchymoses, and epistaxis develop. The diagnosis depends on the exclusion of underlying systemic disorders. The value of assays for detecting antiplatelet antibodies is unclear. In ITP the marrow is normal, although megakaryocytes may be increased in number. 11

In adults, indications for treatment depend on the severity of bleeding and the degree of thrombocytopenia. Asymptomatic patients with platelet counts greater than 40,000/μL can be observed. Patients with platelet counts less than 20,000/μL are usually symptomatic and require treatment. Bleeding associated with ITP is treated with prednisone 1 to 2 mg/kg/day. In 80 to 90% of patients, the platelet count rises to hemostatic levels within 2 to 3 weeks. Intravenous immune globulin (IVIG) concentrates raise the platelet count within 3 to 5 days in most patients and is the most rapidly active agent. Unfortunately, the therapeutic effect is usually transient. Splenectomy improves the platelet count in 70% of patients with ITP and induces sustained remission in approximately 60%. Danazol 200 mg three times per day induces a remission in approximately 40% of cases of chronic ITP.

Other Immune Thrombocytopenias

Antibody-mediated destruction of platelets occurs in *lymphoproliferative disorders* such as chronic lymphocytic leukemia and lymphoma. Immune thrombocytopenia is common in *systemic lupus erythematosus.* Thrombocytopenia associated with antiplatelet antibodies has been reported in patients with *viral* illnesses, including infectious mononucleosis, HIV infection, and CMV infection.

More than 50 *drugs* have been reported to cause immune thrombocytopenia, but infrequently with conclusive confirmation. Quinine, quinidine, sulfa compounds, hydrochlorothiazide, phenytoin, methyldopa, heparin, and digitalis derivatives are among the best documented. The incidence of thrombocytopenia associated with

Table 11–27 ■ DRUGS THAT MAY ALTER HEMOSTASIS

Drugs Reported to Cause Thrombocytopenia

Immune mechanism proposed*

- Quinine/quinidine
- Sulfa compounds
- Ampicillin
- Penicillin
- Thiazide diuretics
- Furosemide
- Chlorthalidone
- Phenytoin
- α-Methyldopa
- Heparin
- Digitalis derivatives
- Aspirin
- Valproic acid
- Ranitidine
- Cimetidine
- Danazol
- Procainamide
- Carbamazepine
- Acetaminophen
- Phenylbutazone
- *p*-Aminosalicylate
- Rifampin
- Acetazolamide
- Anazolene
- Arsenicals

Non-immune mechanisms (hemolytic-uremic syndrome/thrombotic thrombocytopenic purpura)

- Ticlopidine/clopidogrel
- Mitomycin
- Cisplatin
- Cyclosporine

Mechanism undefined

- Gold compounds
- Indomethacin

Drugs That Alter Platelet Function

Primary antiplatelet agents

- Aspirin
- Dextran
- Dipyridamole
- Sulfinpyrazone
- Ticlopidine
- Clopidogrel

Drugs in which inhibition of platelet function is associated with prolongation of the bleeding time

- Non-steroidal anti-inflammatory agents
- β-Lactam antibiotics
- ϵ-Aminocaproic acid ($>$24 g/d)
- Heparin
- Plasminogen activators (streptokinase, urokinase, tissue plasminogen activator)

Drugs That Affect Coagulation Factors

Induction of antibodies inhibiting function

- Lupus anticoagulant†‡
  - Phenothiazines
  - Procainamide
- Factor VIII antibodies
  - Penicillin
- Factor V antibodies
  - Aminoglycosides
- Factor XIII antibodies
  - Isoniazid

Inhibitors of synthesis of vitamin K–dependent clotting factors (Factors II, VII, IX, X; proteins C and S)

- Coumarin compounds
- Moxalactam

Inhibitor of fibrinogen synthesis

- L-Asparaginase‡

*The list is limited to drugs for which there are multiple reports and in vitro or in vivo evidence of antiplatelet antibodies.

†Does not cause bleeding.

‡May cause thrombosis.

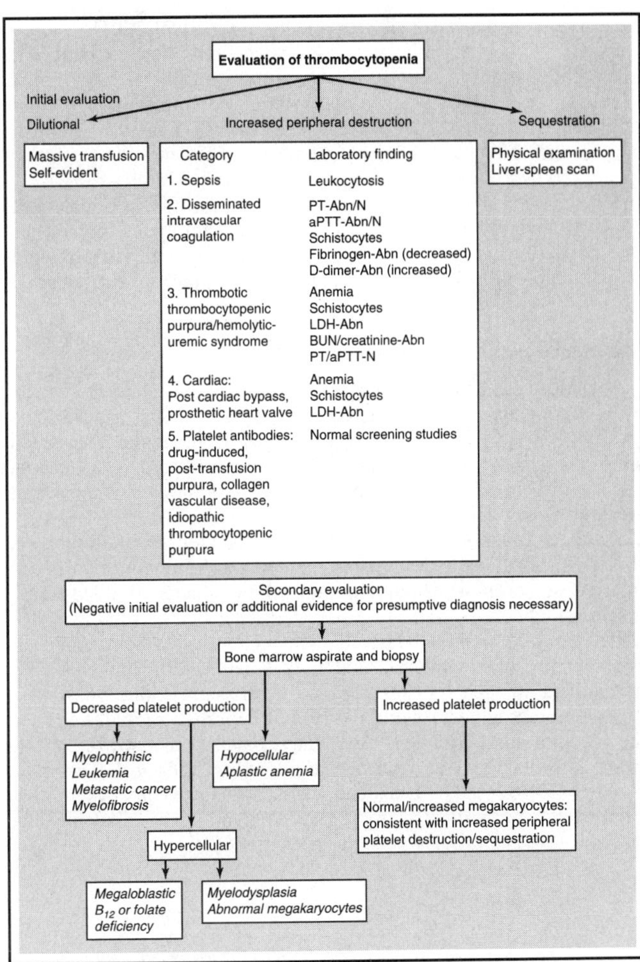

FIGURE 11–6 ■ Evaluation of thrombocytopenia. Abn = abnormal; N = normal; PT = prothrombin time; aPTT = activated partial thromboplastin time; LDH = lactate dehydrogenase; BUN = blood urea nitrogen.

11

heparin therapy appears to be 3 to 5%. If the platelet count falls below 50,000/μL, heparin therapy should be discontinued.

Non-Immune Disorders with Increased Platelet Consumption

Disseminated intravascular coagulation (DIC) results in thrombin formation and the subsequent removal of platelets from the circulation. A rare disease of unknown etiology, *thrombotic thrombocytopenic purpura* (TTP) is characterized by severe thrombocytopenia, microangiopathic hemolytic anemia (>96% of patients), and neurologic abnormalities (>92% of patients). Fever and renal involvement—proteinuria, hematuria, azotemia, and casts—

are present in 98 and 88% of patients, respectively. TTP must be considered when thrombocytopenia and anemia occur acutely with microangiopathic changes of RBCs on the peripheral blood smear (Table 11–28). Although findings in DIC are similar, patients with TTP have minimal changes in coagulation tests. Large-volume plasmapheresis is the treatment of choice for TTP and cures approximately 70% of patients.

Hemolytic-uremic syndrome (HUS) rarely occurs in adults. Like TTP, HUS produces a microangiopathic hemolytic anemia, but thrombocytopenia is mild to moderate and neurologic abnormalities are absent. Unlike TTP, acute renal failure is a prominent feature.

Abnormalities in Platelet Function

Non-steroidal anti-inflammatory agents inhibit platelet function by blocking platelet synthesis of prostaglandins. One aspirin tablet (300 mg) is sufficient to cause this effect. High doses of β-lactam antibiotics such as penicillin and related compounds induce an abnormality in platelet function that persists for 2 to 3 days after the drug is discontinued.

Platelets function abnormally in patients with renal failure and sometimes in liver disease. Abnormal platelet function also occurs in a subset of patients with multiple myeloma or Waldenström's macroglobulinemia.

Patients with essential thrombocythemia and, less commonly, agnogenic myeloid metaplasia and polycythemia vera may have abnormalities of platelet function. In Glanzmann's thrombasthenia, two membrane glycoproteins (GPIIb, GPIIIa) that normally serve as the receptor for fibrinogen in activated platelets are markedly deficient. The diagnosis is confirmed by demonstrating a deficiency of platelet GPIIb and GPIIIa. The platelet count is always normal. Von Willebrand's disease is the most common congenital bleeding disorder that also affects platelet function.

Table 11–28 ■ DISORDERS ASSOCIATED WITH THROMBOCYTOPENIA AND MICROANGIOPATHIC ANEMIA

Thrombotic thrombocytopenic purpura
Hemolytic-uremic syndrome
Disseminated intravascular coagulation
Malignant hypertension
Eclampsia
Vasculitis
Systemic lupus erythematosus
Polyarteritis nodosa
Cavernous hemangioma
(Kasabach-Merritt syndrome)
Disseminated carcinoma
Renal allograft rejection
Prosthetic heart valves
Malignant angioendotheliomatosis

Platelet Transfusions

Platelet transfusions are indicated for patients who are bleeding actively and have either a platelet count lower than 50,000/μL or a qualitative platelet abnormality as manifested by a prolonged bleeding time. Before surgery, platelet counts should be greater than 50,000/μL in most cases and greater than 90,000/μL for procedures such as neurosurgery or ophthalmologic surgery in which any abnormal bleeding may cause excessive morbidity. For invasive procedures such as kidney or liver biopsies, a platelet count over 50,000/μL is probably sufficient, assuming normal platelet function.

When thrombocytopenia is due to decreased production, the platelet count should be maintained at 10,000 to 20,000/μL. When accelerated destruction of platelets exists, transfusion is seldom effective. Patients with ITP frequently tolerate low platelet counts with little bleeding because of the excellent function of the younger platelets available in the circulation.

Vascular Disorders

Normal vascular function is necessary for effective hemostasis. Hereditary hemorrhagic telangiectasia (Osler-Weber-Rendu disease), the most common genetic cause of vascular bleeding, is inherited as an autosomal dominant trait. Its most frequent symptom is spontaneous epistaxis. Telangiectasia occurs most frequently on the face in two thirds of patients, on the mouth in half, and on the cheeks, tongue, nose, and lower lip in approximately one third. Death from intestinal bleeding occurs in 12 to 15% of patients with symptomatic gastrointestinal involvement. Pulmonary arteriovenous fistulas, present in approximately 5% of patients, are manifested by cyanosis, dyspnea, clubbing, and thoracic murmurs. Conjugated estrogen-progestin therapy appears to be efficacious in decreasing the number of bleeding episodes.

Severe vitamin C deficiency results in defective collagen formation in small blood vessels. Bleeding may occur in any tissue but is prominent in the lower extremities and is perifollicular in distribution.

Patients with any of the three types of cryoglobulinemia have purpura as a complication of their disease. Amyloid deposition in the skin and subcutaneous tissue alters the normal structural support for small blood vessels and thereby results in increased vascular fragility. Purpura can occur at any site. Abnormalities in platelet function may also occur with M proteins. Bleeding may be manifested as internal hemorrhage in Ehlers-Danlos syndrome, osteogenesis imperfecta, and pseudoxanthoma elasticum.

For more information about this subject, see *Cecil Textbook of Medicine,* 21st edition. Philadelphia, W.B. Saunders Company, 2000. Chapter 184, Hemorrhagic Disorders: Abnormalities of Platelet and Vascular Function, pages 996 to 1004.

COAGULATION FACTOR DEFICIENCIES

Coagulopathies predominantly result from quantitative defects in biosynthesis of the coagulation factor protein(s), but qualitative defects can also result in bleeding (Table 11–29).

Table 11–29 ■ COAGULATION PROTEINS AND REPLACEMENT THERAPY

COAGULATION PROTEIN DEFICIENCY	INHERITANCE PATTERN	PREVALENCE	MINIMUM HEMOSTATIC LEVEL	REPLACEMENT SOURCES
Factor I (fibrinogen)			100 mg/dL	Cryoprecipitate/fresh-frozen plasma, viral-treated Factor VIII concentrates (intermediate purity)
Afibrinogenemia	Autosomal recessive	Rare (<300 families)		
Dysfibrinogenemia	Autosomal dominant or recessive	Rare (>300 variants)		
Factor II (prothrombin)	Autosomal dominant or recessive	Rare (~25 kindreds)	30% of normal	Fresh-frozen plasma, Factor IX complex concentrates
Factor V (labile factor)	Autosomal recessive	$1/10^6$ births	25% of normal	Fresh-frozen plasma
Factor VII	Autosomal recessive	1/500,000 births	25% of normal	Fresh-frozen plasma, Factor IX complex concentrates, or recombinant Factor VIIa
Factor VIII (antihemophilic factor)	X-linked recessive	1/5000 male births	80–100% for surgery/life-threatening bleeding, 50% for serious bleeding, 25–30% for minor bleeding	Factor VIII concentrates

Von Willebrand's disease (vWD)			>50% vWF antigen and ristocetin cofactor activity	DDAVP for mild-to-moderate vWD (except IIB; variable response to IIA); cryoprecipitate and fresh-frozen plasma (not preferred except in emergencies); Factor VIII concentrates, viral-attenuated, intermediate-purity (preferred for vWD unresponsive to DDAVP and for type III)
Type I and II variants	Usually autosomal dominant	1% prevalence		
Type III	Autosomal recessive	$1/10^6$ births		
Factor IX (Christmas factor)	X-linked recessive	1/30,000 male births	25–50% of normal, depending on extent of bleeding and surgery	Factor IX concentrates; fresh-frozen plasma is not preferred except in dire emergencies
Factor X (Stuart-Prower factor)	Autosomal recessive	1/500,000 births	10–25% of normal	Fresh-frozen plasma or Factor IX complex concentrates
Factor XI (hemophilia C)	Autosomal dominant; severe type is recessive	~4% Ashkenazi Jews; $1/10^6$ general population	20–40% of normal	Fresh-frozen plasma or Factor XI concentrate
Factor XII (Hageman factor), prekallikrein, high-molecular-weight kininogen	Autosomal recessive	Not available	No treatment necessary	
Factor XIII (fibrin stabilizing factor)	Autosomal recessive	$1/3 \times 10^6$ births	5% of normal	Fresh-frozen plasma, cryoprecipitate, or viral-attenuated Factor XIII concentrate

vWF = von Willebrand factor; DDAVP = desmopressin acetate.

The Hereditary Hemophilias

The sex-linked recessive disorders of hemophilia A and B are estimated to occur in approximately 1 in 5000 and 1 in 30,000 male births, respectively. No single mutation is responsible for the hemophilias, and many missense and nonsense point mutations, deletions, and inversions have been described.

The clinical pictures of hemophilia A and B are indistinguishable from each other, with their clinical severity corresponding inversely to the circulating levels of plasma coagulant Factor VIII or IX activity. Individuals with less than 1% of normal Factor VIII or IX activity have severe disease characterized by frequent spontaneous bleeding in joints (hemarthrosis) and soft tissues and by profuse hemorrhage with trauma or surgery. Spontaneous bleeding is uncommon with mild deficiencies of greater than 5% of normal activity; however, excessive bleeding can still occur with trauma or surgery.

Acute hemarthroses produce a tingling or burning sensation, followed by the onset of intense pain and swelling. On physical examination the joint is swollen, hot, and tender to palpation. Narcotic analgesics such as codeine or synthetic derivatives of codeine should be prescribed alone or combined with acetaminophen. Replacement of the deficient clotting factor to normal hemostatic levels rapidly reverses the pain. Swelling and joint immobility improve as the intra-articular hematoma resolves. Recurrent or untreated bleeding results in chronic synovial hypertrophy and eventually damages the underlying cartilage, with subsequent subchondral bone cyst formation, bony erosion, and flexion contractures.

Retroperitoneal hematomas may be clinically confused with appendicitis or hip bleeding. Bleeding involving the tongue or the retropharyngeal space can rapidly produce life-threatening compromise of the airways. Gastrointestinal hemorrhage in hemophiliac patients typically originates from anatomic lesions. Intracranial bleeding is the second most common cause of death in hemophiliac patients after AIDS.

The strategy to minimize or eliminate progressive joint destruction by recurrent hemarthroses is predicated on the concept of primary prophylaxis—the planned administration of clotting factor concentrates two (for Factor IX products) or three (for Factor VIII replacement) times weekly at doses to maintain trough clotting factor activity levels above 1 to 2% of normal. Replacement guidelines are intended to achieve plasma levels of Factor VIII and IX activity of 25 to 30% for minor spontaneous or traumatic bleeding, for example, hemarthroses or persistent hematuria; at least 50% clotting factor activity for the treatment or prevention of severe bleeding, for example, major dental surgery, maintenance replacement therapy following major surgery or trauma; and 80 to 100% activity for any life- or limb-threatening hemorrhagic event, major surgery, trauma, and so on. For each unit of Factor VIII administered per kilogram of body weight, plasma Factor VIII activity will increase about 2% (0.02 U/mL), and for each unit of Factor IX administered per kilogram of body weight, Factor IX activity will increase about 1% (0.01 U/mL). A 70-kg individual with severe hemophilia A or B who required replacement to 100% activity for major surgery should initially receive 3500 U of Factor VIII or 7000 U of Factor IX concentrate, respectively.

Virtually all hemophiliac patients treated before 1985 have been exposed to hepatitis C virus. Approximately 5% of those exposed before 1985 are chronic carriers of hepatitis B surface antigen.

The life expectancy of severe hemophiliac patients approached 62 years by the mid 1980s with the introduction of clotting factor concentrates; however, HIV has tripled the death rate and is currently responsible for over 55% of all hemophilia deaths. Over 75% of patients with hemophilia A and 46% of those with hemophilia B are HIV positive. Otherwise, life expectancy is related to the severity of hemophilia, with the mortality rate of severely affected patients being four to six times greater than that of patients with mild deficiencies.

Alloantibody and Autoantibody Inhibitors to Factors VIII and IX

Alloantibody inhibitors arise predominantly in patients with severe congenital deficiencies of Factors VIII or IX and are suspected when replacement therapy does not provide the usual immediate relief of bleeding symptoms. Low-titer inhibitor patients can easily be overwhelmed by large amounts of human Factor VIII or IX concentrate. Treatment of patients with high-titer inhibitor against Factor VIII or IX is complicated by the observation that no single approach is uniformly successful.

Autoantibody inhibitors occur spontaneously in individuals with previously normal hemostasis (without hemophilias). Although approximately 50% have no obvious underlying cause, the remainder are associated with autoimmune diseases, lymphoproliferative disorders, idiosyncratic drug associations, and pregnancy. Residual clotting factor activities between 3 and 20% of normal are frequently observed in autoantibody patients. The same principles of replacement therapy for alloantibodies also apply to these inhibitors. Porcine Factor VIII concentrate is particularly useful in acquired hemophilia A because very little cross-reactivity usually occurs, even with extremely high titers of anti–human Factor VIII antibodies. Immunosuppressive therapy with steroids and cytotoxic agents is a necessary component of the overall treatment to suppress the inhibitor. High-dose intravenous gamma globulin may be useful adjunctive therapy. For hemorrhagic catastrophes related to either alloantibodies or autoantibodies, extracorporeal plasmapheresis over a staphylococcal protein A column may remove enough of the IgG to allow for replacement therapy with enough factor concentrates to achieve hemostasis.

von Willebrand's Disease

The phenotypic classification of vWD recognizes three major types of the disease based on their multimeric structure and function of the von Willebrand factor (vWF) protein. Type I vWD accounts for up to 75 to 80% of patients and is inherited predominantly via an autosomal dominant mode; a quantitative defect is present in which the vWF structure is normal but vWF antigen and activity are concomitantly reduced. Type II vWD includes approximately 20% of vWD patients, is inherited in either a dominant or recessive pattern, and is characterized by qualitative and quantitative abnormalities in the vWF protein. Up to 30 variants have been described. Type III vWD, an exceedingly rare variant, is characterized by nearly complete absence of circulating vWF.

Most patients with vWD have mild disease that may go undiagnosed until trauma or surgery. Symptomatic individuals manifest easy bruisability and mucosal surface bleeding, including epistaxis and gastrointestinal hemorrhage. Menorrhagia affects 50 to 75% of women. The use of aspirin or non-steroidal anti-inflammatory drugs with antiplatelet aggregation effects may exacerbate the symptoms.

The bleeding time is variably prolonged. The aPTT is also variably increased because of concurrent Factor VIII deficiency; however, a normal aPTT does not exclude the diagnosis. Gene-based assays are the most specific for diagnosing vWF variants.

TREATMENT. The goals of therapy for vWD consist in correcting the deficiencies in vWF protein activity to above 50% of normal and Factor VIII activity to levels appropriate for the clinical situation. Desmopressin acetate (DDAVP) 0.3 μg/kg in 50 mL normal saline infused over a 20-minute period or intranasally at 150 μg per nostril for adults is the recommended treatment and eliminates potential exposure to blood-borne pathogens. The adjunctive use of antifibrinolytic agents such as ϵ-aminocaproic acid is useful following DDAVP therapy for bleeding. Cryoprecipitate is used only in emergency circumstances when no other options are available. Replacement therapy with viral-attenuated, intermediate- or high-purity Factor VIII concentrates is preferred for patients with type I and IIA variants who are unresponsive to DDAVP and for patients with type IIB, IIN, and III disease.

The following important caveats for vWD treatment should be considered: (1) a prolonged bleeding time does not need to be normalized to achieve adequate hemostasis; (2) DDAVP administration should be avoided in patients with type IIB variant vWD; (3) patients with variant type IIN may not manifest a sustained response to DDAVP; (4) patients who respond adequately to intravenously administered DDAVP may not respond adequately to intranasal DDAVP; (5) free water intake, whether intravenous or by mouth, should be severely restricted for 4 to 6 hours after DDAVP administration.

Other Coagulation Factor Deficiencies

FACTOR XI DEFICIENCY (HEMOPHILIA C). Factor XI deficiency is diagnosed in the laboratory by a prolonged aPTT, normal PT, and decreased Factor XI. The clinical bleeding tendencies in Factor XI deficiency are less severe than those seen with severe hemophilia A or B.

CONTACT ACTIVATION FACTORS. Deficiencies of Factor XII, prekallikrein, and high-molecular-weight kininogen will produce in vitro laboratory abnormalities but no clinical bleeding and therefore require no replacement therapy. Counterintuitively, 8 to 10% of individuals with severe Factor XII deficiency ($<1\%$ activity) have experienced premature venous thromboembolic events.

FACTOR XIII DEFICIENCY. Delayed bleeding after surgery and trauma is the hallmark of the disease; however, easy bruisability, poor wound healing with defective scar formation and dehiscence, and hemarthroses are characteristic. Replacement therapy for prophylaxis or treatment of acute bleeding can be accomplished by administering cryoprecipitate, fresh-frozen plasma (FFP), or preferably, plasma-derived Factor XIII concentrate.

DYSFIBRINOGENEMIA AND AFIBRINOGENEMIA. Approximately 300 abnormal fibrinogens have been described. Over 50% of the dysfibrinogenemias are asymptomatic, 25% are associated with a mild hemorrhagic tendency, and 20% predispose individuals to thrombophilia. Concurrent bleeding and thrombosis may also occur. Severe life-threatening hemorrhagic complications can occur at any site. Deficiencies of fibrinogen may be corrected by the administration of FFP or cryoprecipitate; however, viral safety remains an issue. Intermediate-purity Factor VIII concentrates from frozen plasma are preferable alternatives.

FACTOR V DEFICIENCY. Deficiency of Factor V is very uncommon. The severity of the plasma Factor V reduction correlates less well with the risk of clinical bleeding than does the platelet Factor V content in the alpha granules. Transfusions of normal platelets may be preferred over FFP for the treatment of hemorrhagic episodes secondary to congenital or acquired Factor V deficiency. The Factor V Leiden protein, which is responsible for resistance to activated protein C and thrombophilia, does not affect Factor V coagulant activity.

Lupus Anticoagulants

The lupus anticoagulant may be discovered incidentally when routine coagulation assays reveal prolongations in the PT and/or the aPTT, when young women experience recurrent spontaneous miscarriages and/or pregnancy-related thromboembolic events, when young women and elderly men are detected with cerebral arterial thromboses, when patients are affected by systemic lupus erythematosus (20 to 40%) or other autoimmune diseases or lymphoproliferative malignancies, and when patients have been receiving long-term therapy with psychotropic tricyclic medications, for example, chlorpromazine. Lupus anticoagulant can also occur with the active opportunistic infections and malignancies associated with AIDS.

Anticardiolipin antibodies are a subset of the antiphospholipid antibody family. Recent data suggest, however, that anticardiolipin antibody and lupus anticoagulant may represent separate types of antibodies. The pathologic mechanism for thrombotic complications is not clear.

Conventional oral anticoagulation to maintain the International Normalized Ratio (INR) between 2.0 and 3.0 does not effectively prevent recurrent events. Therefore, a more aggressive regimen intended to achieve an INR of 3.0 to 3.5 is recommended.

For more information about this subject, see *Cecil Textbook of Medicine,* 21st edition. Philadelphia, W.B. Saunders Company, 2000. Chapter 185, Coagulation Factor Deficiencies, pages 1004 to 1012.

HEMORRHAGIC DISORDERS: MIXED ABNORMALITIES

DIC, also referred to as consumptive coagulopathy or defibrination, is caused by a wide variety of serious disorders. In most patients, the underlying process dominates the clinical picture, but in some cases (e.g., occult malignancy), DIC may be the initial manifestation of the disorder.

In acute, uncompensated DIC, coagulation factors are consumed at a rate in excess of the capacity of the liver to synthesize them, and platelets are consumed in excess of the capacity of bone marrow megakaryocytes to release them. The resulting laboratory manifestations are a prolonged PT and aPTT, as well as thrombocytopenia. Increased fibrin formation in DIC stimulates the compensatory process of secondary fibrinolysis in which plasminogen activators generate plasmin to digest fibrin (and fibrinogen) into fibrin(ogen) degradation products (FDPs). FDPs are potent circulating anticoagulants. Intravascular fibrin deposition can cause fragmentation of RBCs and thereby lead to the appearance of schistocytes in blood smears; however, frank hemolytic anemia is unusual in DIC. Microvascular thrombosis in DIC can also cause tissue necrosis and end-organ damage.

Infection is the most common cause of DIC. DIC also accompanies obstetric complications, especially in the third trimester. Chronic forms of DIC accompany a variety of malignancies, particularly pancreatic cancer and mucin-secreting adenocarcinomas of the gastrointestinal tract and acute promyelocytic leukemia. Bites from rattlesnakes and other vipers can induce profound DIC. The likelihood and degree of DIC caused by trauma, surgery, and shock are related to the extent of tissue damage and the organs involved. Aortic aneurysms, giant hemangiomas, and other vascular malformations can cause subclinical or clinical DIC.

Low-grade DIC is often asymptomatic and diagnosed only by laboratory abnormalities. Thrombotic complications of DIC occur most often with chronic underlying diseases. Gangrene of the digits or extremities, hemorrhagic necrosis of the skin, and purpura fulminans may also be manifestations of DIC. Bleeding is the most common clinical finding in acute, uncompensated DIC. It tends to be generalized in more severe cases, including widespread ecchymoses and diffuse oozing from mucosal surfaces and orifices.

The laboratory diagnosis of severe, acute DIC is not usually difficult. Consumption and inhibition of the function of clotting factors cause prolongation of the PT, aPTT, and thrombin time. Consumption of platelets causes thrombocytopenia. Secondary fibrinolysis generates increased titers of FDPs.

The coagulopathy of liver failure is often indistinguishable from that of DIC. In thrombotic microangiopathies, including TTP and HUS, the PT, aPTT, thrombin time, and FDPs are generally normal.

Successful treatment of DIC (Table 11–30) requires that the underlying cause be identified and eliminated. Heparin is usually reserved for special forms of DIC, including those manifested by thrombosis or acrocyanosis and those that accompany cancer, vascular malformations, retained dead fetus, and possibly acute promyelocytic leukemia.

Liver Failure

The liver is the principal organ site for the synthesis of coagulation and fibrinolytic factors, and their protein inhibitors. Hepato-

Table 11–30 ■ TREATMENT OF DISSEMINATED INTRAVASCULAR COAGULATION (DIC)

Identify and eliminate the underlying cause
No treatment if mild, asymptomatic, and self-limited
Hemodynamic support, as indicated, in severe cases
Blood component therapy
  Indications: Active bleeding or high risk of bleeding
    Fresh-frozen plasma
    Platelets
    In some cases, consider cryoprecipitate, antithrombin III
Drug therapy
  Indications: Heparin for DIC manifested by thrombosis or acrocyanosis; antifibrinolytic agents generally contraindicated except with life-threatening bleeding and failure of blood component therapy
  Heparin
  Antifibrinolytic agents (generally contraindicated)

cytes produce all of the clotting factors except vWF. Most forms of advanced liver disease are accompanied by some degree of DIC. Quantitative and qualitative abnormalities of platelets also contribute to the bleeding diathesis of liver failure. Bleeding complications in patients with advanced liver disease can be very severe and even fatal and directly account for about 20% of the deaths associated with hepatic failure. The most common hemorrhagic complication is gastrointestinal bleeding.

Both the PT and aPTT are often prolonged. In general, patients with DIC have more marked decreases in levels of Factor VIII and increases in titers of FDPs, particularly D-dimers, than do those with liver failure.

It is usually recommended that attempts be made to correct PT prolongations of over 3 seconds and platelet counts below 70,000/μL before surgical interventions. The most effective treatment is FFP and platelet transfusions.

For more information about this subject, see *Cecil Textbook of Medicine,* 21st edition. Philadelphia, W.B. Saunders Company, 2000. Chapter 186, Hemorrhagic Disorders: Mixed Abnormalities, pages 1013 to 1016.

THROMBOTIC DISORDERS: HYPERCOAGULABLE STATES

Primary Hypercoagulable States

In most patients with primary hypercoagulable states, discrete clinical thrombotic complications appear to be precipitated by acquired prothrombotic events (e.g., pregnancy, use of oral contraceptives, surgery, trauma, immobilization), many of which are the secondary hypercoagulable states (Table 11–31).

Inherited quantitative or qualitative deficiency of *antithrombin III* leads to increased fibrin accumulation and a lifelong propensity to thrombosis. Among all patients seen with venous thromboembolism, antithrombin deficiency is detected in only about 1%, but it is found in about 2.5% of selected patients with recurrent thrombosis and/or thrombosis at a younger age (<45 years).

Protein C deficiency is found in 3 to 4% of patients with venous

Table 11–31 ■ THE PRIMARY HYPERCOAGULABLE STATES

Antithrombin (III)/Heparin Disorders
Antithrombin deficiency
Heparin cofactor II deficiency
Protein C/Protein S Disorders
Protein C deficiency
Protein S deficiency
Activated protein C resistance
Factor V Leiden
Thrombomodulin dysfunction
Prothrombin Gene Mutation
Fibrinolytic Disorders
Hypoplasminogenemia
Dysplasminogenemia
Plasminogen activator deficiency
Dysfibrinogenemia
Hyperhomocysteinemia
Cystathionine β-synthase deficiency
Remethylation pathway defects
Acquired hyperhomocysteinemia
Pyridoxine, cobalamin, folate deficiency

thromboembolism. More than 160 mutations are known to cause protein C deficiency.

Protein S is the principal cofactor of activated protein C (APC), and therefore its deficiency mimics that of protein C. The prevalence of protein S deficiency among patients evaluated for venous thromboembolism (2 to 3%) is comparable to that of protein C deficiency.

The great majority of subjects with functional *activated protein C resistance* have a single, specific point mutation in the Factor V gene, termed *Factor V Leiden.* Heterozygosity for the autosomally transmitted Factor V Leiden increases the risk of thrombosis by a factor of 5 to 10, whereas homozygosity increases the risk by a factor of 50 to 100. APC resistance is found in 10 to 64% of patients with venous thromboembolism.

A prothrombin gene mutation has been associated with elevated plasma levels of prothrombin and an increased risk of venous thrombosis. This mutation is found in 6 to 18% of patients with venous thromboembolism, which makes it second only to Factor V Leiden as a genetic risk factor for venous thrombosis.

Adults with mild to moderate hyperhomocysteinemia have venous or arterial thrombotic manifestations. Acquired causes most commonly involve nutritional deficiencies of the cofactors required for homocysteine metabolism, including pyridoxine, cobalamin, and folate. The mechanism of homocysteine-induced thrombosis and atherogenesis involves complex and probably multifactorial effects on the vessel wall. Deep vein thrombosis (DVT) of the lower extremities and pulmonary embolism are frequent clinical manifestations. More unusual sites of venous thrombosis include superficial thrombophlebitis and mesenteric and cerebral vein thrombosis. Arterial thrombosis involving the coronary, cerebrovascular, and peripheral circulations also is increased.

Laboratory diagnosis requires testing for each of the disorders individually because no general screening test is available to determine whether a patient may have such a condition. The scope and timing of laboratory testing for primary hypercoagulable states should be individualized. Patients with arterial thrombosis should generally not be tested for any of these disorders except hyperhomocysteinemia.

In general, testing for these disorders is not recommended immediately after a major thrombotic event. All these tests are optimally performed in clinically stable patients at least 2 weeks after completing the 3- to 6-month period of oral anticoagulation following a thrombotic episode. When testing is indicated in patients in whom interruption of prophylactic oral anticoagulation is considered too risky, protein C and protein S levels can be determined after warfarin therapy has been discontinued under heparin coverage for at least 2 weeks.

The initial treatment of acute venous thrombosis or pulmonary embolism in patients with primary hypercoagulable states is not different from that in those without genetic defects. Recommendations for long-term management are compromised at this point by the lack of data from rigorously controlled clinical trials. Following a single episode of thrombosis, patients with inherited hypercoagulable states should probably receive indefinite or lifelong anticoagulation if their initial episodes were life-threatening or occurred in unusual sites of if they have more than one prothrombotic genetic abnormality. In the absence of these characteristics, particularly if the initial episode was precipitated by a transient acquired prothrombotic situation (e.g., pregnancy, postoperative state, immobilization), it is reasonable at this time to discontinue warfarin therapy after 6 months and administer subsequent prophylactic anticoagulation only during high-risk periods.

Women with thrombophilia who have had previous thrombosis—and probably also asymptomatic women with thrombophilia—should receive prophylactic anticoagulation throughout pregnancy and for 4 to 6 weeks post partum. LMWH is presently the anticoagulant of choice, and low-molecular-weight heparin appears to be a safe alternative.

Because warfarin-induced skin necrosis is a very rare problem, screening of all patients for inherited protein C or protein S deficiency, conditions that are known to predispose to this complication, is not indicated before starting warfarin therapy. Most cases can be avoided by not initiating warfarin therapy with high loading doses and by concomitant coverage with heparin.

Vitamin supplementation with folate, pyridoxine, and cobalamin can normalize elevated blood levels of homocysteine, but it is not known whether such treatment reduces the risk of thrombosis. The recommended daily doses are folate 1 mg, pyridoxine 100 mg, and cobalamin 0.4 mg.

Secondary Hypercoagulable States

The secondary hypercoagulable states are diverse, mostly acquired disorders that predispose patients to thrombosis by complex, multifactorial pathophysiologic mechanisms.

Certain malignant tissues may stimulate thrombosis directly by elaborating procoagulant substances that initiate a systemic process of chronic DIC. Hypercoagulability appears to be most prominent in patients with pancreatic cancer, adenocarcinomas of the gastrointestinal tract or lung, and ovarian cancers. The most common thrombotic manifestations are DVT and pulmonary embolism. Trousseau's syndrome, characterized by migratory superficial thrombophlebitis of the upper or lower extremities, is strongly linked to cancer. Non-bacterial thrombotic endocarditis involves fibrin-platelet vegetations on heart valves, which produce clinical manifestations by systemic embolization. Because the valve vegetations are often too small to be detected by auscultation of murmurs or by echocardiography, the diagnosis should be suspected in patients with systemic embolic signs, including acute stroke syndromes. Both Trousseau's syndrome and non-bacterial thrombotic endocarditis are highly associated with laboratory evidence of DIC. Many cancer patients are difficult to anticoagulate and may be resistant to warfarin prophylaxis.

Thrombosis and, paradoxically, bleeding are major causes of morbidity and mortality in the myeloproliferative disorders. In addition to DVT and pulmonary embolism, hepatic vein thrombosis (Budd-Chiari syndrome) and portal and other intra-abdominal venous thromboses are associated with myeloproliferative disorders and PNH.

The pathophysiology of hypercoagulability associated with pregnancy involves a progressive state of DIC throughout the course of pregnancy. DVT and pulmonary embolism are the most common thrombotic complications.

For more information about this subject, see *Cecil Textbook of Medicine,* 21st edition. Philadelphia, W.B. Saunders Company, 2000. Chapter 187, Thrombotic Disorders: Hypercoabulable States, pages 1016 to 1021.

ANTITHROMBOTIC THERAPY

Anticoagulant Therapy

Low-molecular-weight heparin (LMWH) given subcutaneously (1 mg/kg every 12 hours) effectively substitutes for dose-adjusted unfractionated heparin for all indications. Because standard (unfractionated) heparin must be given parenterally, with regular monitoring of its anticoagulant effects and frequent adjustment of dosage, its use is largely limited to in-hospital settings. LMWHs produce less bleeding than standard heparin. LMWHs also exhibit greater bioavailability, a longer plasma half-life, and a more predictable anticoagulant response than standard heparin does, which allows LMWHs to be administered subcutaneously twice daily without laboratory monitoring. Heparin-associated thrombocytopenia occurs in about 1 to 3% of treated patients. LMWH is associated with one tenth the frequency of inducing heparin-associated thrombocytopenia. The diagnosis may be confirmed by demonstrating platelet activation of heparin-induced antibiotics in the patient's plasma. In patients with severe thrombocytopenia, heparin therapy should be stopped and an alternative direct thrombin inhibitor used, such as hirudin, bivalirudin, or argatroban. Alopecia and osteoporosis also complicate heparin therapy after prolonged use.

Because LMWH requires no monitoring and has a longer elimination time, it is suited for out-of-hospital management of acute DVT. LMWHs are expected to displace standard heparin as they become more cost-competitive.

Immediate treatment with LMWH or heparin benefits patients with DVT or pulmonary embolism (Table 11–32). LMWH may be started as acute treatment in outpatients (Table 11–33).

Prophylactic Anticoagulation

Moderate-risk general surgery patients who are older than 40 years and undergoing major surgery without additional risk factors should be treated prophylactically with low-dose heparin (5000 U subcutaneously every 12 hours). Low-dose subcutaneous heparin begun before surgery and continuing until the patient is ambulatory reduces the incidence of venous thrombosis by two thirds and pulmonary embolism by half. Patients older than 40 years who are undergoing major surgery and have additional risk factors should receive low-dose subcutaneous heparin (5000 U every 8 hours) or LMWH every 12 hours.

Patients undergoing hip surgery should receive prophylaxis with LMWH, adjusted-dose heparin (to prolong the aPTT in the upper half of the normal range), or moderate-dose warfarin (to maintain the INR at 2.0 to 3.0). Recent controlled clinical trials demonstrate

Table 11–32 ■ ANTICOAGULANT THERAPY FOR DEEP VENOUS THROMBOSIS AND PULMONARY EMBOLISM

Initiate Therapy with Heparin

Administer LMWH at doses indicated for 'Acute Treatment' in Table 11–33; no aPTT monitoring required

Alternative 1: Administer IV heparin and adjust based according to aPTT results

Alternative 2: Administer heparin SC q 12 hr beginning with an initial dose of 18,000 U; check aPTT after 4 hr and adjust subsequent doses to prolong aPTT to 1.5–2.5× control; monitor and maintain range for at least 5–7 days

Maintenance Anticoagulation

Oral anticoagulants

1. Give warfarin 5–10 mg, during first hospital day
2. Check PT daily
3. Adjust dose to prolong PT to INR of 2–3 (1.3–1.5× control with most rabbit brain thromboplastins)
4. Discontinue heparin after minimum of 5 d when PT reaches desired range
5. Continue warfarin as outpatient for at least 3–6 mo

Heparin

Heparin SC q 12 hr in a dose to prolong the mid-interval aPTT to 1.5× control

LMWH = low-molecular-weight heparin; aPTT = activated partial thromboplastin time; PT = prothrombin time; INR = International Normalized Ratio.

Table 11–33 ■ RECOMMENDED DOSES OF COMMERCIAL LOW-MOLECULAR-WEIGHT HEPARINS

	RECOMMENDED DOSE (INTERNATIONAL ANTI-Xa UNITS)		
AGENT	General Surgery Prophylaxis	Orthopedic Surgery Prophylaxis	Acute Treatment
Enoxaparin	2000 U/day SC	4000 U/day SC *or* 3000 U SC bid	7000 U SC bid*
Dalteparin	2500 U/day SC	2500 U SC bid *or* 5000 U/day SC	8400 U SC bid*
Nadroparin	3100 U/day SC		12,300 U SC bid
Tinzaparin (Innohep)	3500 U/day SC	50 U/day/kg SC	12,250 U/day SC*
Ardeparin		50 U/kg SC bid	
Danaparoid†		750 U SC bid	1250 U SC bid

ICU = Institute Choay units; 3 ICU = 1 IU.
*Weight-adjusted dose; stated dose for 70-kg patient.
‡Danaparoid sodium is a heparinoid.

that subcutaneous hirudin 15 mg twice daily reduces thromboembolic complications after orthopedic surgery more effectively than does heparin or LMWH. Patients undergoing intracranial neurosurgical procedures or urologic surgery historically have not received anticoagulants but were treated with intermittent pneumatic compression only. One randomized trial, however, showed that LMWH was beneficial in neurosurgical patients.

Low-dose heparin is recommended for the prophylaxis of DVT and pulmonary embolism in medical patients at prolonged bedrest, such as patients with acute myocardial infarction or heart failure. Similarly, prophylaxis should be provided for patients with ischemic stroke and lower-extremity paralysis in the form of low-dose heparin or LMWH.

Pregnant patients with a history of previous venous thromboembolic disease are at increased risk for DVT and pulmonary embolism; these patients should be given low-dose subcutaneous heparin (5000 U twice daily) throughout their pregnancy. Women who have DVT during pregnancy should receive full-dose intravenous heparin by continuous infusion for 5 to 7 days or subcutaneous LMWH twice daily, followed by twice-daily adjusted-dose subcutaneous heparin until term. Pregnant patients with mechanical heart valves or atrial fibrillation and documented systemic embolization are often treated with twice-daily LMWH or adjusted-dose subcutaneous heparin from the time pregnancy is diagnosed until delivery.

Because drug interactions affect the dose of warfarin needed to maintain optimal therapy, great care is required to maintain therapeutic INR control in patients receiving other medications, particularly drugs used for changing symptoms. The introduction of any new medication prompts an assessment of its effects on the INR.

Anticoagulant-Induced Bleeding

The major risk of anticoagulant therapy is bleeding secondary to excessive anticoagulation. Patients treated with standard doses of either heparin or warfarin have a 2 to 4% per year frequency of bleeding episodes requiring transfusion. The risk of a fatal hemorrhage is about 0.2% per year for patients taking oral anticoagulants. The risk of major bleeding is increased in patients older than 65 years; in patients with a history of stroke, gastrointestinal bleeding, atrial fibrillation, and co-morbid conditions such as uremia and anemia; and with infrequent monitoring. Reversal of heparin is achieved by protamine sulfate.

Management of bleeding in patients receiving warfarin depends on the seriousness of the bleeding episode. If the INR is outside the therapeutic range but less than 5.0, the patient is not bleeding, and no invasive procedures are planned, several doses of warfarin are omitted and the drug is recommenced at a lower dose. If the INR is between 5.0 and 9.0 and the patient is not bleeding or more rapid reversal is needed to prepare for some invasive procedure, the oral administration or intravenous injection of 1 mg of vitamin K often restores the INR to the therapeutic range within 24 hours. If the INR is over 9.0, oral administration or an intravenous dose of 5 mg of vitamin K is recommended, with repeat dosing indicated if the INR remains prolonged at 12 to 24 hours. For more rapid reversal or in patients with an INR greater than 20.0, 10 mg of intravenous vitamin K by slow infusion should be given and the INR checked every 6 hours. Vitamin K may need to be repeated every 12 hours and supplemented with FFP transfusion or factor concentrate. With serious bleeding, replacement with factor concentrates of vitamin K–dependent clotting factors is indicated in addition to supplemental intravenous vitamin K (10 mg repeated every 12 hours until the INR is corrected).

During the first trimester of pregnancy, warfarin therapy is associated with a fetal skeletal embryopathy. Women receiving warfarin should be advised against pregnancy because of this risk. If pregnancy develops, full-dose subcutaneous heparin should be substituted for warfarin. Poisoning with warfarin has occurred in children.

For more information about this subject, see *Cecil Textbook of Medicine,* 21st edition. Philadelphia, W.B. Saunders Company, 2000. Chapter 188, Antithrombotic Therapy, pages 1021 to 1028.

CHAPTER 12

ONCOLOGY

The American Cancer Society (ACS) has recommended a series of cancer screening procedures for asymptomatic individuals (Table 12–1). Not all experts agree, but the ACS recommendations are a well-considered and useful guide.

A tumor reaches the size of clinical detectability when it contains about 10^9 cells, weighing about 1 g and occupying a volume of about 1 mL. A three-log increase to 10^{12} cells, 1 kg, and 1000 mL is often lethal. Below 10^9 cells, the tumor is usually undetectable, but it has already undergone at least 30 doublings, and only 10 further doublings will produce the 1 kg of tumor.

Most chemotherapy acts by damaging DNA, so it tends to be most effective in rapidly growing tumors such as acute leukemia. The sensitivity or resistance to chemotherapy or irradiation, however, probably has as much or more to do with the specific biochemical and metabolic features of the cancer.

MANAGEMENT OF THE PATIENT WITH CANCER

The initial therapeutic goal is to cure the patient. If permanent cure is not possible, the physician must not abandon the patient but rather should aim for a secondary goal—a long, qualitatively satisfactory remission. If and when this second goal is no longer possible, the tertiary level of therapeutic intent is to obtain a remission of any kind and duration. When the possibility of remission of any type becomes remote, the fourth goal is to control the disease and symptoms by the judicious use of palliative therapeutic measures. The objective in this final stage is comfortable terminal care.

The first diagnostic principle is that adequate tissue must be obtained to establish the specific diagnosis and subtype of cancer. The rare exceptions are instances in which a biopsy might be life-threatening and the anatomic location is virtually pathognomonic of a specific histology; two notable examples are brain tumors and anterior mediastinal tumors that compress the trachea and blood vessels. A second diagnostic principle is to establish the extent of the disease (Table 12–2).

There are four principal therapeutic modalities for cancer. *Surgery* is the oldest and most definitive when the tumor is localized. *Radiation therapy* is most useful for localized tumors that cannot be resected at all or without serious morbidity and for tumors, such as Hodgkin's disease, that tend to spread to predictable contiguous sites. *Chemotherapy* most often consists of a combination of drugs, which is almost always more effective than the sequential use of

For more information about this subject, see *Cecil Textbook of Medicine,* 21st edition. Philadelphia, W.B. Saunders Company, 2000. Part XIV: Oncology, pages 1029 to 1081.

Table 12–1 ■ SUMMARY OF AMERICAN CANCER SOCIETY RECOMMENDATIONS FOR THE EARLY DETECTION OF CANCER IN ASYMPTOMATIC PEOPLE

	POPULATION		
TEST OR PROCEDURE	**Sex**	**Age (yr)**	**Frequency**
Sigmoidoscopy, preferably flexible	M & F	≥50	Every 3–5 yr
Fecal occult blood test	M & F	≥50	Every yr
Digital rectal examination	M & F	≥40	Every yr
Prostate examination*	M	≥50	Every yr
Papanicolaou test	F	All women who are or who have been sexually active, or have reached age 18, should have an annual Papanicolaou test and pelvic examination. After a woman has had 3 or more consecutive satisfactory normal annual examinations, the Papanicolaou test may be performed less frequently at the discretion of her physician.	
Pelvic examination	F	18–40	Every 1–3 yr with Papanicolaou test
		>40	Every yr
Endometrial tissue sample	F	At menopause, if at high risk†	At menopause and thereafter at the discretion of the physician
Breast self-examination	F	≥20	Every mo
Breast clinical examination	F	20–40	Every 3 yr
		>40	Every yr
Mammography‡	F	40–49	Every 1–2 yr
		≥50	Every yr
Health counseling and cancer checkups§	M & F	>20	Every 3 yr
	M & F	>40	Every yr

*Annual digital rectal examination and prostate-specific antigen should be performed on men 50 years and older. If either is abnormal, further evaluation should be considered.

†History of infertility, obesity, failure to ovulate, abnormal uterine bleeding, or unopposed estrogen or tamoxifen therapy.

‡Screening mammography should begin by age 40.

§To include examination for cancers of the thyroid, testes, prostate, ovaries, lymph nodes, oral region, and skin.

From Cancer Facts and Figures—1998. Atlanta, American Cancer Society, 1998.

single agents. Chemotherapy is used (1) as a definitive treatment, as in leukemia and some lymphomas; (2) as a principal form of treatment, as in testicular cancer and Ewing's sarcoma; or (3) as an adjuvant to another modality, such as amputation for osteosarcoma or surgical resection for breast or bowel cancer. *Biologic therapy* for cancer includes, in addition to bone marrow transplantation, biologic response modifiers such as lymphokines or monoclonal

Table 12–2 ■ SIMPLIFIED GENERIC CANCER STAGING SYSTEM

Stage 1	Localized. Usually confined to the organ of origin. Usually curable with locally effective measures such as surgery or irradiation.
Stage 2	Regional. Extends beyond organ of origin but remains nearby, in lymph nodes, for example. Often curable by local measures alone or in combination (surgery ± irradiation) or by a local modality with chemotherapy.
Stage 3	Extensive. Has extended beyond regional site of origin, crossing several tissue planes or extending more distantly via lymphatics or blood. Also may be confined to an organ or region, but be unresectable because of anatomic extent or location. This stage is used rather than stage 2 or stage 4 depending on the usefulness of local and systemic treatment modalities and the likelihood of cure for that specific cancer.
Stage 4	Widely disseminated. Often involves the bone marrow or multiple distant organs. Rarely curable with current armamentarium.

antibodies. Supportive care includes management of infectious, metabolic, and cardiopulmonary disorders that frequently occur in patients undergoing aggressive treatment or surgical procedures.

12

The first measure of success is survival without recurrence of tumor. The second is resumption of a normal life.

For more information about this subject, see *Cecil Textbook of Medicine,* 21st edition. Philadelphia, W.B. Saunders Company, 2000. Chapter 189, Introduction to Oncology, pages 1029 to 1032.

GENETICS OF CANCER

Molecular Oncology

Data have identified predictable mutations in the *p53* gene associated with aflatoxin exposure in hepatocellular carcinoma and with ultraviolet light exposure in skin cancers. Cancer susceptibility genes for colon cancer (*APC, MSH2, MLH1*), for breast cancer (*BRCA1* and *BRCA2*), for retinoblastoma (*Rb*), for the Li-Fraumeni syndrome (*p53*), for the von Hippel-Lindau syndrome (*VHL*), for the multiple endocrine neoplasia syndrome (*RET*), and for neurofibromatosis (*NF1*) have already been cloned and can be used for direct screening of cancer susceptibility (Table 12–3).

Tumor Markers

An increasing number of serum tumor markers have been validated for the purpose of assessing prognosis and response to therapy. Tumor markers also may substantially precede other evidence of disease progression or recurrence (Table 12–4).

For more information about this subject, see *Cecil Textbook of Medicine,* 21st edition. Philadelphia, W.B. Saunders Company, 2000. Chapter 191, Oncogenes and Suppressor Genes: Genetic Control of Cancer; and Chapter 192, Tumor Markers, pages 1035 to 1042.

Table 12–3 ■ SOME GENES INVOLVED IN CANCER SUSCEPTIBILITY

DISORDER	GENE
Familial retinoblastoma	*Rb*
Li-Fraumeni syndrome	*p53*
Familial breast and ovarian cancer	*BRCA1*
Familial breast cancer	*BRCA2*
Cowden's disease	*PTEN*
Familial adenomatous polyposis	*APC*
Hereditary non-polyposis colorectal cancer (HNPCC)	*MSH2, MLH1, PMS1, PMS2*
von Hippel-Lindau syndrome	*VHL*
Familial papillary renal cell carcinoma	*MET*
Nevoid basal cell carcinoma	*PTCH*
Familial melanoma	*p16*
MEN-I	*MEN1*
MEN-II	*RET*
Neurofibromatosis	*NF1* and *NF2*
Ataxia-telangiectasia	*ATM*
Wilms' tumor	*WT-1*

MEN-I, MEN-II = multiple endocrine neoplasia, types I and II.

THE EPIDEMIOLOGY OF CANCER

It was estimated that in 1998 about 1.25 million Americans will have developed and nearly 600,000 will have died of cancer (Fig. 12–1). For nearly all cancers, the incidence rates are higher among men than women, the exceptions being gallbladder and thyroid cancers. Rates of most cancers, particularly those deriving from epithelial tissue, rise steadily with advancing age, often exponentially. Racial differences in cancer occurrence are sometimes marked. Total cancer incidence during 1990 to 1994 was higher among black than white males by 26%, whereas rates were higher among white than black females by 3%.

There has been nearly a doubling in the incidence of melanoma and a 50% rise in non-Hodgkin's lymphomas among whites since the early 1970s. In the United States, a sharp rise in the incidence of prostate cancer occurred in the late 1980s, owing mainly to the increased detection of early tumors because of expanded screening with prostate-specific antigen testing.

Cigarette smoking is the dominant cause of the leading cancer (i.e., lung cancer) in the United States and many other Western nations. Cigarette smoking also is a principal cause of cancers of the oral cavity and pharynx, esophagus, larynx, and renal pelvis, and is a major contributor to cancers of the pancreas, bladder, and kidney.

Alcohol combines with tobacco to cause cancers of the oral cavity and pharynx, esophagus, and larynx. Alcoholic beverages also have been implicated in the etiology of liver and rectal cancers.

Asbestos exposure has counted for the largest number of occupational cancers. Radon and its daughter products are another group of potent carcinogens. Among chemicals considered to be causally

Table 12–4 ■ USE OF SERUM TUMOR MARKERS FOR SCREENING, PROGNOSIS, MONITORING RESPONSE TO THERAPY, AND DETECTING RECURRENCE

TUMOR	MARKER(S)	UTILITY OF MARKERS			
		Screening	Prognosis	Monitoring	Recurrence
Colorectal	CEA	No	Yes	Yes	Yes
Ovary	CA-125	No	No	Yes	Yes
Testicle	hCG, AFP	No	In some studies	Yes	Yes
Prostate	PSA	Yes?	Yes	Yes	Yes
Breast	CA 15-3, CEA	No	No	Yes	Yes
Non-Hodgkin's lymphoma	LDH	No	Yes	No	Yes
Myeloma	β_2-M	No	Yes	Yes	Yes
Hepatoma	AFP	Yes, in high-risk patient*	No	Yes	Yes

CEA = carcinoembryonic antigen; hCG = human chorionic gonadotropin; AFP = alpha-fetoprotein; PSA = prostate-specific antigen; LDH = lactate dehydrogenase; β_2-M = β_2-microglobulin.

*Screening studies have been useful in Asian patients with evidence of previous hepatitis infection. Controlled trials are lacking. In the United States and Europe, patients with cirrhosis are often followed with AFP and ultrasound without definitive data from clinical trials.

Leading Sites of New Cancer Cases and Deaths—1998 Estimates*

Cancer Cases by Site and Sex: Male	Cancer Cases by Site and Sex: Female	Cancer Deaths by Site and Sex: Male	Cancer Deaths by Site and Sex: Female
Prostate 184,500	Breast 178,700	Lung 93,100	Lung 67,000
Lung 91,400	Lung 80,100	Prostate 39,200	Breast 43,500
Colon & rectum 64,600	Colon & rectum 67,000	Colon & rectum 27,900	Colon & rectum 28,600
Urinary bladder 39,500	Endometrium (uterus) 36,100	Pancreas 14,000	Pancreas 14,900
Non-Hodgkin's lymphoma 31,100	Ovary 25,400	Non-Hodgkin's lymphoma 13,000	Ovary 14,500
Melanoma of the skin 24,300	Non-Hodgkin's lymphoma 24,300	Leukemia 12,000	Non-Hodgkin's lymphoma 11,900
Oral cavity 20,600	Melanoma of the skin 17,300	Esophagus 9,100	Leukemia 9,600
Kidney 17,600	Urinary bladder 14,900	Urinary bladder 8,400	Endometrium (uterus) 6,300
Leukemia 16,100	Pancreas 14,900	Stomach 8,100	Brain 6,000
Stomach 14,300	Cervix (uterus) 13,700	Liver 7,900	Stomach 5,600
All Sites 627,900	All Sites 600,700	All Sites 294,200	All Sites 270,600

*Excluding basal and squamous cell skin cancer and in situ carcinomas except urinary bladder.
American Cancer Society, Surveillance Research, 1998.

FIGURE 12–1 ■ Leading sites of cancer incidence and death—1998 estimates. (From Cancer Facts and Figures—1998. Atlanta, American Cancer Society, 1998.)

associated with cancer in humans, nearly one half are medications, including drugs used in cancer treatment.

Strong evidence indicates that diet and nutrition can influence cancer risk. Clearest are the inverse associations between risk of certain epithelial cancers, particularly oral, esophageal, stomach, and lung cancers, and intake of fresh fruits and vegetables.

Several viral agents have been associated with human cancer. Hepatitis B virus (HBV) is the primary cause of hepatocellular carcinoma in China. Human papillomavirus (HPV) is the etiologic agent in a high percentage of cases of cervical cancer.

For more information about this subject, see *Cecil Textbook of Medicine,* 21st edition. Philadelphia, W.B. Saunders Company, 2000. Chapter 190, Cancer Prevention; and Chapter 193, The Epidemiology of Cancer, pages 1032 to 1035 and 1042 to 1047.

"ECTOPIC" HORMONE PRODUCTION

Humoral Hypercalcemia of Malignancy

Hypercalcemia is one of the most common hormonal syndromes associated with cancer. An elevated parathyroid hormone (PTH) level in the context of hypercalcemia should prompt further evaluation for parathyroid disease. However, in the majority of cancer patients with hypercalcemia, the intact serum parathyroid hormone (iPTH) value will be suppressed, indicating that the malignancy is generating the hypercalcemia.

PARATHYROID HORMONE–RELATED PROTEIN. Parathyroid hormone–related protein (PTHrp) is normally involved in chondrocytic and dermatologic differentiation. Eight of the first 16 amino acids are homologous with PTH. Ectopic production of PTHrp by a wide variety of tumors is one of the most common causes of hypercalcemia associated with malignancy. The clinical syndrome is nearly identical to that observed with hyperparathyroidism and includes increased osteoclast-mediated bone resorption as well as an increase in renal tubular calcium resorption and a decrease in phosphorus resorption. The only significant clinical difference between PTHrp and PTH-mediated hypercalcemia is the finding of increased serum calcitriol (1,25-dihydroxycholecalciferol) in hyperparathyroidism versus low or normal values in PTHrp-mediated hypercalcemia. PTHrp production is most commonly associated with squamous cell carcinomas, although production has been observed in other types of tumors, including breast, neuroendocrine, renal, melanoma, and prostate tumors.

INCREASED PRODUCTION OF CALCITRIOL. Increased production of calcitriol occurs in a high percentage of patients with lymphoma. Other granulomatous conditions such as sarcoid, berylliosis, and tuberculous or fungal infections may also cause this syndrome. Other clinical features include a suppressed iPTH level, an increased or normal phosphorus level, hypercalciuria, and no evidence of bone metastasis. An elevated serum calcitriol concentration is found in approximately one half of hypercalcemic cancer patients.

Bone metastases are frequently associated with local production of cytokines, PTHrp, or other substances that cause increased bone resorption. Indeed, the distinctions between humoral hypercalcemia of malignancy and localized osteolysis have become blurred because of evidence that tumors such as breast carcinoma or myeloma cause localized osteolysis by local production and secretion of PTHrp.

TREATMENT. Management should focus initially on reversing dehydration and increasing urine calcium excretion by infusion of normal saline solution at rates of 100 to 300 mL/hour. A patient with a serum calcium concentration >13 mg/dL (3.25 mmol/L), altered mental status, or renal dysfunction should also be treated with bisphosphonate (pamidronate 60 to 90 mg/4 hours intravenously [IV]), glucocorticoids (prednisone or methylprednisolone 40 to 60 mg/day), gallium nitrate 200 mg/m^2/day infused for 7 days, or salmon calcitonin 100 to 200 units IV or subcutaneously [SC] every 6 to 12 hours, alone or in combination. PTHrp-mediated or localized osteolysis is most responsive to bisphosphonates or gallium nitrate; vitamin D–mediated hypercalcemia is most responsive to glucocorticoid therapy. Long-term management is focused on therapy of the underlying malignancy.

Ectopic ACTH Secretion

Inappropriate secretion of corticotropin (ACTH) is a rare but important cause of morbidity and mortality in cancer patients. It can be caused by two different mechanisms: expression of the proopiomelanocortin (POMC) gene by a tumor or ectopic expression of corticotropin-releasing hormone (CRH). ACTH production occurs in a broad spectrum of tumors, but it is most commonly associated with small cell carcinoma of the lung (SCCL) or more classic neuroendocrine tumors such as pulmonary carcinoid, islet cell adenomas or carcinomas, and pheochromocytoma.

Hypercorticism associated with ectopic ACTH syndrome may present with classic features of Cushing's syndrome. In other patients, particularly those with rapidly growing SCCL, the clinical picture may be dominated by profound hypokalemic metabolic alkalosis and hypertension.

The finding of a marked elevation of the plasma ACTH concentration (>100 pg/mL) should prompt a search for an ectopic source of ACTH. In a patient with a plasma ACTH value greater than 10 pg/mL but less than 100 pg/mL, more detailed evaluation is appropriate. The difference between a pituitary and an ectopic source may require stimulation of ACTH secretion by CRH combined with measurement of ACTH in blood of the inferior petrosal sinus. Lack of an increase in the inferior petrosal sinus ACTH concentration (more than three times the peripheral ACTH) following peripheral CRH stimulation should prompt a search for an ectopic source. ACTH production from an ectopic source is not generally suppressed by high-dose dexamethasone.

TREATMENT. Hypercortisolism can be managed by removal of the tumor or by metyrapone 1 to 4 g/day orally (PO), aminoglutethimide 250 mg PO four times a day with upward titration, or ketoconazole 200 to 400 mg PO twice a day. Replacement glucocorticoid therapy is needed to prevent adrenal insufficiency. Cytotoxic chemotherapy generally should be delayed, if possible, until the serum cortisol level is normalized, because of the high rate of infection in neutropenic patients with hypercortisolism.

Human Chorionic Gonadotropin Production

Production of the α-subunit of human chorionic gonadotropin (hCG) occurs in a variety of pituitary and non-pituitary tumors and does not cause any discernible clinical syndrome. Production of intact hCG occurs commonly in trophoblastic tumors (choriocarcinomas, testicular embryonal carcinomas, and seminomas) and less commonly in other tumors such as lung and pancreas tumors. Clinical syndromes include gynecomastia and hyperthyroidism.

TREATMENT. Therapy for gynecomastia is directed toward removal or treatment of the underlying tumor. Hyperthyroidism is treated by thioamide therapy, followed by therapy for the underlying tumor.

Hypoglycemia

Three different clinical syndromes cause most cancer-related hypoglycemia. The first is production of insulin by an islet cell tumor. A second cause, insufficient gluconeogenesis to maintain the plasma glucose concentration in the fasting state, is due to near-complete replacement of the liver by metastatic tumor. A third cause of hypoglycemia is increased concentration of insulin-like growth factor-II (IGF-II), a ligand that interacts with the insulin receptor in large abdominal tumors, most commonly fibrosarcomas, hemangiopericytomas, or hepatomas. The patient is at greatest risk during periods of fasting, most commonly during sleeping.

TREATMENT. Therapy should focus on surgical excision or antineoplastic therapy. Initial therapy of hypoglycemia is focused on frequent meals. Continuous infusion of 20% dextrose through a central line may be required, especially during sleeping hours. In patients with insulin-producing or large retroperitoneal tumors, glucagon infusion of 0.5 to 2.0 mg/hour stimulates hepatic gluconeogenesis and prevents hypoglycemia. In patients with large retroperitoneal tumors, treatment with growth hormone 3 to 6 μg/kg SC or glucocorticoids 20 to 40 mg/day may reverse hypoglycemia.

Syndrome of Inappropriate Antidiuretic Hormone Production (SIADH)

Ectopic production of vasopressin by head and neck tumors (3%), SCCL (15%), and other lung carcinomas (1%) causes a clinical syndrome characterized by hyponatremia, hypo-osmolality, excessive urine sodium excretion, and an inappropriately high urine osmolality. Primary brain tumors, hematologic neoplasms, skin tumors, and gastrointestinal, gynecologic, breast, and prostate cancers, and sarcomas are rare causes of this syndrome.

TREATMENT. Fluid restriction may be effective for short-term management. Treatment with demeclocycline 150 to 300 mg/day can block the effects of vasopressin on the kidney and is the most effective long-term therapy.

For more information about this subject, see *Cecil Textbook of Medicine,* 21st edition. Philadelphia, W.B. Saunders Company, 2000. Chapter 194, Endocrine Manifestations of Tumors: "Ectopic" Hormone Production, pages 1047 to 1050.

NON-METASTATIC EFFECTS OF CANCER: THE NERVOUS SYSTEM

Paraneoplastic syndromes, also called "remote effects of cancer on the nervous system," refer to neurologic dysfunction caused by cancer but not ascribable to such well-defined secondary effects of cancer as infection, coagulation abnormalities, nutritional and metabolic disorders, or side effects of therapy. The etiology of most or all remote effects is autoimmune.

Paraneoplastic syndromes are usually classified by the anatomic site of neurologic disability (Table 12–5). However, it is common for more than one anatomic site to be involved.

In *subacute motor neuronopathy* there is progressive painless asymmetrical lower motor neuron weakness of the legs and arms. In *subacute necrotic myelopathy,* rapidly ascending sensory and motor loss is present, usually to the midthoracic level; the patient becomes paraplegic and incontinent within hours or days. Characteristic of carcinoma is *subacute sensory neuronopathy,* marked by loss of sensation with relative preservation of motor power. More common than sensory neuronopathy is a *distal sensorimotor polyneuropathy* characterized by motor weakness, sensory loss, and absence of distal reflexes in the extremities. A *polyneuritis* clinically and pathologically indistinguishable from acute post-infectious polyneuropathy (Guillain-Barré syndrome) also complicates cancers. Typical *dermatomyositis* or *polymyositis* may occur as a remote effect of cancer.

Myasthenia gravis is associated with thymomas but not usually with other systemic tumors. The *Lambert-Eaton myasthenic syndrome* is characterized by weakness and fatigability of proximal muscles, particularly of the pelvic girdle and thighs. The cranial nerves and respiratory muscles are usually spared. The proximal muscles are weak, but strength increases over several seconds of sustained contraction. The diagnosis is made by electromyographic studies. Most patients harbor P/Q-type voltage-gated calcium channel antibodies in their serum. The illness responds to 3,4-diaminopyridine in doses up to 100 mg/day.

Nervous System Injury from Therapeutic Radiation

Acute encephalopathy may follow large radiation doses to the brain. *Early delayed reactions* appear 6 to 16 weeks after therapy and persist for days to months. *Early delayed myelopathy* follows radiation therapy to the neck or upper part of the thorax and is characterized by Lhermitte's sign (an electric shock–like sensation radiating into various parts of the body when the neck is flexed). *Late delayed radiation injury* appears months to years after radiation therapy and may affect any part of the nervous system. *Late delayed myelopathy* is characterized by progressive paralysis, sensory changes, and sometimes pain. *Late delayed neuropathy* may affect any cranial or peripheral nerve.

For more information about this subject, see *Cecil Textbook of Medicine,* 21st edition. Philadelphia, W.B. Saunders Company, 2000. Chapter 195, Non-Metastatic Effects of Cancer: The Nervous System, pages 1051 to 1054.

Table 12–5 ■ PARANEOPLASTIC SYNDROMES OF THE NERVOUS SYSTEM

Brain and Cranial Nerves

Limbic encephalitis
Brain stem encephalitis
Cerebellar degeneration
Opsoclonus-myoclonus
Paraneoplastic visual syndromes
  Cancer-associated retinopathy
  Optic neuritis

Spinal Cord

Necrotizing myelopathy
Myelitis
Motor neuron syndrome
Subacute motor neuronopathy

Dorsal Root Ganglia

Paraneoplastic sensory neuronopathy

Peripheral Nerves

Autonomic neuropathy
Acute sensorimotor neuropathy
  Polyradiculoneuropathy (Guillain-Barré syndrome)
  Brachial neuritis
Chronic sensorimotor neuropathy
  Sensorimotor neuropathies associated with plasma call dyscrasias
Vasculitic neuropathy
Neuromyotonia

Neuromuscular Junction and Muscle

Lambert-Eaton myasthenic syndrome
Myasthenia gravis
Polymyositis/dermatomyositis
Acute necrotizing myopathy
Cachectic myopathy
Carcinoid myopathy
Myotonia

Multiple Levels of Involvement or Uncertain Site

Encephalomyelitis*
Stiff-man syndrome
Carcinomatous neuromyopathy

Italics indicate that in some groups of patients (e.g., children with opsoclonus, postmenopausal women with cerebellar dysfunction), the neurologic disorder is associated with a tumor in more than 50% of instances.

*Can include cerebellar symptoms, autonomic dysfunction, and sensory neuronopathy.

NON-METASTATIC EFFECTS OF CANCER: THE SKIN

Pruritus, or itching, may be an important clue to Hodgkin's disease, lymphocytic leukemia, polycythemia vera, myeloid metaplasia, carcinoid, and less commonly, carcinomas. *Erythroderma,* or exfoliative dermatitis, is a cutaneous reaction with redness, edema, scaling, and lichenification. In 10% of cases it is associated with malignancy, especially lymphomas, leukemia, and mycosis fungoides.

12

Figurate erythemas are red, persistent, gyrate, serpiginous, and annular bands with a fine trailing scale. The lesions have been associated with breast, stomach, bladder, prostate, cervix, tongue, and uterine cancer. *Urticarial-like lesions* may precede the development of leukemia by many months.

Acanthosis nigricans is characterized by soft, velvety, verrucous, brown hyperpigmentation with skin tags in the body folds, especially those of the neck, axilla, and groin. When it occurs in patients older than 40 years, it is often a sign of an underlying malignant tumor, usually adenocarcinoma.

For more information about this subject, see *Cecil Textbook of Medicine,* 21st edition. Philadelphia, W.B. Saunders Company, 2000. Chapter 196, Non-Metastatic Effects of Cancer: The Skin, pages 1054 to 1057.

NON-METASTATIC EFFECTS OF CANCER: OTHER SYSTEMS

The clinical syndrome of *cancer cachexia* includes weight loss, anorexia, muscle atrophy, immune dysregulation (resulting in anergy), and sometimes organ atrophy. Tumor necrosis factor-α (TNF-α), also known as cachectin, is postulated to be the major cytokine released from macrophages and mediates this syndrome. Parenteral nutrition or nutritious supplements may be offered but are not often helpful. High doses (400 to 800 mg/day of the liquid formulation) of the progestational hormone megestrol acetate can improve appetite in a significant percentage of cancer patients. Corticosteroids can also be considered.

The *impaired immunosuppression* observed in cancer patients is associated with increased risk for the development of infections. Immune abnormalities include a decrease in the number of T lymphocytes (with no effect on B-cell numbers).

Anemia is seen in patients with cancer and may be secondary to chronic disease, red blood cell aplasia, bone marrow invasion, blood loss, chemotherapy, radiation therapy, nutritional deficiencies, or autoimmune or microangiopathic hemolysis. Various cytokines produced by tumors, especially interleukin-1 (IL-1) and TNF-α, inhibit messenger RNA (mRNA) synthesis of erythropoietin.

Systemic *activation of coagulation* may result in disseminated intravascular coagulation, superficial venous thrombophlebitis (Trousseau's syndrome), marantic endocarditis, or thrombotic microangiopathy. Tumor cells may release procoagulant materials such as tissue factor-like substances that activate Factor X. Anticoagulant therapy should be initiated cautiously. Chronic therapy may include warfarin or low-molecular-weight heparin on an outpatient basis, although the long-term prognosis is dependent on the primary tumor's response to cytotoxic therapy.

Paraneoplastic *leukemic reactions* can occur in patients with solid tumors or hematologic malignancies and can be associated with fever. Granulocyte colony-stimulating factor (G-CSF) production has been observed in a number of malignancies (malignant fibrous histiocytoma, nasopharyngeal carcinoma, transitional cell carcinoma of the urinary bladder) and is probably the cause.

Cancer-associated erythrocytosis is most frequently seen in malignant and benign conditions of the kidney (renal cell carcinoma, Wilms' tumor, cystic kidney, and hydronephrosis) or the liver (hepatoma). Pheochromocytomas, uterine fibroids, sarcomas, and aldosterone-secreting tumors are also associated with cancer-associated erythrocytosis. This paraneoplastic syndrome is associated with increased levels of endogenous erythropoietin in 50% or fewer of patients; in some cases, cancer-associated erythrocytosis may be secondary to the overproduction of androgens, prostaglandins, and other, yet unidentified substances.

A paraneoplastic *cancer-associated thrombocytosis* is seen in patients with Hodgkin's disease, non-Hodgkin's lymphoma, leukemias, and other solid malignancies and may be related to the overproduction of thrombopoietin(s). Despite the elevated platelet count, secondary thrombocytosis is not generally associated with clinical evidence of thrombotic or bleeding disorders.

Nephrotic syndrome in the setting of malignancy can be due to direct kidney involvement by the cancer, renal vein thrombosis, or a paraneoplastic syndrome. Paraneoplastic nephrotic syndrome is most commonly seen in association with Hodgkin's disease and is usually characterized by lipoid nephrosis (minimal glomerular nephrosis). Other glomerular lesions may be associated with non-Hodgkin's lymphoma, colon cancer, bronchogenic carcinoma, and prostate cancer. Deposition of tumor-associated antigen-antibody complexes can cause membranous glomerulonephritis. *Paraneoplastic hepatopathy,* also known as Stauffer's syndrome, is characterized by hepatic dysfunction, fever, and weight loss and is most commonly seen in non-metastatic renal cell carcinoma.

Pulmonary osteoarthropathy consists of symmetrical clubbing of the nails, active synovitis, and periosteal inflammation of the long bones (often manifested as "arthritis" of the elbows, wrists, knees, or ankles). The bilateral nature of the disease suggests a cytokine-mediated component. The classic triad of clubbing, synovitis, and periostitis may appear at different times in the clinical course. Although the joints of the lower extremities may be painful, red, and swollen, physical examination may reveal that the "arthritis" is discomfort caused by pain in the adjacent long bone. Plain radiography may reveal the periosteal elevations. Bone scans appear to be more sensitive than plain films and may confirm the diagnosis. Arthritic symptoms may be treated with aspirin and/or non-steroidal anti-inflammatory drugs. Vagotomy often results in analgesia within days to weeks. Atropine may also be helpful. Surgery of the primary malignancy may improve the articular complaints, sometimes within hours. Chemotherapy or radiotherapy may provide a gradual beneficial effect.

For more information about this subject, see *Cecil Textbook of Medicine,* 21st edition. Philadelphia, W.B. Saunders Company, 2000. Chapter 197, Non-Metastatic Effects of Cancer: Other Systems, pages 1057 to 1059.

CANCER THERAPY

The major clinical features of cancer to be considered in developing a treatment plan include (1) specific histologic diagnosis of the neoplasm, (2) tumor burden and extent of specific organ involvement (stage), and (3) biologic characteristics and other prognostic factors relevant to the specific type of cancer.

Increasingly, immunohistochemical analysis helps distinguish among various morphologically "undifferentiated" neoplasms. Electron microscopy sometimes can help. Distinctive markers include immunohistochemistry (e.g., overexpression of cyclin D in mantle cell lymphoma), serum or urinary tumor markers (e.g., β-hCG, alpha-fetoprotein, carcinoembryonic antigen, CA-125, myeloma proteins, urinary 5-hydroxyindole acetic acid), karyotype, or molecular analysis.

Most staging systems assess the size of the primary tumor and define regional lymph node involvement as well as the presence or absence of distant metastatic disease. Increasingly, staging can be accomplished by using non-invasive imaging procedures. The temptation to use a variety of redundant and expensive tests should be avoided.

For many tumor types, histopathologic features, such as grade of tumor cell differentiation, are important, with a less differentiated or undifferentiated phenotype indicating a more aggressive neoplasm. For some sites, other biologic factors are of greater value than histologic grade.

Three primary therapeutic approaches dominate the treatment of cancer: surgery, radiation therapy, and medical therapy. A fourth modality, biologic therapy (cytokines, antibodies, vaccines), is beginning to add another dimension to treatment programs.

Cancer surgery is most useful in establishing a tissue diagnosis, in excising the primary tumor with clear surgical margins free of tumor, and in determining the extent of cancer with staging procedures. Surgery also plays an important role in the management of some patients with more extensive cancer. In ovarian cancer, when the gynecologic oncologist "debulks" peritoneal and omental spread and leaves the patient with minimal residual disease, patients become better candidates for systemic chemotherapy.

The basic unit of ionizing irradiation is the gray (Gy), which has superseded the rad (1 Gy = 100 rads) (Table 12–6). Radiation therapy has important palliative as well as potentially curative applications. One of the former is for bone pain due to metastatic involvement of the skeleton. Several classes of compounds are under study as radiosensitizers to enhance the cytotoxic effects of radiation on tumor cells.

Table 12–6 ■ TOLERANCE OF NORMAL TISSUES TO IRRADIATION

TISSUE	TOXIC EFFECT	LIMITING DOSE (Gy)*
Bone marrow	Aplasia	2.5
Lung	Pneumonitis, fibrosis	15.0
Kidney	Nephrosclerosis	20.0
Liver	Hepatitis	25.0
Spinal cord	Infarction, necrosis	45.0
Intestine	Ulceration, fibrosis	45.0
Heart	Pericarditis, myocarditis	45.0
Brain	Infarction, necrosis	50.0
Skin	Dermatitis, sclerosis	55.0

*Radiation in 2.0-Gy fractions to the whole organ for 5 days weekly produces a 5% incidence of the listed toxicities at the limiting doses listed.

Curative medical therapy has been developed for a series of relatively uncommon disseminated neoplasms, and useful palliative therapy has been developed for some common forms of cancer (Table 12–7). Anticancer drugs can be classified as either cell cycle specific (CCS) or cell cycle non-specific (CCNS) (Table 12–8). Endocrine agents also have cyclic activity, because they block the transition of tumor cells from G_1 to the S phase. However, certain endocrine agents (e.g., tamoxifen, progestins) are considered to suppress growth rather than kill tumor cells. Cellular killing with cytotoxic agents follows first-order kinetics, with a given dose of drug killing only a fraction of the tumor cells. Optimal results for most tumor types sensitive to chemotherapy have been achieved with drug combinations, often employing CCNS and CCS agents possessing different mechanisms of action.

Most drug resistance is considered to result from the high spontaneous mutation rate of cancer cells. The most important is multidrug resistance (MDR), mediated by a cell membrane glycoprotein (the P-glycoprotein), which is thought to function as an energy-dependent efflux pump that actively extrudes a variety of cytotoxic agents from the cell. A series of non-cytotoxic drugs has been identified to reverse drug resistance mediated by P-glycoprotein (e.g., verapamil, cyclosporine). In the long run, such chemosensitizers may find their major use in preventing development of MDR expression. Chemosensitivity assays appear to predict drug

Table 12–7 ■ RESPONSIVENESS OF CANCER TO CHEMOTHERAPY

Cure (>30%) of Advanced Disease

Choriocarcinoma
Acute lymphocytic leukemia (childhood)
Malignant lymphoma (Hodgkin's disease, diffuse high-grade or intermediate-grade non-Hodgkin's lymphoma)
Hairy cell leukemia
Testicular cancer
Childhood solid tumors (embryonal rhabdomyosarcoma, Ewing's sarcoma, Wilms' tumor)
Acute myelocytic leukemia
Acute lymphocytic leukemia (adult)
Promyelocytic leukemia

Significant Palliation, Some Cures of Advanced Disease (5–30%)

Ovarian cancer
Bladder cancer
Small cell lung cancer
Gastric cancer

Palliation, Probably Increased Survival

Breast cancer
Multiple myeloma
Head and neck cancer

Adjuvant Treatment Leading to Increased Cure

Breast cancer
Colon cancer
Osteogenic sarcoma
Early-stage large cell lymphoma

Table 12–8 ■ RELATIONSHIP TO TUMOR CELL CYCLE TO ACTIVITY OF MAJOR CLASSES OF CYTOTOXIC ANTICANCER DRUGS

CELL CYCLE SPECIFIC (CCS) AGENTS	CELL CYCLE NON-SPECIFIC (CCNS) AGENTS
Antimetabolites (cytarabine, fluorouracil, methotrexate, mercaptopurine, hydroxyurea)	Alkylating agents (busulfan, cyclophosphamide, mechlorethamine, melphalan, thiotepa, chlorambucil)
Anthracyclines (doxorubicin, daunorubicin)	Antibiotics (dactinomycin, mitomycin)
Bleomycin	Platinum compounds (cisplatin, carboplatin)
Camptothecins (irinotecan, topotecan)	Nitrosoureas (BCNU, CCNU)
Plant alkaloids (vincristine, vinblastine, etoposide, taxol)	Dacarbazine
	L-Asparaginase

resistance but are somewhat less accurate for predicting which drugs will be useful for an individual patient.

The IV route is preferable for most cytotoxic anticancer drugs because it ensures adequate plasma levels while minimizing compliance problems. Regional administration of chemotherapy can be effective for several tumor sites, for example, hepatic artery infusion of 5-fluorodeoxyuridine or 5-fluorouracil (5-FU) for metastic colon cancer limited to the liver. Intraperitoneal drug administration can induce remissions of established metastatic disease. Methotrexate, cytarabine, and thiotepa can be given by the intrathecal route to prevent meningeal leukemia and treat central nervous system leukemia or lymphoma or meningeal carcinomatosis.

Whenever possible, confirmation of response should be obtained pathologically through the use of restaging procedures. Many patients achieve only a partial response, defined as a reduction of tumor burden by 50% or greater. Patients achieving partial responses generally have palliation of symptoms.

Cytotoxic Anticancer Drugs

Safe and effective cytotoxic cancer chemotherapy requires considerable understanding of the pharmacology and toxicology of the various drugs. Therefore, it is wise to use effective and well-established combination protocols (Table 12–9).

ALKYLATING AGENTS. The major acute side effects of alkylating agents are gastrointestinal (nausea and vomiting) and hematologic (myelosuppression). Most cause local skin and subcutaneous tissue necrosis when infiltrated into the skin.

Cyclophosphamide (Cytoxan) is effective in treatment of both hematologic malignancies and solid tumors. Cyclophosphamide produces a less severe pattern of myelosuppressive toxicity than other alkylating agents. Other toxicities include alopecia and immunosuppression. Both cyclophosphamide and a related analogue, *ifosfamide* (Ifex), can cause hemorrhagic cystitis. Bladder toxicity can be blocked by administration of the uroprotective agent *mesna* (Mesnex).

Table 12–9 ■ COMMON COMBINATION CHEMOTHERAPY REGIMENS

ABBREVIATION	DRUGS EMPLOYED	INDICATION
MOPP	Mustargen, vincristine (Oncovin), prednisone, procarbazine	Hodgkin's disease
ABVD	Doxorubicin (Adriamycin), bleomycin, vinblastine, dacarbazine	Hodgkin's disease
CHOP	Cyclophosphamide, hydroxydaunomycin (doxorubicin), vincristine (Oncovin), prednisone	Non-Hodgkin's lymphomas
CMF	Cyclophosphamide, methotrexate, 5-fluorouracil	Breast cancer
CAF	Cyclophosphamide, doxorubicin (Adriamycin), 5-fluorouracil	Breast cancer
M-VAC	Methotrexate, vinblastine, doxorubicin (Adriamycin), cisplatin	Bladder cancer
PVB	Cisplatin (Platinol), vinblastine, bleomycin	Testicular cancer
VAD	Vincristine, doxorubicin (Adriamycin), dexamethasone	Multiple myeloma

Chlorambucil (Leukeran) has antitumor activity similar to that of cyclophosphamide. It is used primarily in the treatment of chronic lymphocytic leukemia, low-grade lymphomas, macroglobulinemia, and polycythemia vera.

Melphalan (Alkeran) is commonly used in the treatment of multiple myeloma and ovarian cancer. *Busulfan* (Myleran) has specificity for myeloid neoplasms and appears to have less antitumor activity in other forms of cancer.

Carmustine (BCNU) and *lomustine* (CCNU) have some activity against primary brain tumors and also are useful in the management of Hodgkin's disease and multiple myeloma. Delayed prolonged myelosuppression can result.

Cisplatin and *carboplatin* are used for testicular, ovarian, head and neck, and lung cancer. Large doses cause renal toxicity and a progressive neuropathy.

Antimetabolites

Cytarabine (cytosine arabinoside, Cytosar-U, ara-C) is particularly useful in acute non-lymphocytic leukemia. Both standard and high-dose ara-C can produce severe myelosuppression. With the high-dose regimen, chemical conjunctivitis is common.

Gemcitabine (Gemzar) is approved for use in the treatment of advanced pancreatic carcinoma. Gemcitabine significantly improves disease-related symptoms in approximately 25% of patients, and a modest increase in survival was demonstrated in patients with pancreatic carcinoma when compared with treatment with 5-FU. Reversible myelosuppression is the dose-limiting toxicity.

Fluorouracil is used to treat a variety of solid tumors, including cancers of the head and neck, esophagus, breast, and colon. It acts synergistically with a variety of agents, including platinum compounds and radiation therapy. Both the gastrointestinal toxicity and the antitumor activity of 5-FU can be enhanced by administration of leucovorin, which increases the binding of fluorodeoxyuridine phosphate to thymidylate synthase. Recent studies showed that 6 months of treatment with 5-FU and leucovorin in the adjuvant setting is the regimen of choice for patients with colorectal cancer. Both 5-FU and floxuridine (5-FUDR) can be given by hepatic artery infusion to treat patients with colorectal carcinoma with metastases confined to the liver. A limitation is that either 5-FU or 5-FUDR can induce a chemical hepatitis and biliary sclerosis with jaundice.

Thioguanine (6-TG) has some uses in acute non-lymphocytic leukemia, whereas *mercaptopurine* (6-MP) is used primarily in acute lymphoblastic leukemia, particularly in childhood. Patients must have their doses reduced to 25% of their standard doses if they are also receiving the xanthine oxidase inhibitor allopurinol.

Fludarabine (Fludara, 5-fluoroadenosine monophosphate) is the single most active agent available for the treatment of chronic lymphocytic leukemia and also exhibits some antitumor activity in other indolent lymphomas and macroglobulinemia. The major toxicity is myelosuppression.

Methotrexate (MTX) is useful primarily for acute lymphoblastic leukemia, SCCL, bladder cancer, head and neck cancer, and breast cancer. Major toxicities are to bone marrow, gastrointestinal mucosa, and, to a lesser extent, skin. Chronic extended use occasionally leads to liver fibrosis and cirrhosis. The toxic effects on the rapidly dividing tissues can be circumvented by administering the reduced folate leucovorin (folinic acid) within 36 hours after MTX administration.

PLANT ALKALOIDS. Both *vinblastine* and *vincristine* provide antitumor activity in leukemias and lymphomas, as well as in selected solid tumors, including SCCL and breast cancer. Whereas the primary toxicity of vinblastine is hematopoietic, vincristine's major toxicity affects peripheral nerves, resulting in sensorimotor and autonomic neuropathies. The neurotoxicity subsides slowly after the drug is discontinued, with improvement requiring months, especially if motor function is impaired.

Etoposide (VP-16, VePesid) is used primarily to treat metastatic testicular cancer in combination with cisplatin and bleomycin. Etoposide also exerts potent effects against SCCL, lymphomas, and monocytic leukemia. The main side effect is myelosuppression, although gastrointestinal toxicity and alopecia also can occur.

Paclitaxel (Taxol) has been approved for the treatment of breast cancer and ovarian cancer and is also widely used for other epithelial tumors (head and neck, esophagus, non-SCCL). The drug may cause hypersensitivity reactions (e.g., hypotension, dyspnea, bronchospasm, and urticaria). Other toxicities include neutropenia, myalgias, and peripheral neuropathy.

ANTITUMOR ANTIBIOTICS. *Daunorubicin* (daunomycin) is active in the treatment of acute leukemia. *Doxorubicin* (Adriamycin) has a broader spectrum of antitumor activity, including both hematologic malignancies and a variety of solid tumors such as carcinoma of the breast and thyroid, lymphoma, and myeloma, as well as osteogenic and soft tissue sarcomas. The most common acute toxicities of the anthracyclines include alopecia, nausea, vomiting, mucositis, and myelosuppression. A dose-dependent, delayed, and potentially irreversible cardiomyopathy with reduced cardiac contractility can develop in patients who receive large cumulative doses of doxorubicin or daunorubicin. Periodic monitoring for cardiac effects is normally initiated when a patient has received a total doxorubicin dose of 350 to 400 mg/m^2. Doxorubicin should be discontinued if the left ventricular ejection fraction falls by 15% and to below 50%.

The major uses of *bleomycin* are in combination therapy to treat carcinomas of the testis and squamous cell carcinomas of the head and neck, cervix, skin, penis, and rectum. It is also used in combination regimens (ABVD) for treatment of lymphomas. Acute toxicities include anaphylactoid reactions and fever associated with hypotension and dehydration. The most serious chronic reaction to bleomycin is pulmonary fibrosis related to the cumulative dose of drug and manifested by cough, dyspnea, and bilateral basilar infiltrates on chest radiography. If the pulmonary diffusion capacity falls abnormally, bleomycin should be discontinued. This toxicity may be irreversible.

Mitomycin (Mutamycin, mitomycin C) has been used in combination with irradiation to treat patients with cancer of the head and neck. Mitomycin's clinical spectrum of antitumor activity includes breast, lung, gastrointestinal, genitourinary, and gynecologic cancers. The major toxicity is delayed myelosuppression. Occasionally, mitomycin can induce interstitial pneumonitis, nephrotoxicity, or hemolytic-uremic syndrome.

TOPOISOMERASE 1 INHIBITORS. *Irinotecan* (CPT-11, Camptosar) has been approved for use in the treatment of patients with colorectal cancer. The principal dose-limiting toxicities are nonhematologic, in particular diarrhea. Severe neutropenia may also occur.

Topotecan (Hycamtin) is approved for use in previously treated patients with ovarian cancer. Topotecan also has activity in other tumors, including hematologic malignancies, SCCL, neuroblastoma, and rhabdomyosarcoma. The dose-limiting and most common toxicity is myelosuppression, especially neutropenia.

MISCELLANEOUS AGENTS. *Procarbazine* (Matulane) has antitumor activity in Hodgkin's disease and in non-Hodgkin's lymphomas, lung cancer, and brain tumors. Patients taking procarbazine may develop hypertension if they ingest tyramine-rich foods such as ripe cheese, wine, and bananas. Disulfiram-like reactions are also seen. Procarbazine also produces azoospermia and anovulation.

Dacarbazine (DTIC) is used in combination chemotherapy for Hodgkin's disease (ABVD, doxorubicin [Adriamycin], bleomycin, and dacarbazine) for soft tissue sarcomas in combination with doxorubicin and other agents, and in single-agent chemotherapy for metastatic melanoma. It causes severe nausea and vomiting.

Hydroxyurea (Hydrea) is used primarily to treat chronic myeloid leukemia and polycythemia vera, but it also has some use in head and neck cancer and metastatic melanoma and as a radiosensitizer. Its major toxicity is to the bone marrow. Gastrointestinal side effects of nausea and vomiting are also common with high-dose therapy.

Mitoxantrone (Novantrone) is a second-line agent for treatment of acute leukemia in relapse but is also useful in the treatment of breast cancer and lymphoma. Gastrointestinal side effects and cardiac toxicity occur.

Asparaginase (Crasnitin, Elspar) is used to treat lymphoblastic leukemias and some lymphomas. Asparaginase toxicity can produce abnormal liver function tests as well as hypoalbuminemia and reductions in plasma levels of clotting factors and insulin.

Management of Toxicity

Doses of myelosuppressive agents often must be adjusted downward to avoid serious or life-threatening side effects. It is useful to check counts between treatment courses, particularly to determine the nadir of absolute granulocyte count (AGC). Falls of AGC below 1000/μL represent a potentially fatal risk. In general, if the AGC immediately before the next course of chemotherapy is less than 2000/μL, the dose of myelosuppressive drugs should be reduced by 50%. With an AGC of less than 1500/μL, doses should be reduced by 75%, and if less than 1000/μL, the drug should be withheld until hematologic recovery occurs. It is also important to make downward dosage adjustments for specific drugs when altered hepatic or renal function plays a major role in drug metabolism.

Endocrine Agents

Endocrine therapy appears generally to work through cytostatic rather than cytotoxic mechanisms and usually requires long-term suppression. Pharmacologic doses of *estrogen* have therapeutic effects in cancers of the prostate and the breast. For breast cancer, the antiestrogen *tamoxifen* (Nolvadex) is better tolerated than high-dose estrogen therapy. *Raloxifene,* also an estrogen antagonist, has been shown to reduce breast cancer risk without increasing the incidence of uterine cancer, which is a concern with tamoxifen.

Progestins are useful in palliative management of metastatic breast or endometrial cancer and can cause tumor regression in endocrine-sensitive disease. In addition to its antitumor effects, megestrol acetate improves appetite in some patients with cancer-induced cachexia.

Glucocorticoids (e.g., prednisone, methylprednisolone, dexamethasone) are useful in treating lymphoid malignancies and may also potentiate the effects of cytotoxic agents in these tumor types as well as in breast cancer and perhaps other neoplasms. The glucocorticoids play an important role in treating complications of cancer (hypercalcemia, cerebral edema).

Aminoglutethimide inhibits the first step in adrenal steroid synthesis. Aminoglutethimide is useful in the palliative treatment of recurrent breast cancer in hormone receptor–positive patients. It can also be used in second-line endocrine therapy for metastatic prostate cancer.

Both *leuprolide acetate* (Lupron) and *goserelin acetate* (Zoladex), which are synthetic analogues of gonadotropin-releasing hormone (GnRH) and luteinizing hormone–releasing hormone (LHRH) agonists, reduce testicular androgen synthesis in men and ovarian estrogen production in women. The effectiveness of GnRH agonists is enhanced by administration in combination with an antiandrogen (flutamide), and the combination has been reported to be more effective than a GnRH agonist alone in patients with stage D metastatic prostate cancer. This form of "medical orchiectomy" is more expensive but acceptable to patients who decline surgical orchiectomy.

Biologic Therapy

The biologic agents have also been termed *biologic response modifiers. Recombinant interferon-alfa-2b* (Intron A, Roferon-A), is useful for single-agent treatment of selected hematologic malignancies and solid tumors. Interferon alfa 2b inhibits the synthesis of a number of proteins in sensitive tumor target cells. Hairy cell leukemia is the tumor most sensitive to interferon alfa 2b. For Kaposi's sarcoma, far more aggressive and toxic schedules are required and can cause anorexia, weight loss, failure in concentration, and profound weakness. Interferon alfa 2b is also useful in the treatment of chronic myeloid leukemia, multiple myeloma, some of the low-grade non-Hodgkin's lymphomas, and in some patients with metastatic melanoma or renal cell carcinoma.

Interleukin-2 (IL-2, aldesleukin, Proleukin) has been approved for therapeutic use in renal cancer and can induce tumor regression in 10 to 20% of patients with renal carcinoma or melanoma. Common side effects are tachycardia and a significant drop in arterial blood pressure.

Antitumor Antibody Therapy

Rituximab (Rituxan) is a genetically engineered chimeric murine-human monoclonal antibody directed against the CD-20 antigen found on the surface of normal and malignant B lymphocytes. Approximately 50% of patients with relapsed or refractory low-grade lymphoma get a partial or complete remission lasting 10 to 12 months.

The *bone marrow growth factors* are glycoproteins that not only result in cell proliferation but also activate differentiation and cell trafficking. These proteins include G-CSF, granulocyte-macrophage colony-stimulating factor (GM-CSF), and epoetin alfa (Epogen, EPO). G-CSF or GM-CSF can shorten the duration of granulocytopenia, the frequency of infectious complications, and the duration of hospitalization after chemotherapy.

All-*trans*-retinoic acid is the first effective differentiation agent introduced into routine clinical care. It causes a high percentage of complete remissions in patients with acute promyelocytic leukemia.

Another attractive target for anticancer drug is antiangiogenesis treatments.

For more information about this subject, see *Cecil Textbook of Medicine,* 21st edition. Philadelphia, W.B. Saunders Company, 2000. Chapter 198, Principles of Cancer Therapy, pages 1060 to 1074.

ONCOLOGIC EMERGENCIES

Fever and Neutropenia

One of the most common oncologic emergencies is fever (a single temperature of 38.5° C [101.3° F] or three temperatures of 38° C [100.4° F] within a 24-hour period) and neutropenia (absolute neutrophil count $<1000/mm^3$). Neutropenic cancer patients have an increased risk of systemic infection and may rapidly develop sepsis. Emergent empiric antibiotic therapy is crucial.

The febrile, neutropenic patient usually presents with few signs or symptoms other than fever. The absence of an adequate number of leukocytes may make the detection of an active infection difficult. The oral cavity should be inspected for evidence of mucositis and lesions suggestive of anaerobic, viral (especially herpes simplex), and fungal (especially *Candida* species) infection. Examination of soft tissue and skin, especially at catheter sites, may show early cellulitis or septic phlebitis. A perirectal abscess should be excluded by careful palpation of the anorectal area for induration, fluctuation, or tenderness.

Before initiation of antibiotic therapy, cultures should be obtained and sent for isolation of bacteria and fungi. Blood cultures must be obtained both from the port of an indwelling central catheter and from peripheral veins. Biopsies of cutaneous lesions may be especially helpful. A lumbar puncture should be performed when suggestive clinical signs or symptoms exist.

TREATMENT. The patient should be started without delay on broad-spectrum antibiotics that include coverage for *Pseudomonas* species and other gram-negative organisms. Many antibiotic regimens have been evaluated in prospective studies, and there is no clearly superior regimen. Emerging antimicrobial resistance at an individual institution may dictate the antibiotics. Suggested regimens are (1) monotherapy with a third- or fourth-generation cephalosporin (cefepime 2 g every 8 hours, or ceftazidime 1 to 2 g every 8 hours IV), (2) a semisynthetic penicillin (piperacillin 3 to 4 g every 4 hours IV) plus an aminoglycoside (gentamicin or tobramycin 2 mg/kg loading dose followed by one to three divided doses daily depending on renal function), or monotherapy with imipenem 50 mg/kg divided every 6 hours IV. If a specific organism is suspected, appropriate antibiotics should be added to the initial regimen. For patients with mucositis, periodontal infections, or perianal infections, anaerobic coverage and either metronidazole or clindamycin should be started while awaiting culture results. Antifungal agents such as fluconazole should be given to patients who present with suspected oral thrush or esophagitis, but these agents do not replace amphotericin B in the treatment of documented or suspected invasive fungal infections.

If fever persists after the initiation of antibiotics, cultures and diagnostic studies should be repeated and the spectrum of antibiotic coverage should be broadened. If the patient remains febrile for 5 to 7 days, empiric antifungal therapy should be started with amphotericin B 0.25 to 1.0 mg/kg/day IV. If neutropenic patients remain febrile despite broad-spectrum therapy, diagnostic possibilities include a second bacterial isolate, superinfection with gram-positive organisms, abscess, anaerobic infection, *Clostridium difficile* enteritis, atypical organisms, fungi, viruses, and drug fever.

If a causative organism or a specific infection is discovered, specific therapy should be initiated; however, broad-spectrum antibiotics should not be discontinued because there is a significant chance of developing infection with a second isolate when antibiotic therapy is narrowed. Patients with documented infections require treatment for a full, usually 2-week, course of antibiotic therapy. If the patient is afebrile and no specific infection has been identified, antibiotics may be discontinued when the absolute neutrophil count exceeds 1000/mm^3. Antibiotics should be continued until the neutropenia resolves in the patient who remains neutropenic despite becoming afebrile because otherwise clinical deterioration or recurrent fever will develop in a significant proportion of these patients.

In general, the patient should remain hospitalized and receive IV antibiotics until the neutropenia resolves. However, there is a trend toward early discharge with outpatient oral or IV antibiotics in low-risk patients.

The prophylactic use of G-CSF or GM-CSF reduces the duration of neutropenia and decreases the frequency of febrile neutropenia, but a survival benefit has not been demonstrated. Randomized clinical trials of therapeutic G-CSF or GM-CSF also have not demonstrated a clinically significant benefit.

Spinal Cord Compression

Back or neck pain can be a harbinger of spinal cord compression, most commonly in lung cancer, breast cancer, lymphoma, and prostate cancer. Typically, midline back pain progresses to radicular pain followed by weakness, sensory loss, paralysis, and/or loss of sphincter control at or below the level of the lesion. Of patients with paraplegia or loss of sphincter tone due to metastatic or primary spinal cancer, fewer than 15% regain function.

EVALUATION AND TREATMENT. Patients who show signs of spinal cord compression require immediate treatment with dexamethasone 10 mg IV plus 4 to 6 mg every 6 hours followed by emergent evaluation. About 60 to 80% of patients with spinal cord compression will have plain film spine radiographs showing erosion or loss of pedicles, partial or complete collapse of vertebral bodies, or a paraspinous mass. Patients with no neurologic findings and no plain film abnormalities usually may be expeditiously evaluated as outpatients; the exception is patients with lymphoma, who more frequently may have epidural tumor without plain film abnormalities. The evaluation of patients with neurologic abnormalities should proceed directly to magnetic resonance imaging (MRI) with gadolinium enhancement. A screening MRI of the entire spine is preferable because malignancies (especially lung, breast, and prostate) often produce multiple noncontiguous bone metastases which should be included in any planned radiation therapy.

Palliative radiation therapy is the treatment of choice for patients who have slowly evolving neurologic symptoms, incomplete block, cauda equina involvement, or widely metastatic disease. Surgery is recommended for the non-terminal patient if a tissue diagnosis is needed; for rapidly developing neurologic signs; if neurologic dysfunction progresses despite radiation treatment; if there is recurrent spinal cord compression in an area of previous radiation therapy; or if there is spinal instability. The patient's prognosis is related to the tempo of the underlying cancer, the presence of other metastases, and other medical problems.

Intracranial Metastases

Headache, altered mental status, seizures, or a focal neurologic examination in cancer patients may signal intracranial metastases (most commonly melanoma and cancers of the lung and breast). The differential diagnosis includes iatrogenic causes (chemotherapy agents, narcotic analgesics, hypnotics, and antiemetics), metabolic disorders (hypercalcemia, hyponatremia, hypoglycemia, hyperviscosity, hepatic encephalopathy), paraneoplastic syndromes (subacute cerebral degeneration, dementia, limbic encephalitis, optic neuritis, progressive multifocal leukoencephalopathy), strokes (coagulation abnormalities, Trousseau's syndrome), sepsis, and intracranial metastases. A careful history and physical examination guide decisions for further evaluation. In acutely ill patients, cranial CT with contrast medium enhancement should be performed to define the presence and characteristics of the intracerebral lesion. MRI is more sensitive in defining metastatic lesions and differentiating between vascular and malignant lesions and should be considered as an alternative to CT. If no mass lesion is demonstrable, leptomeningeal carcinomatosis should be considered as the cause of neurologic signs and symptoms and sought by examination of cerebrospinal fluid.

TREATMENT. If signs of increased intracranial pressure exist with or without impending herniation, IV dexamethasone should be administered to lessen cerebral edema. Radiation therapy for intracranial metastasis is usually palliative. A surgically accessible solitary lesion in a patient with controlled systemic disease merits surgical removal followed by postoperative radiation therapy.

Superior Vena Cava Syndrome

Superior vena cava (SVC) syndrome is usually caused by extrinsic compression (90%), but it can also be due to fibrosis, thrombosis, or invasion of the SVC. The most common malignancies are lung cancer and lymphoma. Signs include cyanosis; edema; venous engorgement of the head, neck, arms, chest, and upper abdomen; varying degrees of airway obstruction; pleural and pericardial effusions; and tracheal edema. Symptoms, which frequently worsen when the patient lies down or leans forward, may include fullness or stuffiness in the ears or nose, visual disturbances, facial swelling, shortness of breath, cough, chest pain, voice changes (hoarseness), dysphagia, headache, stupor, seizures, and syncope.

TREATMENT. Immediate therapy is indicated for impending airway obstruction (stridor) or increased intracranial pressure (stupor, seizure), particularly in a thrombocytopenic patient. However, given the vast array of benign causes of SVC syndrome and the frequency of chemosensitive malignancies such as SCCL and lymphomas, its cause should be determined while the patient is closely observed and managed symptomatically.

In most cases, radiation therapy remains the primary treatment. About 85% of patients improve within 3 weeks. Corticosteroids may improve cerebral or laryngeal edema.

The increasing use of subclavian catheters to deliver chemotherapy has increased the frequency of SVC thromboses. Low-dose warfarin 1 to 2 mg/day may prevent such thrombosis. Fibrinolytic therapy should be considered for patients with catheter-associated thrombosis who have recently developed SVC syndrome if there is not a high risk of bleeding. After successful fibrinolysis, heparinization and subsequent warfarin therapy should be instituted to prevent recurrent SVC syndrome and to maintain the indwelling catheter.

Pericardial Disease

Cardiac tamponade (page 127) may be caused by primary tumors of the pericardium (mesothelioma, sarcoma, and teratoma) or, more frequently, by metastatic disease from breast, lung, leukemia, lymphoma, melanoma, and epidemic or non-epidemic Kaposi's sarcoma. Symptoms are non-specific and include shortness of breath, chest pain, cough, hoarseness, nausea, abdominal pain, hiccups, and anxiety. Two-dimensional echocardiography is the preferred diagnostic study.

TREATMENT. Pericardiocentesis is life-saving. Once a malignancy has been established, the most common approach is a subxiphoid pericardial window. However, patients with malignant pericardial tamponade (especially those with solid tumors) often have such a poor prognosis that surgical approaches are not pursued. After placement of a pigtail catheter, sclerosis of the pericardial space may be considered with various chemotherapeutic agents, radioisotopes, or doxycycline.

Hemoptysis

Major hemoptysis (≥200 mL in 24 hours) or massive hemoptysis (≥1000 mL in 24 hours) associated with respiratory compromise should be considered an emergency. The first intervention is to place the patient on his or her side with the bleeding lung down. Correction of coagulopathy and thrombocytopenia, repletion of blood volume, and determination of the site and cause of bleeding are undertaken simultaneously. Flexible bronchoscopy can determine the site and cause of bleeding. If vigorous suctioning is needed, a rigid bronchoscope should be used. Endobronchial tamponade using an 8F Fogarty catheter is a temporizing procedure. Surgical resection should be considered if the patient can tolerate the procedure. Bronchial artery angiography and embolization is another alternative therapy. Another treatment option for non-emergent situations is neodymium:yttrium-aluminum-garnet (Nd:YAG) laser-induced coagulation.

Airway Obstruction

Airway obstruction by an intrinsic or extrinsic malignancy is an emergency, and management depends on the tempo of narrowing, its location, previous treatment, and the type of tumor (most commonly lung cancer). Corticosteroids should be given to lessen edema. Obstruction at or above the larynx and high tracheal region should first be relieved by tracheostomy with subsequent radiation therapy or surgery performed in a non-emergency setting. A stent placed under fluoroscopic guidance has become a preferred method of palliation. The Nd:YAG laser has been useful in treating high-grade, incomplete, centrally obstructing airway lesions.

Tumor Lysis Syndrome

Tumor lysis syndrome is a metabolic emergency that can be anticipated and prevented. Rapid tumor lysis is usually encountered upon initiation of chemotherapy for rapidly proliferating malignancies such as high-grade lymphomas or acute leukemias. Tumor lysis causes rapid and severe hyperkalemia, hyperuricemia, hyperphosphatemia, and hypocalcemia.

TREATMENT. If possible, IV hydration should begin before the administration of chemotherapy. To avoid uric acid precipitation in the renal tubules, the urine should be alkalinized with 0.25 normal sodium chloride containing two ampules (100 mEq) of sodium bicarbonate; additional bicarbonate is titrated to maintain the urine pH between 7 and 8, and acetazolamide 250 mg PO once or twice daily may be administered. Urinary output between 100 to 200 mL/hour should be maintained. Allopurinol should be administered before chemotherapy. Hyperkalemia must be treated aggressively. Hypocalcemia will occasionally require therapy with IV calcium.

Hemorrhagic Cystitis

Patients who have received or are receiving cyclophosphamide or ifosfamide may develop life-threatening hemorrhagic cystitis. The best management entails prevention by maintaining a high urinary output to decrease the concentration of metabolites in the bladder and by correcting any coagulation defect. Systemic use of mesna prevents mucosal irritation by detoxifying the metabolites within the bladder.

For more information about this subject, see *Cecil Textbook of Medicine,* 21st edition. Philadelphia, W.B. Saunders Company, 2000. Chapter 199, Oncologic Emergencies, pages 1074 to 1078.

APPROACH TO THE PATIENT WITH METASTATIC CANCER, PRIMARY SITE UNKNOWN

Cancers may first become manifest with visceral or nodal metastases without an obvious primary lesion. Patients presenting in this fashion are said to have metastatic cancer, primary site unknown (MCPSU). A complete history and physical examination, blood cell counts, a chemistry screening panel, tests for occult blood in urine and stool, mammography in women, and routine histologic evaluation of the diagnostic pathologic specimen should be performed.

From 2 to 12% of all cancer patients present in this fashion. The most common explanation is that the primary tumor is simply too small to be detected. Other possibilities include prior surgical excision, hemorrhagic infarction with resulting necrosis and scarring, and spontaneous regression.

Routine light microscopic examination will reveal adenocarcinoma in approximately 40% of MCPSU patients, undifferentiated carcinoma or malignant neoplasm in 40%, squamous carcinoma in 10%, and, in fewer than 5% each, melanoma, neuroblastoma, neuroendocrine tumor, or other cancers.

More specialized studies (Table 12–10) may be useful in diagnosing undifferentiated carcinomas or malignant neoplasms. The first clinical manifestation most often occurs in the lung or pleural space, liver, bone, or lymph nodes. The most common ultimately detected primary sites of cancer arise in the pancreas, lung, colon,

Table 12–10 ■ IMMUNOHISTOCHEMICAL TECHNIQUES IN CANCER DIAGNOSIS

ANTIBODY REACTIVITY	LIKELY DIAGNOSIS
Leukocyte common antigen	Lymphoma
S-100 antigen	Melanoma, sarcoma
Epithelial membrane antigen	Carcinoma
Cytokeratin	Carcinoma
Prostate-specific antigen	Prostate cancer
Thyroglobulin	Thyroid cancer
Human chorionic gonadotropin	Germ cell tumor
Alpha-fetoprotein	Germ cell tumor, hepatoma
Gross cystic disease protein	Breast cancer

and hepatobiliary organs. In a minority of patients, the primary site is not apparent even at autopsy. Discovery of the primary tumor will be beneficial to a small minority of patients.

In most cases, CT scans of the abdomen and chest have a high yield but will detect only a poorly treatable malignancy, such as pancreatic or non SCCL. In patients with middle and upper cervical adenopathy in whom biopsy reveals squamous or poorly differentiated carcinoma, complete endoscopic examination with blind biopsies and CT scan to identify areas of submucosal thickening may disclose a primary cancer of the upper aerodigestive tract. Patients with supraclavicular adenopathy more often prove to have an adenocarcinoma that is likely to originate in the lung, breast, or (principally in the left fossa) the gastrointestinal tract. Adenocarcinoma presenting as isolated axillary adenopathy most likely originates in the breast in the female, with lung cancer another possibility in both sexes. Any suspicion of gynecologic neoplasm should lead to abdominal and pelvic CT or pelvic ultrasonography. Approximately 85% of MCPSU patients will present with visceral metastases; no effective systemic therapy is available for the great majority.

Treatment

In patients who, after the staging outlined earlier, have all known tumor confined to a single lymph node region, the disease should be approached aggressively. Squamous and undifferentiated carcinoma in the middle to upper cervical nodes is often managed with radical neck dissection and irradiation. Isolated axillary adenopathy in women with biopsy-proven adenocarcinoma is usually treated as if it were breast cancer. Men and women with squamous or undifferentiated carcinoma confined to axillary nodes should be considered for node dissection because about 20% of such patients so treated will live 5 or more years after surgery. In women with isolated malignant ascites, laparotomy with maximum feasible resection of tumor masses, provided they are confined to the peritoneal cavity, is often appropriate.

In younger men with predominant midline nodal presentations and minimal visceral tumor, historical evidence of rapid tumor growth, or response to previous chemotherapy, the still incompletely characterized syndrome of "poorly differentiated carcinoma of unknown primary site" should be considered. This syndrome, although not yet well defined, is of importance because a fraction of patients with some or all of the above characteristics obtain complete remissions, sometimes durable, with cisplatin-based chemotherapy programs similar to those employed in men with testicular cancer.

Palliative or supportive care is usually the major focus of management in MCPSU patients with visceral metastases, because most have widely disseminated cancer for which no effective systemic treatment is available. However, palliative irradiation, for example, of bone metastases, is often effective in ameliorating associated pain.

Prognosis

The prognosis of the great majority of patients with MCPSU is poor. Five-year survival is reported to be 25 to 50% for patients whose tumor is confined to peripheral lymph nodes and less than 3% for all other patients.

For more information about this subject, see *Cecil Textbook of Medicine,* 21st edition. Philadelphia, W.B. Saunders Company, 2000. Chapter 200, Approach to the Patient with Metastatic Cancer, Primary Site Unknown, pages 1078 to 1081.

CHAPTER 13

METABOLIC DISEASES

APPROACH TO THE PATIENT WITH METABOLIC DISEASE

Here we invoke a genetic approach through the use of predictive genetic testing to identify and prevent irreversible damage from an inborn error of metabolism. The goal is to diagnose the disorder and intervene to prevent damage by a return to metabolic homeostasis before the disease is irreversible. Genetic screening of symptomatic and pre-symptomatic individuals is used to accomplish this objective. Once the disorder is diagnosed, if its pathophysiology is understood, intervention can restore metabolic homeostasis and prevent progressive disease.

Non-selected screening of a pre-symptomatic population is performed to identify homozygous affected individuals and to prevent death, mental retardation, and other irreversible clinical manifestations (Table 13–1).

Selective screening of symptomatic newborns, children, and adults is performed to identify inherited disorders that may be preventable or ameliorated, not only in the patient but in extended family members at risk as well.

Selective and non-selective genetic screening in pregnant women is achieved by fetal sonography, chorionic villus biopsy, or amniocentesis coupled with biochemical, chromosomal, or molecular analyses of cultured fetal cells (Table 13–2).

Screening selected populations at risk for environmental hazards is generally applied to the adult population. Pharmacogenetic disorders fall into this category and include screening plasma pseudocholinesterase concentrations preoperatively to detect pseudocholinesterase deficiency and prevent death from succinyldicholine, and

Table 13–1 ■ PRINCIPLES FOR NON-SELECTIVE GENETIC SCREENING

The disorder should produce a high burden to the affected individual yet be preventable.
Methods for screening, retrieval, diagnosis, and management must be practical and available to the target population as a whole.
The inheritance and pathogenesis of the disease should be understood and genetic counseling should be available.
The benefit-to-cost ratio of the program should be greater than 1.
Patients' rights should be protected (voluntariness, informed consent, confidentiality).
Sensitivity and specificity should be high for the methods used.

For more information about this subject, see *Cecil Textbook of Medicine,* 21st edition. Philadelphia, W.B. Saunders Company, 2000. Part XV: Metabolic Diseases, pages 1082 to 1139.

Table 13–2 ■ GENETIC APPROACHES TO THERAPY

Genetic Counseling: Prospective Therapy

Diagnosis, risk assessment, informational transfer, support for resource allocation

Reproductive alternatives: Contraception, abstinence, artificial insemination, in vitro fertilization, risk taking with or without prenatal monitoring

Environmental Engineering

Avoiding the offending agent
Supplemental physical, speech, developmental therapy
Nutritional management
- Limit toxic precursor
- Provide deficient product
- Detoxify through alternative metabolic route
- Provide feedback inhibitor
- Provide supraphysiologic amounts of vitamin precursor
- Induce protein (enzyme) production
- Chemoprevention

Protein and Enzyme Replacement

Infuse protected pure enzyme
Provide clotting factors and peptide hormones
Transplantation (prospective)
- Organ transplant
- Bone marrow transplant

Genetic Engineering

Somatic gene therapy
- Random insertion
- Homologous recombination (site specific)

Germline therapy

---

determining α_1-antitrypsin genotypes in individuals exposed to dust to prevent occupation-related, early-onset emphysema from α_1-antitrypsin deficiency.

Screening for asymptomatic heterozygotes in a "high-risk" population is another preventive approach to inborn errors of metabolism. The objective is to detect reproductive couples who carry high-burden recessive genes and provide genetic counseling and reproductive alternatives in high-risk matings.

For more information about this subject, see *Cecil Textbook of Medicine,* 21st edition. Philadelphia, W.B. Saunders Company, 2000. Chapter 201, Approach to the Patient with Metabolic Disease, pages 1082 to 1084.

THE HYPERLIPOPROTEINEMIAS

Hyperlipidemia, abnormal elevation of plasma cholesterol and/or triglyceride levels, is one of the most common clinical problems that confronts the physician in daily practice (Table 13–3).

Physiology of Lipoprotein Transport

Lipoproteins are complex macromolecules that transport nonpolar lipids through the aqueous environment of plasma (Table 13–4) and are metabolized in the liver (Fig. 13–1).

Table 13–3 ■ APOLIPOPROTEIN CHARACTERISTICS

APOPROTEIN	LIPOPROTEINS	FUNCTION
Apo B-100	VLDL, IDL, LDL	Secretion of VLDL from liver; structural protein of VLDL, IDL, and LDL, ligand for LDL receptor
Apo B-48	Chylomicrons, remnants	Secretion of chylomicrons from intestine
Apo E	Chylomicrons, VLDL, IDL, HDL	Ligand for binding of IDL and remnants to LDL receptor and LRP
Apo A-I	HDL, chylomicrons	Structural protein of HDL Activator of LCAT
Apo A-II	HDL, chylomicrons	Unknown
Apo C-II	Chylomicrons, VLDL, IDL, HDL	Activator of LPL
Apo C-III	Chylomicrons, VLDL, IDL, HDL	Inhibitor of LPL activity

VLDL = very-low-density lipoproteins; IDL = intermediate-density lipoproteins; LDL = low-density lipoproteins; HDL = high-density lipoproteins; LRP = LDL receptor–related protein; LCAT = lecithin-cholesterol acyltransferase; LPL = lipoprotein lipase.

Hyperlipoprotein Resulting Primarily in Hypercholesterolemia

FAMILIAL HYPERCHOLESTEROLEMIA AND FAMILIAL DEFECTIVE APOLIPOPROTEIN B. Familial hypercholesterolemia (FH) is a common autosomal dominant disorder due to absence of or defective low-density lipoprotein (LDL) receptors, resulting in decreased capacity to remove plasma LDLs. Familial defective apolipoprotein B (apo B) is an autosomonal dominant disorder in which the ligand-binding region of apo B is defective, also leading to delayed plasma LDL clearance. In both disorders LDL cholesterol levels are strikingly increased, frequently associated with characteristic xanthomas in the Achilles tendons, the patellar tendons, the extensor tendons of the hands, and by the presence of xanthelasma. It is frequently associated with early coronary artery disease (CAD).

POLYGENIC HYPERCHOLESTEROLEMIA. The cause of the hypercholesterolemia is unknown, but it is likely due to the conver-

Table 13–4 ■ CHARACTERISTICS OF MAJOR LIPOPROTEIN CLASSES

LIPOPROTEIN CLASS	DENSITY (g/mL)	MAJOR LIPID
Chylomicron and remnants	≪1.006	Dietary triglycerides
VLDL	<1.006	Endogenous triglycerides
IDL	1.006–1.019	Cholesteryl esters, triglycerides
LDL	1.019–1.063	Cholesteryl esters
HDL	1.063–1.210	Cholesteryl esters, phospholipids
Lp(a)	1.055–1.085	Cholesteryl esters

Lp(a) = lipoprotein little A antigen; for other abbreviations, see Table 13–3.

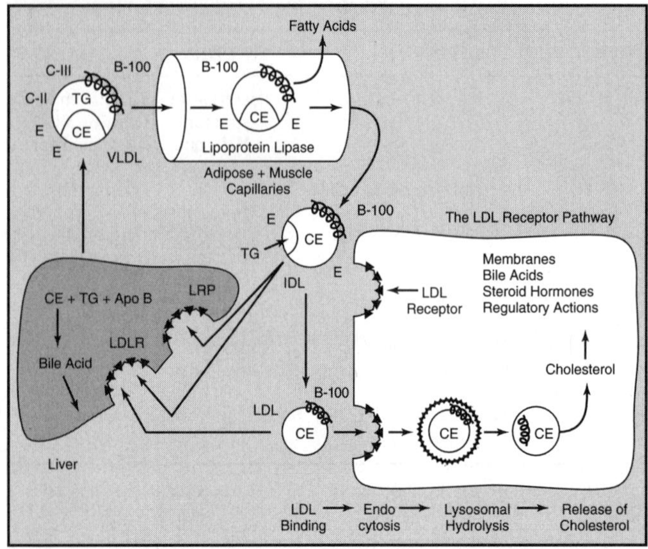

FIGURE 13–1 ■ Simplified scheme of metabolism of apolipoprotein B (Apo B)–containing lipoproteins. In the liver, triglyceride (TG), cholesteryl esters (CE), and apolipoprotein B-100 (B-100) are packaged and released into plasma as very-low-density lipoproteins (VLDL). In capillary beds, lipoprotein lipase hydrolyzes TG to release free fatty acids. The TG-depleted particle is termed an intermediate-density lipoprotein (IDL). The particle is further metabolized to CE-rich low-density lipoprotein (LDL). A major fraction of IDL particles is removed from plasma by hepatic receptors, both by LDL receptors (LDLR) and LDL receptor–related protein (LRP). A portion of IDL is converted to LDL, which is then removed from plasma by LDLR on liver and peripheral cells. Uptake of LDL through the LDLR pathway leads to regulation of cholesterol synthesis and LDLR synthesis. (Modified from Witztum JL: Current approaches to drug therapy for the hypercholesterolemic patient. Circulation 80:1101, 1989. By permission of the American Heart Association, Inc.)

gence of several subtle alterations that affect regulation of LDL levels.

FAMILIAL HYPERALPHALIPOPROTEINEMIA. Occasionally, patients are seen who have mildly elevated total cholesterol levels due to elevated high-density lipoprotein (HDL) cholesterol.

Individuals with hyperalphalipoproteinemia do not have any unusual clinical features, and they have been reported to have slightly increased longevity because of a decreased incidence of CAD.

FAMILIAL HYPERTRIGLYCERIDEMIA. Individuals with this condition have marked hypertriglyceridemia, normal to low LDL levels, and marked decreases in HDL cholesterol levels.

Most experts would not treat patients with isolated hypertriglyceridemia (e.g., triglyceride levels of 250 to 500 mg/dL) if they come from families without evidence of increased atherosclerosis.

DYSBETALIPOPROTEINEMIA. Also known as broad beta disease or type III familial hyperlipoproteinemia, this is a condition in which there is abnormal accumulation of cholesterol-rich intermediate-density lipoprotein (IDL)–type particles, commonly termed β-very-low-density lipoproteins (β-VLDLs). This disorder is due to interaction of (1) an autosomal recessive defect in apolipoprotein E (apo E) that leads to abnormal remnant catabolism and (2) and independent aggravating environmental factor (e.g., obesity, diabetes, pregnancy) or genetic factor (familial combined hyperlipidemic) leading to overproduction of apo B–containing lipoproteins.

FAMILIAL COMBINED HYPERLIPIDEMIA. Among patients with myocardial infarction, a significant number have an apparently dominantly inherited pattern of hyperlipoproteinemia that is expressed by a variable lipoprotein phenotype.

OTHER FORMS OF HYPERTRIGLYCERIDEMIA. Mild hypertriglyceridemia is one of the most commonly encountered hyperlipidemias. Although many patients with hypertriglyceridema will fit into one of the categories noted earlier, there are many other patients with triglyceride levels of 400 to 2000 mg/dL who do not seem to fall into any of those categories. They may have a family history of hypertriglyceridemia and/or quite commonly have one of the secondary forms of hypertriglyceridemia, such as that due to excess alcohol use or diabetes mellitus.

Hyperlipoproteinemia and Atherosclerosis

The etiology of atherosclerosis is multifactorial. Reducing plasma LDL cholesterol levels sharply reduces the risk of subsequent clinical CAD in both patients with pre-existing CAD and in patients free of CAD.

There is no doubt about the atherogenicity of LDLs. Patients with FH have strikingly premature atherosclerosis.

Practical Management of Hyperlipidemia

In almost all cases, lowering LDL levels is achieved first by dietary intervention and then, if necessary, by adding drug therapy. Dietary cholesterol and saturated fats both lead to suppression of hepatic LDL receptor activity, and therefore reduction of these dietary components leads to up-regulation of hepatic LDL receptors and lowered plasma cholesterol levels (Table 13–5).

Regulation of hepatic LDL receptor activity also appears to underlie mechanisms by which many commonly used hyperlipidemic drugs affect plasma cholesterol levels (Fig. 13–2). Bile acid–binding resins work by binding bile acids in the intestine and promoting their subsequent loss in the stool. A second agent, in combination with a bile sequestrant, is frequently used and leads to synergistic lowering of LDL levels. For example, nicotinic acid,

Table 13–5 ■ BLOOD CHOLESTEROL LEVELS (mg/dL)

	DESIRABLE	BORDERLINE	HIGH
Total blood cholesterol	<200	200–239 (borderline high)	>240
LDL	<130	130–159	>160

LDL = low-density lipoprotein.

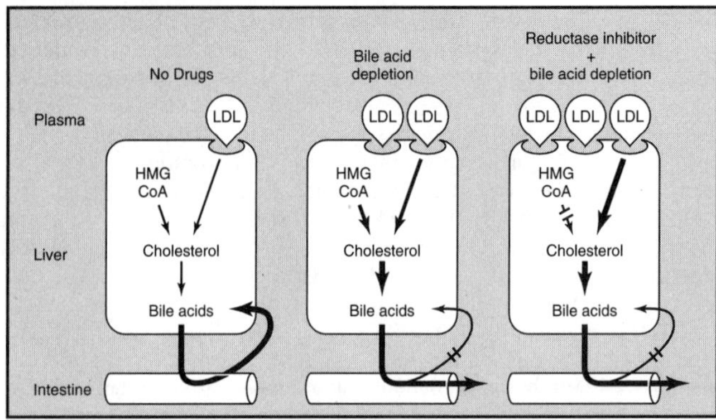

FIGURE 13–2 ■ Mechanisms by which a bile acid–binding resin and a hepatic hydroxymethylglutaryl–coenzyme A (HMG-CoA) reductase inhibitor lower plasma low-density lipoprotein (LDL) levels. (From Brown MS, Goldstein JL: A receptor-mediated pathway for cholesterol homeostasis. Science 232:34, 1986. Copyright 1986 by the American Association for the Advancement of Science.)

which effectively inhibits release of lipoproteins from the liver, is quite effective when combined with a bile acid–binding resin. Even more effective is the use of an hepatic hydroxymethylglutaryl–coenzyme A (HMG-CoA) reductase inhibitor. The therapeutic goals for treatment of hypercholesterolemia are noted in Table 13–6.

For more information about this subject, see *Cecil Textbook of Medicine,* 21st edition. Philadelphia, W.B. Saunders Company,

Table 13–6 ■ **THERAPEUTIC GOALS FOR TREATMENT OF HYPERCHOLESTEROLEMIA**

LDL CHOLESTEROL (mg/dL)	PATIENT CATEGORIES
<130	Moderate risk for CAD Patients with no family history of CAD and no other CAD risk factors Young adults with familial hypercholesterolemia Adults with familial hypercholesterolemia and no other risk factors
<100	High risk for CAD With family history of CAD or ≥2 CAD risk factors Adult familial hypercholesterolemia patients with family history of CAD or ≥1 risk factors Patient with existing CAD Patient after CABG Patient with low HDL cholesterol and family history of CAD

LDL = low-density lipoprotein; HDL = high-density lipoprotein; CAD = coronary artery disease; CABG = coronary artery bypass graft surgery.

2000. Chapter 206, The Hyperlipoproteinemias, pages 1090 to 1100.

THE PORPHYRIAS

Porphyrias are caused by deficiencies of specific enzymes (Fig. 13–3) of the heme biosynthetic pathway and, when clinically expressed, are associated with striking accumulations of heme pathway intermediates (Table 13–7). Most porphyrias are inherited, but other factors are important in determining their severity. These conditions are most prevalent and more often manifested in adults than are most metabolic diseases and are likely to be encountered by physicians in many disciplines. Drugs may play a rôle in causing porphyrias (Table 13–8).

Two major types of clinical manifestations are characteristic of porphyrias. *Neurologic effects* occur in porphyrias characterized by accumulation of the porphyrin precursors δ-aminolevulinic acid (ALA) and porphobilinogen (PBG). *Cutaneous photosensitivity* occurs in types of porphyria in which porphyrins accumulate. Laboratory screening may be necessary (Table 13–9).

For more information about this subject, see the corresponding material in *Cecil Textbook of Medicine,* 21st edition. Philadelphia, W.B. Saunders Company, 2000. Chapter 219, The Porphyrias, pages 1123 to 1130.

WILSON'S DISEASE

Wilson's disease (hepatolenticular degeneration) is a rare, potentially fatal disorder of copper toxicity characterized by progressive liver disease, neurologic deterioration, or both.

In Wilson's disease, biliary excretion of copper is reduced to approximately 20% of normal, and copper progressively accumulates in the liver.

Ceruloplasmin is an α_2-globulin glycoprotein that carries over 80% of the copper present in human plasma. It has amine oxidase activity, by which the holoenzyme can be assayed, and may play a role in copper transport from the liver to other tissues. This process appears to be impaired in Wilson's disease; 95% of patients have reduced ceruloplasmin levels despite having normal amounts of other copper enzymes.

In general, one third of patients with Wilson's disease have liver disease, one third have neurologic impairment, and one third have both. Because copper initially accumulates in the liver, patients with hepatic symptoms are younger, as a rule, than those with extrahepatic symptoms.

Treatment

Adult doses of D-penicillamine are 1 g/day in two to four doses away from meals, although up to 3 g/day has been given. The dose is titrated every 1 or 2 months so that urinary copper losses are 2 mg/day in the first year or two of therapy and 1 mg/day thereafter.

For irreversible liver disease, orthotopic liver transplantation has proved curative in over 50 patients with Wilson's disease; the

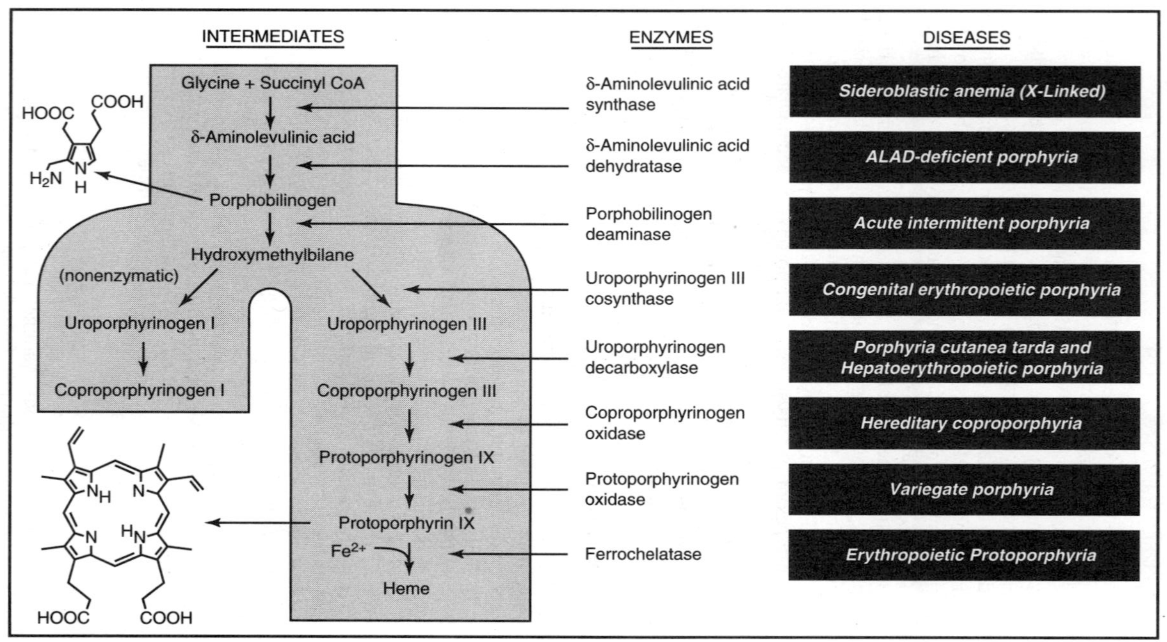

INTERMEDIATES
ENZYMES
DISEASES
Glycine + Succinyl CoA
δ-Aminolevulinic acid
Porphobilinogen
Hydroxymethylbilane
(nonenzymatic)
Uroporphyrinogen I
Coproporphyrinogen I
Uroporphyrinogen III
Coproporphyrinogen III
Protoporphyrinogen IX
Protoporphyrin IX
Fe2+
Heme
HOOC
COOH
H2N
N
H
δ-Aminolevulinic acid synthase
δ-Aminolevulinic acid dehydratase
Porphobilinogen deaminase
Uroporphyrinogen III cosynthase
Uroporphyrinogen decarboxylase
Coproporphyrinogen oxidase
Protoporphyrinogen oxidase
Ferrochelatase
Sideroblastic anemia (X-Linked)
ALAD-deficient porphyria
Acute intermittent porphyria
Congenital erythropoietic porphyria
Porphyria cutanea tarda and Hepatoerythropoietic porphyria
Hereditary coproporphyria
Variegate porphyria
Erythropoietic Protoporphyria

FIGURE 13–3 ■ Intermediates and enzymes of the heme biosynthetic pathway and the major diseases of porphyrin metabolism that have been associated with deficiencies of specific enzymes. The initial and last three enzymes are mitochondrial and the other four are cytosolic. Heme is synthesized from glycine and succinyl coenzyme A (CoA). Intermediates in the pathway include δ-aminolevulinic acid (an amino acid), porphobilinogen (a pyrrole), and hydroxymethylbilane (a linear tetrapyrrole). Uroporphyrinogen III cosynthase catalyzes the closure of hydroxymethylbilane, with inversion of one of the pyrroles, to form a porphyrin macrocycle, uroporphyrinogen III. (Non-enzymatic closure occurs without inversion of this pyrrole to form uroporphyrinogen I, which is not metabolized beyond coproporphyrinogen I.) The next two enzymes result in decarboxylation of six of the eight side chains of uroporphyrinogen III, with sequential formation of hepta-, hexa-, and pentacarboxyl porphyrinogens, coproporphyrinogen III, tricarboxyl porphyrinogen, and protoporphyrinogen IX. The final two enzymes catalyze the oxidation of protoporhyrinogen IX to protoporphyrin IX and the insertion of ferrous iron into the porphyrin macrocycle to form heme (iron protoporphyrin IX). With the exception of protopophyrin IX, all porphyrin intermediates are in their reduced forms (hexahydroporphyrins or porphyrinogens). Chemical structures of two intermediates are shown. ALAD = aminolevulinic acid dehydrase.

Table 13–7 ■ THE THREE MOST COMMON HUMAN PORPHYRIAS AND THEIR MAJOR DIFFERENTIATING FEATURES

DISORDER	INITIAL SYMPTOMS	EXACERBATING FACTORS	MOST IMPORTANT SCREENING TESTS	TREATMENT
Acute intermittent porphyria	Neurovisceral (acute)	Drugs (mostly P-450 inducers), progesterone, dietary restriction	Urinary porphobilinogen	Heme, glucose
Porphyria cutanea tarda	Blistering skin lesions (chronic)	Iron, alcohol, estrogens, hepatitis C virus, halogenated hydrocarbons	Plasma (or urine) porphyrins	Phlebotomy, low-dose chloroquine
Erythropoietic protoporphyria	Painful skin and swelling (mostly acute)		Plasma (or erythrocyte) porphyrins	β-Carotene

Table 13–8 ■ DRUGS CONSIDERED UNSAFE AND SAFE IN ACUTE INTERMITTENT AND VARIEGATE PORPHYRIA AND HEREDITARY COPROPORPHYRIA

UNSAFE	SAFE
Barbiturates*	Narcotic analgesics
Sulfonamide antibiotics*	Aspirin
Meprobamate* (also mebutamate,* tybutamate*)	Acetaminophen
Carisoprodol*	Phenothiazines
Glutethimide*	Penicillin and derivatives
Methyprylon	Streptomycin
Ethchlorvynol*	Glucocorticoids
Phenytoin*	Bromides
Mephenytoin	Gabapentin
Succinimides (ethosuximide, methsuximide)	Insulin
Carbamazepine*	Atropine
Clonazepam	Cimetidine
Primidone*	Ranitidine*†
Valproic acid*	Erythropoietin*†
Pyrazolones (aminopyrine, antipyrine)	? Estrogens*‡
Griseofulvin*	
Ergots	
Metoclopramide*	
Rifampin*	
Pyrazinamide*	
Diclofenac and possibly other NSAIDs*	
Progesterone and synthetic progestins*	
Danazol*	
Alcohol	

NSAIDs = non-steroidal anti-inflammatory drugs.

*Porphyria is listed as a contraindication, warning, precaution, or adverse effect in U.S. labeling for these drugs. For drugs listed here as unsafe, absence of such cautionary statements in U.S. labeling does not imply lower risk.

†Although porphyria is listed as a precaution in U.S. labeling, these drugs are regarded as safe by other sources.

‡There is little evidence that estrogens alone are harmful in acute porphyrias. They have been implicated as harmful mostly from experience with estrogen-progestin combinations and because they can exacerbate porphyria cutanea tarda.

13

survival rate for the procedure approximates 70%. Dietary copper restriction can be helpful and consists of avoiding shellfish and liver.

For more information about this subject, see the corresponding material in *Cecil Textbook of Medicine,* 21st edition. Philadelphia, W.B. Saunders Company, 2000. Chapter 220, Wilson's Disease, pages 1130 to 1132.

IRON OVERLOAD (HEMOCHROMATOSIS)

Hemochromatosis is a state of iron overload that results in parenchymal tissue damage. In persons of European descent, the disorder is most often *hereditary (primary) hemochromatosis. Secondary hemochromatosis* occurs in a variety of chronic anemias caused by ineffective erythropoiesis, as in thalassemia major, or as the result of multiple transfusions or one of the less frequent conditions listed in Table 13–10.

Table 13–9 ■ FIRST-LINE LABORATORY TESTS FOR SCREENING FOR PORPHYRIAS AND SECOND-LINE TESTS FOR FURTHER EVALUATION WHEN INITIAL TESTING IS POSITIVE

	SYMPTOMS SUGGESTING PORPHYRIA	
TESTING	**Acute Neurovisceral Symptoms**	**Cutaneous Photosensitivity**
First-line	Urinary ALA, PBG, and total porphyrins (quantitative, random urine)	Total plasma porphyrins*
Second-line	Urinary ALA, PBG, and total porphyrins† (quantitative, 24-hr urine) Total fecal porphyrins† Erythrocyte PBG deaminase Total plasma porphyrins*	Erythrocyte porphyrins Urinary ALA, PBG, and total porphyrins† (quantitative, 24-hr urine) Total fecal porphyrins‡

ALA = δ-aminolevulinic acid; PBG = porphobilinogen.
*The preferred method is by direct fluorescent spectrophotometry.
†Urinary and fecal porphyrins are fractionated only if the total is increased.

Table 13–10 ■ DISORDERS ASSOCIATED WITH IRON OVERLOAD

- Hereditary hemochromatosis
- Chronic anemias
  - Thalassemia major
  - Sideroblastic anemia
    - Hereditary sideroblastic anemia
    - Refractory anemia with ringed sideroblasts
  - Congenital dyserythropoietic anemia
- Exogenous iron overload
  - Transfusion-dependent anemia
  - Chronic oral iron ingestion (in absence of iron deficiency)
- African (Bantu) hemochromatosis
- Porphyria cutanea tarda
- Portacaval shunt
- Juvenile hemochromatosis
- Neonatal hemochromatosis
- Congenital atransferrinemia

Iron accumulates over decades, as ferritin and hemosiderin, in nearly all cells of the body. Tissue damage that leads to morbidity occurs in the liver, thyroid, hypothalamus, heart, pancreas, gonads, and joints. This leads to cirrhosis of the liver, hypothyroidism, hypothalamic hypogonadism, cardiomyopathy, diabetes mellitus, arthralgias, and deforming arthritis. There is pigment deposition in skin, principally melanin. Cardiac deposition of ferritin and hemosiderin causes cardiac arrhythmias and impaired contractility of cardiac muscle.

Clinically, a number of signs and symptoms may be manifested and laboratory findings may be conclusive (Table 13–11).

The treatment of hemochromatosis is by repeated phlebotomy. This is the most efficient, least inconvenient, and least expensive way to remove excess iron from the body (Fig. 13–4).

For more information about this subject, see *Cecil Textbook of Medicine,* 21st edition. Philadelphia, W.B. Saunders Company, 2000. Chapter 221, Iron Overload (Hemochromatosis), pages 1132 to 1135.

Table 13–11 ■ CLINICAL AND LABORATORY MANIFESTATIONS OF HEMOCHROMATOSIS

SYMPTOMS	SIGNS	ABNORMAL LABORATORY FINDINGS
None (common)	Alopecia	Increased serum iron concentration
Fatigue	Hyperpigmentation	Serum transferrin saturation >60%
Weakness	Tender, swollen joints	Increased serum ALT or AST level
Arthralgia	Cardiac arrhythmia	Increased blood glucose level
Abdominal pain	Cardiomegaly	Abnormal glucose tolerance
Impotence	Hepatomegaly	Low serum testosterone level
Amenorrhea	Splenomegaly	Low serum estrogen and progesterone levels
Dyspnea	Pleural effusion	Low FSH and LH levels
Abdominal swelling	Ascites	Low serum T_4, high TSH levels
Weight loss	Spider telangiectases	Azoospermia
	Signs of hypothyroidism	Thrombocytopenia
	Testicular atrophy	Macrocytosis
		Electrocardiographic abnormalities
		Echocardiographic abnormalities
		Radiographic and imaging abnormalities

ALT = alanine aminotransferase; AST = aspartate aminotransferase. FSH = follicle-stimulating hormone; LH = luteinizing hormone; T_4 = thyroxine; TSH = thyrotropin.

13

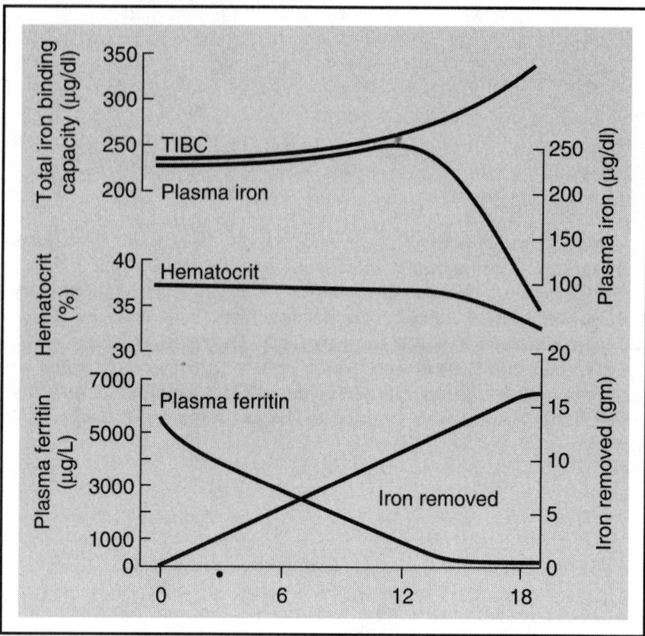

FIGURE 13–4 ■ Serial changes in the hematrocrit, serum (plasma) iron concentration, total iron-binding capacity (TIBC), and serum (plasma) transferrin concentration in a patient with hereditary hemochromatosis during phlebotomy therapy. (N.B. Although shown as plasma iron and ferritin in the illustration, serum specimens are used for these assays, since EDTA-anticoagulated specimens do not have measurable plasma iron by most commonly used methods.) EDTA = ethylenediaminetetraacetic acid. (From Bothwell TH, Carlton RW, Cook JD, et al: Idiopathic haemochromatosis. *In* Iron Metabolism in Man. Oxford, Blackwell Scientific, 1979.)

CHAPTER 14

NUTRITIONAL DISEASES

NUTRITIONAL ASSESSMENT

Nutritional assessment in clinical medicine has three primary goals: (1) to identify the presence and type of malnutrition, (2) to define health-threatening obesity, and (3) to devise suitable diets as prophylaxis against disease later in life. A wide variety of signs and symptoms may indicate nutritional inadequacy (Table 14–1).

The most useful element in the physical examination is body weight, which is expressed as a relative value to evaluate the patient in relation to the healthy population. Weight and height are easily obtained, and standards for comparison have been established (Table 14–2).

PROTEIN-ENERGY MALNUTRITION

The term *protein-energy malnutrition* has been used to describe macronutrient deficiency syndromes (Table 14–3), which include kwashiorkor, marasmus, and nutritional dwarfism in children, and wasting associated with illness or injury in children and adults. Primary protein-energy malnutrition is caused by lack of access to adequate nutrient intake and usually affects children and elderly persons. Secondary protein-energy malnutrition is caused by illnesses that alter appetite, digestion, absorption, or nutrient metabolism and can be divided into three general, but often overlapping categories: (1) diseases that affect gastrointestinal tract function, (2) wasting protein disorders, and (3) critical illnesses. Gastrointestinal disease can cause protein-energy malnutrition by pre-mucosal (lymphatic obstruction) defects.

Protein-Energy Malnutrition in Children (Table 14–4)

MARASMUS. Weight loss and marked depletion of subcutaneous fat and muscle mass are the characteristic features in children with marasmus. Loss of fat and muscle makes ribs, joints, and facial bones prominent. The skin is thin and loose and lies in folds.

KWASHIORKOR. The word "kwashiorkor" comes from the Ga language of West Africa and can be translated as "disease of the displaced child" because it was commonly seen after weaning. The presence of peripheral edema distinguishes children with kwashiorkor from those with marasmus and nutritional dwarfism.

For more information about this subject, see in *Cecil Textbook of Medicine,* 21st edition. Philadelphia, W.B. Saunders Company, 2000. Part XVI: Nutritional Diseases, pages 1140 to 1178.

Table 14–1 ■ CLINICAL SIGNS AND SYMPTOMS OF NUTRITIONAL INADEQUACY IN ADULT PATIENTS

	CLINICAL SIGN OR SYMPTOM	NUTRIENT
General	Wasted, skinny	Calorie
	Loss of appetite	Protein-energy, zinc
Skin	Psoriasiform rash, eczematous scaling	Zinc, vitamin A, EFA
	Pallor	Folate, iron, vitamin B_{12}, copper
	Follicular hyperkeratosis	Vitamin A, vitamin C
	Perifollicular petechiae	Vitamin C
	Flaking dermatitis	Protein-energy, niacin, riboflavin, zinc
	Bruising	Vitamin C, vitamin K
	Pigmentation changes	Niacin, protein-energy
	Scrotal dermatosis	Riboflavin
	Thickening and dryness of skin	Linoleic acid
Head	Temporal muscle wasting	Protein-energy
Hair	Sparse and thin, dyspigmentation	Protein
	Easy to pull out	Protein
	Corkscrew hairs	Vitamin C
Eyes	History of night blindness (also impaired visual recovery after glare)	Vitamin A, zinc
	Photophobia, blurring, conjunctival inflammation	Riboflavin, vitamin A
	Corneal vascularization	Riboflavin
	Xerosis, Bitot spots, keratomalacia	Vitamin A
Mouth	Glossitis	Riboflavin, niacin, folic acid, vitamin B_{12}, pyridoxine
	Bleeding gums	Vitamin C, riboflavin
	Cheilosis	Riboflavin, pyridoxine, niacin
	Angular stomatitis	Riboflavin, pyridoxine, niacin
	Hypogeusia	Zinc
	Tongue fissuring	Niacin
	Tongue atrophy	Riboflavin, niacin, iron
	Nasolabial seborrhea	Pyridoxine

Neck	Goiter	Iodine
	Parotid enlargement	Protein
Thorax	Thoracic rosary	Vitamin D
Abdomen	Diarrhea	Niacin, folate, vitamin B_{12}
	Distention	Protein-energy
	Hepatomegaly	Protein-energy
Extremities	Edema	Protein, thiamine
	Softening of bone	Vitamin D, calcium, phosphorus
	Bone tenderness	Vitamin D
	Bone ache, joint pain	Vitamin C
	Muscle wasting and weakness	Protein, calorie, vitamin D, selenium, sodium chloride
	Muscle tenderness, muscle pain	Thiamine
Nails	Spooning	Iron
	Transverse lines	Protein
Neurologic	Tetany	Calcium, magnesium
	Paresthesias	Thiamine, vitamin B_{12}
	Loss of reflexes, wristdrop, footdrop	Thiamine
	Loss of vibratory and position sense	Vitamin B_{12}
	Ataxia	Vitamin B_{12}
	Dementia, disorientation	Niacin
Blood	Anemia	Vitamin B_{12}, folate, pyridoxine
	Hemolysis	Phosphorus, vitamin E

EFA = essential fatty acids.
Modified from Russell RM: Nutritional assessment. *In* Wyngaarden JB, Smith LH Jr, Bennett JC: Cecil Textbook of Medicine, 19th ed. Philadelphia, 1992, WB Saunders, pp 1151–1155.

Table 14–2 ■ DESIRABLE WEIGHT IN POUNDS IN RELATION TO HEIGHT FOR ADULT MEN AND WOMEN 25 YEARS AND OLDER*

MEN, MEDIUM FRAME				WOMEN, MEDIUM FRAME			
Height		Weight lb		Height		Weight (lb)	
ft	in.	Range	Midpoint	ft	in.	Range	Midpoint
				4	8	93–104	98.5
				4	9	95–107	101
				4	10	98–110	104
				4	11	101–113	107
				5	0	104–116	110
5	1	113–124	118.5	5	1	107–119	113
5	2	116–128	122	5	2	110–123	116.5
5	3	119–131	125	5	3	113–127	120
5	4	122–134	128	5	4	117–132	124.5
5	5	125–138	131.5	5	5	121–136	128.5
5	6	129–142	135.5	5	6	125–140	132.5
5	7	133–147	140	5	7	129–144	136.5
5	8	137–151	144	5	8	133–148	140.5
5	9	141–155	148	5	9	137–152	144.5
5	10	145–160	153	5	10	141–156	148.5
5	11	149–165	157				
6	0	153–170	161.5				
6	1	157–175	166				
6	2	162–180	171				
6	3	167–185	176				

*Corrected to nude weights and heights by assuming 1-in. heel for men, 2-in. heel for women, and indoor clothing weight of 5 and 3 lb for men and women, respectively. Adapted from the Metropolitan Life Insurance Company Statistical Bulletin 4:1, 1959.

Table 14–3 ■ CLASSIFICATION OF PROTEIN-ENERGY MALNUTRITION IN ADULTS

BODY MASS INDEX (kg/m^2)	NUTRITIONAL STATUS
≥18.5	Normal
17.0–18.4	Mildly malnourished
16.0–16.9	Moderately malnourished
<16.0	Severely malnourished

THE EATING DISORDERS

The eating disorders are a group of psychiatric disorders characterized by aberrant eating patterns and disturbed attitudes about the importance of body weight and shape, specifically, the evaluation of self-worth based on weight. Anorexia nervosa (Table 14–5) and bulemia (Table 14–6) are two problems often seen in clinical practice. The long-term treatment goal for both disorders is to ameliorate the psychological and behavioral patterns that promote and maintain aberrant eating habits and the attitudinal disturbances. A second goal is to address the medical complications that accompany these behavioral and psychological patterns, particularly for anorexia nervosa, where weight restoration is a primary emphasis in the initial treatment.

OBESITY

About 97 million adult Americans (55% of those aged 20 to 75 years) are overweight or obese (Table 14–7). The percentage of adult men who are overweight or obese (59.4%) is somewhat greater than that of women (50.7%) (Fig. 14–1). A way to classify

Table 14–4 ■ FEATURES OF PROTEIN-ENERGY MALNUTRITION SYNDROMES IN CHILDREN

FEATURE	KWASHIORKOR	MARASMUS	NUTRITIONAL DWARFISM
Weight for age (% of expected)	60–80	<60	<60
Weight for height	Normal or decreased	Markedly decreased	Normal
Edema	Present	Absent	Absent
Mood	Irritable when picked up Apathetic when alone	Alert	Alert
Appetite	Poor	Good	Good

Table 14–5 ■ DSM-IV DIAGNOSTIC CRITERIA FOR ANOREXIA NERVOSA

A. Refusal to maintain body weight at or above a minimally normal weight for age and height (e.g., weight loss leading to maintenance of body weight less than 85% of that expected or failure to make expected weight gain during period of growth resulting in body weight less than 85% of that expected).
B. Intense fear of gaining weight or becoming fat even though underweight.
C. Disturbance in the way in which one's body weight or shape is experienced, undue influence of body weight or shape on self-evaluation, or denial of the seriousness of the current low body weight.
D. In post-menarchal females, amenorrhea, i.e., the absence of at least three consecutive menstrual cycles. (A woman is considered to have amenorrhea if her periods occur only following hormone, e.g., estrogen, administration.)

Specify type:

Restricting type: During the current episode of anorexia nervosa, the person has not regularly engaged in binge-eating or purging behavior (i.e., self-induced vomiting or the misuse of laxatives, diuretics, or enemas).

Binge-eating/purging type: During the current episode of anorexia nervosa, the person has regularly engaged in binge-eating or purging behavior (i.e., self-induced vomiting or the misuse of laxatives, diuretics, or enemas).

Used by permission from the American Psychiatric Association: Diagnostic and Statistical Manual of Mental Disorders: DSM-IV, 4th ed, Washington, DC, American Psychiatric Association, 1994.

overweight is by computing the body mass index (BMI):

$$\text{BMI} = \text{kg}/(\text{height in meters})^2$$

or

$$\text{BMI} = \text{lb}/(\text{height in inches})^2 \times 703.1$$

REGIONAL DISTRIBUTION OF ADIPOSE TISSUE. Fat mass is distributed differently in men and women. The android, or male, pattern is characterized by fat distributed predominantly around the waist and on the upper body, whereas the gynecoid, or female, pattern shows fat predominantly in the lower body, that is, the lower abdomen, buttocks, hips, and thighs. Central or upper body fat has a significantly worse prognosis for morbidity and mortality than does lower body fat. Abdominal or android fatness carries a greater risk for hypertension, cardiovascular disease, hyperinsulinemia, diabetes mellitus, gallbladder disease, stroke, and cancer of the breast and endometrium. It also carries a greater risk for overall mortality. Because more men than women have the android distribution, they are more at risk for most of these conditions. Also, women who deposit their excess fat in a more android manner have a greater risk than women whose fat distribution is more gynecoid. Reducing a normal number of enlarged fat cells to normal size is easier than reducing large numbers of the smaller cells in the lower body hyperplastic depot to normal or below-normal

Table 14–6 ■ DSM-IV DIAGNOSTIC CRITERIA FOR BULIMIA NERVOSA

A. Recurrent episodes of binge eating. An episode of binge eating is characterized by both of the following:
   1. Eating, in a discrete period (e.g., within any 2-hr period), an amount of food that is definitely larger than most people would eat during a similar period and under similar circumstances.
   2. A sense of lack of control over eating during the episodes (e.g., a feeling that one cannot stop eating or control what or how much one is eating).

B. Recurrent inappropriate compensatory behavior to prevent weight gain such as self-induced vomiting; misuse of laxatives, diuretics, enemas, or other medication; fasting; or excessive exercise.

C. The binge-eating and inappropriate compensatory behaviors both occur, on average, at least twice a week for 3 mo.

D. Self-evaluation is unduly influenced by body shape and weight.

E. The disturbance does not occur exclusively during episodes of anorexia nervosa.

Specify type:

Purging type: During the current episode of bulimia nervosa, the person has regularly engaged in self-induced vomiting or the misuse of laxatives, diuretics, or enemas.

Non-purging type: During the current episode of bulimia nervosa, the person has used other inappropriate compensatory behaviors, such as fasting or excessive exercise, but has not regularly engaged in self-induced vomiting or the misuse of laxatives, diuretics, or enemas.

Used by permission from the American Psychiatric Association: Diagnostic and Statistical Manual of Mental Disorders: DSM-IV, 4th ed. Washington, DC, American Psychiatric Association, 1994.

Table 14–7 ■ CLASSIFICATION OF OVERWEIGHT AND OBESITY BY BODY MASS INDEX (BMI)

	OBEISTY	BMI (kg/m^2)
Underweight		<18.5
Normal		18.5–24.9
Overweight		25.0–29.9
Obesity	I	30.0–34.9
	II	35.0–39.9
Extreme obesity	III	≥40

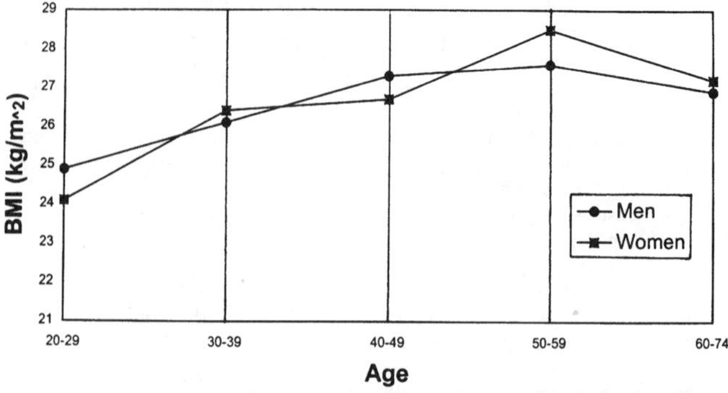

FIGURE 14–1 ■ Weight change with aging for men and women. BMI = body mass index. (Adapted from National Center for Health Statistics: JAMA 272:208, 1994.)

size. This may explain the weight loss difficulties of many women with lower body obesity.

OBESITY AND THE ENDOCRINE SYSTEM. Although obesity has often been described as an "endocrine" disease, fewer than 1% of obese patients have any measurable endocrine dysfunction. Hypothalamic, pituitary, thyroid, adrenal, ovarian, and possibly pancreatic endocrine syndromes have been related to obesity.

TREATMENT. The three approaches to weight control are diet, exercise, and drugs. In general, drugs affect the appetite modestly. Anorectic drugs act centrally through brain catecholamine, dopamine, or serotonin pathways. For example, the derivates of amphetamine seem to produce anorexia through stimulating the central hypothalamic neurochemical pathways in which norepinephrine and/or dopamine is the principal neurotransmitter. Very often patients, and sometimes physicians, have unrealistic goals of what can be accomplished. One pound of fat is equivalent to 4000 kcal/day. Losing 1 lb takes 10 days.

ENTERAL NUTRITION

Enteral nutrition is the provision of liquid formula diets into the gastrointestinal tract. There may be specific medical indications for enteral nutrition (Table 14–8). Diarrhea is the most common complication, (Table 14–9).

Table 14–8 ■ INDICATIONS FOR THE USE OF ENTERAL NUTRITION IN ADULT MEDICAL PATIENTS

Protein-energy malnutrition with anticipated significantly decrased oral intake for at least 7 d
Anticipated significantly decreased oral intake for 10 d
Severe dysphagia
Massive small bowel resection (used in combination with total parenteral nutrition)
Low-output (<500 mL/d) enterocutaneous fistula

Table 14–9 ■ CAUSES OF DIARRHEA IN TUBE-FED PATIENTS

Common Causes Unrelated to Tube Feeding

Elixir medications containing sorbitol
Magnesium-containing antacids
Antibiotic-induced sterile gut
Pseudomembranous colitis

Possible Causes Related to Tube Feeding

Inadequate fiber to form stool bulk
High fat content of formula (in the presence of fat malabsorption syndrome)
Bacterial contamination of enteral products and delivery systems (causal association with diarrhea not documented)
Rapid advancement in rate (after the gastrointestinal tract is unused for prolonged periods)

Unlikely Causes Related to Tube Feedings

Formula hyperosmolality (proved not to be a cause of diarrhea)
Lactose (absent from nearly all enteral feeding formulas)

Table 14–10 ■ DESIGN OF PARENTERAL NUTRITION PROGRAMS: EXAMPLES

Non-obese patient weighing 60 kg; assume basal Harris-Benedict equation estimate of daily caloric requirements of 1250 kcal/d

A. Patient characteristics:
   1. Euvolemic, normal urine output, and no unusual gastrointestinal losses; therefore, appropriate initial estimate of daily fluid requirement is 30 mL/kg body weight
   2. Moderately stressed with normal renal and hepatic function; therefore, appropriate to provide 1.2 g protein per kg body weight
   3. Non-obese; therefore, appropriate to provide Harris-Benedict estimate plus 20% for calories, i.e., 1250 plus 20% = 1500 kcal

B. Program design:
   1. Fluid requirement: 30 mL × body weight; 30 × 6 = 1800 mL
   2. Caloric requirement: Harris-Benedict estimate + 20%; 1250 + 250 = 1500 kcal
   3. Protein requirement for moderately stressed patient: 1.2 g/kg body weight; 60 × 1.2 = ≈70 g protein. 70 g protein × 4 kcal/g protein = 280 kcal
   4. Fat requirement: 30% of total calories; 30% × 1500 kcal = 450 kcal
   5. Carbohydrate requirement: caloric requirement minus the sum of protein and fat calories; 1500 − (280 plus 450 kcal) = 770 kcal. 770 kcal carbohydrate divided by kcal/g carbohydrate (3.4) = ~225 g carbohydrate
   6. Therefore, consider the following PN formula: 1.5 L amino acids, 5%, dextrose, 15%, plus 250 mL of 20% fat emulsion, which provides 1750 mL, 1565 kcal, 75 g protein, 225 g carbohydrate, and 500 fat calories. Note that amino acids, 5%, equals 50 g protein per liter
   7. If institution uses 3-in-1 admixture compounding (amino acids plus dextrose plus fat in one container and stock solutions of amino acids, 10%, dextrose, 70%, and lipid, 20%), a comparable PN program would be 1.5 L amino acids, 5%, dextrose, 15%, fat, 3.5%

C. Similar patient characteristics except patients volume-expanded:
   1. Consider the following fluid-restricted PN formula: 1 L of amino acids, 7%, dextrose, 20%, plus 250 mL 20% fat emulsion which provides 1250 mL, 1460 calories, 70 g protein, 200 g carbohydrate, and 500 fat calories

PN = parenteral nutrition.

14

PARENTERAL NUTRITION

The term *parenteral nutrition* should be used in place of intravenous hyperalimentation. Parenteral nutrition provides amino acids (nitrogen), dextrose (carbohydrate), fat, electrolytes, minerals, trace elements, vitamins, and water by central vein (central parenteral nutrition) or by peripheral vein (peripheral parenteral nutrition) (Table 14–10). The enteral route should always be selected for the provision of nutrition in malnourished patients with a functional gastrointestinal tract because the bowel atrophies when nutrients are provided exclusively by vein.

CHAPTER 15

ENDOCRINE DISEASES

NEUROENDOCRINOLOGY AND THE NEUROENDOCRINE SYSTEM

Neuroendocrinology refers to the general area of endocrinology in which the nervous system interacts with the endocrine system to link aspects of cognitive and non-cognitive neural activity with metabolic and hormonal homeostatic activity. Neural cells that can secrete hormones, that is, *neurosecretory* cells, serve as the final common pathway linking the brain with the endocrine system. The *neurohypophyseal* neurons originate from the paraventricular and supraoptic nuclei, traverse the hypothalamic-pituitary stalk, and release vasopressin and oxytocin from nerve endings in the posterior pituitary. The *hypophysiotropic* neurons, localized in specific hypothalamic nuclei, project their axons to the median eminence to secrete their peptide and bioamine releasing and inhibiting hormones into the proximal end of the hypothalamic-pituitary portal vessels (Fig. 15–1).

The neuroendocrine system operates through a series of feedback loops that control pituitary and target organ hormone levels precisely (Fig. 15–2).

DISEASES OF THE HYPOTHALAMUS. Diseases may affect the hypothalamus by being localized to the hypothalamus, by being part of more generalized central nervous system (CNS) disease such as neurosarcoidosis, or by indirect means such as by causing hydrocephalus (Table 15–1). Furthermore, hormonal changes mediated by functional alterations in hypothalamic regulation may occur in a variety of psychiatric disorders or systemic illnesses.

For more information about this subject, see *Cecil Textbook of Medicine,* 21st edition. Philadelphia, W.B. Saunders Company, 2000. Chapter 235, Neuroendocrinology and the Neuroendocrine System, pages 1198 to 1207.

ANTERIOR PITUITARY

The pituitary is divided into anterior and posterior lobes, with the anterior lobe composing about 80% of the gland. There are six primary cell types that produce the major anterior pituitary hormones (Table 15–2), and folliculostellate cells, which do not produce the classic hormones but may have paracrine functions. The pituitary gland integrates the influences of an array of positive and negative signals to modulate hormone secretion within a narrow

15

For more information about this subject, see *Cecil Textbook of Medicine,* 21st edition. Philadelphia, W.B. Saunders Company, 2000. Part XVII: Endocrine Diseases, pages 1179 to 1317.

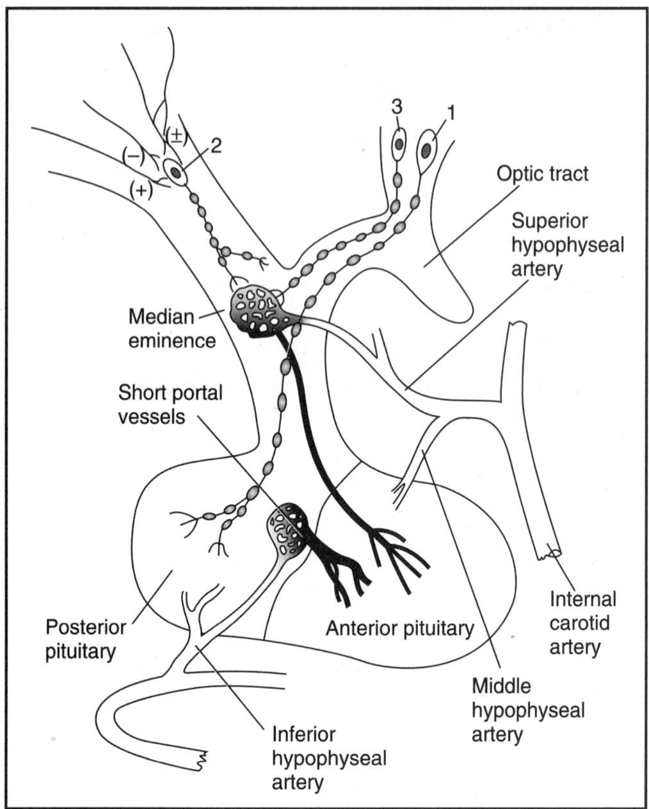

FIGURE 15–1 ■ Neuroendocrine organization of the hypothalamus and pituitary gland. The posterior pituitary is fed by the inferior hypophyseal artery and the hypothalamus by the superior hypophyseal artery, both branches of the internal carotid artery. A small portion of the anterior pituitary also receives arterial blood from the middle hypophyseal artery. Most of the blood supply to the anterior pituitary is venous by way of the long portal vessels, which connect the portal capillary beds in the median eminence to the venous sinusoids in the anterior pituitary. Hypophysiotropic neuron 3 in the parvocellular division of the paraventricular nucleus and neuron 2 in the arcuate nucleus are shown to terminate in the median eminence on portal capillaries. These neurons of the tuberoinfundibular system secrete hypothalamic-releasing and -inhibiting hormones into the portal veins for conveyance to the anterior pituitary gland. Neuron 2 is innervated by monoaminergic neurons. Note that the multiple inputs to such neurons, using neuron 2 as an example, can be (a) stimulatory, (b) inhibitory, or (c) neuromodulatory, in which another neuron may affect neurotransmitter release. Neuron 1 represents a peptidergic neuron originating in the magnocellular division of the paraventricular nucleus or supraoptic nucleus and projects directly to the posterior pituitary by way of the hypothalamic-neurohypophyseal tract. (Courtesy of Ronald M. Lechan, M.D., and modified from Lechan RM: Neuroendocrinology of pituitary hormone regulation. Endocrinol Metab Clin North Am 16:475, 1987, with permission.)

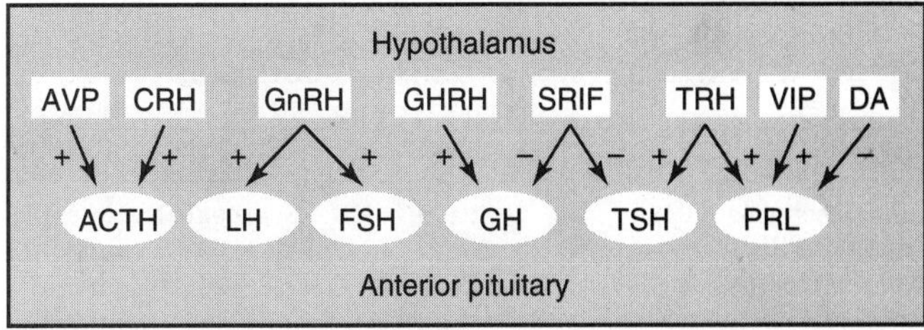

FIGURE 15–2 ■ Interrelationships between hypothalamic and pituitary hormones. Plus signs indicate stimulatory effects and minus signs indicate inhibitory effects. AVP = arginine vasopressin; CRH = corticotropin-releasing hormone; GnRH = gonadotropin-releasing hormone; GHRH = growth hormone–releasing hormone; SRIF = somatotropin release–inhibiting factor [somatostatin]; TRH = thyrotropin-releasing hormone. VIP = vasoactive intestinal polypeptide; DA = dopamine; ACTH = adrenocorticotropic hormone; LH = luteinizing hormone; FSH = follicle-stimulating hormone; TSH = thyroid-stimulating hormone; PRL = prolactin.

Table 15–1 ■ ETIOLOGY OF HYPOTHALAMIC DISEASE

10–25 Years

Tumors: craniopharyngioma, pituitary tumors, glioma hamartoma, dysgerminoma, histiocytosis X, leukemia, dermoid, lipoma, neuroblastoma
Trauma
Subarachnoid hemorrhage, vascular aneurysm, arteriovenous malformation
Inflammatory diseases: meningitis, encephalitis, sarcoidosis, tuberculosis
Disease associated with midline brain defects: agenesis of corpus callosum
Chronic hydrocephalus or increased intracranial pressure

25–50 Years

Nutritional: Wernicke's disease
Tumors: glioma, lymphoma, meningioma, craniopharyngioma, pituitary tumors, angioma, plasmacytoma, colloid cysts, ependymoma, sarcoma, histiocytosis X
Inflammatory diseases: sarcoidosis, tuberculosis, viral encephalitis
Subarachnoid hemorrhage, vascular aneurysms, arteriovenous malformation
Damage from pituitary radiation therapy

50 Years and Older

Nutritional: Wernicke's disease
Tumors: sarcoma, glioblastoma, lymphoma, meningioma, colloid cysts, ependymoma, pituitary tumors
Vascular: infarct, subarachnoid hemorrhage, pituitary apoplexy
Infectious diseases: encephalitis, sarcoidosis, meningitis

Adapted from Plum F, Van Uitert R: Non-endocrine diseases of the hypothalamus. *In* Reichlin S, Baldessarini RJ, Martin JB (eds): The Hypothalamus. New York, Raven Press, 1978, p 415.

Table 15–2 ■ FEATURES OF THE MAJOR ANTERIOR PITUITARY HORMONES

HORMONE	SERUM HALF-LIFE (min)*	CELL TYPE	TARGET GLAND
Growth hormone (GH)	20	Somatotroph	Multiple
Prolactin (PRL)	20	Lactotroph	Breast
Adrenocorticotopic hormone (ACTH)	8	Corticotroph	Adrenal
Thyroid-stimulating hormone (TSH)	50	Thyrotroph	Thyroid
Luteinizing hormone (LH)	50	Gonadotroph	Gonad
Follicle-stimulating hormone (FSH)	220	Gonadotroph	Gonad

*The serum half-lives assume single-compartment monoexponential decay.

range (Table 15–3). A variety of tests have been developed to measure pulmonary insufficiency (Table 15–4).

PITUITARY TUMORS. Pituitary tumors are classified according to the hormones that they produce and their size: microandenomas, less than 10 mm in diameter; macroadenomas, more than 10 mm in diameter; and macroadenomas with extrasellar extension (Table 15–5).

GROWTH HORMONE EXCESS: ACROMEGALY AND GIGANTISM. Growth hormone (GH)–producing pituitary tumors involve the neoplastic proliferation of somatotrophs and account for 10 to 15% of pituitary tumors (see Table 15–5). GH-secreting tumors cause acromegaly (Table 15–6) in adults and gigantism in children in whom GH excess occurs before epiphyseal closure. The most

Table 15–3 ■ FACTORS THAT REGULATE PITUITARY HORMONE SECRETION

HORMONE*	RELEASING FACTORS	INHIBITING FACTORS†
GH	GHRH	Somatostatin, IGF-1
PRL	TRH, VIP, E_2	Dopamine
ACTH	CRH, vasopressin	Cortisol
TSH	TRH	T_4, T_3, somatostatin, dopamine
LH	GnRH	E_2, testosterone
FSH	GnRH, activin	Inhibin, E_2, testosterone

GHRH = growth hormone–releasing hormone; IGF-1 = insulin-like growth factor-1 (formerly called somatomedin C); TRH = thyrotropin-releasing hormone; VIP = vasoactive intestinal peptide; E_2 = estradiol; CRH = corticotropin-releasing hormone; T_4 = thyroxine; T_3 = triiodothyronine.

*For abbreviations, see Table 15–2.

†The gonadal steroids E_2 and testosterone exert much of their inhibitory effects on gonadotropin secretion at the hypothalamic level.

Table 15–4 ■ TESTS OF PITUITARY INSUFFICIENCY

HORMONE	TEST	INTERPRETATION
Growth hormone (GH)	*Insulin tolerance test:* Regular insulin 0.05–0.15 U/kg is given IV and blood is drawn at −30, 0, 30, 45, 60, and 90 min for measurement of glucose and GH	If hypoglycemia occurs (glucose < 40 mg/dL), GH should increase to >7 mg/L
	L-Dopa test: 10 mg/kg PO with GH measurements at 0, 30, 60, and 120 min	Normal response is GH > 7 mg/L
	L-Arginine test: 0.5 g/kg (max 30 g) IV over 30 min with GH measurements at 0, 30, 60, and 120 min	Normal response is GH > 7 mg/L
ACTH	**Insulin tolerance test:* Regular insulin 0.05–0.15 U/kg is given IV and blood is drawn at −30, 0, 30, 45, 60, and 90 min for measurement of glucose and cortisol	If hypoglycemia occurs (glucose < 40 mg/dL), cortisol should increase by >7 mg/dL or to >20 μg/dL
	CRH test: 1 μg/kg ovine CRH IV at 8 A.M. with blood samples drawn at 0, 15, 30, 60, 90, 120 min for measurement of ACTH and cortisol	In most normals, the basal ACTH increases 2- to 4-fold and reaches a peak (20–100 pg/mL); ACTH responses may be delayed in cases of hypothalamic dysfunction; cortisol levels usually reach 20–25 μg/dL
	ACTH stimulation test: ACTH 1-24 (Cosyntropin) 0.25 mg IM or IV; cortisol and aldosterone are measured at 0, 30, and 60 min; a 3-d ACTH stimulation test consists of ACTH 1-24 0.25 mg given IV over 8 hr each day	A normal response is cortisol > 18 μg/dL and aldosterone response of >4 ng/dL above baseline; in suspected hypothalamic-pituitary deficiency, 3-d ACTH test should result in urinary full cortisol increase

Table continued on following page

15

Table 15–4 ■ TESTS OF PITUITARY INSUFFICIENCY *Continued*

HORMONE	TEST	INTERPRETATION
TSH	*Basal thyroid function tests:* Free T_4, free T_3, TSH	Low free thyroid hormone levels in the setting of TSH levels that are not appropriately increased
	TRH test: 200–500 μg IV with measurements of TSH at 0, 20, and 60 min	TSH should increase by more than 5 mU/L unless thyroid hormone levels are increased; peak may be delayed if hypothyroidism due to hypothalamic disease
LH, FSH	*Basal levels of LH, FSH, testosterone, estrogen*	Basal LH and FSH should be increased in postmenopausal women; low testosterone levels in conjunction with low or low-normal LH and FSH are consistent with gonadotrpin deficiency.
	GnRH test: GnRH (100 μg) IV with measurements of serum LH and FSH at 0, 30, and 60 min	In most normal persons, LH should increase by 10 IU/L and FSH by 2 IU/L; normal responses are variable, and repeated stimulation may be required
	Clomiphene test: Clomiphene citrate (100 mg) is given PO for 5 d; serum LH and FSH are measured on d 0, 5, 7, 10, and 13	A 50% increase should occur in LH and FSH, usually by d 5
Multiple hormones	*Combined anterior pituitary test:* GHRH (1 μg/kg), CRH (1 μg/kg), GnRH (100 μg), TRH (200 μg) are given sequentially IV; blood samples are drawn at 30, 15, 30, 60, 90, and 120 min for measurements of GH, ACTH, LH, FSH, and TSH	Combined or individual releasing hormone responses must be evaluated in the context of basal hormone values and may not be diagnostic

*Insulin tolerance tests in suggested pituitary insufficiency can be dangerous because counter-regulatory hormones are missing.

TRH = thyrotropin-releasing hormone; TSH = thyroid-stimulating hormone; ACTH = adrenocorticotropic hormone; T_4 = thyroxine; T_3 = triiodothyronine; LH = luteinizing hormone; FSH = follicle-stimulating hormone; GnRH = gonadotropin-releasing hormone; GHRH = growth hormone–releasing hormone; CRH = corticotropin-releasing hormone.

Table 15–5 ■ PREVALENCE OF DIFFERENT TYPES OF PITUITARY ADENOMAS

TYPE OF PITUITARY ADENOMA	DISORDER	HORMONE PRODUCED	PREVALENCE (%)
Somatograph	Acromegaly/ gigantism	Growth hormone	10–15
Lactotroph (prolactinoma)	Hypogonadism, galactorrhea	Prolactin	25–40
Corticotroph	Cushing's disease	ACTH	10–15
Gonadotroph	Mass effects, hypopituitarism	FSH and LH	10–15
Thyrotroph	Hyperthyroidism	TSH	<3
Nonfunctioning/ null cell	Mass effects, hypopituitarism	None	10–25

ACTH = adrenocorticotropic hormone; FSH = follicle-stimulating hormone; LH = luteinizing hormone; TSH = thyroid-stimulating hormone.

reliable test for acromegaly is the glucose tolerance test (Table 15–7).

CUSHING'S DISEASE. *Cushing's disease* results from a pituitary adenoma that causes excess production of corticotropin (adrenocorticotropic hormone, ACTH). A number of clinical features specifically distinguish Cushing's disease (Table 15–8). Diagnosis of *Cushing's syndrome* is often a challenge, requiring determination as to whether a patient truly has cortisol excess (Table 15–9).

Thyroid-Stimulating Hormone

Central forms of hypothyroidism include secondary hypothyroidism, which is caused by thyroid-stimulating hormone (TSH) deficiency, and tertiary hypothyroidism, which is caused by thyrotropin-releasing hormone (TRH) deficiency. Three different types of

Table 15–6 ■ CLINICAL FEATURES OF ACROMEGALY

CLINICAL FEATURES	NO. OF SUBJECTS	YEARS OR FREQUENCY
Age at diagnosis	885	42 yr
Delay to diagnosis	680	8.7 yr
Sex (% male)	1331	48%
Acral/facial changes	595	98%
Oligo/(a)menorrhea (females)	366	72%
Hyperhidrosis	751	64%
Headaches	825	55%
Paresthesias/carpal tunnel syndrome	725	40%
Impotence (males)	355	36%
Hypertension	630	28%
Goiter	705	21%
Visual field defects	993	19%

From Molitch ME: Clinical manifestations of acromegaly. Endocrinol Metab Clin North Am 21:597, 1992.

Table 15–7 ■ SELECTED TESTS OF EXCESS PITUITARY FUNCTION

HORMONE	TEST	INTERPRETATION
Growth hormone (GH)	*Basal IGF-1*	Elevated IGF-1 levels are consistent with acromegaly when interpreted in the context of age and nutritional status
	Oral glucose suppression test: After 75-g glucose load, GH is measured at −30, 0, 30, 60, 90, 120 min	GH should be suppressed to <2 μg/L in normals; GH may paradoxically increase in acromegaly
	TRH test: TRH 200 μg is given IV with serum GH measurements at 0, 20, 60 min	GH is not stimulated by TRH in most normals; a GH increase of 10 μg/L or >50% of baseline is consistent with acromegaly, but it can also occur in other disorders; the test is most useful for evaluating surgical cure
Prolactin (PRL)	*Basal PRL levels*	Elevated PRL (>200 μgL) is consistent with a prolactinoma; when PRL levels are between 20–200 μg/L, other causes of hyperprolactinemia should be considered
ACTH	*Measurement of 24-hr urine free cortisol*	Elevated urine free cortisol level is suggestive of Cushing's syndrome, but it has several other causes as well
	Overnight dexamethasone suppression test: Dexamethasone 1 mg PO at midnight followed by 8 A.M. plasma cortisol	In normal persons A.M. cortisol should be suppressed to <5 μg/dL; normal dexamethasone suppression excludes Cushing's syndrome; several other disorders can cause failure to suppress normally
	Low-dose dexamethasone suppression test: Dexamethasone 0.5 mg q6h for 8 doses with basal and end-of-treatment measurements that may include 24-hr urine collections for free cortisol or 17-hydroxysteroids and A.M. plasma cortisol and ACTH	17-Hydroxysteroids should be suppressed to <4 mg/24 hr; urine free cortisol should be <20 μg/24 hr; serum cortisol should be suppressed to <6 μg/dL; failure to suppress cortisol production is consistent with diagnosis of Cushing's syndrome
	High-dose dexamethasone suppression test. Dexamethasone 2 mg q6h for 8 doses with basal and end-of-treatment measurements that may include 24-hr urine collections for free cortisol or 17-hydroxysteroids and A.M. plasma cortisol and ACTH	The high-dose test is intended to distinguish Cushing's disease (pituitary adenoma), ectopic ACTH production, and adrenal adenoma; the 50% suppression of 17-hydroxysteroids or 90% suppression of urine free cortisol production is suggestive of Cushing's disease; <50% suppression suggests ectopic ACTH or adrenal adenoma; low ACTH levels are consistent with adrenal adenoma

	CRH test: Ovine CRH 1 μg/kg is administered IV and ACTH and cortisol are drawn at −15, 0, 15, 30, 60, 90, and 120 min	In Cushing's disease, there is usually a 50% increase in ACTH and a 20% increase in cortisol; adrenal adenoma is associated with suppressed ACTH; ectopic ACTH is associated with high basal ACTH and cortisol levels that are not affected by CRH
	Petrosal sinus ACTH sampling: The inferior petrosal sinus is catheterized, ideally bilaterally, and plasma ACTH is compared with simultaneous peripheral samples; the sampling can be done in conjunction with CRH stimulation	In Cushing's disease, the ACTH petrosal sinus–periphery ratio is ≥ 2; in ectopic ACTH, the ratio is < 1.5
TSH	*Basal thyroid function tests*	An inappropriate normal or elevated TSH in the setting of increased free thyroid hormone levels is consistent with a TSH-producing tumor or other causes of inappropriate TSH secretion
	Free α-subunit level	Elevated free α-subunit level associated with inappropriately elevated TSH is suggestive of a TSH-producing tumor
FSH, LH	*Basal FSH, LH, testosterone*	Increased LH and testosterone levels in males are consistent with LH-secreting tumors; elevated FSH and low-normal testosterone is suggestive of an FSH-producing tumor if primary gonadal failure is not present; in females, assessment of excess hormone secretion is difficult because of changes during menstrual cycle and at menopause
	TRH test: TRH 200 μg is given IV with measurements of serum FSH, LH, FSH β- and LH β-subunits at 0, 20, 60 min	Stimulation of LH, FSH, or their free β-subunits is suggestive of a gonadotropin-producing adenoma

IGF = insulin-like growth factor; TRH = thyrotropin-releasing hormone; ACTH = adrenocorticotropic hormone; CRH = corticotropin-releasing hormone; TSH = thyroid-stimulating hormone; FSH = follicle-stimulating hormone; LH = luteinzing hormone.

Table 15–8 ■ CLINICAL FEATURES OF CUSHING'S DISEASE

General

- Obesity (centripetal distribution)
- "Moon facies" and mild proptosis
- Increased supraclavicular fat and "buffalo hump"
- Hypertension

Skin

- Hyperpigmentation
- Facial plethora
- Hirsutism
- Violaceous striae and thin skin
- Capillary fragility and easy bruising
- Acne
- Edema

Musculoskeletal

- Muscle weakness (proximal)
- Osteoporosis and back pain

Reproductive

- Decreased libido
- Oligo(a)menorrhea

Neuropsychiatric

- Depression
- Irritability and emotional lability
- Psychosis

Metabolic

- Hypokalemia and alkalosis
- Hypercalciuria and renal stones
- Glucose intolerance or diabetes mellitus
- Impaired wound healing
- Impaired resistance to infection
- Granulocytosis and lymphopenia

Tumor Mass Effects

- Headache
- Visual field loss
- Hypopituitarism

congenital TSH deficiency are caused by genetic mutations. Acquired, central forms of hypothyroidism are often associated with other pituitary hormone deficiencies and usually there is no goiter because of low TSH levels. Suspicion of central hypothyroidism should prompt measurements of thyroxine (T_4), triiodothyronine (T_3), and TSH, as well as other pituitary hormones.

TSH-SECRETING TUMORS. These are rare and account for between 1 and 3% of pituitary tumors. The clinical features of TSH-secreting tumors resemble those of Graves' disease except that features of autoimmunity, such as ophthalmopathy, are absent. Diffuse goiter is present in the majority of patients with TSH-producing tumors, and the 24-hour uptake of radioiodine is elevated.

For more information about this subject, see *Cecil Textbook of Medicine*, 21st edition. Philadelphia, W.B. Saunders Company, 2000. Chapter 237, Anterior Pituitary, pages 1208 to 1225.

Table 15–9 ■ TESTS USED IN THE DIFFERENTIAL DIAGNOSIS OF CUSHING'S SYNDROME*

ETIOLOGY	OVERNIGHT DEXAMETHASONE SUPPRESSION TEST	PLASMA ACTH	LOW-DOSE DEXAMETHASONE	HIGH-DOSE DEXAMETHASONE	CORTICOTROPIN-RELEASING HORMONE STIMULATION OF ACTH	PETROSAL-PERIPHERAL ACTH RATIO
Normal	Suppression	Normal	Suppression		Normal	
Pituitary	No suppression	Normal or high	No suppression	Suppression	Normal or increased	>2
Ectopic	No suppression	High or normal	No suppression	No suppression	No response	<1.5
Adrenal	No suppression	Low	No suppression	No suppression	No response	

*Classic responses are indicated. Certain cases of ectopic adrenocorticotropic hormone (ACTH) production are suppressed by high-dose dexamethasone or are stimulated by corticotropin-releasing hormone. In these cases, petrosal sinus sampling is the most reliable method for distinguishing pituitary and ectopic sources of ACTH.

POSTERIOR PITUITARY

VASOPRESSIN AND REGULATION OF OSMOLALITY. The primary physiologic action of vasopressin is its function as a water-retaining hormone. The central sensing system (osmostat) for control of release of vasopressin is anatomically discrete located in a small area of the hypothalamus just anterior to the third ventricle.

Diabetes Insipidus

Diabetes insipidus is the excretion of a large volume of hypotonic, insipid (tasteless) urine, usually accompanied by polyuria and polydipsia. *Hypothalamic diabetes insipidus* is the inability to secrete (and usually to synthesize) vasopressin in response to increased osmolality. *Nephrogenic diabetes insipidus* is a disorder in which an otherwise normal kidney is unable to respond to vasopressin. *Primary polydipsia* is a primary disorder of thirst stimulation. Ingested water produces a mild decrease in serum osmolality that turns off the secretion of vasopressin.

TREATMENT. The best therapeutic agent is the vasopressin agonist desmopressin. Desmopressin is different from vasopressin in that the terminal amino group of cystine has been removed to prolong the duration of action and D-arginine is substituted for L-arginine in position 8 to decrease the pressor effect.

The prognosis of properly treated diabetes insipidus is excellent. When the diabetes insipidus is secondary to a recognized disease process, it is that disease that determines the ultimate prognosis.

For more information about this subject, see *Cecil Textbook of Medicine,* 21st edition. Philadelphia, W.B. Saunders Company, 2000. Chapter 238, Posterior Pituitary, pages 1225 to 1231.

THE THYROID

A feedback loop involving the hypothalamus, pituitary, and thyroid gland regulates the glandular secretion of thyroid hormone (Fig. 15–3).

Evaluation of Patients with Thyroid Disease

Techniques employed to measure thyroid hormone values by radioimmunoassay or enzyme-coupled immunoassays are rapidly changing. Serum thyroid hormone concentrations in normals and patients with thyroid disease are noted in Table 15–10. Various causes of increased T_4 levels can be seen in Table 15–11.

Thyrotoxicosis

Thyrotoxicosis occurs (Table 15–12) when tissues are exposed to excess amounts of thyroid hormone, resulting in specific metabolic changes and pathophysiologic alterations in organ function (Table 15–13). *Hyperthyroidism* denotes increased formation and release of thyroid hormone from the thyroid gland, whereas thyrotoxicosis describes the clinical syndrome that results. The most frequent cause of thyrotoxicosis is *Graves' disease,* accounting for 60 to 90% of cases and occurring among women with a frequency of 1.9%. Men experience one tenth of the occurrence in women.

Graves' disease carries the hallmarks of excess formation and

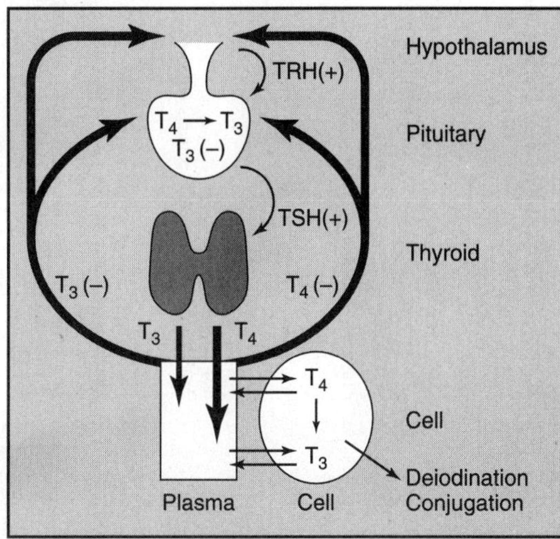

FIGURE 15–3 ■ Hypothalamic-pituitary-thyroid interrelationship. Thyrotropin-releasing hormone (TRH) exerts a positive stimulatory effect on thyroid-stimulating hormone (TSH) secretion, which stimulates thyroid hormone formation. Thyroxine (T_4) is the primary thyroid secretory product, which is converted in the cells of specific organs, such as kidney and liver, to triiodothyronine (T_3).T_3 is the most biologically active thyroid hormone and is inactivated by further deiodination or conjugation and biliary excretion.

secretion of thyroid hormone and diffuse goiter. Additional characteristics include exophthalmos, dermopathy (especially pretibial myxedema), and rarely thyroid acropachy. These supplementary manifestations seldom appear together and often run a divergent time course. Severe thyrotoxicosis should be treated aggressively (Table 15–14). 15

Hypothyroidism

Hypothyroidism is the clinical syndrome that results from decreased secretion of thyroid hormone from the thyroid gland. It most frequently represents a disease of the gland itself (primary hypothyroidism) but can also be caused by pituitary disease (sec-

Table 15–10 ■ SERUM THYROID HORMONE VALUES IN NORMAL PERSONS AND PATIENTS WITH THYROID DISEASE

	NORMAL	HYPERTHYROID	HYPOTHYROID
T_4 (μg/dL)	4.5–12.5	>12.5	<4.5
Free T_4 (ng/dL)	0.9–2	>2	<0.9
T_3 (ng/dL)	80–220	>220	<80
TSH (μU/mL)	0.3–6	<0.3	>6

T_4 = thyroxine; T_3 = triiodothyronine; TSH = thyroid-stimulating hormone.

Table 15–11 ■ CAUSES OF INCREASED SERUM TOTAL THYROXINE (T_4) CONCENTRATION

THYROID STATE CONDITION	T_4	FREE T_4	T_3	TSH	COMMENTS
Hyperthyroid State	H	H	H or N	L	High T_4 combined with hypermetabolic state and hyperthyroidism
Euthyroid State					
Binding abnormalities					
T_4-binding globulin levels increased	H	N	H	N	Autosomal dominant
T_4 binding to albumin increased (familial dysalbuminemic hyperthyroxinemia)	H	N,H*	N	N	*Same "free T_4" methods lead to erroneous results
T_4 binding by transthyretin increased (familial)	H	N	N	N	
T_4 antibodies present	H	N,H	N,L,*H*	N	*Method-based anti–T_3 antibody may also be present
Drug effects					
Inhibitors of 5′-deiodinase					
Oral cholecystographic contrast agents (ipodate, iopanoate)	H	H	L	H	Inhibition of T_3 formation
Amiodarone	H	H	L	L,N	
Propranolol	H	N	L,N	N,H	Only with large doses
Heparin	H	N,H	N	N	Temporary after IV doses
T_4 administration	H	H	N	L	Mild hyperthyroxinemia in patients on T_4 replacement
Various disorders					
Non-thyroidal illness syndrome	H,N	N,L	L	N,L,H	
Hyperemesis gravidarum	H	H,N	N	L	During early part of pregnancy; remits
Acute psychiatric illness	H,N	H,N	N	L	During acute phase; remits without treatment
Extrathyroidal deiodinase defect	H	H	N	N	A few case reports but not completely documented
Thyroid hormone resistance syndrome (pituitary and generalized)	H	H	H	H	In generalized resistance syndrome, hypothyroid features can be present, especially related to central nervous system development. If only pituitary resistance, thyrotoxic symptoms

H = high; N = normal; L = low; T_3 = triiodothyronine; TSH = thyroid-stimulating hormone.
*Sequence indicates frequency of occurrence; for example, free T_4 = H,N—more frequently free T_4 is high, but normal levels can also be encountered.

Table 15–12 ■ CAUSES OF THYROTOXICOSIS

Dependent on Increased Thyroid Hormone Production

Dependent on increased occupancy of the thyroid-stimulating hormone (TSH) receptor by:
- Thyroid-stimulating immunoglobuin (TSI)
  - Graves' disease
  - Hashimoto's thyroiditis
- Human chorionic gonadotropin (hCG)
  - Hydatiform mole
  - Choriocarcinoma
- TSH
  - TSH-producing pituitary tumor

Autonomous overproduction of thyroid hormone (independence of TSH)
- Toxic adenoma (TSH receptor mutant)
- Toxic multinodular goiter
- Follicular cancer (rare)

Jodbasedow effect (excess iodine-induced hyperthyroidism)

Independent of Increased Thyroid Hormone Production

Increased thyroid hormone release
- Subacute granulomatous thyroiditis (painful)
- Subacute lymphocytic thyroiditis (painless)

Non-thyroidal source of thyroid hormone
- Thyrotoxicosis factitia
- "Hamburger" thyrotoxicosis
- Ectopic production by:
  - Ovarian teratoma (struma ovarii)
  - Metastasis of follicular cancer

ondary hypothyroidism) or hypothalamic disease (tertiary hypothyroidism) (Table 15–15). The different causes of hypothyroidism lead to similar symptoms (Table 15–16). 15

Diagnosis is based on measurement of thyroid hormone levels (Fig. 15–4).

Myxedema coma, whether spontaneous or caused by cold expo-

Table 15–13 ■ TISSUE-SPECIFIC SIGNS AND SYMPTOMS OF THYROTOXICOSIS

TISSUE	SYMPTOMS AND SIGNS
Central nervous system	Nervousness and emotional lability Fine tremor of hands
Cardiovascular	Palpitations, tachycardia, atrial fibrillation, increased difference between systolic and diastolic blood pressure
Gastrointestinal	Hyperdefecation, gastrointestinal hypermotility, diarrhea
Muscle	Proximal muscle weakness, muscle atrophy, hyperreflexia
Skin	Warm moist smooth skin, onycholysis, fine hair, hair loss, excessive perspiration
Metabolic	Heat intolerance, weight loss usually with increased appetite
Thyroid	Enlargement of nodule(s)

Table 15–14 ■ MANAGEMENT OF THYROID STORM

Inhibition of Thyroid Hormone Formation and Secretion

PTU, 400 mg q8h PO or by nasogastric tube
Sodium iodide, 1 g IV in 24 hr, or saturated solution of KI, 5 drops q8h

Sympathetic Blockade

Propranolol 20–40 mg q4–6h, or 1 mg IV slowly (repeat doses until heart rate slows); not indicated in patients with asthma or congestive heart failure that is not rate-related

Glucocorticoid Therapy

Hydrocortisone 50–100 mg IV q6h

IV fluids (depending on indication: glucose, electrolytes, multivitamins)
Temperature control (cooling blankets, acetaminophen; avoid salicylates)
O_2 if required
Digitalis for congestive failure and to slow ventricular response; pentobarbital for sedation
Treatment of precipitating event (e.g., infection)

PTU = propylthiouracil.

Table 15–15 ■ CAUSES OF HYPOTHYROIDISM

Primary Hypothyroidism

Insufficient amount of thyroid tissue
- *Destruction of tissue by autoimmune process*
  - Hashimoto's thyroiditis (atrophic and goitrous forms)
  - Graves' disease—end-stage
- *Destruction of tissue by iatrogenic procedures*
  - ^{131}I therapy
  - Surgical thyroidectomy
  - External radiation
- *Destruction of tissue by infiltrative processes*
  - Amyloidosis, lymphoma, scleroderma

Defects of thyroid hormone biosynthesis
- Congenital enzyme defects
- Congenital mutations in TSH receptor
- Iodine deficiency or excess
- Drug-induced: thionamides, lithium, sulfonamides, interleukins, tumor necrosis factor, others

Secondary Hypothyroidism

Pituitary
- Panhypopituitarism (e.g., neoplasm, radiation, surgery, Sheehan's syndrome)
- Isolated TSH deficiency

Hypothalamic
- Congenital
- Infeciton
- Infiltration (sarcoidosis, granulomas)

Transient Hypothyroidism

Silent and subacute thyroiditis
Thyroxine withdrawal

Generalized Resistance to Thyroid Hormone

TSH = thyroid-stimulating hormone.

Table 15–16 ■ TISSUE-SPECIFIC SIGNS AND SYMPTOMS OF HYPOTHYROIDISM

TISSUE	SIGNS AND SYMPTOMS
Central nervous system	Forgetfulness, stoic appearance, myxedematous dementia, cerebellar ataxia
Cardiovascular	Bradycardia, pericardial effusion, hypertension
Respiratory	Depressed ventilatory drive, pleural effusion, sleep apnea
Gastrointestinal	Constipation, hypomotility
Muscle	Delayed tendon reflexes, muscle stiffness and cramps, increased muscle volume weakness
Skin	Dry, rough, hyperkeratosis; non-pitting puffiness due to mucopolysaccharide deposits
Metabolic	Basal metabolic rate decreased, cold intolerance, decreased T_4 and drug turnover, weight gain

T_4 = thyroxine.

sure, is a special clinical condition. Treatment (Table 15–17) should be initiated immediately, and if T_4 and TSH levels cannot be readily obtained, therapy may be started on clinical suspicion.

Thyroiditis

Thyroiditis includes infectious and autoimmune inflammatory disease of the thyroid. Thyroiditis is divided into acute (suppurative), subacute painful (granulomatous), subacute painless (lymphocytic), chronic lymphocytic (Hashimoto's), and chronic fibrous (Riedel's) thyroiditis. Postpartum thyroiditis is classified as a variant of subacute painless lymphocytic thyroiditis.

15

Non-Toxic Diffuse and Nodular Goiter

The term *non-toxic* or *simple goiter* indicates an increase in the mass of the thyroid gland resulting from excessive replication of benign thyroid epithelial cells. The aim of therapy (Fig. 15–5) is to

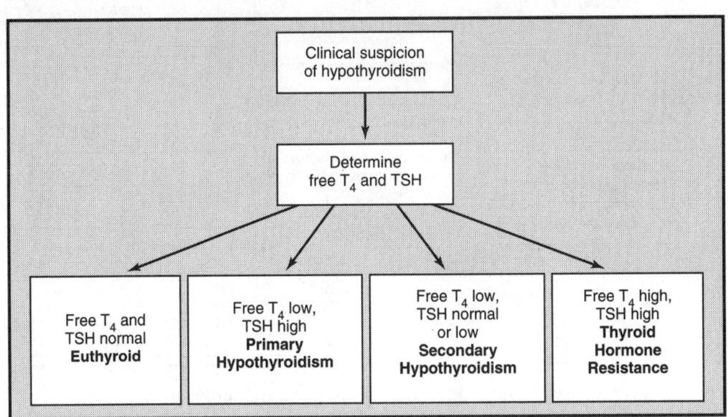

FIGURE 15–4 ■ Diagnostic approach to hypothyroidism.

Table 15–17 ■ TREATMENT OF MYXEDEMA COMA

Thyroid Hormone Administration

T_4 300 μg over 5–10 min initially, followed by T_4 100 μg IV q24h until oral T_4 therapy can be started

Alternatively, T_3 10 μg IV q4h until oral T_4 therapy can be started

Glucocorticoid Administration

Hydrocortisone 100 mg IV bolus followed by 25 mg q6h by IV drip

Cover to conserve heat

IV fluids, electrolytes, and glucose to correct electrolyte abnormalities and hypoglycemia

Tracheal intubation and mechanical ventilation as required

Treat precipitating conditions (infection)

Avoid sedatives, narcotics, and overhydration

T_4 = thyroxine.

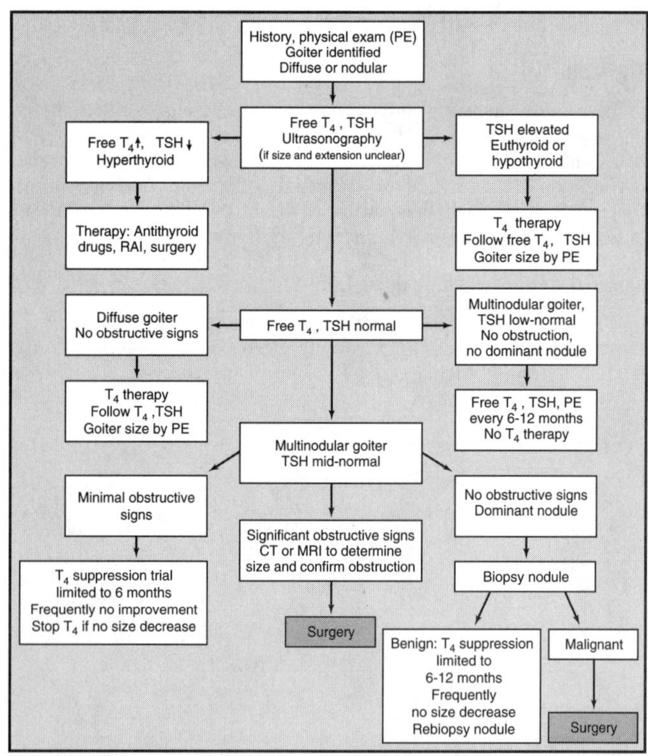

FIGURE 15–5 ■ Evaluation and management of patients with non-toxic diffuse and nodular goiter and undetermined thyroid status. RAI = radioactive iodine; CT = computed tomography; MRI = magnetic resonance imaging.

decrease the size of the thyroid, relieve pressure-induced symptoms, and achieve a euthyroid state.

Thyroid Cancer

Thyroid cancer surgery should be performed by an experienced thyroid surgeon. Iodine-131 ablation is used in patients who undergo near-total thyroidectomy, especially if the primary lesion is a papillary cancer greater than 2 cm in diameter or a follicular cancer. One day after surgery, patients are started on T_3 (Cytomel 25 μg every day or twice a day) and maintained on this dose of T_3 for 4 to 6 weeks. T_3 has a half-life of 1 day and the patient becomes hypothyroid much more quickly than with T_4 treatment. After the TSH has attained levels of at least 40 μU/mL, a scanning dose of 3 mCi of ^{123}I is administered. If a small remnant of thyroid tissue is left in the bed of the thyroid, an ablative dose of 29 mCi of ^{131}I is administered. Identification of a larger amount of thyroid tissue or lymph node metastases leads to the administration of a higher dose of ^{131}I, ranging from 75 to 125 mCi according to the amount of remaining tissue.

When patients become hypothyroid for radioactive iodine (RAI) scanning, it is important to obtain a thyroglobulin level: elevated levels indicate that a sizable mass of thyroid tissue was left after surgery. Patients who had considerable thyroid tissue left or tumor spread to lymph nodes should be rescanned 6 months after the initial scan to ensure that the initial RAI treatment ablated all thyroid tissue.

For more information about this subject, see *Cecil Textbook of Medicine,* 21st edition. Philadelphia, W.B. Saunders Company, 2000. Chapter 239, The Thyroid, pages 1231 to 1250.

THE ADRENAL CORTEX

Provocative Tests of Adrenal Function.

Three provocative tests of adrenal function are in common use. The *ACTH simulation test* is the most reliable screening test for adrenal hypofunction. It is also the standard method by which suspected enzymatic deficiencies in adrenal steroidogenesis are examined. The test is performed by administering 250 μg of synthetic ACTH (Cortrosyn) intravenously and measuring the serum steroids of interest 45 and 60 minutes later. The normal adrenal gland produces plasma cortisol concentrations greater than 20 μg/dL in response to this challenge. *Corticotropin-releasing hormone,* the 41–amino acid hypothalamic secretagogue for ACTH, is a useful test for separating ACTH-dependent from ACTH-independent hypercortisolism and is an essential component of the inferior petrosal sinus sampling procedure for localizing the site of ACTH secretion. The test is performed by infusing corticotropin-releasing hormone 1 μg/kg intravenously over a period of 1 minute and measuring the ACTH response between 3 and 30 minutes thereafter.

The *dexamethasone suppression test* is widely used to screen for adrenal hyperfunction. The test has so many false-positive and false-negative results (sensitivity and specificity of about 0.8), however, that it is superseded by the tests mentioned above. The test retains some value in the differential diagnosis of mineralocorticoid excess. Many iterations of this test are available, the simplest being dexamethasone 0.5 mg administered by mouth every 6 hours for 2 days.

Plasma and urine aldosterone and plasma renin activity are important tests to evaluate states of apparent mineralocorticoid excess and deficiency.

The differential diagnosis of congenital adrenal hyperplasia requires the measurement of specific steroid biosynthetic intermediates that accumulate proximal to the responsible enzymatic deficiencies in the steroid biosynthetic cascade. The most commonly measured are 17-hydroxyprogesterone (21-hydroxylase deficiency) and 11-deoxycortisol (11-hydroxylase deficiency). These steroids are most reliably measured in the context of an ACTH stimulation test, as described above.

Adrenal Hyperfunction

Four syndromes of adrenal hyperfunction are differentiated: Cushing's syndrome, hypokalemic metabolic alkalosis, masculinization, and feminization. These syndromes result from the excessive secretion of cortisol, mineralocorticoid, androgen, and estrogen, respectively. These disorders can occur in isolation or, more commonly, in combination with one or more of the others.

GLUCOCORTICOID EXCESS—CUSHING'S SYNDROME. Cushing's syndrome is caused by glucocorticoid excess. The "classic" syndrome is defined clinically (Table 15–18). The causes of Cushing's syndrome can be divided into ACTH-dependent and ACTH-independent causes (Table 15–19). Ectopic secretion of ACTH from a neoplasm not of pituitary origin is one example of ACTH-dependent Cushing's syndrome (Table 15–20). Renin-angiotensin–independent mineralocorticoid excess is another form of disease and may take an independent (Table 15–21) or dependent (Table 15–22) form.

Adrenal Hypofunction

A broad specturm of signs and symptoms can herald the presence of glucocorticoid deficiency (Table 15–23).

PRIMARY ADRENAL INSUFFICIENCY. The most common cause of primary adrenal insufficiency worldwide is tuberculosis. The most common cause of adrenal insufficiency in the industrialized West is an autoimmune process, usually as part of the polyglandular deficiency syndrome. In this disorder, an autoimmune "adrenalitis" leads to destruction of the adrenal cortex. This disease has two forms, types I and II (Table 15–24).

MINERALOCORTICOID DEFICIENCY. The clinical manifestations of mineralocorticoid deficiency include hyponatremia, hyperkalemia, and mild metabolic acidosis. The diagnosis of isolated hypoaldosteronism depends on the demonstration of an inappropriately low circulating aldosterone level (Table 15–25).

For more information about this subject, see *Cecil Textbook of Medicine,* 21st edition. Philadelphia, W.B. Saunders Company, 2000. Chapter 240, The Adrenal Cortex, pages 1250 to 1257.

Table 15–18 ■ CLINICAL FEATURES OF GLUCOCORTICOID EXCESS

FEATURE	FREQUENCY (%)
Weight gain	90
"Moon facies"	75
Hypertension	75
Violaceous striae	65
Hirsutism	65
Glucose intolerance	65
Proximal muscle weakness	60
Plethora	60
Menstrual dysfunction	60
Acne	40
Easy bruising	40
Osteopenia	40
Dependent edema	40
Hyperpigmentation	20
Hypokalemic metabolic alkalosis	15

Table 15–19 ■ CAUSES OF CUSHING'S SYNDROME

ACTH-Dependent Causes

ACTH-secreting pituitary tumor (Cushing's disease)
Non-pituitary ACTH-secreting neoplasm (ectopic ACTH syndrome)

ACTH-Independent Causes

Adrenal adenoma
Adrenal carcinoma
Micronodular adrenal disease
Factitious or surreptitious glucocorticoid administration

ACTH = adrenocorticotropic hormone.

15

Table 15–20 ■ COMMON CAUSES OF ECTOPIC ADRENOCORTICOTROPIC HORMONE SECRETION

Small cell carcinoma of the lung	50%
Endocrine tumors of foregut origin	35%
Thymic carcinoid	
Islet cell tumor	
Medullary carcinoma, thyroid	
Bronchial carcinoid	
Pheochromocytoma	5%
Ovarian tumors	2%

Table 15–21 ■ COMMON CAUSES OF RENIN-ANGIOTENSIN–INDEPENDENT MINERALOCORTICOID EXCESS

Aldosterone-secreting adenoma
Adrenal cancer
Congenital adrenal hyperplasia
- 11-Hydroxylase deficiency
- 17-Hydroxylase deficiency

11β-Hydroxysteroid dehydrogenase deficiency
Licorice intoxication
Glucocorticoid-suppressible hyperaldosteronism

Table 15–22 ■ COMMON CAUSES OF RENIN-ANGIOTENSIN–DEPENDENT MINERALOCORTICOID EXCESS

- Vomiting
- Diuretics
- Edematous disorders
  - Congestive heart failure
  - Hepatic cirrhosis
  - Nephrotic syndrome
- Renal ischemia
- Bartter's syndrome
- Renin-secreting tumors

Table 15–23 ■ CAUSES OF GLUCOCORTICOID DEFICIENCY

ACTH-Independent Causes

- Tuberculosis
- Autoimmune (idiopathic)
- Other rare causes
  - Fungal infection
  - Adrenal hemorrhage
  - Metastases
  - Sarcoidosis
  - Amyloidosis
  - Adrenoleukodystrophy
  - Adrenomyeloneuropathy
  - HIV infection
  - Congenital adrenal hyperplasia
  - Medications (ketoconazole, OP′DDD)

ACTH-Dependent Causes

- Hypothalamic-pituitary-adrenal suppression
  - Exogenous
    - Glucocorticoid
    - ACTH
  - Endogenous—cure of Cushing's syndrome
- Hypothalamic-pituitary lesions
  - Neoplasm
    - Primary pituitary tumor
    - Metastatic tumor
  - Craniopharyngioma
  - Infection
    - Tuberculosis
    - Actinomycosis
    - Nocardiosis
- Sarcoid
- Head trauma
- Isolated ACTH deficiency

ACTH = adrenocorticotroic hormone; HIV = human immunodeficiency virus; OP′DDD = *ortho, para′*-dichlorodiphenyldichloroethane.

Table 15–24 ■ POLYENDOCRINE DEFICIENCY SYNDROMES

FEATURE	TYPE I	TYPE II
Age of onset	12 yr	24 yr
Adrenal insufficiency	+	+
Diabetes mellitus	−	+
Autoimmune thyroid disease	−	+
Hypoparathyroidism	+	−
Mucocutaneous candidiasis	+	−
Hypogonadism	+	±
Chronic active hepatitis	+	−
Pernicious anemia	+	−
Vitiligo	+	+

THE ADRENAL MEDULLA, CATECHOLAMINES, AND PHEOCHROMOCYTOMA

Catecholamines are released from the adrenal medulla into the circulation through the adrenal vein. Norepinephrine from sympathetic neurons is released pre-synaptically and acts as a cell-to-cell neurotransmitter.

Pheochromocytoma

Pheochromocytoma is a chromaffin cell neoplasm that typically causes symptoms and signs of episodic catecholamine release, including paroxysmal hypertension. The tumor is an unusual cause of hypertension and accounts for, at most, 0.1 to 0.2% of cases of high blood pressure (Table 15–26).

ANATOMIC LOCALIZATION. The tumor location must be known to plan the proper surgical route. Ninety-five per cent of pheochromocytomas are in the abdomen, and the great majority of these can be visualized by one of three modalities: computed tomography (CT), magnetic resonance imaging (MRI), or metaiodobenzylguanidine (MIBG) scintigraphy. CT and MRI are highly sensitive, although non-specific because they visualize any mass

Table 15–25 ■ CAUSES OF ISOLATED HYPOALDOSTERONISM

Renin-Angiotensin–Dependent

Hyporeninemic hypoaldosteronism
Autonomic neuropathy
Prostaglandin synthesis inhibitors

Renin-Angiotensin–Independent

Inhibition of aldosterone synthesis
- Heparin
- Cyclosporine
- Calcium channel blockers

Following resection of an aldosterone-secreting adenoma
18-Hydroxylase deficiency
Aldosterone resistance (pseudohypoaldosteronism)

Table 15–26 ■ DIAGNOSTIC APPROACH TO PHEOCHROMOCYTOMA

- Clinical clues or "tip-offs"
  - History
    - Paroxysmal symptoms (classic triad is headache, diaphoresis, palpitations)
    - History of extraordinarily labile or refractory hypertension
    - Family history of pheochromocytoma, von Hippel-Lindau syndrome, or multiple endocrine neoplasia
    - Incidental adrenal abnormality on abdominal imaging test (rarely)
  - Physical examination
    - Labile, refractory hypertension
    - Orthostatic hypotension
    - von Hippel-Lindau syndrome—or multiple endocrine neoplasia–associated findings (retinal angiomas, thyroid enlargement, mucosal neuromas)
- Biochemical confirmation (only after clue or tip-off; begin with urinary tests)
  - Urinary catecholamines and metabolites (24-hr sample or 2-hr sample after a paroxysm; metanephrines, the initial screening test)
  - Plasma catecholamines (if urinary values are equivocal; take care to obtain a basal, resting sample)
  - Clonidine suppression test (if plasma catecholamines are in the equivocal 1000–2000 pg/mL range)
  - Plasma chromogranin A (storage vesicle protein released with catecholamines; also elevated by renal failure)
- Anatomic localization (only after biochemical confirmation)
  - By morphology (most sensitive, less specific)
    - Computed tomography (the imaging test most frequently obtained)
    - Magnetic resonance imaging (may have advantages for extra-adrenal tumors)
  - By function (most specific, less sensitive)
    - Radiolabeled metaiodobenzylguanidine scanning (accumulates in functioning chromaffin tissue)

lesion, not just pheochromocytomas. MIBG scanning is highly specific for chromaffin tissue, although somewhat less sensitive than CT or MRI.

MANAGEMENT. ***PREOPERATIVE PREPARATION AND DRUG TREATMENT.*** Once pheochromocytoma has been diagnosed, the patient is prepared for surgery with adrenergic blockade for a period of 1 to 4 weeks. α-Blockade is usually accomplished with oral phenoxybenzamine, an irreversible, non-competitive antagonist that acts predominantly at α_1-receptors. The drug is begun at 5 mg twice daily, and the dose is adjusted gradually upward by increments of 10 mg every 1 to 4 days to a maximum of 50 to 100 mg twice daily. The usual dose range required is 30 to 80 mg/day.

If blood pressure or tachyarrhythmias, including sinus tachycardia, are not fully controlled by α-blockade, β-blockade is instituted with oral propranolol 10 to 40 mg four times daily. β-Blockade must not be undertaken before α-blockade has been instituted.

If combined management with α- plus β-adrenergic antagonists is not fully effective, the tyrosine hydroxylase inhibitor α-methylparatyrosine is added at an oral dose of 0.25 to 1.0 g four times daily. Its use may be complicated by sedation, fatigue, anxiety, diarrhea, or extrapyramidal reactions.

OPERATIVE AND PERIOPERATIVE MANAGEMENT. In the postoperative period, several problems occur with some frequency:

1. *Hypotension.* Most commonly, hypotension results from hypovolemia and responds to saline infusion; several liters may be required, often with the guidance of central pressure measurements. After volume repletion, norepinephrine can be infused if needed.
2. *Hypertension.* Plasma catecholamine levels remain elevated for several days after complete pheochromocytoma resection. Even 2 weeks postoperatively, up to one fourth of patients still have hypertension. At this time the differential diagnosis includes residual unresected tumor, essential hypertension, or hypertension secondary to renal damage caused by prior hypertension. A urine collection for catecholamines, obtained at least 1 to 2 weeks after tumor resection, will clarify matters.
3. *Hypoglycemia.* After correction of catecholamine excess, insulin release may be increased and end-organ responsiveness to insulin augmented, resulting in hypoglycemia. Hypoglycemia may masquerade as refractory hypotension. Infusion of glucose (5% dextrose in water or saline) during the intraoperative and immediate postoperative period is useful.

The Incidental Adrenal Mass ("Incidentaloma")

Up to 2% of all abdominal CT scans (as well as 9% of autopsies) incidentally discover minimal adrenal gland abnormalities. Rarely do these lesions require further attention.

For more information about this subject, see *Cecil Textbook of Medicine,* 21st edition. Philadelphia, W.B. Saunders Company, 2000. Chapter 241, The Adrenal Medulla, Catecholamines, and Pheochromocytoma, pages 1257 to 1262.

DIABETES MELLITUS

In the United States the number of diagnosed cases of diabetes mellitus has increased substantially in the last half of the 20th century. Diabetes mellitus is the fourth most common reason for patient contact with a physician, accounts for about 15% of health care costs in the United States and is a major cause of premature disability and mortality (Table 15–27).

Pathogenesis

Type 1 diabetes produces profound beta cell failure with secondary insulin resistance, whereas type 2 diabetes causes less severe insulin deficiency and a more severe impairment in insulin action. Given the similarity in the overall picture, it is not surprising that both forms of diabetes share many pathophysiologic features. However, despite the apparent phenotypic similarity, the underlying

Table 15-27 ■ CLASSIFICATION OF DIABETES

Clinical Diabetes

I. Type 1 diabetes, formerly called insulin-dependent diabetes mellitus (IDDM) or "juvenile-onset diabetes"
   A. Immune-mediated
   B. Idiopathic
II. Type 2 diabetes, formerly called non–insulin-dependent diabetes (NIDDM) or "adult-onset diabetes"
III. Other specific types
   A. Genetic defects of β-cell function (e.g., maturity-onset diabetes of the young [MODY] types 1–3 and point mutations in mitochondrial DNA)
   B. Genetic defects in insulin action
   C. Disease of the exocrine pancreas (e.g., pancreatitis, trauma, pancreatectomy, neoplasia, cystic fibrosis, hemochromatosis, fibrocalculous pancreatopathy)
   D. Endocrinopathies (e.g., acromegaly, Cushing's syndrome, hyperthyroidism, pheochromocytoma, glucagonoma, somatostatinoma, aldosteronoma)
   E. Drug- or chemical-induced (e.g., glucocorticosteroids, thiazides, diazoxide, pentamidine, thyroid hormone, phenytoin [Dilantin], β-agonists, oral contraceptives)
   F. Infections (e.g., congenital rubella, cytomegalovirus)
   G. Uncommon forms of immune-mediated diabetes (e.g., 'stiff-man' syndrome, anti–insulin receptor antibodies)
   H. Other genetic syndromes (e.g., Down, Klinefelter's, Turner's syndromes; Huntington's disease, myotonic dystrophy, lipodystrophy, ataxia-telangiectasia)
IV. Gestational diabetes mellitus

Risk Categories

I. Impaired fasting glucose
II. Impaired glucose tolerance

pathogenetic mechanisms leading to type 1 and type 2 diabetes are strikingly different.

TYPE 1 DIABETES. Type 1 diabetes results from an interplay of genetic, environmental, and autoimmune factors that selectively destroy insulin-producing beta cells.

TYPE 2 DIABETES. Hyperglycemia in type 2 diabetes results from an undefined genetic defect(s) (concordance rates in identical twins are nearly 100%), the expression of which is modified by environmental factors. Inasmuch as hyperglycemia itself impairs

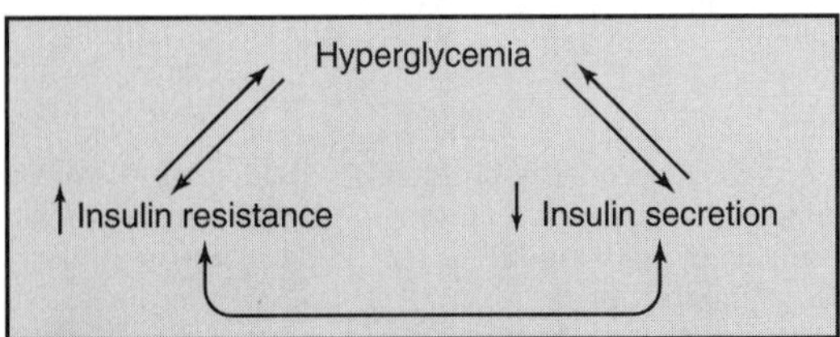

FIGURE 15-6 ■ Elevations of circulating glucose initiate a vicious circle in which hyperglycemia begets more severe hyperglycemia.

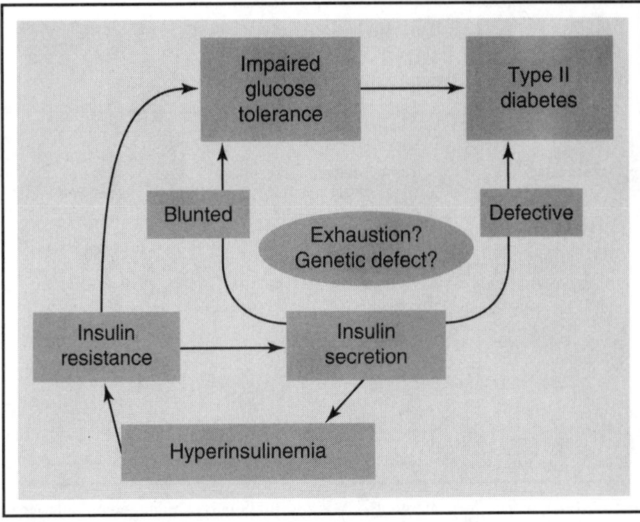

FIGURE 15–7 ■ A proposed sequence of events leading to the development of type 2 diabetes: insulin resistance resulting from genetic influences, central obesity, inactivity, or a combination of these factors leads over time to a progressive loss of the beta cell's capacity to compensate for this defect.

insulin secretion and action, a phenomenon termed "glucose toxicity" is sometimes used (Figs. 15–6 and 15–7).

15

Treatment

Treatment of diabetes mellitus involves changes in lifestyle, and pharmacologic intervention with insulin or oral glucose-lowering drugs. Although therapeutic strategies may differ for the two types of the disease, the short-term and long-term goals of treatment are identical (Table 15–28). A comprehensive management plan should be drafted for each patient (Fig. 15–8).

TYPE 1 DIABETES. A variety of highly purified insulin preparations are commercially available that differ mainly in their time of onset and duration of action (Table 15–29). Therapeutic regimens

Table 15–28 ■ TREATMENT GOALS IN DIABETES

Short-term
- Restore metabolic control to as close to normal as possible
- Improve sense of well-being

Long-term
- Minimize risk of diabetic complications
  - Accelerated atherosclerosis
  - Microangiopathy (retinopathy, nephropathy)
  - Neuropathy

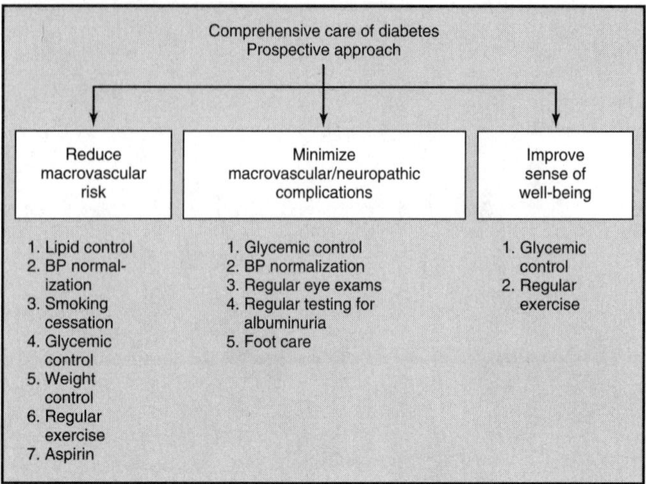

FIGURE 15–8 ■ The key elements of a comprehensive management plan for patients with diabetes.

may be adjusted to fit the patient (Fig. 15–9), and lifestyle modifications are important (Table 15–30).

TYPE 2 DIABETES. In most type 2 diabetic patients, diet and exercise are the key or only therapeutic interventions required to restore metabolic control. However, several new classes of oral glucose-lowering agents are available for these patients (Table 15–31).

Complications of Diabetes

Diabetic ketoacidosis may herald the onset of type 1 diabetes, but it most often occurs in established diabetic patients as a result of an intercurrent illness, an inappropriate reduction in insulin dosage, or missed injections (especially in adolescents). The goals of therapy are to reverse the metabolic disturbance and replace fluid and electrolyte deficits.

For more information about this subject, see *Cecil Textbook of Medicine,* 21st edition. Philadelphia, W.B. Saunders Company, 2000. Chapter 242, Diabetes Mellitus, pages 1263 to 1285.

HYPOGLYCEMIA AND PANCREATIC ISLET CELL DISORDERS

HYPOGLYCEMIA. Hypoglycemia is a clinical syndrome of diverse causes in which low levels of plasma glucose eventually lead to neuroglycopenia. During acute insulin-induced hypoglycemia in healthy persons, autonomic symptoms are recognized at a threshold of approximately 60 mg/dL (3 nmol/L) and impairment of brain function manifested by neuroglycopenic symptoms occurs at a threshold of approximately 50 mg/dL (2.8 nmol/L). It is useful to review a classification based on clinical characteristics of hypogly-

Table 15–29 ■ INSULIN PREPARATIONS: TIME COURSE OF ACTION AFTER SUBCUTANEOUS ADMINISTRATION

CLASS	PREPARATION	ONSET OF EFFECT	PEAK EFFECT (hr)	DURATION OF ACTION (hr)
Rapid-acting	Regular	30 min	2–4	5–8
	Lispro	10–15 min	1–2	3–4
Intermediate-acting	NPH or Lente	1–2 hr	6–10	16–24
Long-acting	Ultralente	4–6 hr	8–20	24–28

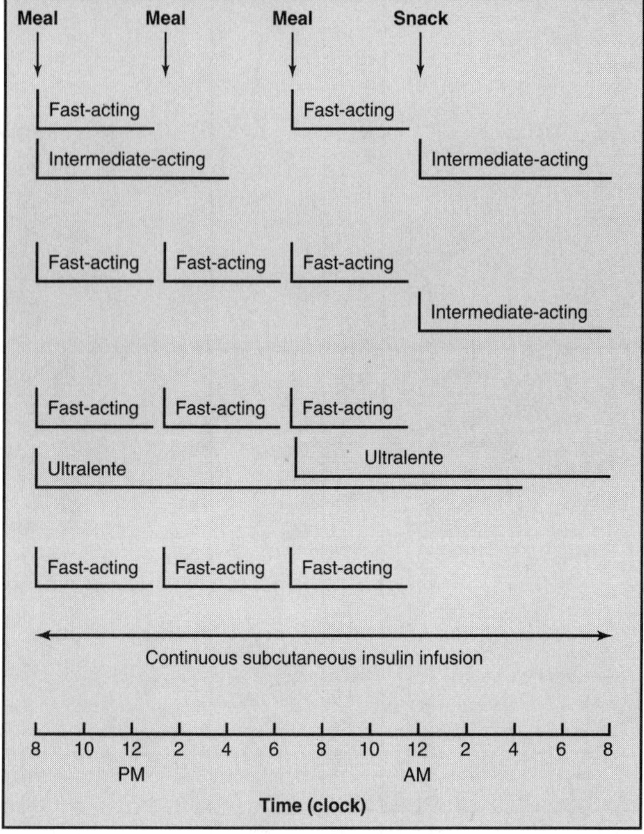

FIGURE 15–9 ■ Several intensive insulin regimens commonly used in the treatment of diabetes. Each is designed to provide a continuous supply of insulin around the clock and to make extra insulin available at the time of meals, thereby simulating more closely the normal physiologic pattern of insulin secretion.

cemic disorders (Table 15–32). A prolonged supervised (72-hour) fast is the classic diagnostic test (Table 15–33).

ISLET CELL TUMORS. Tumors of the endocrine pancreas generally are malignant. Functioning islet cell tumors are commonly associated with one of five widely recognized syndromes (Table 15–34).

For more information about this subject, see *Cecil Textbook of Medicine,* 21st edition. Philadelphia, W.B. Saunders Company, 2000. Chapter 243, Hypoglycemia/Pancreatic Islet Cell Disorders, pages 1285 to 1292.

Table 15–30 ■ LIFESTYLE MODIFICATIONS FOR PATIENTS WITH DIABETES

Diet prescription
1. Weight reduction, gain, or maintenance (as appropriate)
2. Carbohydrates: 45–60% (depending on severity of diabetes and triglyceride levels)
3. Restriction of saturated fat (to <10% of calories)
4. Increased monounsaturated fat (depending on need to limit carbohydrate)
5. Decreased cholesterol intake to <200 mg/d
6. Sodium restriction in patients prone to hypertension

*Exercise prescription**
1. Aerobic strongly preferred; avoid heavy lifting, straining, and Valsalva maneuvers that raise blood pressure
2. Intensity: increase pulse rate to at least 120–140, depending on age and cardiovascular state of the patient
3. Frequency: 3–4 d/wk
4. Duration: 20–30 min preceded and followed by stretching and flexibility exercises for 5–10 min

*Limitations are imposed by pre-existing coronary or peripheral vascular disease, proliferative retinopathy, peripheral or autonomic neuropathy, and poor glycemic control.

MULTIPLE-ORGAN SYNDROMES: POLYGLANDULAR DISORDERS

Polyglandular Neoplasia

MULTIPLE ENDOCRINE NEOPLASIA TYPE I (MEN-I). MEN-I is an autosomal dominant disorder involving characteristically the parathyroid glands, the pancreatic islets, and the anterior pituitary.

MULTIPLE ENDOCRINE NEOPLASIA TYPES IIA AND IIB. MEN-IIA is an autosomal dominant disease that presents as medullary carcinoma of the thyroid, pheochromocytoma, and, less commonly, hyperparathyroidism. MEN-IIB is closely related to MEN-IIA because it also presents with medullary carcinoma of the thyroid and pheochromocytoma but also with a number of abnormalities not found in MEN-IIA. These include mucosal neuromas of the tongue, lips, eyelids, and gastrointestinal tract and a marfanoid habitus. Hyperparathyroidism rarely occurs in MEN-IIB. MEN-IIB is less common than MEN-IIA; both diseases are rarer than MEN-I.

15

Autoimmune Polyglandular Dysfunction

Organ-specific autoimmune disease, characterized by lymphocytic infiltration and organ-specific autoantibodies, commonly results in endocrine hypofunction or hyperfunction (Table 15–35).

For more information about this subject, see *Cecil Textbook of Medicine,* 21st edition. Philadelphia, W.B. Saunders Company, 2000. Chapter 244, Multiple Organ Syndromes: Polyglandular Disorders, pages 1292 to 1295.

Table 15–31 ■ CHARACTERISTICS OF ORAL GLUCOSE-LOWERING AGENTS

AGENT	TOTAL DAILY DOSE (mg/d)	DOSES PER DAY	DURATION OF ACTION (hr)
Sulfonylureas			
First generation			
Chlorpropamide	100–750	1	60
Tolazamide	100–1000	1–2	12–14
Tolbutamide	500–3000	2–3	6–12
Second generation			
Glimepiride	1–8	1	24
Glyburide	1.25–20	1–2	Up to 24
Glyburide micronized	0.75–12	1–2	Up to 24
Glipizide	2.5–40	1–2	Up to 24
Glipizide GITS	5.0–20	1	24
Biguanide			
Metformin	500–2550	2–3	Up to 24
Thiazolidinedione			
Troglitazone	400–600	1	24
Pioglitazone	15–45*	1	24
Rosiglitazone	4–8*	1–2	Up to 24
α-Glucosidase Inhibitors			
Acarbose	75–300	3†	NA
Miglitol	75–300	3†	NA
Benzoic Acid Derivatives			
Repaglinide	1–16	3†	Short

GITS = gastrointestinal therapeutic system; NA = not available.
*Pending FDA approval
†To be taken with meals.

MULTIPLE-ORGAN SYNDROMES: CARCINOID SYNDROME

Clinical Manifestations

Carcinoid tumors typically have a slow rate of growth, and many patients with carcinoid syndrome survive for a decade after the disease is recognized. For much of the duration of the illness, morbidity results largely from the endocrine functions of the tumor. Death usually is caused by cardiac or hepatic failure and by complications associated with tumor growth.

VASODILATOR PAROXYSMS. Cutaneous flushing is the most common clinical feature.

TELANGIECTASIA. Some patients also develop telangiectasia, primarily on the face and neck.

GASTROINTESTINAL SYMPTOMS. Intestinal hypermotility with borborygmi, cramping, and explosive diarrhea may accompany the flushing.

CARDIAC MANIFESTATIONS. Plaquelike thickening of the endocardium of the valvular cusps and cardiac chambers occurs primarily on the right side of the heart.

PULMONARY SYMPTOMS. Bronchoconstriction occurs, usually most pronounced during flushing attacks.

Table 15–32 ■ CLINICAL CLASSIFICATION OF HYPOGLYCEMIC DISORDERS

I. Patient appears healthy*
  A. No coexistent disease
    1. Drugs
      a. Ethanol
      b. Salicylates
      c. Quinine
      d. Haloperidol
    2. Insulinoma
    3. Islet hyperplasia/nesidioblastosis
    4. Factitial hypoglycemia from insulin or sulfonylurea
    5. Severe exercise
    6. Ketotic hypoglycemia
  B. Compensated coexistent disease
    1. Drugs
      a. Dispensing error
      b. Disopyramide
      c. β-Adrenergic blocking agents
      d. Sulfhydryl- or thiol-containing drugs with autoimmune insulin syndrome
      e. Unripe ackee fruit and undernutrition
II. Patient appears ill
  A. Drugs
    1. Pentamidine and *Pneumocystis pneumonia*
    2. Sulfamethoxazole-trimethoprim and renal failure
    3. Propoxyphene and renal failure
    4. Quinine and cerebral malaria
    5. Quinine and malaria
    6. Topical salicylates and renal failure
  B. Predisposing illness
    1. Small-for-gestational-age infant
    2. Beckwith-Wiedemann syndrome
    3. Erythroblastosis fetalis
    4. Infant of diabetic mother
    5. Glycogen storage disease
    6. Defects in amino acid and fatty acid metabolism
    7. Reye's syndrome
    8. Cyanotic congenital heart disease
    9. Hypopituitarism
    10. Isolated growth hormone deficiency
    11. Isolated ACTH deficiency
    12. Addison's disease
    13. Galactosemia
    14. Hereditary fructose intolerance
    15. Carnitine deficiency
    16. Defective type 1 glucose transporter in the brain
    17. Acquired severe liver disease
    18. Large non–β-cell tumor
    19. Sepsis
    20. Renal failure
    21. Congestive heart failure
    22. Lactic acidosis
    23. Starvation
    24. Anorexia nervosa
    25. Postoperative removal of pheochromocytoma
    26. Insulin receptor antibody hypoglycemia
  C. Hospitalized patient
    1. Diseases predisposing to hypoglycemia
    2. Total parenteral nutrition and insulin therapy
    3. Cholestyramine resin (Questran) interference with glucocorticoid absorption
    4. Shock

*Mutations in the β-cell sulfonylurea receptor gene, glutamate, dehydrogenase gene, and glucokinase gene are rare causes of hyperinsulinemic hypoglycemia usually manifested in infancy or childhood.

Table 15–33 ■ DIAGNOSTIC INTERPRETATION OF THE RESULTS OF A 72-HOUR FAST*

	SIGNS AND SYMPTOMS	GLUCOSE† (mg/dL)	INSULIN‡ (μU/mL)	C-PEPTIDE§¶ (nmol/L)	PROINSULIN§‖ (pmol/L)	β-HYDROXYBUTRYATE (mmol/L)	CHANGE IN GLUCOSE** (mg/dL)	SULFONYLUREA IN PLASMA
Normal	No	≥40	<6	<0.2	<5	>2.7	<25	No
Insulinoma	Yes	≤45	≥6††	≥0.2	≥5	≤2.7	≤25	No
Factitious hypoglycemia from insulin	Yes	≤45	≥6‡‡	<0.2	<5	≤2.7	≥25	No
Sulfonylurea-induced hypoglycemia	Yes	≤45	≥6	≥0.2	≥5	≤2.7	≥25	Yes§§
Hypoglycemia mediated by insulin-like growth factor	Yes	≤45	≤6	<0.2	<5	≤2.7	≥25	No
Non–insulin-mediated hypoglycemia	Yes	≤45	<6	<0.2	<5	>2.7	<25	No
Inadvertent feeding during the fast	No	≤45	<6	<0.2	<5	≤2.7	≥25	No
Non-hypoglycemic disorder	Yes	≥40	<6	<0.2	<5	>2.7	<25	No

*Measurements are made at the point the decision is made to end the fast.

†Sequential plasma glucose measurements in the hypoglycemic range fluctuate. Plasma glucose levels ≤45 mg/dL at the time a decision is made to end the fast may rise to as much as 56 mg/dL when the fast is actually ended approximately 1 hour later. Plasma glucose levels may be as low at 40 mg/dL during prolonged fasting in normal women.

‡Measured by double-antibody radioimmunoassay (lower limit of detection, 5 μU/mL) using ICMA criterion is ≥3 μU/mL.

§In normal subjects plasma insulin, C-peptide, and proinsulin levels may be higher if the plasma glucose level is >60 mg/dL.

¶Measured by the immunochemiluminometric technique (lower limit of detection, 0.033 nmol/L).

‖Measured by the immunochemiluminometric technique (lower limit of detection, 0.2 pmol/L).

**In response to intravenous glucagon (peak value minus value at end of fast).

††Ratios of insulin to glucose are of no diagnostic value in patients with insulinomas.

‡‡Plasma insulin levels may be very high (>100 μU/mL or even ≥1000 μU/mL) in factitious hypoglycemia produced by insulin.

§§Unlike the first generation of sulfonylurea drugs, which were easily measured, second-generation drugs are difficult to measure.

Reprinted with permission from Service FJ: Hypoglycemia disorder. N Engl J Med 332:1144, 1995.

Table 15–34 ■ CHARACTERISTICS OF FUNCTIONING ISLET CELL CARCINOMAS

SYNDROME	CLINICAL PRESENTATION	BIOCHEMICAL DIAGNOSIS	RATE OF MALIGNANCY (%)	METASTASES AT DIAGNOSIS (%)	LOCALIZATION (RADIOGRAPHIC)	ECTOPIC SITES (NON-PANCREATIC)
Insulinoma	Neuroglycopenia Adrenergic response	Blood glucose ≤45 mg/dL Insulin >6 μU/mL Absence of insulin antibodies Nl/elevated C-peptide	<10	<10	US, spiral CT, selective calcium stimulation test	Rare
Zollinger-Ellison syndrome	Dyspepsia/ulcer Diarrhea	Elevated basal gastrin Elevated basal acid output Positive secretin test	50–60	50–80	US, CT, angio, PVS	Duodenum Rarely other
WDHA (VIPoma)	Profuse, secretory diarrhea Hypokalemia Hypo(a)chlorhydria, hypercalcemia, hyperglycemia	Elevated VIP	50	50	CT, occasionally angio, PVS	Retroperitoneum Lung
Glucagonoma	Dermatitis Diabetes Weight loss Anemia	Elevated glucagon	75	60–70	CT	Rare
Somatostatinoma	Diabetes Cholelithiasis Diarrhea Steatorrhea	Elevated somatostatin	90–100	50–75	CT	Duodenum

WDHA = watery diarrhea, hypokalemia, achlorhydria; VIP = vasoactive intestinal peptide; US = ultrasonography; angio = angiography; PVS = portal venous sampling; CT = computed tomography.

Modified from Grant CS: Surgical management of malignant islet cell tumors. World J Surg 17:498–503, 1993.

Table 15–35 ■ CLINICAL FEATURES OF AUTOIMMUNE POLYGLANDULAR SYNDROMES

	TYPE 1	TYPE 2
Mucocutaneous candidiasis	Very common	Not seen
Hypoparathyroidism	Common	Rare
Addison's disease	Common	Common
Primary hypogonadism	Common	Occurs
Autoimmune thyroid disease	Rare	Common
Autoimmune diabetes	Occurs	Common
Hypophysitis	Occurs	Occurs
Autoimmune hepatitis	Occurs	Not seen
Pernicious anemia	Occurs	Occurs
Vitiligo	Occurs	Occurs
Malabsorption syndrome	Occurs	Occurs in celiac disease
Alopecia	Common	Occurs
Myasthenia gravis	Not seen	Occurs
Keratopathy	Common	Not seen
Tympanic membrane calcification	Common	Not seen
Inheritance	Autosomal recessive	HLA association
Age at onset	Usually childhood	Usually adulthood

The Endocrine Function of Carcinoid Tumors

SEROTONIN. The most constant biochemical feature of carcinoid tumors is the presence of tryptophan hydroxylase, which catalyzes the formation of 5-hydroxytryptophan (5-HTP) from tryptophan.

Diagnosis

The diagnostic hallmark of carcinoid syndrome is overproduction of 5-hydroxyindoles accompanied by increased excretion of urinary 5-hydroxyindoleacetic acid (5-HIAA). Normally, excretion of 5-HIAA does not exceed 9 mg/day. Ingestion of foods containing serotonin may complicate the biochemical diagnosis of carcinoid syndrome; both bananas and walnuts contain enough serotonin to produce abnormally elevated urinary excretion of 5-HIAA after their ingestion. When dietary 5-hydroxyindoles are excluded, urinary excretion of 25 mg of 5-HIAA daily is diagnostic of carcinoid.

Treatment

Treatment of the carcinoid syndrome is directed toward (1) pharmacologic therapy for humorally mediated symptoms and (2) the reduction of tumor mass.

The discovery that somatostatin can prevent the flushing and other endocrine manifestations of the carcinoid syndrome has provided the basis for a major advance in the treatment of these patients. One of the somatostatin analogues, octreotide, has been found to markedly improve the flushing and other endocrine manifestations of most patients with carcinoid syndrome. Octreotide is administered at intervals of approximately 8 hours, usually beginning with 75 to 150 μg and titrating upward until maximum inhibition of flushing and other symptoms is achieved, which usually occurs at single doses of 750 μg or less.

A concerted strategy consisting of removal of the primary tumor, reduction in tumor bulk, and the administration of octreotide (with or without interferon alfa) can lead to considerable amelioration of symptoms and improvement in quality of life, and also is intended to reduce the release of the humoral substances that engender the cardiac lesions.

For more information about this subject, see *Cecil Textbook of Medicine,* 21st edition. Philadelphia, W.B. Saunders Company, 2000. Chapter 245, Multiple Organ Syndromes: Carcinoid Syndrome, pages 1295 to 1297.

THE TESTIS AND MALE SEXUAL FUNCTION

A wide variety of causes may be found for testicular failure or male infertility (Table 15–36). The approach to the diagnosis of an infertile couple includes management of both the male and female partners (Fig. 15–10).

Table 15–36 ■ CAUSES OF PRIMARY TESTICULAR FAILURE AND END-ORGAN RESISTANCE

Congenital disorders
- Chromosomal disorders
  - Klinefelter's and related syndromes (e.g., XXY, XXY/XY, XYY, XX males)
- Testosterone biosynthetic enzyme defects
- Myotonia dystrophy
- Developmental disorders
  - Prenatal diethylstilbestrol syndrome
  - Cryptorchidism

Acquired defects
- Orchitis
  - Mumps and other viruses
  - Granulomatous (e.g., tuberculosis, leprosy)
  - Human immunodeficiency virus
- Infiltrative diseases (i.e., hemochromatosis, amyloidosis)
- Surgical, traumatic injuries, and torsion of testis
- Irradiation
- Toxins (i.e., alcohol, fungicides, insecticides, heavy metals, cottonseed oil, DDT and other environmental estrogens)
- Drugs
  - Cytotoxic agents
  - Inhibition of testosterone synthesis and antiandrogens (e.g., ketoconazole, cimetidine, flutamide, cyproterone, spironolactone)
  - Ethanol and recreational drugs
- Autoimmune testicular failure
  - Isolated
  - Associated with other organ-specific disorders (i.e., Addison's disease, Hashimoto's thyroiditis, insulin-dependent diabetes)
- Systemic diseases (e.g., cirrhosis, chronic renal failure, sickle cell disease, acquired immunodeficiency syndrome, amyloidosis)

Androgen resistance syndromes

5α-Reductase deficiency

15

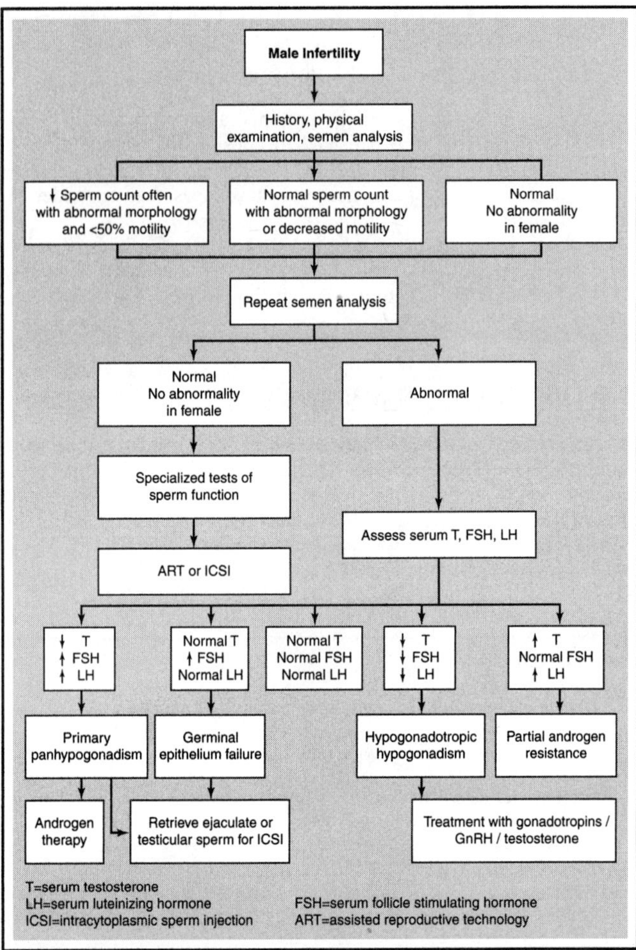

FIGURE 15–10 ■ Algorithmic approach to the diagnosis and treatment of male infertility.

CLINICAL MANAGEMENT OF ERECTILE DYSFUNCTION. ***ORAL MEDICATIONS FOR ERECTILE DYSFUNCTION.*** Trazodone possesses both serotonin and α_2-adrenergic antagonistic properties. It appears to be moderately effective in approximately one third of patients. Oral sildenafil has been approved by the U.S. Food and Drug Administration (FDA) and rapidly has become the most widely used new drug for this disorder. Sildenafil is a competitive and more selective inhibitor of cyclic guanosine monophosphate (GMP) phosphodiesterase-5 (the primary phosphodiesterase in cavernosal tissue).

For more information about this subject, see *Cecil Textbook of Medicine,* 21st edition. Philadelphia, W.B. Saunders Company, 2000. Chapter 247, The Testis and Male Sexual Function, pages 1306 to 1317.

CHAPTER 16

WOMEN'S HEALTH

MENSTRUAL CYCLE AND FERTILITY

Characteristics of the Menstrual Cycle

Between menarche at approximately age 12 years and the menopause at about age 51 years, the reproductive organs of normal women undergo a series of closely coordinated changes at approximately monthly intervals that together constitute the normal menstrual cycle (Fig. 16–1).

Abnormalities of the Reproductive Years

DYSMENORRHEA AND ENDOMETRIOSIS. Dysmenorrhea, perhaps the most common of all gynecologic disorders, affects about 50% of postpubertal women. Dysmenorrhea can be classified as primary or secondary.

Primary dysmenorrhea occurs only in ovulatory cycles.

In *secondary dysmenorrhea* there is a pathologic cause for the dysmenorrhea. Endometriosis is the most common cause in severe cases. Other possible causes include pelvic inflammatory disease, congenital abnormalities such as atresia of a portion of the distal genital tract and cystic duplication of the paramesonephric ducts, and cervical stenosis.

Premenstrual syndrome (PMS) is a complex of physical and/or emotional symptoms that occur repetitively in a cyclic fashion before menstruation and that diminish or disappear with menstruation (Table 16–1).

16

ABNORMAL UTERINE BLEEDING. ***DIFFERENTIAL DIAGNOSIS.*** The causes of abnormal uterine bleeding in the reproductive years include complications from the use of oral contraceptive preparations; complications of pregnancy (especially threatened, incomplete, or missed abortion and ectopic pregnancy); coagulation disorders (most commonly idiopathic thrombocytopenic purpura and von Willebrand's disease); and pelvic disease such as intrauterine polyps, leiomyomas, and tumors of the vagina and cervix. Clear cell adenocarcinoma of the vagina or cervix may occur in women exposed to diethylstilbestrol (DES) during fetal life as a result of maternal ingestion.

Dysfunctional uterine bleeding, abnormal uterine bleeding with no demonstrable organic genital or extragenital cause (75% of cases), is most frequently associated with anovulation. All cases of abnormal bleeding should be evaluated, with special emphasis on the amount and duration of blood loss. Even profuse bleeding in

---

For more information about this subject, see *Cecil Book of Medicine,* 21st edition. Philadelphia, W.B. Saunders Company, 2000. Part XVIII: Women's Health, pages 1318 to 1382.

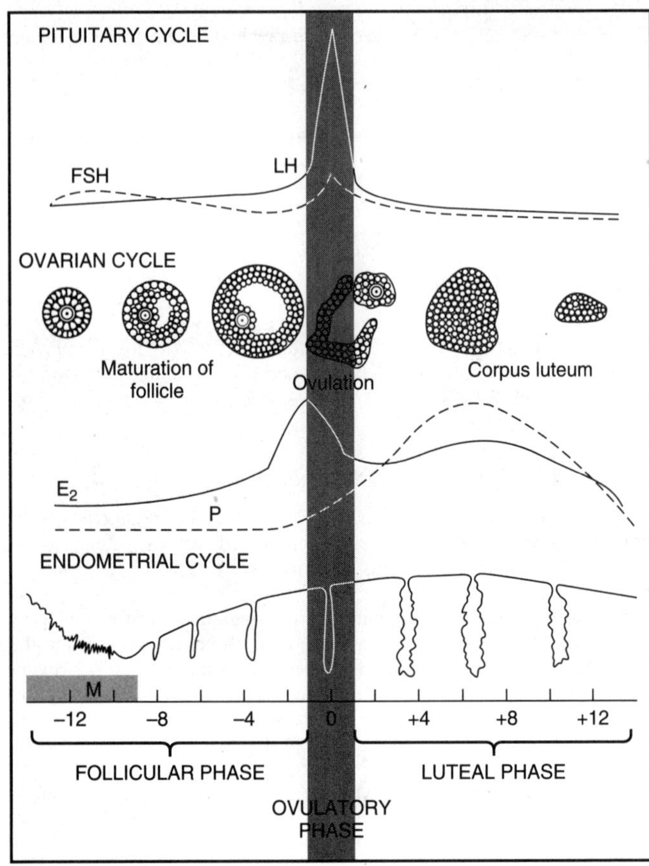

FIGURE 16–1 ■ The idealized cyclic changes observed in gonadotropins, estradiol (E_2), progesterone (P), and uterine endometrium during the normal menstrual cycle. The data are centered on the day of the luteinizing hormone (LH) surge (day 0). Days of menstrual bleeding are indicated by M. FSH = follicle-stimulating hormone. (Reprinted with permission from Endocrine and Metabolism Continuing Education Quality Control Program, 1982. Copyright American Association for Clinical Chemistry, Inc.)

anovulatory women can almost always be successfully treated by administering one combination oral contraceptive pill every 6 hours for 5 to 7 days. Bleeding should cease within 24 hours, but patients should be warned to expect heavy bleeding 2 to 4 days after stopping therapy.

AMENORRHEA. Amenorrhea is the absence of menstruation for 3 or more months in women with past menses (*secondary amenorrhea*) or the absence of menarche by the age of 16 years regardless of the absence or presence of secondary sex characteristics (*primary amenorrhea*) (Table 16–2).

Chronic anovulation, the most frequent form of amenorrhea en-

Table 16–1 ■ COMMON SYMPTOMS OF CYCLIC PREMENSTRUAL SYNDROME

Somatic Symptoms	
Abdominal bloating	Constipation or diarrhea
Acne	Headache
Alcohol intolerance	Peripheral edema
Breast engorgement and tenderness	Weight gain
Clumsiness	
Emotional and Mental Symptoms	
Anxiety	Insomnia
Change in libido	Irritability
Depression	Lethargy
Fatigue	Mood swings
Food cravings (especially salt and sugar)	Panic attacks
	Paranoia
Hostility	Violence toward self and others
Inability to concentrate	Withdrawal from others
Increased appetite	

countered in women of reproductive age, implies that functional ovarian follicles remain and that cyclic ovulation can be induced or reinitiated with appropriate therapy (Table 16–3).

For more information about this subject, see *Cecil Textbook of Medicine,* 21st edition. Philadelphia, W.B. Saunders Company, 2000. Chapter 250, Menstrual Cycle and Fertility, pages 1327 to 1340.

PREGNANCY: HYPERTENSION AND OTHER COMMON MEDICAL PROBLEMS

Hypertension

16

Hypertension is the most common medical problem during pregnancy, with a prevalence of 7 to 12%. Hypertension during pregnancy can be classified as (1) preeclampsia, (2) transient gestational

Table 16–2 ■ CAUSES OF AMENORRHEA

Disorders of Sexual Differentiation
Distal genital tract obstruction (müllerian agenesis and dysgenesis)
Gonadal dysgenesis
Ambiguity of external genitalia (male and female pseudohermaphroditism)
Other Peripheral Causes
Pregnancy
Gestational trophoblastic disease
Amenorrhea traumatica (Asherman's syndrome)
Chronic Anovulation or Ovarian Failure
Due to CNS-hypothalamic-pituitary dysfunction
Due to inappropriate feedback (e.g., polycystic ovary syndrome)
Due to thyroid and adrenal disorders
Presumptive ovarian failure (i.e., primary hypogonadism)

Table 16–3 ■ CAUSES OF CHRONIC ANOVULATION

- I. Chronic anovulation of hypothalamic-pituitary origin
  - A. Hypothalamic chronic anovulation
    1. Psychogenic
    2. Exercise-associated
    3. Associated with diet, weight loss, and/or malnutrition
    4. Anorexia nervosa and bulimia
    5. Pseudocyesis
  - B. Forms of isolated gonadotropin deficiency (including Kallmann's syndrome)
  - C. Due to hypothalamic-pituitary damage
    1. Pituitary and parapituitary tumors
    2. Empty-sella syndrome
    3. Following surgery
    4. Following irradiation
    5. Following trauma
    6. Following infection
    7. Following infarction
  - D. Idiopathic hypopituitarism
  - E. Hypothalamic-pituitary dysfunction or failure with hyperprolactinemia (multiple causes)
  - F. Due to systemic diseases
- II. Chronic anovulation due to inappropriate feedback (i.e., polycystic ovary syndrome)
  - A. Excessive extraglandular estrogen production (i.e., obesity)
  - B. Abnormal buffering involving sex hormone–binding globulin (including liver disease)
  - C. Functional androgen excess (adrenal or ovarian)
  - D. Neoplasms producing androgens or estrogens
  - E. Neoplasms producing chorionic gonadotropin
- III. Chronic anovulation due to other endocrine and metabolic disorders
  - A. Adrenal hyperfunction
    1. Cushing's syndrome
    2. Congenital adrenal hyperplasia (female pseudohermaphroditism)
  - B. Thyroid dysfunction
    1. Hyperthyroidism
    2. Hypothyroidism
  - C. Prolactin and/or growth hormone excess
    1. Hypothalamic dysfunction
    2. Pituitary dysfunction (microadenomas and macroadenomas)
    3. Drug-induced
  - D. Malnutrition

Modified from Rebar RW: Chronic anovulation: *In* Serra GB (ed.): The Ovary. New York, Raven Press, 1983, p 217.

or pregnancy-induced hypertension, (3) chronic hypertension, and (4) chronic hypertension plus preeclampsia. *Pregnancy associated hypertension* is a more genetic term and includes preeclampsia and transient gestational hypertension. During a normal pregnancy, blood pressure declines during the first and second trimesters, rising to pre-pregnancy levels near term. Because of the initial blood pressure decrement, when readings before pregnancy are not known, an elevation during the third trimester could represent either pre-existing or pregnancy-associated hypertension.

Preeclampsia usually develops during the third trimester, often after 32 weeks. Its incidence varies in different groups of women, with a prevalence of 6 to 10% in Western countries. In addition to hypertension, criteria for preeclampsia are rapid weight gain (>2 kg/week), generalized edema, and proteinuria (>0.3 g/24 hours or >1+ on a random specimen). Among women with eclampsia (preeclampsia plus seizures), 20% did not have proteinuria and 40% did not have edema. Hypertension without other manifestations of preeclampsia is termed *transient gestational* or *pregnancy-induced hypertension.* Hypertension in pregnancy may be managed with medication (Table 16–4).

Cardiac Disease

The prevalence of heart disease during pregnancy is approximately 1%. In Western countries, congenital lesions have surpassed rheumatic heart disease as its most common etiology. Pregnancy is proarrhythmic, and both atrial and ventricular ectopy increase. Certain cardiac abnormalities pose unique considerations. For women with Marfan syndrome, pregnancy's connective tissue changes and hyperdynamic state can increase the risk for aortic dissection. *Peripartum cardiomyopathy* is defined as onset of a global dilated cardiomyopathy during the third trimester to 6 months post partum. Its prevalence is 1 in 4000 pregnancies.

Thromboembolic Disease

Thromboembolism (deep venous thrombosis and pulmonary emboli) is uncommon during pregnancy, with a prevalence of 1 per 2000 pregnancies.

Asthma

Asthma is the most common chronic respiratory illness during pregnancy, with a prevalence of 1 to 7%. Management is similar to that in non-pregnant patients (Table 16–5).

Thyroid Disorders

Pregnancy alters certain indices of maternal thyroid function. Thyroxine-binding globulin increases during pregnancy, leading to an elevation of total thyroxine and a decreased triiodothyronine resin uptake. However, free thyroxine and the calculated thyroid index accurately reflect thyroid function during pregnancy. Thyroid-stimulating hormone levels are altered only slightly and remain a useful means of screening for hypothyroidism.

Diabetes Mellitus

Diabetes is present during 3% of all pregnancies. More than 90% of pregnant women with diabetes have *gestational diabetes mellitus* (GDM), defined as glucose intolerance detected during pregnancy. Risk factors for GDM include obesity, age older than 35 years, family history of type 2 diabetes, and prior delivery of a large (>9 lb) infant.

Hepatic Disease

Most liver function tests are unchanged by pregnancy. Jaundice occurs in approximately 1 in 2000 pregnancies. The pregnancy-

Table 16–4 ■ ANTIHYPERTENSIVE DRUG USE DURING PREGNANCY*

MEDICATION	SAFETY OF USE DURING PREGNANCY	COMMENTS
Methyldopa (central sympatholytic)	++++	Extensive use; best-studied antihypertensive used during pregnancy. It reduces vascular resistance while preserving maternal cardiac output and uteroplacental perfusion.
α- and β-Blockers (labetalol)	++++	Agents block both α- and β-receptors. α-Blocking results in vasodilation (including uteroplacental blood vessels), and β-blockade prevents reflex tachycardia. Cardiac output is unchanged.
β-Blockers (atenolol, pindolol, metoprolol, oxprenolol)	+++	Probably safe for third-trimester use, but neonatal bradycardia, respiratory distress, and hypoglycemia have been reported. Use earlier in gestation may result in intrauterine growth retardation.
Hydralazine (direct arterial vasodilator)	++++	Extensively used during pregnancy. It causes vascular dilatation and a reflex tachycardia. Primarily used parenterally for acute management of hypertension or with methyldopa or a β-blocker for treatment of pregnancy-associated hypertension.
Calcium channel blockers (nifedipine most commonly used, owing to its having primarily peripheral effects)	+++	Probably safely used in the third trimester. Their use maintains uteroplacental perfusion; may also have tocolytic effects. Avoid use with magnesium sulfate, because combination risks profound hypotension.
Diuretics	±	Use during pregnancy is controversial. Often discontinued as blood pressure decreases, early in pregnancy. If used before pregnancy, it can be continued, but its use should not be initiated during pregnancy.
Clonidine	++	Although it has been used safely, it is not a first-line antihypertensive agent during pregnancy. It has the potential for rebound when discontinued abruptly.
Angiotensin-converting enzyme inhibitors and angiotensin II receptor antagonists	0	Use is contraindicated during pregnancy, because miscarriage, fetal death, malformations, and neonatal renal failure can result. No reports of adverse effects from brief use, limited to the first trimester.

*Drugs listed have established effects during pregnancy. Antihypertensive agents not listed may be safe during pregnancy; however, until that is known, those drugs should be switched to one of the safely used listed agents.

Table 16–5 ■ DRUG TREATMENT OF ASTHMA DURING PREGNANCY

THERAPY	COMMENTS
Desensitization or immunotherapy ("allergy shots")	Do not begin desensitization during pregnancy, but ongoing therapy can be continued
Disodium cromoglycolate	Less than 10% of drug is absorbed; no reported adverse effects from use during pregnancy
Aminophylline	Distribution and clearance altered during pregnancy, and levels should be checked monthly; it crosses the placenta, and, rarely, neonatal toxicity has been reported, despite therapeutic maternal levels
β-Agonists	Use is safe during pregnancy; rare report of tocolytic effects
Inhaled corticosteroids	Regular use reduces asthma exacerbations during pregnancy
Oral corticosteroids	May be used safely, when indicated; 90% of prednisone is inactivated by the placenta, reducing fetal exposure; betamethasone does not undergo placental 11-oxidation and is the preferred corticosteroid when promoting fetal lung maturation
Anticholinergics	Experience is limited, but use is believed to be safe

associated causes of jaundice are intrahepatic cholestasis of pregnancy, preeclampsia, and the HELLP syndrome (*h*emolysis, *e*levated *l*iver enzymes, and *l*ow *p*latelet count), acute fatty liver of pregnancy, and hepatic rupture. Each typically presents in the third trimester. During the first trimester, hyperemesis gravidarum also may cause jaundice. However, its clinical manifestations usually suggest this diagnosis and abnormalities resolve within days of improved nutrition.

16

Human Immunodeficiency Virus

Pregnant women are at risk of transmitting HIV to their newborns, with approximately 25% of exposed infants becoming infected unless intervention occurs. A treatment recommendation put forth by the Pediatric AIDS Clinical Trials Group is noted in Figure 16–2.

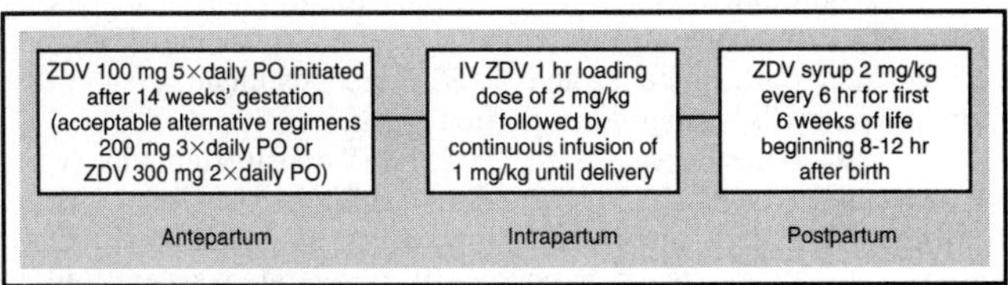

FIGURE 16–2 ■ PACTG 076 zidovudine (ZDV) regimen for prevention of mother-to-infant transmission of HIV.

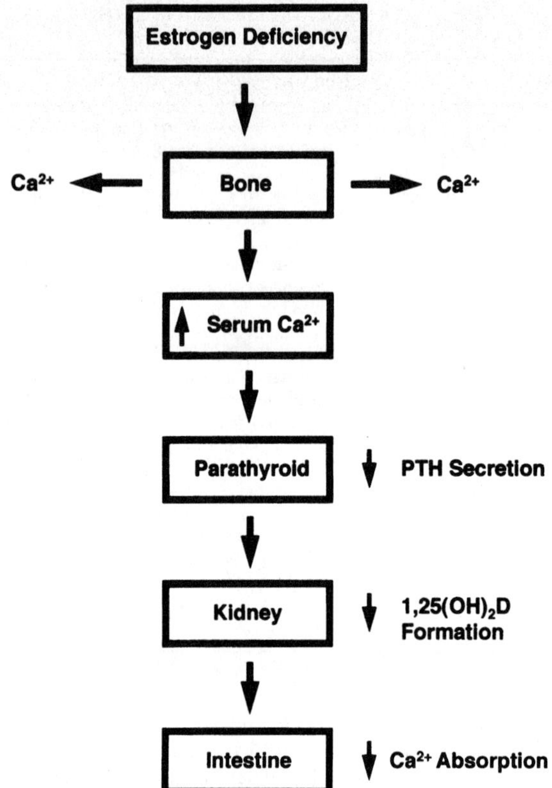

FIGURE 16–3 ■ Physiologic alterations in women with type I ("postmenopausal") osteoporosis. PTH = parathyroid hormone.

For more information about this subject, see *Cecil Textbook of Medicine,* 21st edition. Philadelphia, W.B. Saunders Company, 2000. Chapter 253, Pregnancy: Hypertension and Other Common Medical Problems; and Chapter 254, HIV in Pregnancy, pages 1351 to 1358.

OSTEOPOROSIS

Osteoporosis affects 20 million Americans and leads to approximately 1.3 million fractures in the United States each year. During their lifetime, women lose about 50% of their trabecular bone and 30% of their cortical bone, and 30% of all postmenopausal white women eventually sustain osteoporotic fractures.

After peak bone density is reached, bone density remains stable for years and then declines. Bone loss begins before menses cease in women, although the precise time of onset is unknown. Once menses cease, the rate of bone loss is accelerated severalfold in women. A subset of women in whom osteoporosis is more severe than expected for their age are said to have type I or "postmeno-

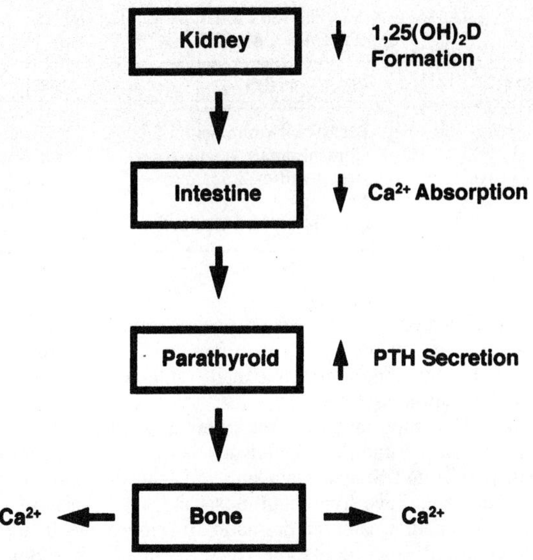

FIGURE 16–4 ■ Physiologic alterations in women with type II ("senile") osteoporosis.

pausal" osteoporosis. Clinically, type I osteoporosis often presents as vertebral "crush" fractures or Colles' fractures.

The osteopenia that results from normal aging, which occurs in both women and men, has been termed *type II* or *"senile" osteoporosis* (Figures 16–3 and 16–4).

Treatment

16

At present, it is not possible to reverse established osteoporosis. Most postmenopaual women consume less than 500 mg of calcium each day, far below the U.S. recommended dietary allowance (RDA) of 1000 to 1500 mg. Overall, it appears that calcium therapy is somewhat beneficial in both early and late postmenopausal women.

Estrogen replacement therapy inhibits osteoclastic bone resorption. It prevents both cortical and trabecular bone loss in estrogen-deficient women and is effective if administered orally or topically. Although the beneficial effects of estrogen replacement therapy on bone mass are well established, fewer than 15% of postmenopausal women in the United States take estrogen replacement. The decision to treat with estrogen is influenced by other factors and should be individualized. Tamoxifen, a mixed estrogen receptor antagonist and agonist, prevents bone loss from the spine and proximal femur in women with breast cancer and lowers serum low-density lipoprotein cholesterol levels.

Several bisphosphonates have been reported to increase bone mineral density in postmenopausal women, although alendronate is the only bisphosphonate that has been approved by the Food and Drug Administration (FDA) for prevention of bone loss or treat-

Table 16–6 ■ SCREENING RECOMMENDATIONS (AMERICAN CANCER SOCIETY)

AGE GROUP	EXAMINATION	FREQUENCY
20–39 yr	Breast self-examination	Every month
	Clinical breast examination	Every 3 yr
40 yr and over	Breast self-examination	Every month
	Mammography	Every year
	Clinical breast examination	Every year

ment of established osteoporosis in postmenopausal women. Calcitonin is approved by the FDA for treatment of late postmenopausal women with low bone mineral density and is available for both parenteral and intranasal use.

Vitamin D is important for absorption of calcium from the gastrointestinal tract. Vitamin D deficiency is common yet rarely diagnosed in the United States. Data indicate that over half of general medical inpatients have hypovitaminosis D. Small doses of vitamin D (800 IU/day) plus calcium dramatically reduce the incidence of hip fractures and other non-spine fractures in elderly women with hypovitaminosis D.

For more information about this subject, see *Cecil Textbook of Medicine,* 21st edition. Philadelphia, W.B. Saunders Company, 2000. Chapter 257, Osteoporosis, pages 1366 to 1373.

BREAST CANCER AND DIFFERENTIAL DIAGNOSIS OF BENIGN NODULES

Breast cancer is the most common cancer affecting American women. In the United States in 1998, 180,000 new cases of breast cancer were diagnosed and 44,000 women died of breast cancer.

Table 16–7 ■ INFORMATION RESOURCES

WEB ADDRESS OR NUMBER	DESCRIPTION
1-800-4-CANCER	Access number for the NCI Cancer Information Service.
http://cancernet.nci.nih.gov	Information service of the NCI. Includes PDQ and summaries on treatment, screening, prevention, supportive care, and ongoing clinical trials. Also access to CANCERLIT, NCI's bibliographic database.
http://www.nabco.org	The National Alliance of Breast Cancer Organizations is the leading non-profit resource for information about breast cancer events and activities and has links to other key sites.
http://www.breastcancernet.net	Excellent general site with many helpful links.

NCI = National Cancer Institute; PDQ = Physician Data Query.

Breast cancer will occur in 12.5% of women (one of every eight women) during their lifetime and accounts for 32% of cases of female cancer. Regular screening is recommended (Table 16–6).

EVALUATING A BREAST MASS. Most breast masses, especially those found in young premenopausal women, are benign. All breast masses require evaluation. In a premenopausal woman, if the mass is small and likely to be a cyst, it can be observed for 2 to 4 weeks until after the next menstrual period. If the mass persists, biopsy is indicated; all masses in postmenopausal women require prompt investigation.

Mammograms and/or ultrasound evaluation may help characterize a mass as well as detect abnormalities in non-involved breast tissues, but all persistent masses require biopsy—even when all imaging studies are normal.

OBTAINING INFORMATION. Never has high-quality medical information been more accessible to the practicing clinician. The Internet has now become a major resource for a wealth of up-to-date information derived from multiple sources (Table 16–7).

For more information about this subject, see *Cecil Textbook of Medicine,* 21st edition. Philadelphia, W.B. Saunders Company, 2000. Chapter 258, Breast Cancer and Differential Diagnosis of Benign Nodules, pages 1373 to 1380.

CHAPTER 17

DISEASES OF BONE AND BONE MINERAL METABOLISM

MINERAL AND BONE HOMEOSTASIS

Total calcium concentration in blood is tightly regulated so that typical diurnal fluctuations are not more than 5% from the mean value. Calcium in blood is divided among protein-bound, complexed, and ionized fractions (Fig. 17–1). Protein binding of calcium in blood is principally to albumin, and this binding is decreased by acid pH. The ionized calcium fraction is the focus for metabolic control by the parathyroid gland, and measurements of ionized calcium in blood give the most valid index of pathologic disruptions of calcium homeostasis. Phosphate and magnesium in blood are principally unbound.

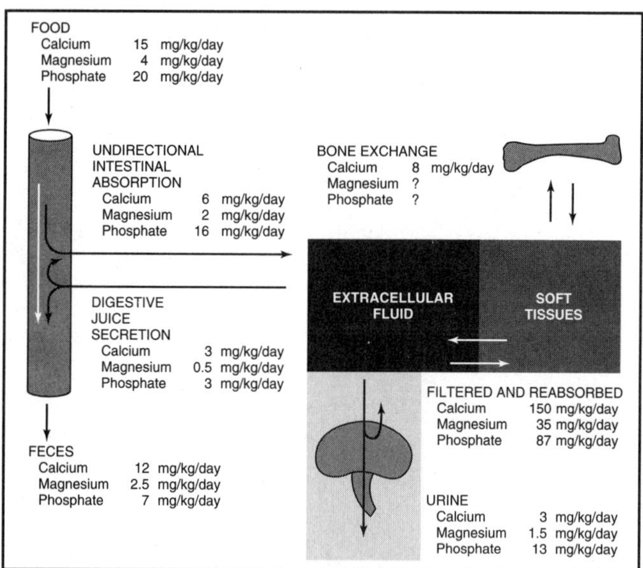

FIGURE 17–1 ■ Typical mineral fluxes in adults. (Modified from Aurbach GD, Marx SJ, Spiegel AM: Pazathyroid hormone, calcitonin, and the calciferols. *In* Wilson JD, Foster DW [eds]: Williams Textbook of Endocrinology, 7th ed. Philadelphia, WB Saunders, 1985, p 1144.)

For more information about this subject, see *Cecil Textbook of Medicine,* 21st edition. Philadelphia, W.B. Saunders Company, 2000. Part XIX: Diseases of Bone and Bone Mineral Metabolism, pages 1383 to 1422.

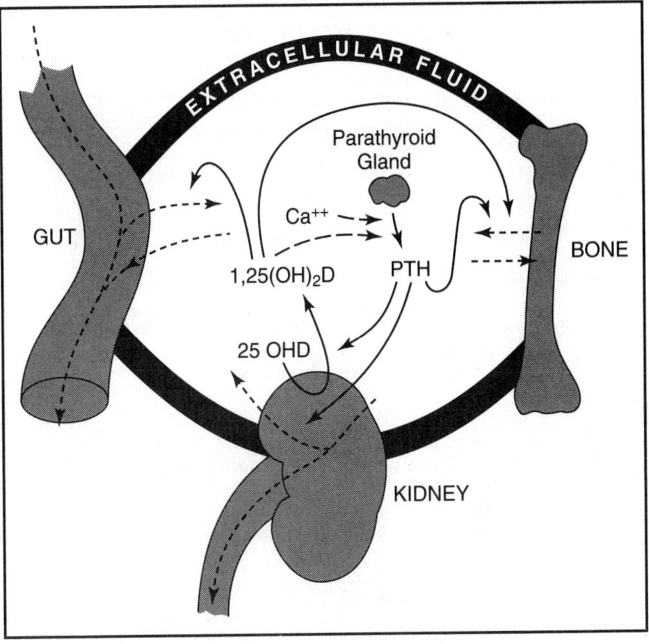

FIGURE 17–2 ■ Integrated control of secretion and actions of parathyroid hormone (PTH) and calcitriol (1α,25[OH]$_2$ vitamin D = 1α,25[OH]$_2$D) with emphasis on calcium fluxes. Solid lines show secretion and targets of PTH and calcitriol..

ADAPTATIONS TO DISRUPTIONS OF MINERAL METABOLISM. Two principal calciotropic hormones, parathyroid hormone (PTH) and 1α,25-dihydroxyvitamin D [1α,25(OH)$_2$D], interact with each other and with multiple target tissues to control the metabolism of calcium, phosphate, and, to a lesser degree, magnesium (Fig. 17–2). 17

OSTEOMALACIA AND RICKETS

Rickets and osteomalacia are diseases characterized by defective bone and cartilage mineralization in children and defective bone mineralization in adults. Clinical manifestations and syndromes in which rickets and osteomalacia are featured are noted in Table 17–1.

Rickets and osteomalacia caused by disorders of the vitamin D endocrine system comprise a wide variety of calciopenic diseases. The variable biochemical abnormalities associated with these disparate disorders are summarized in Table 17–2.

For more information about this see *Cecil Textbook of Medicine,* 21st edition. Philadelphia, W.B. Saunders Company, 2000. Chapter 263, Osteomalacia and Rickets, pages 1391 to 1398.

Table 17–1 ■ THE RICKETS AND OSTEOMALACIA SYNDROMES

I. Disorders of the vitamin D endocrine system
  A. Decreased bioavailability of vitamin D
    1. Deficient endogenous production
    2. Nutritional deficiency
    3. Loss of vitamin D metabolites
  B. Vitamin D malabsorption
    1. Gastrointestinal disorders
    2. Pancreatic insufficiency
    3. Hepatobiliary disease
  C. Abnormal vitamin D metabolism
    1. Impaired hepatic 25-hydroxylation of vitamin D
    2. Impaired renal 1α-hydroxylation of 25-hydroxyvitamin D
  D. Target organ resistance to vitamin D and metabolites
II. Disorders of phosphate homeostasis
  A. Dietary
    1. Low phosphate intake
    2. Ingestion of phosphate-binding antacids
  B. Impaired renal tubular phosphate reabsorption
    1. Hereditary
    2. Acquired
      a. Tumor-induced osteomalacia (oncogenous osteomalacia)
      b. Sporadic hypophosphatemic osteomalacia
  C. General renal tubular disorders
    1. Fanconi's syndrome type I
    2. Fanconi's syndrome type 2
III. Metabolic acidosis
  A. Distal renal tubular acidosis
IV. Disorders of calcium homeostasis: Dietary calcium deficiency
V. Abnormal bone matrix
VI. Primary mineralization defects
VII. Mineralization inhibitors
  A. Etidronate
  B. Fluoride
  C. Aluminum

THE PARATHYROID GLANDS, HYPERCALCEMIA, AND HYPOCALCEMIA

Normally, there are four parathyroids, averaging 120 mg in total weight, but as many as 5% of normal persons may have more than four glands.

Assay of Parathyroid Hormone in Plasma

Normally, the concentration of biologically active PTH circulating in plasma is quite low (<50 pg/mL). Total urinary cyclic adenosine monophosphate (cAMP) excretion (normalized to creatinine clearance by simultaneously measuring serum and urinary creatinine) is an easily measured and sensitive index of circulating PTH bioactivity.

Hypercalcemia (Table 17–3 and 17–4)

Malignancies can cause hypercalcemia through two non-mutually exclusive mechanisms. First, local osteolytic hypercalcemia is

Table 17–2 ■ BIOCHEMICAL ABNORMALITIES OF THE CALCIOPENIC RACHITIC AND OSTEOMALACIC DISORDERS

	VDDR	CRF	HVDDR 1	HVDDR 2	HP	PSH
Biochemical Findings						
Calcium	⇓	⇓	⇓	⇓	⇓	⇓
Phosphorus	N/⇓	⇑	N/⇓	N/⇓	⇑	⇑
Alkaline phosphatase	⇑	⇑	⇑	⇑	N/⇑	N/⇑
Parathyroid hormone	⇑	⇑	⇑	⇑	⇓	⇑
2(OH)D	⇓	N/⇓	N	N	N	N
$1\alpha,25(OH)_2D$	⇑	⇓	⇓	⇑	⇓	⇓
Renal Function						
Urinary phosphorus	⇑	⇓	⇑	⇑	⇓	⇓
Urinary calcium	⇓	⇓	⇓	⇓	⇓	⇓
Gastrointestinal Function						
Calcium absorption	⇓	⇓	⇓	⇓	⇓	⇓
Phosphorus absorption	⇓	⇓	⇓	⇓	⇓	⇓

VDDR = Vitamin D–deficiency rickets (including sunlight or nutritional deficiency, vitamin D malabsorption, inhibition of 25-hydroxylation); CRF = chronic renal failure; HVDDR 1 = hereditary vitamin D–dependent rickets type 1; HVDDR-2 = hereditary vitamin D–dependent rickets type 2; HP = hypoparathyroidism; PSH = pseudohypoparathyroidism; N = normal; ⇓ = decreased; ⇑ = increased; N/⇓ = normal or decreased; and N/⇑ = normal or increased.

Table 17–3 ■ CAUSES OF HYPERCALCEMIA

Parathyroid hormone–mediated causes
- Primary hyperparathyroidism
  - Sporadic, familial (multiple endocrine neoplasia type I and II)
- Familial hypocalciuric hypercalcemia*
- Ectopic secretion of parathyroid hormone by tumors (very rare)

Non-parathyroid hormone–mediated causes
- Malignancy-associated
  - Local osteolytic hypercalcemia
  - Humoral hypercalcemia of malignancy
- Vitamin D–mediated
  - Vitamin D intoxication
  - Excessive production of 1α,25(OH)$_2$D in granulomatous disorders
- Other endocrinopathies
  - Thyrotoxicosis
  - Hypoadrenalism

Immobilization with increased bone turnover, e.g., Paget's disese
Acute renal failure with rhabdomyolysis
Calcium carbonate ingestion (milk-alkali syndrome)
Jansen-type metaphyseal chondrodysplasia (activating mutation of parathyroid hormone receptor)

*Parathyroid hormone secretion in necessary for hypercalcemia but is not the primary defect.

caused by tumor metastatic to bone. Second, humoral hypercalcemia of malignancy is caused by tumor-secreting factors in the circulation that act systemically to increase bone resorption. Hypercalcemia is caused by unregulated formation of 1α,25(OH)$_2$D in granuloma-associated macrophages. Normally, 1-hydroxylation

Table 17–4 ■ DIAGNOSTIC APPROACH TO HYPERCALCEMIA

1. Distinguish parathyroid hormone (PTH)–mediated forms of hypercalcemia from non–PTH-mediated forms: *PTH immunoassay (preferably two-site type) is the definitive test.*
2. If the PTH level is elevated, primary hyperparathyroidism is the most likely diagnosis: *Family history for hypercalcemia should be checked to distinguish sporadic from familial (multiple endocrine neoplasia syndromes and hypocalciuric hypercalcemia) disease. Marginal elevation in PTH levels, particularly in young, asymptomatic individuals, should prompt urine calcium measurement to exclude familial hypocalciuric hypercalcemia. In patients with coexisting malignancy, selective venous sampling can be done to exclude ectopic PTH secretion, but the latter is extremely rare.*
3. If PTH is low or undetectable, further laboratory tests (in addition to complete history, physical, and radiologic studies) are needed to distinguish among the various forms of non–PTH-mediated forms of hypercalcemia: *Increased urinary cAMP excretion suggests tumor secretion of PTH-related peptide (direct radioimmunoassays for this peptide are now available). Increased 1α,25(OH)$_2$D suggests granulomatous disease (including some types of lymphoma).*

cAMP = cyclic adenosine monophosphate.

Table 17–5 ■ CAUSES OF HYPOCALCEMIA

Hypoparathyroidism

Deficient parathyroid hormone secretion
- Idiopathic (autoimmune)
- Parathyroid hormone gene mutation
- Activating calcium-sensing receptor mutation (autosomal dominant hypoparathyroidism)
- Surgical
- Infiltrative (iron overload, Wilson's disease)

Functional
- Hypomagnesemia
- Transient postoperative

Deficient parathyroid hormone action (hormone resistance)
- Pseudohypoparathyroidism types Ia and Ib

Normal or Increased Parathyroid Hormone Function

Renal failure
Intestinal malabsorption
Acute pancreatitis
Osteoblastic metastases
Vitamin D deficiency or resistance

takes place in the kidney and is sensitive to feedback suppression by high serum calcium levels. Unregulated synthesis of $1\alpha,25(OH)_2D$ in patients with granulomatous diseases renders them hypersensitive to vitamin D (from the diet or through sun exposure).

Hypocalcemia

Hypocalcemia is an abnormal reduction in serum ionized calcium concentration (Table 17–5). It is associated with certain typical signs and symptoms, most prominent of which is neuromuscular excitability. Acute asymptomatic hypocalcemia requires emergency treatment in the form of intravenous calcium infusion. Definitive resolution of the disorder requires treating the underlying disease.

For more information about this subject, see *Cecil Textbook of Medicine,* 21st edition. Philadelphia, W.B. Saunders Company, 2000. Chapter 264, The Parathyroid Glands, Hypercalcemia, and Hypocalcemia, pages 1398 to 1406.

CALCITONIN AND MEDULLARY THYROID CARCINOMA

The main biologic effect of calcitonin (CT) is to decrease bone resorption by inhibiting the osteoclast. This effect decreases the concentration of blood calcium, with a nadir directly related to bone turnover. This property of CT makes it an effective drug for hyperresorptive diseases, such as Paget's disease, osteoporosis, and hypercalcemia. In addition to its role in skeletal physiology and treatment, CT is a serum and tumor marker for medullary thyroid carcinoma (MTC), which is the signal tumor of multiple endocrine neoplasia (MEN) type II and its variants (Table 17–6).

For more information about this subject, see *Cecil Textbook of Medicine,* 21st edition. Philadelphia, W.B. Saunders Company,

Table 17–6 ■ COMPONENTS OF MULTIPLE ENDOCRINE NEOPLASIA TYPE II (MEN-II) AND THEIR FREQUENCY BASED ON AVERAGE FIGURES FROM THE LITERATURE

COMPONENT	MEN-IIA (%)	MEN-IIB (%)
Medullary thyroid carcinoma	97	90
Pheochromocytoma	30	45
Hyperparathyroidism	50	Rare
Mucosal neuroma syndrome	—	100

2000. Chapter 265, Calcitonin and Medullary Thyroid Carcinoma, pages 1406 to 1409.

RENAL OSTEODYSTROPHY

Renal osteodystrophy is a metabolic bone disease that develops secondary to chronic failure of the kidneys' excretory and endocrine functions. Renal osteodystrophy encompasses a wide variety of derangements in mineral and bone metabolism.

Incidence and Prevalence

The earliest histologic abnormalities of bone are seen after a relatively mild reduction in the glomerular filtration rate (creatinine clearances between 70 and 40 mL/minute). Histologic changes are found in virtually all patients with end-stage renal disease (ESRD). The incidence of ESRD in the United States is 56,600 patients per year (215 per million per year) and the prevalence is 218,000 patients (825 per million).

Pathogenesis

In advanced renal failure a variety of factors have been identified as direct stimulators of PTH secretion, including hypocalcemia, low levels of circulating calcitriol (the active vitamin D metabolite), and more recently, hyperphosphatemia. However, most patients with mild chronic renal failure exhibit increased serum PTH levels without alterations in serum levels of calcium, phosphorus, and calcitriol.

When the glomerular filtration rate reaches levels of less than 25% of normal, the serum phosphorus content rises. At this level of reduced renal function, the ability of the remaining nephrons to increase phosphate excretion is exhausted. This results in increased production of PTH and increased parathyroid gland mass.

Patients with ESRD are in a hypogonadal state, and some of them are treated with glucocorticoids, which have an impact on bone metabolism. Patients maintained on chronic dialysis have retention of β_2-microglobulin and alterations in cytokines, growth factors, PTH, and vitamin D receptors that may be involved in the regulation of bone remodeling, thus affecting the histologic pattern of renal osteodystrophy.

Diagnosis

The only unequivocal tool for the exact diagnosis of renal osteodystrophy is bone biopsy for mineralized bone histology after tetracycline double-labeling and aluminum staining. In the absence of bone biopsy, the physician needs to estimate the level of bone turnover, the presence of osteomalacia, and the possibility of bone aluminum toxicity. Abnormalities in serum calcium, phosphorus, and alkaline phosphatase levels indicate severe renal osteodystrophy, but are useless when used alone to indicate bone turnover or osteomalacia. Hypercalcemia may be observed in severe hyperparathyroidism or adynamic bone disease, especially with vitamin D therapy. Hyperphosphatemia is an indication of non-compliance with phosphate binders and/or severe hyperparathyroidism secondary to increased release of phosphorus from bone. High serum levels of alkaline phosphatase are usually seen in both osteomalacia and predominant hyperparathyroidism.

Therapy

Therapeutic intervention should begin before far-advanced bone disease develops, that is, not later than at the time of institution of dialysis. Secondary hyperparathyroidism can be prevented by avoiding deviations of serum phosphorus and calcium levels from normal.

Any therapeutic maneuver that lowers plasma aluminum levels and creates a concentration gradient across the bone–extracelluar fluid membrane will be able to move aluminum from bone to blood.

When adynamic bone disease is not the result of bone aluminum toxicity, measures to avoid oversuppression of PTH and bone turnover are indicated. These measures include discontinuation of vitamin D therapy and reduction in calcium-containing phosphate binders and/or the dialysate calcium content. However, no specific treatment is available for adynamic bone disease at present. Thus preventive measures should be carefully considered because of the morbidity and risk of hypercalcemia associated with this condition.

For more information about this subject, see *Cecil Textbook of Medicine,* 21st edition. Philadelphia, W.B. Saunders Company, 2000. Chapter 266, Renal Osteodystrophy, pages 1409 to 1414.

PAGET'S DISEASE OF BONE (OSTEITIS DEFORMANS)

Paget's disease of bone is a focal disorder of skeletal metabolism in which all the elements of skeletal remodeling (resorption, formation, and mineralization) are increased. Increased bone formation results in the disorganized assembly of collagen, which gives rise to bony enlargement and deformity (Table 17–7).

For more information about this subject, see *Cecil Textbook of Medicine,* 21st edition. Philadelphia, W.B. Saunders Company, 2000. Chapter 267, Paget's Disease of Bone (Osteitis Deformans), pages 1414 to 1416.

Table 17–7 ■ CLINICAL FEATURES AND COMPLICATIONS OF PAGET'S DISEASE

Common
Bone pain—pagetic, articular
Fracture—long bones, vertebral bodies
Neurologic—deafness
Deformity and enlargement of bones
Uncommon
Pain—fissure fracture
Spinal neurologic syndromes
Hypercalciuria of immobilization or fracture
Vascular bleeding from bone during surgery
Extraskeletal (aortic) calcification
Osteosarcoma and other bone tumors
Rare
Cardiovascular disease
Cranial nerve lesions (except VIII)
Brain stem and cerebellar lesions
Hypercalcemia of immobilization
Extramedullary hematopoiesis
Epidural hematoma
Significance uncertain
Gout
Pseudogout
Angioid streaks
Hyperparathyroidism
Urolithiasis

From Kanis JA: Pathophysiology and Treatment of Paget's Disease of Bone, 2nd ed. London, Martin Dunitz, 1998.

CHAPTER 18

DISEASES OF THE IMMUNE SYSTEM

PRIMARY IMMUNODEFICIENCY DISEASES

Approaches to the Patient with Suspected Immunodeficiency

The number of patients suspected of having primary immunodeficiency will far exceed the incidence of these diseases.

In assessing B-cell function, determinations of antibody titers to proteins (such as tetanus and diphtheria toxoids) and polysaccharides (such as pneumococcal antigens) after immunization are the most useful tests. However, the presence of such antibodies does not exclude IgA deficiency, which would also be missed on a serum electrophoretic analysis. The quantification of serum IgA is particularly cost-effective. If the IgA concentration is normal, this finding rules out not only IgA deficiency but also all of the permanent types of agammaglobulinemia, because the IgA level is usually very low or absent in those conditions as well.

The most cost-effective test for assessing T-cell function is an intradermal skin test with 0.1 mL of a 1:1000 dilution of a known potent *Candida albicans* extract. If the test result is positive, as defined by erythema and induration of 10 mm or greater at 48 hours, virtually all primary T-cell defects are excluded and the need for more expensive in vitro tests, such as lymphocyte phenotyping or assessments of responses to mitogens, is obviated.

Killing defects of phagocytic cells, which should be suspected if the patient has problems with staphylococcal or gram-negative infections, can be screened for by tests measuring the neutrophil respiratory burst after phagocytosis or phorbol ester stimulation.

Complement defects can be most effectively screened for in a CH_{50} assay (total serum hemolytic complement), which measures the intactness of the entire complement pathway. If results of these tests are abnormal, or even if they are normal and clinical features of the patient still strongly suggest a host defect, the patient should be evaluated at a center where more definitive immunologic studies can be done before any type of immunologic treatment is begun. 18

For more information about this subject, see *Cecil Textbook of Medicine,* 21st edition. Philadelphia, W.B. Saunders Company, 2000. Chapter 272, Primary Immunodeficiency Diseases, pages 1433 to 1440.

For more information about this subject, see *Cecil Textbook of Medicine,* 21st edition. Philadelphia, W.B. Saunders Company, 2000. Part XX: Diseases of the Immune System, pages 1423 to 1471.

Table 18–1 ■ CLASSIFICATION OF URTICARIA AND ANGIOEDEMA

I. Manifestation of hypersensitivity to a defined agent
   A. Drug reactions
   B. Foods and food additives
   C. Inhaled and contact allergens
II. Presumed immune complex–induced
   A. Collagen disease
   B. Endocrine disease (thyroid disorders)
   C. Serum sickness
   D. Transfusion-induced
   E. Malignancy (tumor antigen–induced)
   F. Infectious agents
   G. Urticarial vasculitis
III. Physical urticarias
   A. Dermatographism
   B. Familial and acquired cold urticaria
   C. Localized heat urticaria
   D. Cholinergic urticaria
   E. Exercise-induced anaphylaxis/urticaria
   F. Delayed pressure urticaria/angioedema
   G. Familial and acquired vibratory angioedema
   H. Solar urticaria
   I. Aquagenic urticaria
IV. Urticaria pigmentosa and systemic mastocytosis
V. Chronic urticaria and angioedema
VI. Defined complement-related disorders
   A. Hereditary angioedema
   B. Acquired C1 inhibitor deficiency
   C. Complement factor I deficiency
VII. Angioedema induced by angiotensin-converting enzyme inhibitors and interleukin-2

URTICARIA AND ANGIOEDEMA

Urticaria is defined as the transient appearance of elevated, erythematous pruritic wheals (hives) or serpiginous exanthem, usually surrounded by an area of erythema. It commonly involves the trunk and extremities, sparing palms and soles, but it may involve any epidermal or mucosal surface (Table 18–1).

For more information about this subject, see *Cecil Textbook of Medicine,* 21st edition. Philadelphia, W.B. Saunders Company, 2000. Chapter 273, Urticaria and Angioedema, pages 1440 to 1445.

ANAPHYLAXIS

The anaphylactic reaction is immune in nature and depends on the formation of IgE antibody, the immunoglobulin responsible for typical allergic reactions. The initial sensitization step induces the formation of IgE specifically directed to the initiating substance. In anaphylaxis, the reaction is systemic, occurs rapidly after administration of minute concentrations of the offending material, and is potentially fatal (Table 18–2).

Table 18–2 ■ AGENTS CAUSING ANAPHYLAXIS

TYPE	COMMON	RARE
Proteins	Venom (Hymenoptera)	Hormones, (insulin, ACTH, vasopressin, parathormone)
	Pollen (ragweed, grass, etc.) Food (eggs, seafood, nuts, grains, beans, cottonseed oil, chocolate) Horse and rabbit serum (antilymphocyte globulin) Latex	Enzymes (trypsin, penicillinase) Human proteins (serum proteins, seminal fluid)
Haptens and other low-molecular-weight substances	Antibiotics (penicillins, sulfonamides, cephalosporins, tetracyclines, amphotericin B, nitrofurantoin, aminoglycosides) Local anesthetics (lidocaine, procaine, etc.)	Vitamins (thiamine, folic acid)
Polysaccharides		Dextrans, iron dextran

ACTH = adrenocorticotropic hormone.

Prevention and Treatment

Patients who have previously experienced anaphylactic episodes should wear a MedicAlert bracelet. The physician must be aware of drugs containing cross-reacting antigens. For example, patients with allergy to sulfa-containing antibiotics should avoid other sulfa-containing substances such as chlorthiazide diuretics, furosemide, sulfonylureas, and dapsone.

Fifteen per cent of allergic patients have a reaction if a cephalosporin is substituted for penicillin because they share the presence of a β-lactam ring. Reactions with second- and third-generation cephalosporins may also occur, but aztreonam is an exception.

If an anaphylactic reaction is encountered, epinephrine given early quickly reverses most manifestations. When administered at a 1:1000 dilution (0.01 mL/kg with a maximum dose of 0.5 mL subcutaneously repeated every 20 minutes as necessary), it is initial treatment once an adequate airway is in place. 18

If any respiratory, vascular, or cardiac complications occur, an intravenous line should be placed promptly and a sample of arterial blood obtained for pH, P_{O_2} and P_{CO_2}. Hypovolemic shock requires rapid intravenous fluid administration. Additionally, 5 mL of a 1:10,000 solution of epinephrine repeated every 5 to 10 minutes can be given intravenously to patients in severe shock. A vasopressor such as dopamine 2 to 20 μg/kg/minute is indicated to manage hypotension unresponsive to volume expansion.

Giving antihistamines at the onset of the acute episode may relieve pruritus, urticaria, and angioedema. Once an intravenous line is placed, diphenhydramine 50 to 100 mg can be given slowly as a bolus.

For more information about this subject, see *Cecil Textbook of*

Table 18–3 ■ STING SYMPTOMS REPORTED BY 245 PATIENTS

SYMPTOM	PERCENT
Cutaneous only	14
Urticaria-angioedema	78
Dizziness-hypotension	61
Dyspnea-wheezing	53
Throat tightness–hoarseness	40
Loss of consciousness	33

Medicine, 21st edition. Philadelphia, W.B. Saunders Company, 2000. Chapter 275, Anaphylaxis, pages 1450 to 1452.

INSECT STING ALLERGY

Stings of insects of the order Hymenoptera have long been recognized as a potential cause of severe, often life-threatening reactions in susceptible individuals (Table 18–3).

Treatment

The treatment of choice for anaphylactic reactions is subcutaneous epinephrine, 1:1000, 0.5 mL initially and repeated twice at 10-minute intervals, if necessary, to reverse the progression of symptoms. Antihistamines and glucocorticoids do not contribute to the management of life-threatening symptoms but may reduce the duration and severity of cutaneous manifestations. Affected persons not yet protected by immunotherapy are advised to carry, and are instructed in the use of, a kit containing a syringe device preloaded with one or two recommended doses of epinephrine.

Venom immunotherapy is successful in virtually all patients. Fewer than 2% of those immunized have any systemic symptoms after a challenge sting. Those with a history of life-threatening reactions should be treated.

For more information about this subject, see *Cecil Textbook of Medicine,* 21st edition. Philadelphia, W.B. Saunders Company, 2000. Chapter 276, Insect Sting Allergy, pages 1452 to 1454.

IMMUNE COMPLEX DISEASES

Immune complex diseases are a group of conditions resulting from inflammation induced in tissues where immune complexes are formed or deposited. The clinical consequences may be local when immune complexes form in the tissues of a specific organ, or systemic when complexes circulate and are widely deposited. A variety of antigens have been associated with the induction of immune complex disease in humans (Table 18–4).

For more information about this subject, see *Cecil Textbook of Medicine,* 21st edition. Philadelphia, W.B. Saunders Company, 2000. Chapter 277, Immune Complex Diseases, pages 1454 to 1457.

Table 18–4 ■ REPRESENTATIVE ANTIGENS KNOWN TO CAUSE IMMUNE COMPLEX DISEASE IN HUMANS

ANTIGENS	SYNDROME
Therapeutic Agents	
Horse serum products	Serum sickness
Antilymphocyte globin	
Snake venom antiserum	
Monoclonal antibody products	
Streptokinase	
Drugs	
Cephalosporins, penicillin, amoxicillin, trimethoprim-sulfamethoxazole, fluoxetine, iron dextran, carbamazepine, and others	
Quinidine, chlorpromazine, sulfonamides	Hemolytic anemia (innocent bystander reaction)
Autologous (Self-) Antigens	
DNA	Vasculitis and glomerulonephritis of systemic lupus erythematosus
IgG, IgM	Vasculitis of rheumatoid arthritis and mixed cryoglobulinemia
Tumor antigens: Colon carcinoma (carcinoembryonic antigen)	Glomerulonephritis
Microbial Antigens	
Hepatitis B	Systemic vasculitis
Plasmodium malariae	
Schistosoma mansoni	Glomerulonephritis
β-Hemolytic streptococci	
Staphylococcus epidermidis	

DRUG ALLERGY

The designation "drug allergy" should be reserved for adverse drug reactions caused by immunologic mechanisms. Although drug allergies are responsible for only a minority of adverse drug effects, the possibility of such reactions is a daily concern of most physicians (Table 18–5). The following criteria should be considered when diagnosing drug allergy:

1. Enough time has elapsed for an immune response. For the initial use of most drugs, sufficient time is at least 7 to 10 days. Reactions with a more rapid onset are considered pseudoallergic or depend on prior sensitization during previous administration of the drug or a cross-reacting agent.
2. The character of the reaction does not suggest a pharmacologic or toxic effect of the drug.
3. The reaction does not appear to be dose dependent and is not caused by drug interaction or abnormalities of absorption or elimination.
4. The reaction has characteristics that suggest a hypersensitivity response, such as skin rash, fever, and eosinophilia.
5. Clinical improvement occurs promptly after use of the suspect drug is discontinued (48–72 hours).

Table 18–5 ■ DRUGS FREQUENTLY CAUSING ALLERGIC AND PSEUDOALLERGIC REACTIONS

Antimicrobials
β-Lactams
Sulfonamides
Vancomycin
Nitrofurantoin
Antituberculous drugs
Quinolones
Anticonvulsants
Phenytoin
Carbamazepine
Barbiturates
Cardiovascular agents
Procainamide
Hydralazine
Quinidine
Methyldopa
ACE inhibitors
Macromolecules
Heterologous antisera
Enzymes
Hormones
Anti-inflammatory agents
Aspirin
Other non-steroidal anti-inflammatory drugs
Gold salts
Penicillamine
Antineoplastic agents
Azathioprine
Procarbazine
Asparaginase
Cisplatin
Other
Allopurinol
Radiographic contrast media
Opiates
Sulfasalazine
Neuromuscular blocking drugs
Antithyroid drugs

ACE = angiotensin-converting enzyme.

Although it is not necessary that all these criteria be met, all should be considered when a patient is evaluated for possible drug allergy.

For more information about this subject, see *Cecil Textbook of Medicine,* 21st edition. Philadelphia, W.B. Saunders Company, 2000. Chapter 279, Drug Allergy, pages 1463 to 1466.

CHAPTER 19

MUSCULOSKELETAL AND CONNECTIVE TISSUE DISEASES

SPECIALIZED PROCEDURES IN THE MANAGEMENT OF PATIENTS WITH RHEUMATIC DISEASES

In any patient with undiagnosed arthritis and an associated joint effusion (Table 19–1), examination of the synovial fluid is mandatory (Table 19–2). Successful joint or bursal aspiration depends on a thorough familiarity with certain principles. Both the physician and the patient must be comfortable. The physician should have some experience and confidence concerning the joint to be tapped.

Testing serum for the presence of *antinuclear antibodies (ANAs)* is useful primarily in the evaluation of suspected systemic lupus erythematosus (SLE) Many different antigen-antibody reactions underlie the various patterns detected by the ANA test, and identification of antibody to a specific antigen is diagnostically useful in several instances (Table 19–3).

For more information about this subject, see *Cecil Textbook of Medicine,* 21st edition. Philadelphia, W.B. Saunders Company, 2000. Chapter 285, Specialized Procedures in the Management of Patients with Rheumatic Diseases, pages 1487 to 1491.

RHEUMATOID ARTHRITIS

Rheumatoid arthritis (RA) is a chronic systemic inflammatory disease predominantly affecting diarthrodial joints and frequently a variety of other organs (Tables 19–4 and 19–5).

THERAPEUTIC MANAGEMENT. Objectives of management include (1) relief of pain and stiffness, (2) reduction of inflammation, (3) minimization of undesirable drug side effects, (4) preservation of muscle strength and joint function, and (5) maintenance of as normal a lifestyle as possible. The basic initial program that achieves these objectives for the great majority of patients consists of (1) adequate rest, (2) adequate anti-inflammatory therapy, and (3) physical measures to maintain joint function. An additional objective is to attempt to modify the disease course with early, aggressive drug therapies. Anti-inflammatory therapy is crucial to the basic program (Table 19–6).

Immunosuppressive agents such as azathioprine, cyclophosphamide, chlorambucil, and cyclosporine have been used to treat espe-

Text continues on page 532

For more information about this subject, see *Cecil Textbook of Medicine,* 21st edition. Philadelphia, W.B. Saunders Company, 2000. Part XXI: Musculoskeletal and Connective Tissue Diseases, pages 1472 to 1562.

Table 19–1 ■ CLASSIFICATION OF RHEUMATIC DISEASE

CATEGORY	PROTOTYPES	USEFUL TESTS	TREATMENTS
Synovitis	Rheumatoid arthritis	Latex, erythrocyte sedimentation rate	Methotrexate
	Autoimmune collagen diseases	ANA test	Prednisone
Enthesopathy	Ankylosing spondylitis	Sacroiliac radiographs	Indomethacin
	HLA-B27 spondyloarthropathies		
Crystal-induced synovitis	Gout	Joint fluid crystal examination	Indomethacin
	Pseudogout	Radiographic chondrocalcinosis Joint fluid crystal examination	Indomethacin
Joint space disease	Septic arthritis	Joint fluid culture	Antibiotics
Cartilage degeneration	Osteoarthritis	Radiographs of affected area	Physical therapy Analgesics
Osteoarticular disease	Avascular bone necrosis	Radiographs, magnetic resonance imaging	Prosthetic joint replacement
Polymyositis	Dermatomyositis Inclusion body myositis	Muscle enzymes, EMG, muscle biopsy	Corticosteroids
Local conditions	Tendinitis	None, radiographs of affected area	Local
General conditions	Fibromyalgia	Erythrocyte sedimentation rate	Fitness exercises

ANA = antinuclear antigen; EMG = electromyogram.

Table 19–2 ■ SYNOVIAL FLUID ANALYSIS

	NON-INFLAMMATORY (GROUP I)	INFLAMMATORY (GROUP II)	PURULENT (GROUP III)	HEMORRHAGIC (GROUP IV)
Color	Yellow	Yellow	Yellow-green	Red
Clarity	Transparent	Translucent	Opaque	Opaque
Leukocyte count (WBC/mL)	<2000	2000–50,000*	>50,000	*
Polymorphonuclear leukocytes (%)	<25	>50	>75	*
Disease examples	Osteoarthritis Trauma Osteochondritis dissecans Osteonecrosis Amyloidosis Scleroderma Systemic lupus† Polymyalgia rheumatica† Hypertrophic pulmonary osteoarthropathy	Rheumatoid arthritis (RA) Reiter's syndrome Crystal synovitis, acute Gout, pseudogout Psoriatic arthritis Viral arthritis Rheumatic fever Behçet's syndrome Lyme disease Some bacterial infections	Bacterial infections Tuberculosis RA (rare) Reiter's syndrome (rare) Pseudogout (rare)	Trauma Neuropathic joint Coagulation disorders Hemophilia von Willebrand's disease Heparin or warfarin Sickle cell disease Chondrocalcinosis Scurvy Tumor, especially pigmented villonodular synovitis, hemangioma

*Wide range; WBC count should be interpreted in light of peripheral blood WBC and RBC counts.
†Sometimes inflammatory.

Table 19–3 ■ ASSOCIATIONS BETWEEN SELECTED NUCLEAR AND CYTOPLASMIC AUTOANTIBODIES AND CERTAIN RHEUMATIC DISEASES

SUBSTRATE AND IMMUNO-FLUORESCENCE PATTERN	ANTIBODY	ANTIGEN	DISEASE ASSOCIATION(S)	COMMENTS
Human Epithelial Cells (Hep-2)				
Homogeneous ANA	Anti-histone	Histones H1, H2A, H2B, H3, H4	Drug-induced lupus (>95%), infectious mononucleosis (5–10%), normals (1–2%)	Low titer (<1:320) in "normals"
Rim ANA	Anti-native DNA	Double-stranded DNA	SLE (50%)	Antibodies to double-stranded DNA, highly specific for SLE; rim ANA is rare pattern on Hep-2 cells
Speckled ANA	Anti-Sm	Non-histone proteins D–G complexed with small nuclear RNAs	SLE (30%)	Highly specific for SLE
	Anti-U1-nRNP	U1 small nuclear ribonucleoprotein	SLE (35%); MCTD (>95%)	High titer in MCTD
	Anti-Ro (SS-A)	Two proteins complexed with small RNAs Y1–Y5	SLE (35%); Sjögren's syndrome (70–80%)	Often missed on Hep-2 ANA; common in ANA-negative lupus
	Anti-La (SS-B)	Single protein + RNA polymerase III transcript	SLE (15%); Sjögren's syndrome (50–70%)	
	Anti-Ku	DNA binding protein	SLE (10%)	May identify SLE/PSS/myositis overlap
	Anti-Scl-70	DNA topoisomerase I	PSS (40–70%); CREST (10–20%)	
Nucleolar ANA	Anti-PM-Scl	Nucleolar protein complex	PSS (3%); PM (8%)	May identify "sclerodermatomyositis" overlap
	Anti-Mi-2	Nuclear protein complex	DM (15–20%)	Rare in PM
	Anti-RNA polymerase I	Subunits of RNA polymerase I	PSS (4%)	

Dividing cell—specific patterns	Anticentromere	Centromere/kinetochore protein	CREST (80%), PSS (30%)	In patients with isolated Raynaud's phenomenon, may predict progression to CREST
	Anti–proliferating cell nuclear antigen	Auxiliary protein of DNA polymerase δ	SLE (3%)	
Cytoplasmic staining	Antisynthetases:			
	Anti–Jo-1	Histidyl tRNA synthetase	PM/DM (18–25%)	Often with ISLD
	Anti–PL-7	Threonyl tRNA synthetase	PM/DM (3%)	Often with ISLD
	Anti–PL-12	Alanyl tRNA synthetase	PM/DM (3%)	Often with ISLD
	Anti-SRP	SRP	PM (4%)	No Raynaud's phenomenon, rare ISLD, poor prognosis
	Antiribosomal P	Large ribosomal subunit	SLE (10%)	May associate with CNS manifestations
	Antimitochondrial	E2 component of pyruvate dehydrogenase complex at inner mitochondrial membrane	Primary biliary cirrhosis (PBC) (90–95%; normals, <1%)	PCB may show CREST, Sjögren's features
Alcohol-Fixed Human Neutrophils				
Cytosol staining	c-ANCA	Serine protease 3 (PR-3)	Wegener's granulomatosis (90%)	
Perinuclear staining	p-ANCA	Myeloperoxidase	Microscopic polyarteritis (necrotizing glomerulonephritis with or without extrarenal small vessel vasculitis); Churg-Strauss syndrome, miscellaneous vasculitides	
	p-ANCA (atypical)	Lysozyme, lactoferrin, cathepsin G, bactericidal/permeability increasing protein (BPI)	Ulcerative colitis (40–80%), Crohn's disease (10–40%), primary sclerosing cholangitis (65–84%)	

ANA = antinuclear antibody; SLE = systemic lupus erythematosus; MCTD = mixed connective tissue disease; PSS = progressive systemic sclerosis (diffuse scleroderma); CREST = *c*alcinosis, *R*aynaud's phenomenon, *e*sophageal dysfunction, *s*clerodactyly, and *t*elangiectasia; PM = polymyositis; DM = dermatomyositis; ISLD = interstitial lung disease; ANCA = antineutrophil cytoplasmic antibody; tRNA = transfer RNA; SRP = signal recognition particle.

Table 19–4 ■ CLASSIFICATION CRITERIA FOR RHEUMATOID ARTHRITIS*

1. Morning stiffness (≥1 hr)
2. Swelling (soft tissue) of ≥3 joints
3. Swelling (soft tissue) of hand joints (PIP, MCP, or wrist)
4. Symmetrical swelling (soft tissue)
5. Subcutaneous nodules
6. Serum rheumatoid factor
7. Erosions and/or periarticular osteopenia in hand or wrist joints seen on radiograph

PIP = proximal interphalangeal; MCP = metacarpophalangeal.

*Criteria 1 to 4 must have been continuous for 6 weeks or longer and criteria 2 to 5 must be observed by a physician. A diagnosis of rheumatoid arthritis requires that four of the seven criteria be fulfilled.

cially severe, unremitting RA. A soluble recombinant tumor necrosis factor-α (TNF-α) receptor, etanercept (Embrel), has recently been approved for use in patients with RA.

Combinations of certain long-lasting agents are increasingly being advocated for severe RA and may prove beneficial in some patients. The likelihood of serious side effects is significantly increased, however, and close consultation with a rheumatologist is strongly recommended.

JUVENILE CHRONIC ARTHRITIS. A chronic arthritis beginning in childhood and for which no underlying cause is apparent has been termed *juvenile rheumatoid arthritis.* Because the majority of these cases do not resemble adult RA, the term *juvenile chronic arthritis* is a more appropriate designation.

Arthritis of systemic onset, or Still's disease, accounts for about 20% of patients. It can begin at any age. Rheumatic factor and ANAs are generally not found.

For more information about this subject, see *Cecil Textbook of Medicine,* 21st edition. Philadelphia, W.B. Saunders Company, 2000. Chapter 286, Rheumatoid Arthritis, pages 1492 to 1499.

THE SPONDYLOARTHROPATHIES

The spondyloarthropathies are a heterogeneous group of disorders that share a number of clinical, radiographic, and genetic features (Table 19–7). Distinctive features permit consideration as a group of related disorders when considering diagnosis and treatment of affected individuals (Fig. 19–1). The disorders include ankylosing spondylitis, Reiter's syndrome (Table 19–8), reactive arthritis, psoriatic arthritis, and the enteropathic arthropathies. Therapeutic options are largely the same for most of the spondyloarthropathies and may be considered together (Fig. 19–2).

For more information about this subject, see *Cecil Textbook of Medicine,* 21st edition. Philadelphia, W.B. Saunders Company, 2000. Chapter 287, The Spondyloarthropathies, pages 1499 to 1507.

Table 19–5 ■ HLA ASSOCIATIONS WITH RHEUMATOID ARTHRITIS (RA)

	HLA TYPES (ALLELES) AND METHODS OF DETECTION			THIRD HYPERVARIABLE REGION AMINO ACID SEQUENCES					
	Alloantisera (DR)	MLC (Dw)	DNA (DRBI)	70	71	72	73	74	MOST COMMON ETHNIC GROUPS
Associated with RA	DR4	Dw4	*0401	Q	K	R	A	A	Whites (western Europe)
	DR4	Dw14	*0404	·	R	·	·	·	Whites (western Europe)
	DR4	Dw15	*0405	·	R	·	·	·	Japanese, Chinese
	DR1	Dw1	*0101	·	R	·	·	·	Asian Indians, Israelis
	DR6 (14)	Dw16	*1402	·	R	·	·	·	Yakima Native Americans
	DR10	—	*1001	R	R	·	·	·	Spanish, Greeks, Israelis
Not associated with RA	DR4	Dw10	*0402	D	E	·	·	·	Whites (eastern Europe)
	DR4	Dw13	*0403	·	R	·	·	E	Polynesians
	DR2	Dw2	*1501	D	A	·	·	·	Whites
	DR3	Dw3	*0301	·	·	·	G	R	Whites

Q = glutamine, K = lysine, R = arginine, A = alanine, D = aspartic acid, E = glutamic acid; · = the same amino acid in that position as DRBI*0401.

Table 19–6 ■ THERAPEUTIC AGENTS USED IN RHEUMATOID ARTHRITIS

Anti-Inflammatory Drugs
Salicylates
Non-steroidal anti-inflammatory drugs
Cyclooxygenase-1 and -2 inhibitors
Corticosteroids
Disease-Modifying Therapies
Antimalarials
Methotrexate
Leflunomide
Sulfasalazine
Gold salts
Penicillamine
Minogeline
Immunosuppressive Agents
Azathioprine
Cyclophosphamide
Chlorambucil
Cyclosporine

INFECTIOUS ARTHRITIS

Infectious arthritis is a topic of great relevance to clinical medicine, and despite major advances in diagnostic approaches and the development of newer and more powerful antibiotics, its impact in terms of human morbidity and mortality has remained unchanged in the past 25 years.

NON-GONOCOCCAL BACTERIAL ARTHRITIS. Early recognition of infection is the most important step in the management of septic arthritis. Arthrocentesis is mandatory in the presence of joint effusion (Table 19–9).

GONOCOCCAL ARTHRITIS. Gonorrhea is the most commonly reported communicable disease in the United States, and disseminated gonococcal infection remains the most common cause of acute septic arthritis is young sexually active persons. Joint pain—monoarthralgia, oligoarthralgia, or polyarthralgia—the most common symptom of disseminated gonococcal infection, occurs in a diffuse, migratory, or additive pattern within a few days of onset. Tenosynovitis, with or without arthritis, commonly develops in the wrists, fingers, ankles, or toes in two thirds of patients. Fever and chills are common. Skin involvement occurs in approximately two thirds of patients.

The major differential diagnosis includes Reiter's syndrome, bacterial arthritis, juvenile rheumatoid arthritis, meningococcemia, bacterial endocarditis, and acute rheumatic fever.

VIRAL ARTHRITIS. The most important viral infections associated with rheumatic complaints are hepatitis viruses, parvovirus, rubella virus, and human immunodeficiency virus (HIV). Hepatitis

Table 19–7 ■ COMPARISON OF THE SPONDYLOARTHROPATHIES

FEATURE	ANKYLOSING SPONDYLITIS	POST-URETHRAL REACTIVE ARTHRITIS	POST-DYSENTERIC REACTIVE ARTHRITIS	ENTEROPATHIC ARTHRITIS	PSORIATIC ARTHRITIS
Sacroiliitis	+++++	+++	++	+	++
Spondylitis	++++	+++	++	++	++
Peripheral arthritis	+	++++	++++	+++	++++
Articular course	Chronic	Acute or chronic	Acute > chronic	Acute or chronic	Chronic
HLA-B27	95%	60%	30%	20%	20%
Enthesopathy	++	++++	+++	++	++
Common extra-articular manifestations	Eye Heart	Eye Gu Oral/GI Heart	GU Eye	GI Eye	Skin Nails Eye
Other names	von Bechterev's, Marie-Strümpell	Reiter's syndrome, SARA, NGU, chlamydial arthritis	Reiter's syndrome	Crohn's disease, ulcerative colitis	

GU = genitourinary; GI = gastrointestinal; SARA = sexually acquired reactive arthritis; NGU = non-gonococcal urethritis.

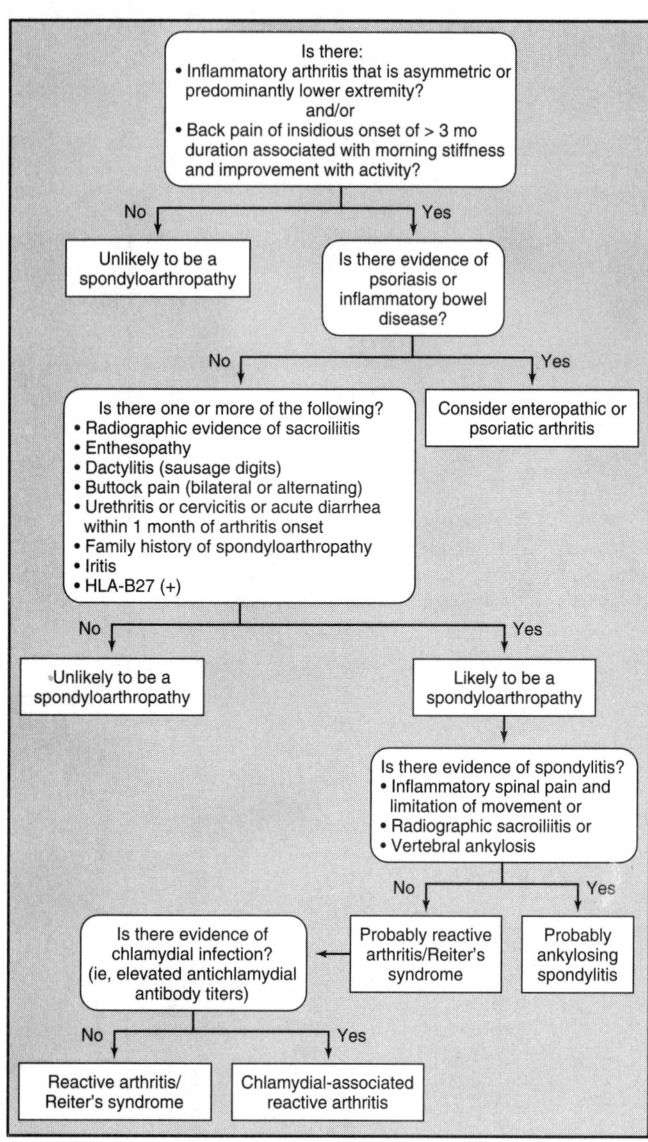

FIGURE 19–1 ■ Algorithm for diagnosis of the spondyloarthropathies.

B and C, and, to a lesser degree, hepatitis A, virus may cause immune complex–mediated rheumatic syndromes.

MISCELLANEOUS FORMS OF INFECTIOUS ARTHRITIS. Other forms of arthritis may occur with Lyme disease or syphilis, or as tuberculous arthritis or fungal arthritis.

For more information about this subject, see *Cecil Textbook of*

Table 19–8 ■ INFECTIOUS ORGANISMS ASSOCIATED WITH THE ONSET OF REITER'S SYNDROME

ENTERIC PATHOGENS	UROGENITAL PATHOGENS
Shigella flexneri (serotypes 2a, 1b)	*Chlamydia trachomatis*
Salmonella typhimurium	*Chlamydia psittaci*
Salmonella enteritidis	*Ureaplasma urealyticum*
Salmonella paratyphi	
Salmonella heidelberg	
Yersinia enterocolitica (serotypes 0:3, 0:8, 0:9)	
Yersinia pseudotuberculosis	
Campylobacter jejuni	
Campylobacter fetus	

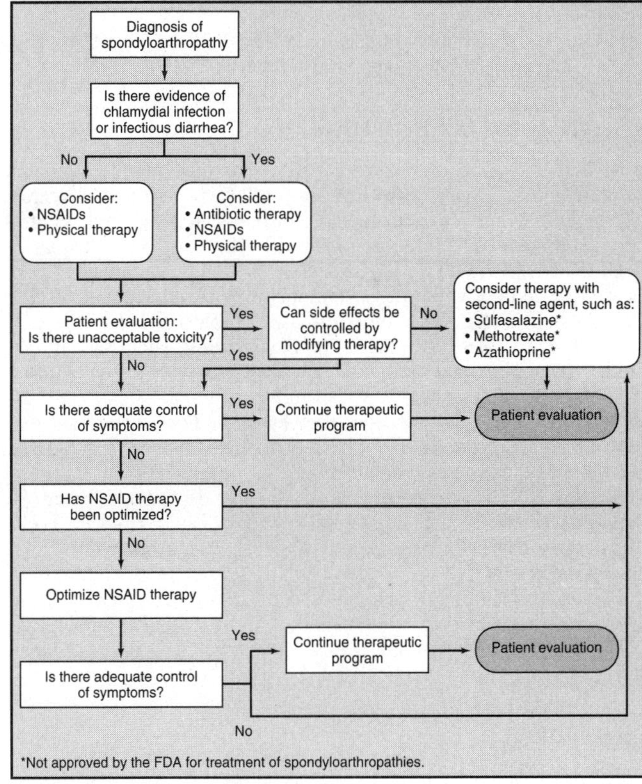

FIGURE 19–2 ■ Treatment algorithm for patients with a spondyloarthropathy. NSAID = non-steroidal anti-inflammatory drug.

19

Table 19–9 ■ MOST COMMON MICROORGANISMS IN ACUTE NON-GONOCOCCAL BACTERIAL ARTHRITIS (ALL AGES)

MICROORGANISM	FREQUENCY (%)
Gram positive	**60–90**
Staphylococcus aureus	50–70
Group B streptococci	15–30
Streptococcus pneumoniae	1–3
Gram negative	**5–25**
Salmonella	
Pseudomonas aeruginosa	
Escherichia coli	
Kingella kingae	
Haemophilus influenzae	
Brucella	
Anaerobes	**1–2**
Fusobacterium necrophorum	
Anaerobic cocci	
Bacteriodes fragilis	

Medicine, 21st edition. Philadelphia, W.B. Saunders Company, 2000. Chapter 288, Infectious Arthritis, pages 1507 to 1509.

SYSTEMIC LUPUS ERYTHEMATOSUS

SLE is a disease of unknown cause that may produce variable combinations of fever, rash, hair loss, arthritis, pleuritis, pericarditis, nephritis, anemia, leukopenia, thrombocytopenia, and central nervous system (CNS) disease (Table 19–10).

CLINICAL MANIFESTATIONS. SLE is highly variable in onset as well as course. The initial symptoms may be non-specific (Table 19–11) and may resemble other diseases (Table 19–12).

DRUG-INDUCED LUPUS. Some medications, such as sulfonamides, penicillin, and oral contraceptives, may exacerbate lupus. Hydralazine and procainamide can induce a lupus-like disease, especially in those who are slow acetylators and/or HLA-DR4 positive. Other medications may possibly induce lupus or just ANAs, but the evidence is less convincing.

MANAGEMENT. Management of SLE is determined based on the organ involved and degree of severity (Table 19–13). Treatment starts conservatively and, if the response is inadequate, becomes more aggressive.

For more information about this subject, see *Cecil Textbook of Medicine,* 21st edition. Philadelphia, W.B. Saunders Company, 2000. Chapter 289, Systemic Lupus Erythematosus, pages 1509 to 1517.

SCLERODERMA

Scleroderma (systemic sclerosis) is a chronic, systemic disease that targets the skin, lungs, heart, gastrointestinal tract, kidneys, and musculoskeletal system. The disorder is characterized by three features: (1) tissue fibrosis; (2) small blood vessel vasculopathy; and

Table 19–10 ■ CRITERIA FOR CLASSIFICATION OF SYSTEMIC LUPUS ERYTHEMATOSUS*

CRITERION	DEFINITION
1. Malar rash	Fixed erythema, flat or raised, over the malar eminences, tending to spare the nasolabial folds
2. Discoid rash	Erythematous raised patches with adherent keratotic scaling and follicular plugging; atrophic scarring may occur in older lesions
3. Photosensitivity	Skin rash as a result of unusual reaction to sunlight, by patient history or physician observation
4. Oral ulcers	Oral or nasopharyngeal ulceration, usually painless, observed by a physician
5. Arthritis	Non-erosive arthritis involving two or more peripheral joints and characterized by tenderness, swelling, or effusion
6. Serositis	a. Pleuritis—convincing history of pleuritic pain or rub heard by a physician or evidence of pleural effusion *or* b. Pericarditis—documented by electrocardiogram or rub or by evidence of pericardial effusion
7. Renal disorder	a. Persistent proteinuria >0.5 g/d or $>3+$ if quantitation not performed b. Cellular casts—may be red blood cell, hemoglobin, granular, tubular, or mixed
8. Neurologic disorder	a. Seizures—in the absence of offending drugs or known metabolic derangements, e.g., uremia, ketoacidosis, or electrolyte imbalance *or* b. Psychosis in the absence of offending drugs or known metabolic derangements, e.g., uremia, ketoacidosis, or electrolyte imbalance
9. Hematologic disorder	a. Hemolytic anemia with reticulocytosis *or* b. Leukopenia $<4000/mm^3$ total on 2 or more occasions c. Lymphopenia $<1500/mm^3$ on 2 or more occasions *or* d. Thrombocytopenia $<100{,}000/mm^3$ in the absence of offending drugs
10. Immunologic disorder	a. Positive tests for antiphospholipid antibodies *or* b. Anti-DNA: antibody to native DNA in abnormal titer *or* c. Anti-Sm: presence of antibody to Sm nuclear antigen *or* d. False-positive serologic test for syphilis known to be positive for at least 6 mo and confirmed by *Treponema pallidum* immobilization or fluorescent treponemal antibody absorption test
11. Antinuclear antibody	An abnormal titer of antinuclear antibody by immunofluorescence or an equivlent assay at any point and in the absence of drugs known to be associated with "drug-induced lupus" syndrome

*The classification is based on 11 criteria. For the purpose of identifying patients in clinical studies, a person shall be said to have systemic lupus erythematosus if any 4 or more of the 11 criteria are present, serially or simultaneously, during any interval of observation.

Table 19–11 ■ CLINICAL FEATURES IN SYSTEMIC LUPUS ERYTHEMATOSUS

	APPROXIMATE FREQUENCY (%)	
MANIFESTATION	**At Onset**	**At Any Time**
Non-Specific		
Fatigue	—	90
Fever	36	80
Weight loss	—	60
Arthralgia/myalgia	69	95
Specific		
Arthritis	—	90
Skin		
Butterfly rash	40	50
Discoid LE	6	20
Photosensitivity	29	58
Mucous ulcers	11	30
Alopecia	—	71
Raynaud's phenomenon	18	30
Purpura	—	15
Urticaria	—	9
Renal	16	50
Nephrosis	—	18
Gastrointestinal	—	38
Pulmonary	3	50
Pleurisy	—	45
Effusions	—	24
Pneumonia	—	29
Cardiac	—	46
Pericarditis	—	48
Murmurs	—	23
ECG changes	—	34
Lymphadenopathy	7	50
Splenomegaly	—	20
Hepatomegaly	—	25
Central nervous system	12	75
Functional	—	Most
Psychosis	—	20
Seizures	—	20
Hematologic	—	90

LE = lupus erythematosus; ECG = electrocardiogram.

(3) a specific autoimmune response associated with autoantibodies (Table 19–14).

Scleroderma patients also have evidence of ongoing autoimmunity, namely, disease-specific autoantibodies (Table 19–15).

No drug or treatment has proved safe and effective in altering the underlying disease process in scleroderma.

Patients with limited scleroderma generally have a normal survival, unless severe pulmonary hypertension is present. Patients with later age at onset, diffuse skin disease, presence of tendon friction rubs, and antitopoisomerase antibody have a worse prognosis.

Table 19–12 ■ DISORDERS RESEMBLING SYSTEMIC LUPUS ERYTHEMATOSUS

COMMON	LESS COMMON
Drug-induced lupus	Polymyositis/dermatomyositis
Scleroderma	Rheumatic fever
Wegener's granulomatosis	Sarcoidosis
Cutaneous (discoid) lupus	Relapsing polychondritis
Rheumatoid arthritis	Weber-Christian disease
Chronic active hepatitis (lupoid hepatitis)	Mixed cryoglobulinemia
Vasculitis	Whipple's disease
Felty's syndrome	Familial Mediterranean fever
Juvenile (rheumatoid) arthritis	
Sjögren's syndrome	
Mixed connective tissue disease	
Fibromyalgia/chronic fatigue syndrome	

For more information about this subject, see the corresponding material in *Cecil Textbook of Medicine,* 21st edition. Philadelphia, W.B. Saunders Company, 2000. Chapter 290, Scleroderma (Systemic Sclerosis), pages 1517 to 1522.

SJÖGREN'S SYNDROME

Sjögren's syndrome is a chronic immune-mediated inflammatory disorder characterized by lymphocytic infiltration of the exocrine glands, especially the lacrimal and salivary glands, associated with the clinical features of keratoconjunctivitis sicca and xerostomia (Table 19–16).

Treatment of dry eyes is largely symptomatic and includes artificial tears and lubricant ointments. Occasionally, patients may re-

Table 19–13 ■ TREATMENT OF SPECIFIC PROBLEMS IN LUPUS

Fever: NSAIDs → antimalarials → steroids
Arthralgia/myalgia: NSAIDs → acetaminophen → amitriptyline
Arthritis: NSAIDs → antimalarials → steroids (alternate-day) or methotrexate
Rashes: sunscreens → topical steroids → antimalarials → injection
Oral ulcers: antimalarials
Raynaud's phenomenon: no smoking, caffeine, decongestants → warm clothing → biofeedback → (long-acting) nifedipine → prazosin
Serositis: indomethacin → steroids
Pulmonary: steroids
Hypertension: diuretics → ACE inhibitors → calcium channel blockers → β-blockers → vasodilators
Thrombocytopenia/hemolytic anemia: steroids → IV gamma globulin → immunosuppressives → splenectomy
Renal disease: steroids → pulse steroids → immunosuppressives
CNS disease
  Organic: steroids → antiseizure drugs → immunosuppressives
  Functional: antianxety/antidepression drugs

NSAIDs = non-steroidal anti-inflammatory drugs; ACE = angiotensin-converting enzyme; CNS = central nervous sytstem.

19

Table 19–14 ■ CRITERIA AND CLASSIFICATION FOR SCLERODERMA (SYSTEMIC SCLEROSIS)

Definite scleroderma. Scleroderma skin changes proximal to the metacarpophalangeal joints or metatarsophalangeal joints *or* (2 of 3): (1) sclerodactyly (scleroderma limited to the fingers); (2) digital pitting scars or loss of finger pad; (3) bi-basilar pulmonary fibrosis

Diffuse cutaneous scleroderma. Scleroderma skin changes above the elbows or knees and/or on the trunk (abdomen or chest)

Limited cutaneous scleroderma. Scleroderma skin changes distal to the elbow, knees, and above the clavicles

- *CREST syndrome.* Subcutaneous *c*alcinosis, *R*aynaud's phenomenon, *e*sophageal dysfunction, *s*clerodactyly, and *t*elangiectasia (3 of 5 must be present)

Overlap syndromes: Diffuse or limited scleroderma plus typical features of one or more of another connective tissue or autoimmune disease

- *Mixed connective tissue disease:* Features of scleroderma, systemic lupus erythematosus, polymyositis, rheumatoid arthritis, and the presence of anti-U1snRNP

Systemic sclerosis sine scleroderma. Systemic features without skin involvement

Undifferentiated connective tissue disease. Features of scleroderma but no definite clinical or laboratory findings to make a definite diagnosis

Localized scleroderma. Asymmetrical plaques of fibrotic skin without systemic disease

- *Morphea.* Limited (single plaque); generalized (multiple plaques)
- *Linear scleroderma.* Longitudinal fibrotic bands
- *Nodular scleroderma.* Keloid-like nodules

quire surgical punctal occlusion by an ophthalmologist to block tear drainage.

Managing the oral component of Sjögren's syndrome requires using saliva substitutes, stimulating salivary flow from functioning acinar tissue with pilocarpine hydrochloride at doses of 5 mg three times daily.

Young women with primary Sjögren's syndrome, especially those with antibodies to Ro (SS-A), should be counseled about the increased risk of delivering a child with neonatal SLE and congenital complete heart block; such women, when pregnant, should be monitored closely by an obstetrician expert in high-risk pregnancies.

For more information about this subject, see *Cecil Textbook of Medicine,* 21st edition. Philadelphia, W.B. Saunders Company, 2000. Chapter 291, Sjögren's Syndrome, pages 1522 to 1524.

THE VASCULITIC SYNDROMES

Vasculitis is a clinicopathologic process characterized by inflammation and necrosis of the blood vessel wall. The vasculitic syndromes are generally thought to result from immunopathogenic mechanisms; however, the evidence for such mechanisms varies among the different syndromes. The heterogeneity and the obvious overlap among the vasculitic syndromes have led to difficulties in classification of this group of diseases (Table 19–17).

For more information about this subject, see *Cecil Textbook of*

Table 19–15 ■ CHARACTERISTICS OF SUBSETS OF SCLERODERMA

Diffuse Scleroderma
Widespread skin thickening involving distal and proximal body
Rapid onset (within 1 yr) of skin and other features following appearance of Raynaud's phenomenon
Significant visceral involvement including the heart, lungs, gastrointestinal tract, or kidneys
High scores on disability and organ damage indices secondary to extensive fibrosis of tissues
Poor prognostic signs include later age at onset, female sex, black or Native American race, absence of Raynaud's phenomenon, presence of large pericardial effusion, or tendon friction rubs
Associated with antinuclear antibodies and the absence of anticentromere antibody
Highly variable disease course but overall poorer prognosis with 10-yr survival of 40–60%
Limited Scleroderma
Limited to no skin thickening
Several-year interval or slow progression of disease from onset of Raynaud's phenomenon
Late visceral disease with unique features of isolated pulmonary hypertension and digital amputations secondary to severe ischemic vascular disease
CREST syndrome is a variant of limited scleroderma
Associated with primary biliary cirrhosis
Associated with anticentromere antibody
Relatively good prognosis with 10-yr survival of >70%

CREST = *c*alcinosus, *R*aynaud's phenomenon, *e*sophageal dysfunction, *s*clerodactyly, *t*elangiectasia.

Medicine, 21st edition. Philadelphia, W.B. Saunders Company, 2000. Chapter 292, The Vasculitic Syndromes, pages 1524 to 1527.

POLYARTERITIS NODOSA GROUP

The lesions of polyarteritis affect arteries of medium and small caliber, especially at bifurcations and branchings. The segmental process involves the media, with edema, fibrinous exudation, fibrinoid necrosis, and infiltration of polymorphonuclear neutrophils, and extends to the adventitia and intima. Finally, the involved segment is replaced by scar tissue with associated intimal thickening and periarterial fibrosis. These changes produce partial occlusion, thrombosis and infarction, and palpable or visible aneurysms with occasional rupture.

19

CLINICAL MANIFESTATIONS AND DIAGNOSIS. Widespread distribution of the arterial lesions produces diverse clinical manifestations that reflect the particular organ systems in which the arterial supply has been impaired. Among the early symptoms and signs of polyarteritis nodosa are fever, weight loss, and pain in viscera and/or the musculoskeletal system. Striking and specific initial signs may relate to abdominal pain, acute glomerulitis, polyneuritis on occasion, or myocardial infarction. Pulmonary manifestations, espe-

Table 19–16 ■ PRELIMINARY CRITERIA FOR THE CLASSIFICATION OF SJÖGREN'S SYNDROME (EUROPEAN COMMUNITY STUDY GROUP)

1. Ocular symptoms: A positive response to at least 1 of these questions:
   a. Have you had daily, persistent, troublesome dry eyes for more than 3 mos?
   b. Do you have a recurrent sensation of sand or gravel in the eyes?
   c. Do you use tear substitutes more than 3 times a day?
2. Oral symptoms: A positive response to at least 1 of these questions:
   a. Have you had a daily feeling of dry mouth for more than 3 mos?
   b. Have you had recurrent or persistently swollen salivary glands as an adult?
   c. Do you frequently drink liquids to aid in swallowing dry foods?
3. Ocular signs: Objective evidence of ocular involvement determined on the basis of a positive result on at least 1 of the following tests:
   a. Schirmer test ($\leq$5 mm in 5 min)
   b. Rose Bengal score ($\geq$4, according to the van Bijsterveld scoring system)
4. Histopathologic features: Focus score of 1 or more on minor salivary gland biopsy (*focus* defined as an agglomeration of at least 50 mononuclear cells; *focus score* defined as the number of foci per 4 mm^2 of glandular tissue)
5. Salivary gland involvement: Objective evidence of salivary gland involvement determined on the basis of a positive result on at least 1 of the following tests:
   a. Salivary scintigraphy
   b. Parotid sialography
   c. Unstimulated salivary flow ($\leq$1.5 mL in 15 min)
6. Autoantibodies: Presence of at least 1 of the following serum autoantibodies:
   a. Antibodies to Ro (SS-A) or La (SS-B) antigens
   b. Antinuclear antibodies
   c. Rheumatoid factor

Exclusion criteria: Pre-existing lymphoma, acquired immunodeficiency syndrome, sarcoidosis, or graft-versus-host disease.

Modified from Vitali C, Bombardieri S, Moutsopoulos HM, et al: Preliminary criteria for the classification of Sjögren's syndrome: Results of a prospective concerted action supported by the European Community. Arthritis Rheum 36:340, 1992.

cially intractable bronchial asthma, would indicate allergic angiitis and granulomatosis rather than classic polyarteritis nodosa.

TREATMENT. Large doses, in the range of prednisone 40 to 60 mg/day, afford symptomatic relief. Dramatic remission with cyclophosphamide 2 mg/kg/day has been observed.

For more information about this subject, see *Cecil Textbook of Medicine,* 21st edition. Philadelphia, W.B. Saunders Company, 2000. Chapter 293, Polyarteritis Nodosa Group, pages 1527 to 1529.

WEGENER'S GRANULOMATOSIS

The classic histopathologic finding in Wegener's granulomatosis is necrotizing granulomatous vasculitis involving small arteries and veins, most reliably found on biopsies of the lung.

Renal biopsies typically show focal segmental glomerulonephri-

Table 19–17 ■ CLINICAL SPECTRUM OF VASCULITIS

Polyarteritis Nodosa Group
Classic polyarteritis nodosa
Allergic angiitis and granulomatosis (Churg-Strauss disease)
Overlap syndrome
Hypersensitivity Vasculitis
Henoch-Schönlein purpura
Serum sickness and serum sickness–like reactions
Vasculitis associated with infectious diseases
Vasculitis associated with neoplasms
Vasculitis associated with connective tissue diseases
Vasculitis associated with other underlying diseases
Congenital deficiencies of the complement system
Granulomatous Vasculitides
Wegener's granulomatosis
Angiocentric immunoproliferative lesions (lymphomatoid granulomatosis)
Giant cell arteritides
Cranial or temporal arteritis
Takayasu's arteritis
Other Vasculitis Syndromes
Mucocutaneous lymph node syndrome (Kawasaki syndrome)
Behçet's disease
Vasculitis isolated to the central nervous system
Thromboangiitis obliterans (Buerger's disease)
Erythema nodosa
Erythema multiforme
Erythema elevatum diutinum
Miscellaneous vasculitides

tis. Biopsy does help exclude other conditions such as SLE, post-streptococcal disease, Goodpasture's syndrome, and cryoglobulinemia.

Wegener's granulomatosis is a multisystem disorder predominantly involving the upper and lower respiratory tracts and the kidneys (Table 19–18).

TREATMENT. Optimal treatment of active Wegener's granulomatosis, particularly with multisystem involvement, including renal disease, entails cyclophosphamide and corticosteroids (Table 19–19). Cyclophosphamide therapy is started at a dose of 1 to 2 mg/kg/day. The dose is adjusted according to blood counts, particularly as corticosteroid use is tapered. The drug is generally continued for approximately 1 year beyond clinical remission. 19

Corticosteroids are used at the time of diagnosis for severe disease, initially at 1 mg/kg/day. Prednisone equivalent doses of 60 mg/day are then tapered to alternate-day therapy over 1 month and then to the lowest possible level to control upper airway and/or musculoskeletal symptoms, preferably discontinuing use of this drug by 3 to 6 months.

For more information about this subject, see *Cecil Textbook of Medicine,* 21st edition. Philadelphia, W.B. Saunders Company, 2000. Chapter 1529, Wegener's Granulomatosis, pages 1529 to 1532.

Table 19–18 ■ CLINICAL MANIFESTATIONS OF WEGENER'S GRANULOMATOSIS

REGION/ORGAN	SIGN OR SYMPTOM
Upper airway (90–95%)	Sinusitis, serous otitis media, rhinitis, nasal ulcerations/septal perforation, epistaxis, oral ulcerations, saddle nose deformity (later), headaches
Lower airway (90–95%)	Cough, dyspnea, hemoptysis, pulmonary infiltrates (may be fleeting or persistent), nodules, cavities, pleural effusions/pleuritis, subglottic stenosis, endobronchial lesions, interstitial lung disease
Kidneys (75%)	Urinary sediment abnormalities (microscopic hematuria, casts, proteinuria), with or without renal insufficiency, nephrotic syndrome, hypertension
Musculoskeletal (70–90%)	Polyarthalgias, myalgias, mono-, oligo-, or polyarthritis (may be in a rheumatoid pattern), myositis, muscle weakness
Eye (50–65%)	Conjunctivitis, scleritis/episcleritis, uveitis, proptosis, nasolacrimal duct obstruction, orbital mass lesions, retinal vasculitis, corneoscleral ulceration
Skin (50%)	Palpable purpura, subcutaneous nodules, petechiae, vesicles, ulcers, Raynaud's phenomenon, digital ischemia, livedo reticularis, necrotic papules, pyoderma gangrenosum–type lesions (rare)
Neurologic (20–25%)	Mononeuritis multiplex, peripheral neuropathy, cranial neuropathy, central nervous system vasculitis (cerebral hemorrhage, cerebritis, syncope, diabetes insipidus)
Cardiac (20%)	Pericarditis, pancarditis, cardiomyopathy, arrhythmias, coronary arteritis
Gastrointestinal (15–30%)	Alkaline phosphatase/aminotransferase elevations, granulomatous hepatitis/triaditis, small bowel vasculitis, ascites, splenic granulomatous vasculitis
Miscellaneous (<1–5%)	Involvement of the breast, prostate, testicle, pinnae, urethra, ureter, lymph nodes, parotid, pulmonary or temporal artery, vagina, other
Constitutional	Fatigue, weight loss, fever, malaise, anorexia

POLYMYALGIA RHEUMATICA AND GIANT CELL ARTERITIS

POLYMYALGIA RHEUMATICA. Polymyalgia rheumatica is characterized by aching and morning stiffness in the shoulder and hip girdles, the proximal ends of the extremities, the neck, and the torso. The mean age at onset is about 70 years, and it nearly always occurs after age 50, with women affected twice as commonly as men (Table 19–20).

GIANT CELL ARTERITIS. Giant cell (temporal) arteritis affects large and medium-sized arteries, especially those branching from the proximal aorta that supply the neck, the extracranial structures of the head, and the arms (Table 19–21).

MANAGEMENT. Therapy for polymyalgia rheumatica is corticosteroids, with an initial daily dose of 10 to 20 mg of prednisone (or the equivalent dose of another corticosteroid).

For more information about this subject, see *Cecil Textbook of Medicine,* 21st edition. Philadelphia, W.B. Saunders Company,

Table 19–19 ■ TREATMENT OF WEGENER'S GRANULOMATOSIS

DRUG	INDICATIONS	INITIAL DOSE	MONITORING	DURATION
Cyclophosphamide	Moderate to severe	1–2 mg/kg/d PO	CBC weekly; keep WBC >3000, PMN >1000, and monitor liver tests; urine cytology and/or cystoscopy if prolonged therapy	Approximately 1 yr beyond clinical remission
	Fulminant	3–4 mg/kg/d IV for 2–3 d, then reduce to 2 mg/kg/day PO or IV		
Corticosteroids	Moderate to severe	1 mg/kg/d prednisone equivalent (IV initially or PO)	Glucose, lipids, bone density	Taper to low dose (5–10 mg/d) or alternate-day therapy over 2 mo
Cyclosporine	Refractory disease, dialysis dependent, patients awaiting renal transplant	3–5 mg/kg/d	BP, chemistries (Cr, Mg)	1 yr beyond clinical remission or until transplant

CBC = complete blood count; WBC = white blood cell count; PMN = polymorphonuclear leukocytes; BP = blood pressure.

Table 19–20 ■ DIFFERENTIAL FEATURES IN POLYMYALGIA RHEUMATICA AND SIMILAR DISORDERS

SIGNS/SYMPTOMS	POLYMYALGIA RHEUMATICA	GIANT CELL ARTERITIS	RHEUMATOID ARTHRITIS	DERMATOMYOSITIS	FIBROMYALGIA
Morning stiffness >30 min	+	±	+*	±	Variable
Headache and/or scalp tenderness	0	+	0	0	Variable
Pain with active joint movement	+	0	+*	0	Inconstant
Tender joints	±	0	+*	0	Tender spots
Swollen joints	±	±	+	0	0
Muscle weakness	±†	0	+*	+	0
Normochromic anemia	+	+	+	0	0
Elevated erythrocyte sedimentation rate	+	+	+	±	0
Elevated serum creatine kinase	0	0	0	+	0
Serum rheumatoid factor	0	0	70%	0	0
Distinct electromyographic abnormality	0	0	0	+	0
Response to non-steroidal anti-inflammatory drug	±	0	+	0	0

0 = absent; + = present; ± = present in minority of cases.
*Associated with affected joints.
†Pain inhibits movement. Disuse atrophy may occur.

Table 19–21 ■ GIANT CELL ARTERITIS: CLINICAL FINDINGS IN 94 PATIENTS

CLINICAL MANIFESTATION	FREQUENCY (%)
Headache	77
Abnormal temporal artery	53
Jaw claudication	51
Scalp tenderness	47
Constitutional symptoms	48
Polymyalgia rheumatica	34
Fever	27
Respiratory symptoms	23
Facial pain	14
Diplopia/blurred vision	12
Transient vision loss	5
Blindness (partial or complete)	13
Hemoglobin <11.0 g/dL	24
Erythrocyte sedimentation rate >40 mm/hr	97

From Machado EBV, Michet CJ, Ballard DJ, et al: Trends in incidence and clinical presentation of temporal arteritis in Olmstead County, Minnesota, 1950–1985. Arthritis Rheum 31:745, 1988.

2000. Chapter 295, Polymyalgia Rheumatica and Giant Cell Arteritis, pages 1532 to 1534.

IDIOPATHIC INFLAMMATORY MYOPATHIES

The term "idiopathic inflammatory myopathy" designates a group of rare diseases of unknown cause that are characterized by symmetrical proximal muscle weakness and non-suppurative inflammation (Table 19–22).

Many patients with idiopathic inflammatory myopathies have circulating autoantibodies. Some are termed "myositis-specific autoantibodies" (Table 19–23).

Table 19–22 ■ CRITERIA USED TO DEFINE IDIOPATHIC INFLAMMATORY MYOPATHY*

1. Symmetrical weakness of limb girdle muscles and anterior neck flexors with or without dysphagia
2. Elevation in serum of skeletal muscle enzymes, especially creatine phosphokinase
3. Electromyographic changes consistent with inflammatory myopathy: short, small polyphasic motor units; fibrillations; positive waves; and bizarre, high-frequency repetitive discharges
4. Muscle biopsy evidence of fiber necrosis, phagocytosis, and regeneration; variation in fiber size; and inflammatory exudate

*Patients are classified as having definite disease with four, probable disease with three, and possible disease with two criteria. These criteria were originally proposed in 1975 by Bohan and Peter to define polymyositis. At that time the term "polymyositis" was used to represent a specific disease, as well as being a general term representing all the recognized forms of inflammatory myopathy.

Table 19–23 ■ MYOSITIS-SPECIFIC AUTOANTIBODIES FOUND IN PATIENTS WITH IDIOPATHIC INFLAMMATORY MYOPATHY

AUTOANTIBODY	CLINICAL ASSOCIATION
Anti-tRNA synthetases	PM with interstitial lung disease, arthritis, and fever; less common in DM
Anti-Jo-1	
Anti-PL-7	
Anti-PL-12	
Anti-OJ	
Anti-EJ	
Anti-SRP	PM with poor prognosis
Anti-MAS	PM after alcoholic rhabdomyolysis
Anti-Mi-2	DM

tRNA = transfer RNA; PM = polymyositis; DM = dermatomyositis.

Certain ANAs may herald an associated connective tissue disease: anti-SM and anti–double-stranded DNA for SLE; anti-SS-A and anti-SS-B for Sjögren's syndrome; anti-centromere for CREST syndrome (*c*alcinosis, *R*aynaud's phenomenon, *e*sophageal dysfunction; *s*clerodactyly, and *t*elangiectasia); and anti-PM-1, anti-Ku, anti-PM-Sc1, and anti-SCL70 for scleroderma.

TREATMENT. During the active stage of the disease, bed rest is essential, and physical therapy with passive range-of-motion exercises should be performed to maintain function and avoid contractures.

Treatment with corticosteroids is empiric but standard. Initially, prednisone is used in single daily doses of 1 to 2 mg/kg. Once remission is attained, steroid use is tapered very gradually, a process that may require up to 2 years.

Immunosuppressive agents are used in patients who do not respond adequately to corticosteroids.

For more information on about this subject, see *Cecil Textbook of Medicine,* 21st edition. Philadelphia, W.B. Saunders Company, 2000. Chapter 296, Idiopathic Inflammatory Myopathies, pages 1534 to 1538.

THE AMYLOID DISEASES

Amyloidosis is not one clinical entity but a group of diverse, structurally driven protein deposition diseases. They are similar in that protein deposition occurs extracellularly and these deposits stain eosinophilic with standard tissue histologic stains, bind Congo red dye, and emit an apple-green birefringence when examined under polarized light microscopy.

PRIMARY (AL) AMYLOIDOSIS. AL amyloid was the first amyloid protein defined biochemically and shown to be identical to the variable region of immunoglobulin light chain (Bence Jones protein). It is associated with plasma cell myeloma (20%) or plasma cell dyscrasias (80%), with involvement of skin and subcutaneous tissue, nerve, liver, spleen, heart, kidney, and lung (Table 19–24).

Table 19–24 ▪ NOMENCLATURE AND CLASSIFICATION OF THE AMYLOIDOSES, 1990

	AMYLOID PROTEIN	CLINICAL STATE(S)	MAJOR ORGAN/TISSUE INVOLVEMENT
Major systemic amyloidoses	1. AA	1. Chronic inflammatory conditions	K, L, S, GI, Sc
		a. Infectious: tuberculosis, osteomyelitis, etc.	H, unusual
		b. Non-infectious: juvenile rheumatoid arthritis, ankylosing spondylitis, Crohn's disease, etc.	N, rare
		2. Familial Mediterranean fever	
	2. AL	Plasma cell dyscrasia	H, L, S, T
		10% multiple myeloma/macroglobulemia	N, GI, Sc
		90% idiopathic; "primary"	
	3. ATTR	Various familial polyneuropathies and cardiomyopathies	N, H, K, E, GI, Sc
Major localized amyloidoses	4. $A\beta_2M$	Chronic dialysis usually >8 yr	B, Sy, Ts
	5. $A\beta$	1. Alzheimer's disease	
		2. Down syndrome	
		3. Hereditary cerebral hemorrhage, Dutch	C, CV
		4. Non-traumatic cerebral hemorrhage of the elderly	
Miscellaneous amyloidoses	6. A Apo AI	Familial polyneuropathy, Iowa	N, K
	7. A Gel	Familial amyloidosis, Finnish	CN, E, skin
	8. A Cys	Hereditary cerebral hemorrhage, Icelandic	C, CV
	9. A Scr	Creutzfeldt-Jakob disease	C
	10. A Cal	Medullary carcinoma of the thyroid	Th
	11. AANF	Atrial amyloid	H
	12. AIAPP	Diabetes mellitus, insulinomas	P

B = bone; C = cerebrum; CN = cranial nerves; CV = cerebral vessels; E = eye; GI = gastrointestinal; H = heart; K = kidney; L = liver; N = nerve; P = pancreas; S = spleen; Sc = subcutaneous tissue; T = tongue; Th = thyroid; Ts = tenosynovium; Sy = synovium.

SECONDARY (AA) AMYLOIDOSIS. In this case the precursor protein is a serum component (serum amyloid A) synthesized in the liver that may increase 100- to 200-fold following an inflammatory stimulus.

Other forms of amyloid are listed in Table 19–24 and resulting diseases depend on the organ in which deposition has occurred.

TREATMENT. AL amyloidosis is treated with chemotherapy as a plasma cell neoplasm. Successful prevention and treatment of the amyloidosis of familial Mediterranean fever with low-dose colchicine 0.6 mg once or twice daily have been dramatic developments in the treatment of AA amyloidosis.

For more information about this subject, see *Cecil Textbook of Medicine,* 21st edition. Philadelphia, W.B. Saunders Company, 2000. Chapter 297, The Amyloid Diseases, pages 1538 to 1540.

GOUT

Gout refers to the *inflammatory arthritis* induced by microscopic *crystals* of monosodium urate monohydrate and to the pathognomonic deposition of aggregated monosodium urate crystals (*tophi*) in various tissues and some organs. Chronic *hyperuricemia* is necessary for the development of gout, although not sufficient (Table 19–25).

MECHANISM OF THE ACUTE GOUTY ATTACK. The neutrophil is an essential mediator of acute inflammation in gout. Gout is usually initially manifested as a fulminating arthritic attack affecting the lower extremity. Over 75% of initial attacks are monarticular; at least half involve the metatarsophalangeal joint of the great toe (podagra). Within minutes to hours the affected joint becomes

Table 19–25 ■ CLASSIFICATION OF HYPERURICEMIA AND GOUT

TYPE
Primary
I. Idiopathic (>99% of primary gout)
A. Normal urinary excretion (80–90% of primary gout)
B. Increased urinary excretion (10–20% of primary gout)
II. Due to specific inherited metabolic defects (>1% of primary gout)
A. PP-ribose-P synthase overactivity
B. Hypoxanthine-guanine phosphoribosyltransferase deficiency
Secondary
I. Glucose-6-phosphatase deficiency
II. Chronic hemolysis; erythroid, myeloid, and lymphoid proliferative disorders
III. Renal mechanisms
A. Familial progressive renal insufficiency
B. Acquired chronic, renal insufficiency
C. Drugs (diuretics; cyclosporine; toxins, including lead)
D. Endogenous metabolic products (lactate, ketoacids, β-hydroxybutyrate)

PP-ribose-P = phosphoribosylpyrophosphate.

hot, dusky red, and exquisitely tender and painful. Very severe attacks may be manifested as fever, leukocytosis, and an increased erythrocyte sedimentation rate, suggestive of infection. Once the attack has broken, recovery is generally rapid and complete. The patient then re-enters an asymptomatic phase, often termed "intercritical" or "interval" gout. Progressive inability to dispose of urate results insidiously in tophaceous crystal deposition in and around joints.

TREATMENT. Salicylates should not be used during an acute attack because of their effects on urate excretion. A general scheme for treatment of gout is set out in Table 19–26.

For more information about this subject, see *Cecil Textbook of Medicine,* 21st edition. Philadelphia, W.B. Saunders Company, 2000. Chapter 299, Gout and Uric Acid Metabolism, pages 1541 to 1548.

CRYSTAL DEPOSITION ARTHROPATHIES

At least three different calcium-containing crystals are now known to be deposited in joints and are associated with a variety of patterns of arthritis, in much the same way as urate crystals cause the various features of gouty arthritis. Definitive diagnosis is made only by aspiration of synovial fluid for identification of crystal type (Table 19–27).

For more information about this subject, see *Cecil Textbook of Medicine,* 21st edition. Philadelphia, W.B. Saunders Company, 2000. Chapter 300, Crystal Deposition Arthropathies, pages 1548 to 1550.

OSTEOARTHRITIS

Osteoarthritis is a disorder of diarthrodial joints characterized clinically by pain and functional limitations, radiographically by osteophytes and joint space narrowing, and histopathologically by alterations in cartilage integrity.

The pattern of joint involvement in osteoarthritis is strikingly affected by age, sex, and previous occupational history (Table 19–28).

TREATMENT. Because no therapy in humans is known to affect the basic disease process (inhibit cartilage degradation or enhance synthesis), medical therapy has focused on providing symptomatic relief. Reliance has been placed on pharmacologic intervention, particularly non-steroidal anti-inflammatory drugs (NSAIDs), as initial therapy at the expense of physical measures that have less morbidity and may provide longer-term benefits. The American College of Rheumatology has recently formulated evidence-based guidelines for progressive, stepwise treatment of patients with knee and hip osteoarthritis that incorporates this approach.

For more information about this subject, see *Cecil Textbook of Medicine,* 21st edition. Philadelphia, W.B. Saunders Company, 2600. Chapter 302, Osteoarthritis (Degenerative Joint Disease), pages 1550 to 1554.

Table 19–26 ■ TREATMENT OF GOUT

ACUTE GOUT	INTERVAL GOUT	LONG-TERM TREATMENT
Therapeutic goal: Terminate acute inflammatory attack.	*Therapeutic goal:* Prevent recurrent attacks.	*Therapeutic goals:* Prevent attacks, resolve tophi, maintain serum urate at ≤6 mg/dL.
NSAIDs (preferred): Indomethacin 50 mg qid, or ibuprofen, 800 mg tid (or other NSAIDs in full doses) *(lower dose in renal insufficiency; contraindicated* with *peptic ulcer disease).* *or*	*Colchicine, oral:* 0.6–1.2 mg/d as prophylaxis against recurrent attacks.	*Colchicine, oral:* 0.6–1.2 mg/d for 1–2 wk before initiating hypouricemic therapy and for several months afterward to prevent recurrent attacks during initial period of hypouricemic therapy.
Colchicine, oral (used infrequently): 0.6–1.2 mg (1–2 tablets), then 0.6 mg (1 tablet) 1–2 hr until attack subsides or until nausea, diarrhea, or GI cramping develops. Maximum total dose, 4–6 mg. If ineffective in 48 hr, do not repeat.	*Hypouricemic agent:* Start only if indicated by frequent attacks, severe hyperuricemia, presence of tophi, urolithiasis, or urate overexcretion.	*Allopurinol:* Dose variable; usually 300 mg once daily, but up to 900 mg may be needed in occasional patient; dose should be reduced to 100 mg/d or every other day in patients with renal insufficiency *or* *Uricosuric agent (reduced efficacy if creatinine clearance <80 mL; ineffective if <30 mL):* Probenecid 0.5–1 g bid, or sulfinpyrazone, 100 mg tid or qid; usually well tolerated, but may cause headache, GI upset, rash.
Colchicine, IV (only if oral medication is precluded); 1–2 mg in 20 mL 0.9% saline infused slowly *(extravasation causes tissue necrosis);* dose may be repeated once in 6 hr. Few GI symptoms with IV use. Maximum total dose, 4 mg per attack. Monitor blood counts. *Steroids (if NSAIDs or colchicine is contraindicated or if oral medication is precluded, e.g., postoperatively):* Triamcinolone acetonide 60 mg IM, *or* ACTH 40 U IM *or* 25 U by slow IV infusion, *or* prednisone, 20–40 mg/d. Intra-articular steroids may be used to treat a single inflamed joint: triamcinolone hexacetonide 5–20 mg, or dexamethasone phosphate 1–6 mg. *Hypouricemic agents:* Of no benefit for inflammatory attack and may initiate recurrent attack. Should not be started until attack has resolved, but *ongoing use should not be interrupted during an attack.*	*Other:* Diet—moderate protein, low fat; avoid excessive alcohol. Treat hypertension if present. High fluid intake to promote uric acid excretion in a dilute urine (for uric acid overexcretors).	*Other:* Diet—moderate protein, low fat; avoid excessive alcohol. Treat hypertension if present. For uric acid overexcretors or when initiating uricosuric agent: high fluid intake, particularly at night, to promote uric acid excretion in a dilute urine. Acetazolamide 250 mg at bedtime may be used to keep urine pH >6.

NSAIDs = non-steroidal anti-inflammatory drugs; GI = gastrointestinal; ACTH = adrenocorticotropic hormone.

Table 19–27 ■ DIFFERENTIAL DIAGNOSTIC FEATURES OF SOME OF THE CRYSTAL-ASSOCIATED ARTHROPATHIES

	CRYSTAL SIZE (μm)	CRYSTAL SHAPE	CRYSTAL BIREFRINGENCE AND ELONGATION	OTHER POINTS	RADIOGRAPH FINDINGS
Calcium pyrophosphate	2–20	Rods, rhomboids	Weak positive	Elderly: consider associated metabolic diseases	Chondrocalcinosis, bony sclerosis
Apatite	2–25	Chunks or globules*	Non-birefringent	Clumps stained with alizarin red S	Soft tissue calcification
Oxalate	2–15	Rods, bipyramids	Positive	Renal failure	Chondrocalcinosis or soft tissue calcification
Monosodium urate	2–20	Rods, needles	Bright negative	Middle-aged men and elderly women	Cysts and erosions; tophi may calcify
Liquid lipid crystals	2–12	Maltese crosses	Positive	Unexplained acute arthritis	
Cholesterol	10–80	Notched rectangles	Positive or negative	May complicate RA and OA	
Depot corticosteroids	4–15	Irregular or rods	Bright positive or negative	Can cause iatrogenic inflammation	
Immunoglobulins, other proteins	3–60	Rods or irregular	Positive or negative	Cryoglobulinemia	
Charcot-Leyden crystals	10–25	Spindles	Positive or negative	Eosinophilic synovitis	

RA = rheumatoid arthritis; OA = osteoarthritis.

*Aggregates are seen by light microscopy. Individual needle-shaped crystals are seen only by electron microscopy.

Table 19–28 ■ CLASSIFICATION OF OSTEOARTHRITIS

Idiopathic (Primary)

Localized
- Hands: Heberden's nodes, erosive interphalangeal arthropathy
- Feet: hallux valgus, hammer toes; talonavicular osteoarthritis
- Knees: medial, lateral, patellofemoral compartments
- Hips: sites of cartilage loss—eccentric (superior), concentric (axial, medial), diffuse
- Spine: zygapophyseal joints, osteophytes, intervertebral disks (spondylosis); ligaments, e.g., disseminated idiopathic skeletal hyperostosis
- Other single sites: shoulder, temporomandibular and carpometacarpal joints

Generalized—includes 3 or more areas listed above

Mineral deposition diseases
- Calcium pyrophosphate deposition disease
- Hydroxyapatite arthropathy
- Destructive disease (e.g., Milwaukee shoulder)

Secondary

Post-traumatic

Congenital or developmental
- Legg-Calvé-Perthes hip dislocation
- Epiphyseal dysplasias
- Articular cartilage disorders associated with a gene deficiency (e.g., association with type II procollagen gene mutation)

Disturbed local tissue structure by primary disease, e.g., ischemic necrosis, tophaceous gout, hyperparathyroid cysts, Paget's disease, rheumatoid arthritis, osteopetrosis, osteochondritis

Miscellaneous additional diseases
- Endocrine: diabetes mellitus, acromegaly, hypothyroidism
- Metabolic: hemochromatosis, ochronosis, Gaucher's disease
- Neuropathic arthropathies
- Miscellaneous: frostbite, Kashin-Bek disease, caisson disease
- Mechanical: obesity, unequal lower extremity length; valgus/varus deformities, ligamentous laxity (including associations with type I procollagen gene mutations of Ehlers-Danlos syndrome)

Compiled in part by the Osteoarthritis Diagnostic Criteria Committee, American Rheumatism Association, 1983.

SYSTEMIC DISEASES IN WHICH ARTHRITIS IS A FEATURE

Arthralgias may represent early symptoms of systemic diseases that could be diagnosed only by the appearance of other clinical signs or by laboratory testing (Table 19–29).

For more information about this subject, see *Cecil Textbook of Medicine,* 21st edition. Philadelphia, W.B. Saunders Company, 2000. Chapter 304, Systemic Diseases in Which Arthritis is a Feature, pages 1556 to 1558.

Table 19–29 ■ LABORATORY TESTS IN THE EVALUATION OF NON-SPECIFIC JOINT SYMPTOMS

TEST	DISEASE
Liver function tests	Primary biliary cirrhosis; hepatitis B and C; chronic active hepatitis
Calcium and phosphorus	Hyperparathyroidism
Serum protein electrophoresis	Hypogammaglobulinemic arthritis; primary amyloidosis; hyperimmunoglobulin D
Serum iron and total iron-binding capacity; ferritin	Hemochromatosis
Lipase or amylase	Pancreatic-arthritis syndrome
Thyroid-stimulating hormone; thyroxine	Thyroid myopathy or arthritis
Complete blood cell count	Leukemia; sickle cell disease
Lipid analysis	Hyperlipidemia-associated arthritis
Partial thromboplastin time; rapid plasma reagin (RPR) or VDRL	Hemophilia Syphilis
Anti–human immunodeficiency virus (HIV)	HIV arthritis
Antiparvovirus antibody	Parvovirus arthritis

CHAPTER 20

INFECTIOUS DISEASES

THE FEBRILE PATIENT

Most febrile patients with a localized infection have pain, tenderness, redness, and swelling at the site of inflammation, and the cause of the fever is readily identified.

FEVER OF UNEXPLAINED ORIGIN. An *unexplained fever* is usually defined in adults as an illness lasting more than 3 weeks with temperatures greater than 101° F (38.3° C) in which a diagnosis has not been made despite a good hospital or office evaluation (Table 20–1).

Table 20–1 ■ CAUSES OF FEVER OF UNKNOWN ORIGIN

Infections
- Abscesses—hepatic, subhepatic, gallbladder, subphrenic, splenic, periappendiceal, perinephric, pelvic, and other sites
- Granulomatous—extrapulmonary and miliary tuberculosis, atypical mycobacterial infection, fungal infection
- Intravascular—catheter-related endocarditis, meningococcemia, gonococcemia, *Listeria, Brucella,* rat-bite fever, relapsing fever
- Viral, rickettsial, and chlamydial—infectious mononucleosis, cytomegalovirus, human immunodeficiency virus, hepatitis, Q fever, psittacosis
- Parasitic—extraintestinal amebiasis, malaria, toxoplasmosis

Non-infectious inflammatory disorders
- Collagen-vascular diseases—rheumatic fever, systemic lupus erythematosus, rheumatoid arthritis (particularly Still's disease), vasculitis (all types)
- Granulomatous—sarcoidosis, granulomatous hepatitis, Crohn's disease
- Tissue injury—pulmonary emboli, sickle cell disease, hemolytic anemia

Neoplastic diseases
- Lymphoma/leukemia—Hodgkin's and non-Hodgkin's lymphoma, acute leukemia, myelodysplastic syndrome
- Carcinoma—kidney, pancreas, liver, gastrointestinal tract, lung, especially when metastatic
- Atrial myxomas
- Central nervous system tumors

Drug fevers
- Sulfonamides, penicillins, thiouracils, barbiturates, quinidine, laxatives (especially with phenolphthalein)

Factitious illnesses
- Injections of toxic material, manipulation or exchange of thermometers

Other causes
- Familial Mediterranean fever, Fabry's disease, cyclic neutropenia

---

For more information about this subject, see *Cecil Textbook of Medicine,* 21st edition. Philadelphia, W.B. Saunders Company, 2000. Part XXII: Infectious Diseases, pages 1563 to 1888.

For more information about this subject, see *Cecil Textbook of Medicine,* 21st edition. Philadelphia, W.B. Saunders Company, 2000. Chapter 311, The Febrile Patient, pages 1564 to 1565.

THE COMPROMISED HOST

"Compromised host" is used to describe patients who have an increased risk for infectious complications as a consequence of a congenital or acquired qualitative or quantitative abnormality in one or more components of the host defense matrix (Table 20–2).

Initial Management of the Neutropenic Patient Who Becomes Febrile

Although gram-negative bacteria still predominate at some institutions, in recent years the trend has been toward more gram-positive infections, which now represent the majority of isolates at many centers. In general, gram-negative infections tend to be more virulent, and early empiric regimens have been formulated to provide protection primarily against these organisms while maintaining a broad spectrum of activity against other potential pathogens.

Although no single best regimen or recipe is known, a number of options are appropriate. Selection of a specific antibiotic regimen depends on many factors, including institutional sensitivity patterns, individual and institutional experience, and clinical variables (Table 20–3).

For more information about this subject, see *Cecil Textbook of Medicine,* 21st edition. Philadelphia, W.B. Saunders Company, 2000. Chapter 314, The Compromised Host, pages 1569 to 1581.

NOSOCOMIAL INFECTIONS

The word *nosocomial* is derived from the Greek *nosos* (disease) and *komeion* (to take care of) and is defined as "belonging or pertaining to a hospital." Infections acquired within a hospital or other health care facility have therefore been termed *nosocomial infections.*

Nosocomial pathogens can originate from either endogenous or exogenous sources. Endogenous pathogens originate from the commensal flora of the patient's skin or gastrointestinal or respiratory tract. Exogenous pathogens are transmitted to the patient from external sources after admission to the hospital (Table 20–4).

For more information about this subject, see *Cecil Textbook of Medicine,* 21st edition. Philadelphia, W.B. Saunders Company, 2000. Chapter 315, Nosocomial Infections, pages 1581 to 1586.

ADVICE TO TRAVELERS

Millions of North Americans and Europeans travel to developing areas of the world each year. Modern air transportation has brought even the most exotic sites within easy reach. Most travelers go for vacation or business and are away for a few weeks or less, but some spend extended periods abroad. In addition, thousands of American troops are deployed at various times in tropical or devel-

Text continues on page 565

Table 20–2 ■ PREDOMINANT PATHOGENS IN COMPROMISED PATIENTS; ASSOCIATION WITH SELECTED DEFECTS IN HOST DEFENSE

HOST DEFENSE IMPAIRMENT/PHAGOCYTIC DYSFUNCTION	BACTERIA	FUNGI	VIRUSES	OTHER
Neutropenia	Gram-negative Enteric organisms *Escherichia coli, Klebsiella pneumoniae, Enterobacter* spp., *Citrobacter* spp. *Pseudomonas aeruginosa* Gram-positive Staphylococci Coagulase-negative, coagulase-positive Streptococci, including viridans enterococci Anaerobes Anaerobic streptococci, *Clostridium* spp., *Bacteroides* spp.	*Candida* spp. *C. albicans* > *C. Tropicalis* > other species *Aspergillus* spp. *A. fumigatus, A. flavus* Other opportunistic fungi *Mucor, Trichosporon*		
Abnormal cell-mediated immunity	*Legionella* *Nocardia asteroides* *Salmonella* spp. Mycobacteria *M. tuberculosis* and atypical mycobacteria Disseminated infection from live bacteria vaccine (BCG)	*Cryptococcus neoformans* *Histoplasma capsulatum* *Coccidioides immitis* *Candida*	Varicella-zoster virus Herpes simplex virus Cytomegalovirus Epstein-Barr virus Herpesvirus 6 Disseminated infection from live virus vaccines (vaccinia, measles, rubella, mumps, yellow fever, live polio)	*Pneumocystis carinii* *Toxoplasma gondii* *Cryptosporidium* *Strongyloides stercoralis*

Immunoglobulin abnormalities	Gram-positive *Streptococcus pneumoniae, Staphylococcus aureus* Gram-negative *Haemophilus influenzae* *Neisseria* spp., enteric organisms		Enteroviruses Disseminated infection from live virus vaccines (vaccinia, measles, rubella, mumps, yellow fever, polio)	*Giardia lamblia*
Complement abnormalities				
C3, C5	Gram-positive *S. pneumoniae,* staphylococci Gram-negative *H. influenzae, Neisseria* spp., Enteric organisms			
C5–C9	*Neisseria* spp. *N. gonorrhoeae, N. meningitidis*			
Anatomic disruption				
Oral cavity	α-Hemolytic streptococci, oral anaerobes *Peptococcus, Peptostreptococcus*	*Candida*	Herpes simplex virus	
Esophagus	Staphylococci, other colonizing organisms	*Candida*	Herpes simplex virus Cytomegalovirus	
Lower gastrointestinal tract	Gram-positive Enterococci Gram-negative Enteric organisms Anaerobes *(Bacteroides fragilis, Clostridium perfringens)*	*Candida*		*S. stercoralis*

Table continued on following page

Table 20–2 ■ PREDOMINANT PATHOGENS IN COMPROMISED PATIENTS; ASSOCIATION WITH SELECTED DEFECTS IN HOST DEFENSE *Continued*

HOST DEFENSE IMPAIRMENT/PHAGOCYTIC DYSFUNCTION	BACTERIA	FUNGI	VIRUSES	OTHER
Skin (IV catheter)	Gram-positive Staphylococci, streptococci *Corynebacterium, Bacillus* spp. Gram-negative *P. aeruginosa,* enteric organisms Mycobacteria *M. fortuitum, M. chelonei*	*Candida* *Aspergillus*		
Urinary tract	Gram-positive Enterococci Gram-negative Enteric organisms *P. aeruginosa*	*Candida*		
Splenectomy	Gram-positive *S. pneumoniae* Gram-negative *Capnocytophaga* *H. influenzae* *Salmonella* (sickle cell disease)			*Babesia*

BCG = bacille Calmette-Guérin.

From Rubin M, Walsh TJ, Pizzo PA: Clinical approach to the compromised host. *In* Hoffman R, Benz EJ Jr, Shattil SJ, et al (eds): Hematology: Basic Principles and Practices, 2nd ed. New York, Churchill Livingstone, 1994.

Table 20–3 ■ MEDICATIONS IN PATIENTS WITH NEUTROPENIA

AGENT	COMMENTS
Antibiotic	
Third-generation cephalosporins	Only ceftazidime and cefepime are appropriate for coverage of *Pseudomonas aeruginosa.*
Carbapenems	If *P. Aeruginosa* is suspected or cultured, an aminoglycoside should be added.
Extended-spectrum penicillins	Because of the potential for resistance, piperacillin, azlocillin, or mezlocillin should be administered with either an aminoglycoside or a third-generation cephalosporin.
Monobactams	Aztreonam is an important alternative for patients allergic to β-lactam antibiotics, but it should be combined with vancomycin for empiric therapy.
Quinolones	Important for gram-negative infection and possibly for use in low-risk patients with neutropenia; to avoid resistance, do not use for prophylaxis.
Vancomycin	Pathogen-directed therapy generally suffices. Empiric use can be restricted to centers with a high incidence of methicillin-resistant *Staphylococcus aureus.* Of concern, strains of vancomycin-resistant enterococci have been described.
Antifungal	
Amphotericin B	Still the best treatment. A dose of 0.6 mg/kg body weight per day suffices for *Candida albicans* and *Cryptococcus,* 1 mg/kg/d is preferred for *Candida tropicalis,* and 1.5 mg/kg/d is preferred for *Aspergillus.*
Lipid preparations of amphotericin	Similar to and slightly greater benefit than amphotericin B with less toxicity albeit more expense.
Ketoconazole	Not an alternative to amphotericin B for empiric therapy. Useful for thrush or esophagitis.
Fluconazole	Very effective for thrush or esophagitis. Of value for systemic mycoses, including hepatosplenic candidiasis; requires additional study.
Itraconazole	Activity against *Aspergillus,* although absorption can be unpredictable.
Antiviral	
Acyclovir	Oral therapy is not advised for severely immunocompromised patients with varicella-zoster infections. For such patients, parenteral therapy (1500 mg/m^2 of body surface area per day in 3 divided doses) is indicated. For patients with herpes simplex, oral or parenteral therapy (750 mg/m^2/d in 3 divided doses) is satisfactory.
Ganciclovir	Of value for cytomegalovirus retinitis, prevention of pneumonitis, and combined with an IV immunoglobulin for pneumonitis.
Foscarnet	Of value for cytomegalovirus retinitis in patients in whom ganciclovir is ineffective.
Antiparasitic	
Trimethoprim-sulfamethoxazole	Best drug for *Pneumocystis carinii* prophylaxis. Not required in all cancer patients. Thrice-weekly schedule is satisfactory (150 mg/m^2/d in 2 divided doses).
Aerosolized pentamidine	Expensive and not as effective as trimethoprim-sulfamethoxazole in adults with HIV infection.

Modified from Pizzo PA: Management of fever in patients with cancer and treatment-induced neutropenia. N Engl J Med 328:1323, 1993. Copyright by the Massachusetts Medical Society.

Table 20–4 ■ PER CENT DISTRIBUTION OF NOSOCOMIAL PATHOGENS BY INFECTION SITE

PATHOGEN*	ALL INFECTION SITES	URINARY TRACT	SURGICAL SITE	BLOOD STREAM	PNEUMONIA	OTHER
Staphylococcus aureus	13	2	20	16	19	18
Escherichia coli	12	24	8	5	4	4
Coagulase-negative staphylococci	11	4	14	31	2	14
Enterococcus spp.	10	16	12	9	2	5
Pseudomonas aeruginosa	9	11	8	3	17	7
Enterobacter spp.	6	5	7	4	11	4
Candida albicans	5	8	3	5	5	4
Klebsiella pneumoniae	5	8	3	5	8	3
Gram-positive anaerobes	4	0	1	1	0	19
Proteus mirabilis	3	5	3	1	2	2

*Pathogens with fewer than 1% of the isolates at all sites are not shown.

oping areas. Proper immunization is essential (Table 20–5). Malaria continues to pose a threat travelers to endemic tropical areas, for whom chemoprophylaxis remains necessary (Table 20–6).

For more information about this subject, see *Cecil Textbook of Medicine,* 21st edition. Philadelphia, W.B. Saunders Company, 2000. Chapter 316, Advice to Travelers, pages 1586 to 1589.

ANTIBACTERIAL THERAPY

Modern antibacterial therapy has markedly reduced the morbidity and mortality of infections, has prevented disease, and has contributed significantly to the development of modern surgery, trauma therapy, and organ transplantation. The broad application of antimicrobial agents in modern medicine has not, however, been problem-free. These agents occasionally cause major adverse reactions, interact with other classes of pharmacologic agents, and exert a major selective pressure for widespread antimicrobial resistance among bacteria (Table 20–7).

For more information about this subject, see *Cecil Textbook of Medicine,* 21st edition. Philadelphia, W.B. Saunders Company, 2000. Chapter 318, Antibacterial Therapy, pages 1591 to 1603.

Table 20–5 ■ IMMUNIZATION OF INTERNATIONAL TRAVELERS

Routine vaccines that should be up-to-date in all travelers
Diphtheria-tetanus
Pertussis (children <7 yr)
Poliomyelitis
Measles
Mumps
Rubella
Haemophilus influenzae (children)
Hepatitis B
Varicella
Vaccines indicated in special populations
Influenza
Pneumococcal
*Vaccines potentially indicated for travelers to developing areas**
Cholera (seldom used)
Hepatitis A (or serum immune globulin)
Japanese B encephalitis
Meningococcus
Poliomyelitis
Rabies
Typhoid
Yellow fever†

*The choice of specific vaccines depends on the itinerary, activities, and duration of travel, as well as cost, efficacy, and potential side effects of the vaccines.

†Required for entry by some countries. See Centers for Disease Control and Prevention: CDC Health Information for International Travel 1999. HHS Publication No. (CDC) 99-8280. Atlanta.

20

Table 20–6 ■ CHEMOPROPHYLAXIS FOR MALARIA*

Travelers to areas with chloroquine sensitive Plasmodium *species*
Chloroquine phosphate 300 mg base (500 mg salt) PO once a week†
Travelers to areas with chloroquine resistance
Mefloquine, 250 mg PO once a week†
or
Doxycycline, 100 mg/d PO†
Prevention of late relapses with Plasmodium vivax *and* Plasmodium ovale‡
Primaquine phosphate 15 mg base (26.3 mg salt) PO each day for 14 d

*Insect repellents, insecticide-impregnated bed nets, and proper clothing are important adjuncts for preventing malaria. Chloroquine has been used extensively and safely in pregnancy, but other prophylactic medications are either contraindicated during pregnancy (doxycycline and primaquine) or their safety is uncertain (mefloquine). No prophylactic regimen guarantees protection, and travelers should be warned about the possibility of malaria during travel or after return.

†Adult dose: start 1 week before departure with chloroquine and mefloquine, 1 to 2 days before with doxycycline, continue during travel and for 4 weeks after return.

‡Occasional relapses have been reported with this regimen. Some experts prescribe primaquine during the last 2 weeks of malaria prophylaxis for travelers with prolonged exposure to *P. vivax* or *P. ovale*. Others avoid primaquine and rely on early detection and treatment of *P. vivax* or *P. ovale* malaria if it occurs.

PNEUMOCOCCAL PNEUMONIA

Pneumococcal pneumonia is an acute, suppurative infection of the lungs produced by an encapsulated bacterium, *Streptococcus pneumoniae* (pneumococcus). It is the most commonly occurring bacterial pneumonia in the world; in the United States, an estimated 150,000 to 570,000 cases occur annually (Table 20–8).

Invasion of the blood stream by pneumococci may lead to serious metastatic disease at a number of extrapulmonary sites (Table 20–9).

The peripheral white blood cell (WBC) count is often two to three times the normal value; however, in alcoholic or immunosuppressed patients, it may be normal or low. Of more value is the WBC differential, which consists predominantly of bands and polymorphonuclear leukocytes (left shift).

Treatment

All patients with suspected pneumococcal pneumonia should be treated as promptly as possible with an effective antimicrobial agent. One should not wait for cultural confirmation of the diagnosis to initiate therapy.

Blood and tissue levels of penicillin G in excess of the minimum inhibitory concentration (MIC) for susceptible strains (<0.1 μg/mL) are easily achieved with doses of 1.2 to 2.4 million U/day. If the infecting strain is of intermediate resistance (MIC ≥ 0.1 to <2.0 μg/mL), as are 15% of isolates, penicillin G can still be used successfully; however, doses approximating 6 to 12 million U/day need to be used, or treat with fluoroquinolone. For patients who are believed to be allergic to penicillin, one may select a first- or second-generation cephalosporin or erythromycin, clindamycin, or a fluoroquinolone.

Text continues on page 571

Table 20–7 ■ PHARMACOLOGIC PROPERTIES OF COMMONLY USED ANTIBIOTICS

CLASS/AGENT	DOSE (ROUTE)*	ORAL FORMU-LATION	PEAK SERUM CONCENTRA-TION (μg/mL)	PROTEIN BINDING (%)	NORMAL SERUM HALF-LIFE (hr)	DOSE ADJUSTMENT		SERUM LEVELS AFFECTED BY DIALYSIS
	Systemic Infection					Hepatic Failure	Renal Failure	
Aminoglycosides								
Amikacin	5–7 mg/kg q8h	—	35	0	2–3	No	Major	Yes (H, P)
Gentamicin	1.7 mg/kg q8h	—	7	0	2–3	No	Major	Yes (H, P)
Netilmicin	1.7 mg/kg q8h	—	7	0	2–3	No	Major	Yes (H, P)
Tobramycin	1.7 mg/kg q8h	—	7	0	2–3	No	Major	Yes (H, P)
Antituberculous Agents								
Ethambutol	15 mg/kg/d (PO)	Yes	2	10	1.5	No	Major	Yes (H, P)
Isoniazid	5 mg/kg/d (PO)	Yes	4.5	10	3	Yes	Minor	Yes (H, P)
Pyrazinamide	10 mg/kg q8h (PO)	Yes	39	—	10	Yes	Yes	Yes (H)
Rifampin	10 mg/kg/d (PO)	Yes	7	70	3	Yes	Minor	No (H)
First-Generation Cephalosporins								
Cefadroxil	15 mg/kg q12 hr (PO)	Yes	16	20	1.2	No	Yes	Yes (H)
Cefazolin	15 mg/kg q8h	—	80	80	2	No	Major	Yes (H), No (P)
Cephalexin	7 mg/kg q6h (PO)	Yes	18	15	1	No	Yes	Yes (H, P)
Cephapirin	30 mg/kg q6h	—	150	50	0.6	No	Yes	Yes (H, P)
Cephradine	30 mg/kg q6h	Yes†	140	10	0.7	No	Yes	Yes (H, P)
Second-Generation Cephalosporins								
Cefaclor	7 mg/kg q6h (PO)	Yes†	13	20	1	No	Yes	Yes (H)
Cefmetazole	30 mg/kg q12h	—	140	65	1.1	No	Yes	Yes (H)
Cefotetan	30 mg/kg q12h	—	230	85	3	No	Major	Yes (H)
Cefoxitin	30 mg/kg q6h	—	150	70	0.7	No	Yes	Yes (H), No (P)
Cefprozil	15 mg/kg q12h (PO)	Yes	10	42	1.2	No	Yes	Yes (H)
Cefuroxime	15–20 mg/kg q12h	—	100	50	1.5	No	Yes	Yes (H, P)
Cefuroxime axetil	7.5 mg/kg q12h (PO)	Yes	9	50	1.2	No	Yes	Yes (H, P)

Table continued on following page

Table 20–7 ■ PHARMACOLOGIC PROPERTIES OF COMMONLY USED ANTIBIOTICS *Continued*

CLASS/AGENT	DOSE (ROUTE)*	ORAL FORMU-LATION	PEAK SERUM CONCENTRA-TION (μg/mL)	PROTEIN BINDING (%)	NORMAL SERUM HALF-LIFE (hr)	DOSE ADJUSTMENT		SERUM LEVELS AFFECTED BY DIALYSIS
	Systemic Infection					Hepatic Failure	Renal Failure	
Third-Generation Cephalosporins								
Cefepime	30 mg/kg q12h	—	193	20	2.1	No	Yes	Yes (H, P)
Cefixime	8 mg/kg/d (PO)	Yes	3.9	67	3.7	No	Yes	No (H, P)
Ceftibuten	3–5 mg/kg q12h (PO)	Yes	9.9	60	2.5	No	Yes	Yes (H)
Cefdinir	5–7 mg/kg q12h (PO)	Yes	2.9	60	1.7	No	Yes	Yes (H)
Cefotaxime	30 mg/kg q6h	—	130	50	1.2	Some	Minor	Yes (H), No (P)
Cefpodoxime proxetil	3–6 mg/kg q12h (PO)	Yes	3.9	25	2.5	No	Yes	Yes (H)
Ceftazidime	30 mg/kg q8h	—	160	60	2	No	Major	Yes (H, P)
Ceftizoxime	30 mg/kg q6–8h	—	130	50	1.3	No	Minor	Yes (H), No (P)
Ceftriaxone	30 mg/kg q12–24h	—	250	90	8	No	No	No (H)
Penicillins								
Amoxicillin	7 mg/kg q6h (PO)	Yes	6	20	1	No	Yes	Yes (H), No (P)
Ampicillin	30 mg/kg q6h	Yes†	100	20	1	No	Yes	Yes (H), No (P)
Cloxacillin	7 mg/kg q6h (PO)	Yes†	9	95	0.5	No	No	No (H, P)
Dicloxacillin	7 mg/kg q6h (PO)	Yes†	18	97	0.5	No	No	No (H, P)
Mezlocillin	50 mg/kg q6h	—	260	50	1	Yes	Major	Yes (H), No (P)
Nafcillin	30 mg/kg q4–6h	—	160	90	0.5	Yes	No	No (H, P)
Oxacillin	30 mg/kg q4–6h	—	200	90	0.5	Yes	No	Yes (H, P)
Penicillin G	3–4 million U q4–6h	Yes†	60	60	0.5	No	Yes	Yes (H), No (P)
Penicillin V	7 mg/kg q6h (PO)	Yes	4	80	1	No	No	Yes (H), No (P)
Piperacillin	40 mg/kg q6h	—	240	50	1	Minor	Major	Yes (H)
Ticarcillin	40 mg/kg q4–6h	—	220	50	1	Minor	Major	Yes (H, P)

Quinolones								
Ciprofloxacin	7 mg/kg q12h (PO)	Yes†	2.0–2.8	30	3	No	Yes	No (H, P)
Lomefloxacin	6 mg/kg q24h	Yes	4	10	8		Yes	No (H, P)
Ofloxacin	6 mg/kg q12h	Yes†	3–5	30	7		Yes	No (H, P)
Levofloxacin	7 mg/kg q24h	Yes	5.7	35	6–8	No	Yes	No (H, P)
Sparfloxacin	400 mg load, 200 mg q24h (PO)	Yes	1.3	45	16–20	No	Yes	No (H)
Grepafloxacin	8.5 mg/kg q24h (PO)	Yes	2.4	50	12	Yes	No	No (H, P)
Trovafloxacin	3–4 mg/kg q24h	Yes	3.1	70	12	Yes	No	No (H, P)
Tetracyclines								
Doxycycline	1.5 mg/kg q12–24h	Yes	1.8–2.9	90	15–20	Avoid	No	No (H, P)
Minocycline	1.5 mg/kg q12–24h	Yes	2.2	90	15	No	Avoid	No (H, P)
Tetracycline	7 mg/kg q6h	Yes†	4	50	7	Avoid	Avoid	No (H, P)
Sulfonamides								
Sulfadiazine	15 mg/kg q6h	Yes	30	50	3	Avoid	Avoid	Unknown
Sulfamethoxazole	12 mg/kg q8h (IV)	Yes	100	50	6	Avoid	Major	Yes (H), No (P)
Trimethoprim (used with sulfamethoxazole)	2.3 mg/kg q8–12h (IV)	Yes	3–9	60	10	No	Avoid	Yes (H), No (P)
Macrolides-Lincosamides								
Azithromycin	4 mg/kg q24h (PO)	Yes†	0.4	50	57 (tissue)	Unknown	Unknown	Unknown
Clarithromycin	7.5 mg/kg q12h (PO)	Yes	2–3	70	7	No	Yes	Yes (H), No (P)
Clindamycin	7 mg/kg q6h	Yes	15	90	2.5	Some	No	No (H, P)
Erythromycin	7 mg/kg q6h (PO)	Yes†	1.8	20	1.5	Some	No	No (H, P)

Table continued on following page

Table 20–7 ■ PHARMACOLOGIC PROPERTIES OF COMMONLY USED ANTIBIOTICS *Continued*

CLASS/AGENT	DOSE (ROUTE)* Systemic Infection	ORAL FORMU-LATION	PEAK SERUM CONCENTRA-TION (μg/mL)	PROTEIN BINDING (%)	NORMAL SERUM HALF-LIFE (hr)	DOSE ADJUSTMENT Hepatic Failure	DOSE ADJUSTMENT Renal Failure	SERUM LEVELS AFFECTED BY DIALYSIS
Other Agents								
Aztreonam	30 mg/kg q8h	—	250	60	2.0	No	Major	Yes (H, P)
Chloramphenicol	7–15 mg/kg q6h (PO)	Yes	8–14	30	1.5	Some	No	Yes (H), No (P)
Imipenem	7.5 mg/kg q6h	—	40	15	1	No	Avoid	Yes (H)
Loracarbef	15 mg/kg q12h (PO)	Yes†	18	25	1.2	No	Yes	Yes (H)
Meropenem	15 mg/kg q8h	—	40		1.0	Unknown	Yes	Yes (H)
Metronidazole	7 mg/kg q6h	Yes	25	20	8	Yes	No	Yes (H), No (P)
Nitrofurantoin	1 mg/kg q6h (PO)	Yes	Nil	60	0.3	No	Avoid	Yes (H)
Spectinomycin	30 mg/kg/d	—	100	0	2	No	Avoid	Unknown
Vancomycin	15 mg/kg q12h	Yes‡	35	10	6	No	Major	No (H, P)
Quinupristin-dalfopristin (30:70)	7.5 mg/kg q8h	—	2.5/6.8§	90/30	0.8/0.6§	Some	No	No (P)

H = hemodialysis; P = peritoneal dialysis.

*Milligrams per kilogram body weight at hour intervals in patients with normal renal function; all doses are parenteral unless specified PO.

†Do not administer with food—absorption is decreased or delayed.

‡Orally administered vancomycin is not absorbed; gastrointestinal tract lumen therapy only.

§Extensive non-enzymatic degradation to active metabolites that are not included.

Table 20–8 ■ RISK FACTORS OR UNDERLYING CONDITIONS PREDISPOSING TO THE DEVELOPMENT OF PNEUMOCOCCAL PNEUMONIA OR SERIOUS PNEUMOCOCCAL INFECTIONS

Age (extremes)
Alcoholism
Bone marrow transplantation
Bronchiectasis
Cerebrovascular occlusions or severe neurologic impairment
Chronic bronchitis
Chronic lymphocytic leukemia
Chronic obstructive pulmonary disease
Cirrhosis or chronic liver disease
Complement deficiency (particularly C′3 and C′4)
Conditions associated with aspiration (e.g., seizures)
Congestive heart failure
Dementia
Diabetes mellitus
Immunologic deficiencies (acquired, hereditary, or iatrogenic)—humoral (IgG or IgA) or cellular (e.g., AIDS)
Institutionalization, homelessness, day care centers
Malignancy (particularly solid tumors of the lung)
Multiple myeloma
Nephrotic syndrome
Neutropenia
Smoking
Splenic dysfunction (e.g., in sickle cell disease) or asplenia
Viral disease, especially influenza

AIDS = acquired immunodeficiency syndrome.

Complications

Empyema develops in approximately 5% of patients with pneumococcal pneumonia, although sterile pleural effusion commonly develops in a larger percentage (up to 30%).

If pneumococcal bacteremia occurs, extrapulmonary complications such as *meningitis, septic arthritis,* and *endocarditis* must be

Table 20–9 ■ CONCURRENT OR COMPLICATING PNEUMOCOCCAL INFECTIONS OCCURRING IN PNEUMOCOCCAL PNEUMONIA

Otitis media
Sinusitis/mastoiditis
Conjunctivitis (suppurative)
Epiglottiditis
Tracheobronchitis
Pleuritis (empyema)
Soft tissue cellulitis (Ludwig's angina)
Pericarditis*
Endocarditis*
Meningitis*
Arthritis (septic)*
Peritonitis (in presence of ascites)*

*Usually blood-borne.

Table 20–10 ■ HUMAN MYCOPLASMA SPECIES

ESTABLISHED PATHOGENS	OPPORTUNISTS	COMMENSALS
M. pneumoniae	*M. salivarium*	*M. buccale*
M. hominis	*M. orale*	*M. faucium*
M. fermentans	*M. genitalium*	*M. lipophilum*
M. urealyticum	*M. pirum*	*M. primatum*
	M. penetrans	*M. spermatophilum*
	M. arginini	*A. laidawii**
	M. felis	*A. oculi**
	M. edwardii	

**Acholeplasma* species.

excluded because their therapy generally requires higher dosages of antibiotics and, in the case of septic arthritis, may require drainage. A spinal tap with examination of cerebrospinal fluid (CSF) should be done if meningitis is suspected, and multiple pre-treatment blood cultures and echocardiography of the heart valves should be obtained if endocarditis is suspected.

The case fatality rate for untreated pneumococcal pneumonia is about 25%, whereas in those treated promptly with an appropriate antibiotic, it may be less than 5%.

For more information about this subject, see *Cecil Textbook of Medicine,* 21st edition. Philadelphia, W.B. Saunders Company, 2000. Chapter 319, Pneumococcal Pneumonia, pages 1603 to 1609.

MYCOPLASMAL INFECTION

The mycoplasmas associated with humans include species from the genera *Mycoplasma, Ureaplasma,* and *Acholeplasma* (Table 20–10). Most patients with *Mycoplasma pneumoniae* infection are older children, adolescents, and young adults with a minor respiratory illness.

Mycoplasma hominis is a commensal of the genitourinary tract, especially in women. It is seen in up to 50% of sexually active

Table 20–11 ■ ANTIBIOTIC SUSCEPTIBILITY

MYCOPLASMA	ERY	TCN	CLN	QUN
M. pneumoniae	sens	sens	res	sens*
M. fermentans	res†	sens	sens	sens
M. hominis	res	sens‡	sens	sens*
U. urealyticum	sens‡	sens‡	res	sens

ERY = erythromycin; TCN = tetracycline; CLN = clindamycin; QUN = quinolones; sens = sensitive; res = resistant.

*Sensitivity to quinolones is adequate for the earlier quinolones, e.g., ciprofloxacin and ofloxacin, but it is greatest for newer agents of this class, e.g., sparfloxacin and trovafloxacin.

†Sensitive to azithromycin and clarithromycin.

‡Some resistance seen.

women and 30% of sexually active men. Antibiotic susceptibility is noted in Table 20–11.

For more information about this subject, see *Cecil Textbook of Medicine,* 21st edition. Philadelphia, W.B. Saunders Company, 2000. Chapter 320, Mycoplasmal Infection, pages 1609 to 1612.

PNEUMONIA CAUSED BY AEROBIC GRAM-NEGATIVE BACILLI

Gram-negative enteric bacilli (GNB) rarely cause pneumonia in previously healthy hosts. These organisms are not highly virulent respiratory pathogens but strike instead individuals whose defense mechanisms have been diminished by acute or chronic disease. The typical patient would be in an intensive-care unit (ICU), intubated, and receiving mechanical ventilation after surgery, trauma, or life-threatening illness (Table 20–12).

For more information about this subject, see *Cecil Textbook of Medicine,* 21st edition. Philadelphia, W.B. Saunders Company, 2000. Chapter 321, Pneumonia Caused by Aerobic Gram-Negative Bacilli, pages 1612 to 1615.

LEGIONELLOSIS

"Legionellosis" is the term used to describe infections caused by bacteria of the genus *Legionella.* The most important of these diseases is pneumonia, called "legionnaires' disease."

Legionnaires' disease is acquired by inhaling aerosolized water containing *Legionella* organisms or possibly by pulmonary aspiration of contaminated water. The contaminated aerosols are derived

Table 20–12 ■ EMPIRIC ANTIBIOTIC THERAPY FOR AEROBIC GRAM-NEGATIVE BACILLARY PNEUMONIA*

Monotherapy

Consider in mild to moderately ill patients in whom *Pseudomonas aeruginosa* is unlikely.

Cefuroxime 1.5 g q8h
Cefotaxime 2 g q8h
Ticarcillin/clavulanate 3.1 g q4h
Piperacillin/tazobactam 4.5 g q6h
Ciprofloxacin 400 mg q12h
Alatrofloxacin, 300 mg q24h

Combination Therapy

Consider in patients with severe illness, immunosuppression, neutropenia, and those with a high likelihood of *P. Aeruginosa*

Aminoglycoside† or ciprofloxacin 400 mg q12h, plus one of the following:

- Ceftazidime 2 g q8h
- Cefepime 2 g q12h
- Piperacillin/tazobactam 4.5 g q6h
- Imipenem/cilastatin 500 mg q6h
- Aztreonam 2 g q8h

Ciprofloxacin 400 mg q12h plus aminoglycoside

*Recommendations for adults with normal renal function.

†Dosages of 5 mg/kg/24 hrs for gentamicin and tobramycin; 15 mg/kg/24 hours for amikacin.

20

Table 20–13 ■ RISK FACTORS FOR LEGIONNAIRES' DISEASE

Altered Local and Systemic Host Defenses
Glucocorticosteroid administration or Cushing's disease (5–10)*
Cytotoxic chemotherapy (5)
Cigarette smoking (2–5)
Diabetes (2)
Male sex or age >50 yr (>2)
AIDS (40)
Immunosuppressive therapy for solid organ transplantation (>2)
Chronic heart or lung disease (>1)
Renal failure requiring dialysis (20)
Lung or hematologic cancer (especially hairy cell leukemia) (7–20)
Increased Chance of Exposure to Environmental *Legionella* Bacteria
Recent travel away from home (2)
Use of domestic well water (2)
Recent plumbing work in home or at work (2)
Exposure to poorly maintained hot tub spas
Recent surgical procedure

*Numbers in parentheses represent the approximate relative risk of acquiring legionnaires' disease over that for someone without the risk, where known.

from humidifiers, shower heads, respiratory therapy equipment, industrial cooling water, and cooling towers (Table 20–13). Erythromycin is the drug of choice (Table 20–14).

For more information about this subject, see Cecil Textbook of Medicine, 21st edition. Philadelphia, W.B. Saunders Company, 2000. Chapter 323, Legionellosis, pages 1616 to 1619.

STREPTOCOCCAL INFECTIONS

Group A Streptococcal Infections

PHARYNGITIS AND THE ASYMPTOMATIC CARRIER. Patients with streptococcal pharyngitis have an abrupt onset of sore throat, submandibular adenopathy, fever, and chilliness, but not usually frank rigors. Cough and hoarseness are rare, but pain on swallowing is characteristic.

SCARLET FEVER. During the last 30 to 40 years, outbreaks of scarlet fever in the Western world have been notably mild, and the illness has been referred to as "pharyngitis with a rash" or "benign scarlet fever."

ERYSIPELAS. Erysipelas is caused exclusively by *Streptococcus pyogenes* and is characterized by an abrupt onset of fiery red swelling of the face or extremities. Distinctive features are well-defined margins, particularly along the nasolabial fold, scarlet or salmon-red rash, rapid progression, and intense pain.

STREPTOCOCCAL PYODERMA (IMPETIGO CONTAGIOSA). Impetigo is most common in patients with poor hygiene or malnutrition. Colonization of the unbroken skin occurs first, and then

Table 20–14 ■ ANTIMICROBIAL DRUG THERAPY FOR LEGIONNAIRES' DISEASE

PATIENT TYPE	DISEASE SEVERITY*	FIRST CHOICES	DOSAGE	ALTERNATIVES	DOSAGE
Normal host	Mild to moderate	Erythromycin†	500 mg–1 g IV, 500 mg PO each 4 times daily for 14–21 d	Levofloxacin†‡	500 mg IV or PO once daily for 7–10 d
		or		*or*	
		Doxycycline	200 mg IV or PO once daily for 14–21 d	Azithromycin†	500 mg IV or PO once daily for 3 d
	Severe	Levofloxacin†‡	500 mg IV or PO once daily for 7–10 d	Azithromycin†	Same dosage as above for 5 d
Immunosuppressed	Any type	Levofloxacin†‡	Same as above	Azithromycin†	Same dosage as above for 5 d

*Severe disease is that causing respiratory failure, bilateral pneumonia, or rapidly worsening pulmonary infiltrates, or the presence of at least two of the following three: blood urea nitrogen ≥30 mg/dL (11 mmol/L); diastolic blood pressure <60 mm Hg; respiratory rate >30/min.

†Approved by the Food and Drug Administration for the treatment of legionnaires' disease.

‡Acceptable alternatives include trovafloxacin† 200 mg once daily IV or orally and ofloxacin 500 mg twice daily IV or orally, both for 7 to 10 days.

intradermal inoculation is usually initiated by minor abrasions or insect bites.

CELLULITIS. Group A streptococcus is the most common cause of cellulitis.

LYMPHANGITIS. Cutaneous infection with bright-red streaks ascending proximally is invariably due to group A streptococcus. Prompt parenteral antibiotic treatment is mandatory because bacteremia and systemic toxicity develop rapidly once streptococci reach the blood stream via the thoracic duct.

NECROTIZING FASCIITIS. Necrotizing fasciitis, originally called "streptococcal gangrene" is a deep-seated infection of the subcutaneous tissue that results in progressive destruction of fascia and fat but may spare the skin itself.

PNEUMONIA. Pneumonia caused by group A streptococcus is most common in women in the second and third decades of life and causes large pleural effusions and empyema that develop rapidly.

STREPTOCOCCAL TOXIC SHOCK SYNDROME. This illness is associated with bacteremia, deep soft tissue infection, shock, multiorgan failure, and death in 30% of cases. (Table 20–15).

Treatment

The recommended antibiotic therapies for group A streptococcal diseases are shown in Table 20–16.

For more information about this subject, see *Cecil Textbook of Medicine,* 21st edition. Philadelphia, W.B. Saunders Company, 2000. Chapter 324, Streptococcal Infections, pages 1619 to 1624.

RHEUMATIC FEVER

Rheumatic fever is an inflammatory disease that occurs as a delayed, non-suppurative sequela of upper respiratory infection with group A streptococci. Its clinical manifestations include polyarthritis, carditis, subcutaneous nodules, erythema marginatum, and chorea in varying combinations. In its classic form the disorder is acute, febrile, and largely self-limited. However, damage to heart valves may be chronic and progressive and cause cardiac disability or death many years after the initial episode (Table 20–17).

Perhaps the most effective strategy for avoiding the mortality and chronic cardiac disability associated with acute rheumatic fever is that of "secondary prevention." The strategy focuses on the group of persons who have already suffered a rheumatic attack and who are inordinately susceptible to a recurrence following an immunologically significant streptococcal upper respiratory infection (Table 20–18).

For more information about this subject, see *Cecil Textbook of Medicine,* 21st edition. Philadelphia, W.B. Saunders Company, 2000. Chapter 325, Rheumatic Fever, pages 1624 to 1630.

INFECTIVE ENDOCARDITIS

Endocarditis is characterized pathologically by the "vegetation," a lesion that results from deposition of platelets and fibrin on the endothelial surface of the heart.

Table 20–15 ■ CLINICAL AND LABORATORY FEATURES OF STREPTOCOCCAL TOXIC SHOCK SYNDROME

Symptoms
- Viral-like prodrome
- Severe pain
- Confusion
- Nausea
- Chills

Signs
- Fever
- Soft tissue swelling and tenderness
- Tachycardia
- Tachypnea
- Hypotension

Laboratory findings
- Hematologic tests
  - Marked left shift
  - Red blood cell hemolysis
  - Thrombocytopenia
- Chemistry tests
  - Azotemia
  - Hypocalcemia
  - Hypoalbuminemia
  - Creatine phosphokinase elevation
- Urinalysis
  - Hematuria
- Blood gases
  - Hypoxia
  - Acidosis
- Radiography
  - ARDS
  - Soft tissue swelling

Complications
- Profound hypotension
- ARDS
- Renal failure
- Liver failure
- Necrotizing soft tissue infections
- Bacteremia
- Death (30%)

ARDS = adult respiratory distress syndrome.

Endocarditis is the result of interaction among (1) host factors that predispose the endothelium to infection, (2) circumstances that lead to transient bacteremia (Table 20–19), and (3) the tissue tropism and virulence of the circulating bacteria. 20

Prosthetic cardiac valves are a major risk factor for endocarditis. Endocarditis occurs in 1 to 5% of patients with prosthetic valves over the lifetime of the valve, with an incidence rate of about 300 to 600 per 100,000 patient-years.

Treatment

Effective antimicrobial therapy for endocarditis optimally requires identification of the specific pathogen and assessment of its susceptibility to various antimicrobial agents. Standardized regi-

Table 20–16 ■ ANTIBIOTIC THERAPY FOR GROUP A STREPTOCOCCAL INFECTIONS

CONDITION	ROUTE	DOSAGES
Pharyngitis and impetigo		
Benzathine penicillin	IM	1.2 million U (>27 kg)
Penicillin G (or V)	PO	200,000 U qid for 10 d
Erythromycin	PO	40 mg/kg/d (up to 1 g/d)
Recurrent streptococcal pharyngitis/tonsillitis		
Same as above		
or		
Ampicillin plus clavulanic acid	PO	20–40 mg/kg/d
Oral cephalosporin		Check PDR
Clindamycin	PO	10 mg/kg/d
Cellutitis and erysipelas		
Penicillin G or V	PO	200,000 U qid for 10 d
Dicloxacillin*	PO	500 mg qid for 10 d (adults)
Necrotizing fasciitis/myositis/streptococcal toxic shock syndrome		
Clindamycin	IV	1800–2100 mg/d (adults)
Penicillin	IV	2 million U q4h (adults)

PDR = *Physicians' Desk Reference.*

*Alternative to penicillin if *Staphylococcus aureus* is of concern. Cephalosporins could be used; however, most (except ceftriaxone) have less activity than penicillin G against streptococci.

mens are recommended for the most common pathogens—viridans streptococci, enterococci, and staphylococci (Table 20–20), although they may not be available for more unusual pathogens.

For more information about this subject, see *Cecil Textbook of Medicine,* 21st edition. Philadelphia, W.B. Saunders Company, 2000. Chapter 326, Infective Endocarditis, pages 1631 to 1640.

STAPHYLOCOCCAL INFECTIONS

Staphylococcus aureus has been recognized since the beginning of the 20th century as one of the most important and lethal human bacterial pathogens. Until the antibiotic era, more than 80% of patients growing *S. aureus* from their blood died; most of those

Text continues on page 583

Table 20–17 ■ THE MANY FACES OF ACUTE RHEUMATIC FEVER: POSSIBLE FEATURES

High fever, prostration, crippling polyarthritis
Lassitude, tachycardia, new cardiac murmurs
Acute pericarditis
Fulminant heart failure
Sydenham's chorea without fever or toxicity
Acute abdominal pain mimicking appendicitis
Varying combinations of the above

Table 20–18 ■ SECONDARY PREVENTION OF RHEUMATIC FEVER (PREVENTION OF RECURRENT ATTACKS)

AGENT	DOSE	MODE
Benzathine penicillin G	1,200,000 U every 4 wk*	Intramuscular
	or	
Penicillin V	250 mg twice daily	Oral
	or	
Sulfadiazine	0.5 g once daily for patients ≤27 kg (60 lb)	Oral
	0.1 g once daily for patients >27 kg (60 lb)	
For individuals allergic to penicillin and sulfadiazine		
Erythromycin	250 mg twice daily	Oral

*In high-risk situations, administration every 3 weeks is justified and recommended. Reproduced by permission of Pediatrics 96:758, copyright American Academy of Pediatrics 1995.

Table 20–19 ■ CIRCUMSTANCES LIKELY TO LEAD TO TRANSIENT BACTEREMIA THAT CAN PRECEDE ENDOCARDITIS

Chemoprophylaxis Recommended for High- and Medium-Risk Patients

- Dental procedures
  - Dental and periodontal procedures known to induce mucosal bleeding
    - Dental extractions
    - Periodontal procedures, including surgery, scaling and root planing, probing, and recall maintenance
  - Dental implant placement and reimplantation of avulsed teeth
  - Endodontic instrumentation or surgery only beyond the apex
  - Subgingival placement of antibiotic fibers or strips
  - Initial placement of orthodontic bands but not brackets
  - Intraligamentary local anesthetic injections
- Respiratory tract
  - Tonsillectomy and adenoidectomy
  - Bronchoscopy with a rigid bronchoscope
  - Surgery on respiratory mucosa
- Genitourinary tract
  - Prostate surgery
  - Cystoscopy or urethral dilation

Chemoprophylaxis Recommended for High-Risk, Optional for Medium-Risk Patients

- Gastrointestinal tract
  - Esophageal dilation or sclerotherapy for esophageal varices
  - Biliary tract surgery
  - Endoscopic retrograde cholangiography with biliary obstruction
  - Surgery on intestinal mucosa

Chemoprophylaxis Optional for High-Risk Patients

- Bronchoscopy with a flexible bronchscope with or without biopsy
- Transesophageal echocardiography
- Endoscopy with or without gastrointestinal biopsy
- Vaginal hysterectomy
- Vaginal delivery

Adapted from Dajani AS, Taubert KA, Wilson W, et al: Prevention of bacterial endocarditis. Recommendations of the American Heart Association. JAMA 277:1794, 1997.

Table 20–20 ■ ANTIBIOTIC THERAPY (ADULT DOSES)[a] FOR INFECTIVE ENDOCARDITIS

REGIMEN — **DOSE AND DURATION[a]**

Highly penicillin-susceptible streptococci (MIC, ≤0.1 μg/mL)

1. Aqueous penicillin 12–18 million U/d IV, cefazolin[b] 1 g IV q8h, ceftriaxone[b] 2 g IV q24h, or vancomycin[c] 15 mg/kg (max 2 g/d unless serum levels are monitored[d]) IV q12h for 4 wk (this regimen is preferred in patients ≥65 yr and those with 8th nerve or renal impairment).
2. Aqueous penicillin, 12–18 million U/d IV, or ceftriaxone[b] 2 g IV q24h, plus streptomycin[e, f] 7.5 mg/kg (max 500 mg/dose) q12h, or gentamicin,[e, f] 1 mg/kg IV or IM q8h for 2 wk (this regimen is appropriate for uncomplicated cases of endocarditis in patients at low risk for adverse events from aminoglycosides. If streptomycin is preferred, susceptibility to high levels of this aminoglycoside must be determined in vitro. Isolates from patients with endocarditis rarely have been reported that are resistant to high levels of streptomycin (MIC, >1000 μg/mL) and lack penicillin-streptomycin synergy in vitro. Endocarditis from these high-level streptomycin-resistant strains that are susceptible to high levels of gentamicin in vitro (MIC, ≤500 μg/mL) can be treated with a penicillin-gentamicin combination).

Relatively penicillin-resistant streptococci (MIC, >0.1 and <0.5 μg/mL)

Aqueous penicillin, 18 million U/d IV, cefazolin[b] 1 g IV q8h, ceftriaxone[b] 2 g IV q24h, or vancomycin[c, g] 15 mg/kg (max 2 g/d unless serum levels are monitored[d]) IV q12h for 4–6 wk, plus streptomycin,[e, f] 7.5 mg/kg (max 500 mg/dose) q12h, or gentamicin[e, f] 1 mg/kg IV or IM q8h for the first 2 wk. (This regimen gives high cure rates for endocarditis secondary to highly penicillin-susceptible streptococci but is now reserved for endocarditis secondary to relatively resistant strains. For patients with streptococcal prosthetic valve endocarditis, a 6-wk course of penicillin plus gentamicin for at least the first 2 wk is recommended.)

Penicillin-resistant streptococci (MIC, ≥0.5 μg/mL), enterococci, or nutritionally variant streptococci or for streptococcal prosthetic valve endocarditis

Aqueous penicillin 18–30 million U/d IV, or vancomycin[c, h] 15 mg/kg (max 2 g/d unless serum levels are monitored[d]) IV q12h, plus streptomycin[e, f] 7.5 mg/kg (max 500 mg/dose) q12h, or gentamicin[e, f] 1 mg/kg IV or IM q8h for 4–6 wk. (Because of technical difficulties in susceptibility testing of nutritionally variant streptococci, many experts recommend treating endocarditis caused by these strains with the standard regimen recommended for enterococci. Six weeks of therapy is recommended for patients with streptococcal prosthetic valve endocarditis or for patients with enterococcal endocarditis and more than 3 mo of symptoms before therapy.)

Methicillin/gentamicin-susceptible staphylococci—uncomplicated[i], Right-sided, native valve only

Nafcillin or oxacillin[j] 2 g q4h IV for 2 wk
with
Gentamicin[e] 1 mg/kg q8h IV/IM for 2 wk

Methicillin-susceptible staphylococci—native valve

Nafcillin or oxacillin[j] 2 g q4h IV for 4–6 wk
with or without
Gentamicin[k] 1 mg/kg q8h IV/IM for the first 3–5 d only

Methicillin-susceptible staphylococci—native valve, penicillin-allergic patient

Cefazolin[b] 2 g IV q8h for 4–6 wk
with or without
Gentamicin[k] 1 mg/kg q8h IV/IM for the first 3–5 d only
or

Vancomycin[c, j] 30 mg/kg/d (max 2 g/d unless serum levels are monitored[d]) divided q12h for 4–6 wk

Methicillin-resistant staphylococci—native valve

Vancomycin 30 mg/kg/d (max 2 g/d unless serum levels are monitored[d]) divided q12h for 4–6 wk

Methicillin-resistant staphylococci—prosthetic device

Vancomycin 30 mg/kg/d (max 2 g/d unless serum levels are monitored[d]) divided q12h for ≥6 wk

plus

Rifampin[l] 300 mg q8h for ≥6 wk

plus

Gentamicin[e, m] 1 mg/kg q8h IV/IM for the first 2 wk

Methicillin-susceptible staphlococci—prosthetic device

Nafcillin or oxacillin[j, n] 2 g q4h IV for ≥6 wk

plus

Rifampin[l] 300 mg q8h for ≥6 wk

plus

Gentamicin,[e, m] 1 mg/kg q8h IV/IM for the first 2 wk

MIC = minimum inhibitory concentration.

[a]Antibiotic doses are for adults with normal renal function.

[b]Cephalosporins or vancomycin could be used in patients with penicillin allergy. However, cephalosporins should not be used in individuals with an immediate-type hypersensitivity reaction (urticaria, angioedema, or anaphylaxis) to penicillin.

[c]Vancomycin is preferred if immediate-type hypersensitivity to penicillin is suspected. Vancomycin use may enhance the nephrotoxicity of gentamicin.

[d]Vancomycin peak serum levels should be obtained 1 hour after completion of a 1- to 2-hour infusion and should be in the range of 30 to 45 μg/mL.

[e]Gentamicin peak serum levels obtained 1 hour after start of a 20- to 30-minute IV infusion or IM injection should be about 3 μg/mL and trough level should be less than 1 μg/mL. The streptomycin peak serum level 1 hour after IM administration is about 20 μg/mL.

[f]The choice of an aminoglycoside should be based on in vitro high-level aminoglycoside susceptibility testing. If the strain is susceptible to high levels of gentamicin, gentamicin is preferred because determination of gentamicin serum levels is more generally available.

[g]When vancomycin is chosen, the addition of gentamicin is not recommended by the American Heart Association.

[h]For treatment of enterococcal endocarditis, penicillin desensitization should be considered if penicillin allergy is not suspected to be of the immediate type; cephalosporins are not acceptable alternatives.

[i]No evidence of metastatic pleuropulmonary or systemic infection or left-sided endocarditis and the isolate is gentamicin susceptible.

[j]Vancomycin is less rapidly bactericidal than antistaphylococcal β-lactam antibiotics, as reflected by slower clearance of staphylococci from the vegetations and blood. Consequently, vancomycin is not effective in the short-course (2-week) regimen and similarly should not be used in other regimens, unless the organism is methicillin resistant or the patient has penicillin allergy that precludes use of a β-lactam antibiotic.

[k]The additional benefit of an aminoglycoside has not been clearly established. Gentamicin should be used only if the isolate is gentamicin susceptible.

[l]Rifampin should be added in cases of rifampin-susceptible staphylococcal endocarditis in the presence of a prosthetic device; combination therapy is essential to prevent the emergence of rifampin resistance.

[m]If the isolate is gentamicin resistant, another aminoglycoside to which the isolate is sensitive should be used. If resistant to all aminoglycosides, a fluoroquinolone to which the isolate is sensitive should be substituted.

[n]Cefazolin or vancomycin should be used in penicillin-allergic patients. Vancomycin is preferred if immediate-type penicillin hypersensitivity is present.

Adapted from Wilson WR, Karchmer AW, Dajani AS, et al: Antibiotic treatment of adults with infective endocarditis due to streptococci, enterococci, staphylococci and HACEK microorganisms. JAMA 274:1706, 1995. © 1995, American Medical Association.

Table 20–21 ■ STAPHYLOCOCCAL SPECIES FOUND ON HUMAN SKIN AND MUCOUS MEMBRANES

COAGULASE-POSITIVE	COAGULASE-NEGATIVE	
S. aureus	*S. epidermidis*	*S. cohnii*
	S. saprophyticus	*S. xylosus*
	S. haemolyticus	*S. auricularis*
	S. warneri	*S. simulans*
	S. capitis	*S. schleiferi*
	S. hominis	*S. lugdanensis*
	S. saccharolyticus	*S. caprae*
		S. pasteuri

Table 20–22 ■ INFECTIONS CAUSED BY *Staphylococcus aureus*

COMMON	LESS COMMON
Furuncle or skin abscess	Cellulitis
Bullous impetigo	Hospital-acquired pneumonia
Surgical wound infection	Brain abscess
Hospital-acquired bacteremia	Empyema
Acute or right-sided bacterial endocarditis	
Hematogenous osteomyelitis	
Septic arthritis	
Pyomyositis	
Renal carbuncle	
Scalded skin syndrome	
Toxic shock syndrome	
Food-borne gastroenteritis (short incubation)	
Botryomycosis	
Paraspinous or epidural abscess	

Table 20–23 ■ DIAGNOSTIC CRITERIA FOR STAPHYLOCOCCAL TOXIC SHOCK SYNDROME

1. Fever (usually $\leq$38.9° C, or 102° F)
2. Rash (diffuse macular erythroderma, sunburn- or scarlet fever–like)
3. Desquamation, 1–2 wk after onset of illness, particularly of palms and soles
4. Hypotension (systolic <90 mm Hg or orthostatic syncope)
5. Involvement of 3 or more of the following organ systems: gastrointestinal (nausea and vomiting), muscular (myalgias), mucous membrane (hyperemia), renal, hepatic, hematologic ($\downarrow$ platelets), central nervous system, or pulmonary (adult respiratory distress syndrome)
6. *S. aureus* infection or mucosal colonization

dying had been healthy with no underlying disease. Although infections caused by coagulase-positive *S. aureus* were generally known to be potentially lethal, coagulase-negative staphylococci had been dismissed as avirulent skin commensals incapable of causing human disease. However, over the past 20 years, coagulase-negative staphylococcal infections have emerged as one of the major complications of medical progress. They are currently the pathogens most commonly isolated from infections of indwelling foreign devices and are the leading cause of hospital-acquired bacteremias in the United States. This ascendancy of staphylococci as pre-eminent nosocomial pathogens also has been associated with a major increase in the proportion of these isolates that are resistant to multiple antimicrobial agents.

S. aureus constitutes a homogeneous species, as determined by biochemical testing and nucleic acid analysis, whereas coagulase-negative staphylococci are sufficiently varied to be assigned to numerous species (Table 20–21). A small percentage of local infections progress to dissemination, where *S. aureus* gains access to the blood. Dissemination is characterized by *bacteremia* and *metastatic infection.*

S. aureus produces three toxins, or classes of toxin, that produce specific syndromes without the need for the organism itself to invade and disseminate (Table 20–22). *Staphylococcal food poisoning* occurs when a pre-formed, heat-stable *enterotoxin* is ingested and interacts with parasympathetic ganglia in the stomach. *Staphylococcal scalded skin syndrome* results from the production of *exfoliative toxin* by *S. aureus.* The variety of *toxic shock syndrome* associated with tampon use in young women is due to toxic shock syndrome toxin (TSST-1) entering into the blood through the vagina and is produced by *S. aureus* organisms that colonize the mucosa (Table 20–23).

COAGULASE-NEGATIVE STAPHYLOCOCCAL INFECTIONS. The major infections caused by coagulase-negative staphylococci are hospital-acquired and involve indwelling foreign devices (Table 20–24).

THERAPY. Antimicrobial agents effective against *S. aureus* are listed in Table 20–25.

For more information about this subject, see *Cecil Textbook of Medicine,* 21st edition. Philadelphia, W.B. Saunders Company, 2000. Chapter 327, Staphylococcal Infections, pages 1641 to 1645.

BACTERIAL MENINGITIS

Meningitis is an inflammation of the arachnoid, the pia mater, and the intervening CSF. The inflammatory process extends throughout the subarachnoid space about the brain and spinal cord and regularly involves the ventricles.

The clinical setting in which meningitis develops may provide a clue to the specific bacterial cause. Meningococcal disease, including meningitis, may occur sporadically and in cyclic outbreaks.

Certain predisposing factors are frequently associated with the development of *pneumococcal meningitis. Acute otitis media* (with or without *mastoiditis*) occurs in about 20% of adult patients. *Pneumonia* is present in about 15% of patients with pneumococcal

Table 20–24 ■ CHARACTERISTICS OF COAGULASE-NEGATIVE STAPHYLOCOCCAL INFECTIONS

1. Hospital-acquired
2. Caused by *S. epidermidis* (70–80%)
3. Resistant to multiple antimicrobial agents (>80% methicillin resistant)
4. Involve indwelling foreign devices (catheters, prosthetic heart valves and joints, vascular grafts)
5. Exhibit a long latent period between device contamination and clinical presentation

meningitis. *Acute pneumococcal sinusitis* is occasionally the initial focus from which infection spreads.

S. aureus meningitis is seen most commonly as a complication of a neurosurgical procedure. Meningitis caused by *gram-negative bacilli* takes one of three forms: neonatal meningitis, meningitis after trauma, or meningitis after neurosurgery. The most frequent causes of bacterial meningitis in patients with neoplastic disease are gram-negative bacilli (particularly, *Pseudomonas aeruginosa* and *Escherichia coli*).

Clinical Manifestations

GENERAL PHYSICAL FINDINGS. Evidence of meningeal irritation (drowsiness and decreased mentation, stiff neck, Kernig's and Brudzinski's signs) is usually present. *The presence of a petechial, purpuric, or ecchymotic rash in a patient with meningeal findings almost always indicates meningococcal infection and requires prompt treatment because of the rapidity with which this infection can progress.*

NEUROLOGIC FINDINGS AND COMPLICATIONS. Cranial nerve abnormalities, involving principally the third, fourth, sixth, or sev-

Table 20–25 ■ ANTIMICROBOBIAL AGENTS EFFECTIVE FOR TREATING *Staphylococcus aureus* INFECTIONS

	RESISTANCE*	
AGENTS	Hospital Acquired	Community Acquired
Penicillin G	>90	>90
Antistaphylococcal penicillins and cephalosporins	30	S
Erythromycin	40	10
Clindamycin	40	10
Trimethoprim-sulfamethoxazole	20	S
Tetracycline	20	10
Minocycline	S	S
Rifampin	S	S
Gentamicin	30	S
Quinolones	30	S
Vancomycin	S	S

S = >95% susceptible.

* Numbers are percentage of isolates from patients with hospital-acquired or community-acquired infections resistant to each agent.

enth nerves, occur in 5 to 10% of adults. Persistent sensorineural hearing loss occurs in 10% of children with bacterial meningitis.

Seizures (focal or generalized) occur in 20 to 30% of patients and may result from readily reversible causes (high fever in infants; penicillin neurotoxicity when large doses are administered intravenously in the presence of renal failure) or, more commonly, from focal cerebral injury.

Papilledema is rare (1%) in bacterial meningitis, even with high CSF pressures.

LABORATORY DIAGNOSIS. ***CEREBROSPINAL FLUID EXAMINATION.*** Initial CSF pressure is usually moderately elevated (200 to 300 mm H_2O in the adult). Striking elevations (>450 mm H_2O) occur in occasional patients with acute brain swelling complicating meningitis in the absence of an associated mass lesion.

GRAM-STAINED SMEAR. By the time of hospitalization, most patients with pyogenic meningitis have large numbers (at least 10^5/mL) of bacteria in the CSF.

CELL COUNT. The cell count in untreated meningitis usually ranges between 100 and 10,000/mm^3, with polymorphonuclear leukocytes predominating initially (≥80%) and lymphocytes appearing subsequently.

GLUCOSE. The CSF glucose is reduced to values of 40 mg/dL or less (or <50% of the simultaneous blood level) in 50% of patients with bacterial meningitis; this finding can be very valuable in distinguishing bacterial meningitis from most viral meningitides or parameningeal infections.

RADIOLOGIC STUDIES. In view of the frequency with which pyogenic meningitis is associated with primary foci of infection in the chest, nasal sinuses, or mastoid, radiographs of these areas should be taken at the appropriate time after antimicrobial therapy begins, when clinically indicated. Computed tomography (CT) is not indicated in most patients with bacterial meningitis. If a mass lesion (cerebral abscess, subdural empyema) is suspected by history, clinical setting, or physical findings (papilledema, focal cerebral signs), then CT should be performed.

Recurrent Meningitis

Repeated episodes of bacterial meningitis generally indicate a host defect, either in local anatomy or in antibacterial and immunologic defenses (e.g., recurrent *Neisseria meningitidis* infections in patients with congenital or acquired deficiencies of complement, particularly late-acting components).

Treatment

Antimicrobial therapy should be begun promptly in this life-threatening emergency. Treatment should be aimed at the most likely causes based on clinical clues (age of the patient, presence of a petechial or purpuric rash, a recent neurosurgical procedure, CSF rhinorrhea) (Tables 20–26 and 20–27).

For more information about this subject, see *Cecil Textbook of Medicine,* 21st edition. Philadelphia, W.B. Saunders Company, 2000. Chapter 328, Bacterial Meningitis, pages 1645 to 1654.

Table 20–26 ■ ANTIMICROBIAL THERAPY OF COMMUNITY-ACQUIRED BACTERIAL MENINGITIS OF KNOWN CAUSE*

	PREFERRED THERAPY			ALTERNATIVE THERAPY		
ORGANISM	**Antimicrobial**	**Adults (24-hr Dose)**	**Children (24-hr Dose)**	**Antimicrobial**	**Adults (24-hr Dose)**	**Children (24-hr Dose)**
Streptococcus pneumoniae						
Penicillin MIC <0.1 μg/mL	Penicillin G	24 million U IV q4h aliquots	300,000 U/kg IV q4h aliquots	Cefotaxime	12 g IV q4h aliquots	200 mg/kg IV q4–6h aliquots
	or Ampicillin	12 g IV q4h aliquots	200–400 mg/kg IV q4h aliquots	*or* Ceftriaxone†	4 g IV q12h aliquots	80–100 mg/kg IV q12h aliquots
				or Vancomycin‡	2 g IV q8–12h aliquots	50 mg/kg IV q6h aliquots
				or Chloramphenicol	4–6 g IV q6h aliquots	75–100 mg/kg IV q6h aliquots
Penicillin MIC 0.1–1.0 μg/mL	Ceftriazone†	4 g IV q12h aliquots	80–100 mg/kg IV q12h aliquots	Vancomycin‡	2 g IV q8–12h aliquots	50 mg/kg IV q6h aliquots
	or Cefotaxime	12 g IV q4h aliquots	200 mg/kg IV q4–6h aliquots	*or* Meropenem§	6 g IV q8h aliquots	40 mg/kg q8h IV (each dose)
Penicillin MIC >1.0 μg/mL	Vancomycin‡,¶	2 g IV q8–12h aliquots	50 mg/kg IV q6h aliquots	Meropenem§	6 g IV q8h aliquots	40 mg/kg q8h IV (each dose)
Neisseria meningitidis	Penicillin G	24 million U IV q4h aliquots	300,000 U/kg IV q4h aliquots	Ceftriaxone† *or* cefotaxime	As above	80–100 mg/kg IV q12h aliquots 200 mg/kg IV q4–6h aliquots
	or Ampicillin	12 g IV q4h aliquots	200–400 mg/kg IV q4h aliquots	*or* Chloramphenicol	4–6 g IV q6h aliquots	75–100 mg/kg IV q6h aliquots

Haemophilus influenzae						
β-Lactamase negative	Ampicillin	12 g IV q4h aliquots	200–400 mg/kg IV q4h aliquots	Third-generation cephalosporin** or chloramphenicol as above		Third-generation cephalosporin** or chloramphenicol as above
β-Lactamase positive	Ceftriaxone†	4 g IV q12h aliquots	80–100 mg/kg IV q12h aliquots	Chloramphenicol as above		75–100 mg/kg IV q6h aliquots
	or Cefotaxime	12 g IV q4h aliquots	200 mg/kg IV q4–6h aliquots			
Listeria monocytogenes	Ampicillin ‖	12 g IV q4h aliquots	200–400 mg/kg IV q4h aliquots	Trimethoprim-sulfamethoxazole	10–20 mg/kg IV†† q6–8h aliquots	10–20 mg/kg IV†† q6h aliquots
	or Penicillin G ‖	24 million U IV q4h aliquots	300,000 U/kg IV q4h aliquots			

MIC = minimum inhibitory concentration.

*Dosages are those for patients with normal renal and hepatic function.

†4 g maximum daily dose.

‡Monitoring of peak and trough serum levels advisable; may need to monitor CSF levels if patient not responding well and, if levels are low, may need to increase daily dose temporarily by 0.5–1.0 g in adults or add adjuvant intrathecal vancomycin as in treatment of methicillin-resistant *Staphylococcus aureus* meningitis.

§Use may be associated with seizures, but much less so than with imipenem.

‖Addition of IV gentamicin to be considered.

¶Addition of rifampin should be considered.

**Ceftriaxone or cefotaxime.

††Dosage based on trimethoprim component of the combination.

Modified from Swartz MN: Acute bacterial meningitis. *In* Gorbach SL, Bartlett JG, Blacklow NR (eds): Infectious Diseases, 2nd ed. Philadelphia, WB Saunders, 1998.

Table 20–27 ■ INITIAL THERAPY FOR COMMUNITY-ACQUIRED PURULENT MENINGITIS OF UNKNOWN CAUSE IN ADULTS

AGE	LIKELY PATHOGENS	PREFERRED DRUG	ALTERNATIVE DRUGS
Immunocompetent			
3 mo–18 yr	*Streptococcus pneumoniae*, *Neisseria meningitidis*, *Haemophilus influenzae*	Cefotaxime or ceftriaxone* plus vancomycin‡	Ampicillin* plus chloramphenicol
18–50 yr	*S. pneumoniae*, *N. meningitidis*	Cefotaxime or ceftriaxone* ± ampicillin† plus vancomycin‡	Vancomycin plus chloramphenicol
>50 yr	*S. pneumoniae*, *N. meningitidis*, *L. monocytogenes*	Cefotaxime or ceftriaxone* plus ampicillin plus vancomycin‡	Cefotaxime* plus trimethoprim-sulfamethoxazole
Impaired cellular immunity	*L. monocytogenes*, gram-negative bacilli	Ampicillin plus ceftazidime plus vancomycin‡	Trimethoprim-sulfamethoxazole plus meropenem or chloramphenicol
Cerebrospinal fluid leak, basilar skull fracture	*S. pneumoniae*, *N. meningitidis*, *H. influenzae*, various streptococci	Cefotaxime* plus vancomycin‡	Vancomycin plus chloramphenicol

*When *S. pneumoniae* is suspected in communities where highly penicillin-resistant or cephalosporin-resistant *S. pneumoniae* has occurred (or is likely), vancomycin should be added.
†If clinical features suggest *L. monocytogenese*.
‡Vancomycin is given in situations of undiagnosed purulent meningitis. It is stopped if not indicated when resistance studies are returned.

MENINGOCOCCAL INFECTIONS

N. meningitidis is the causative agent in meningococcal infections. It has become the most common cause of bacterial meningitis in American children since the use of *Haemophilus influenzae* type b protein-capsular polysaccharide conjugate vaccine.

N. meningitidis can cause endemic and epidemic infection. At the present time, meningococcal infection is endemic in the United States, with approximately 2500 cases per year reported to the Centers for Disease Control and Prevention (CDC). This gives a case rate of approximately 1 in 10^5 total population. The case fatality rate is approximately 12%.

Acute systemic infection can be manifested clinically by three syndromes: (1) meningitis, (2) meningitis with meningococcemia, and (3) meningococcemia without obvious signs of meningitis. It must be remembered that patients with meningococcemia may not necessarily have meningeal signs, but from 50 to 80% will have petechiae on presentation. An examination of the mucosal surfaces of the soft palate and ocular and palpebral conjunctiva for petechiae must be done.

TREATMENT OF SYSTEMIC MENINGOCOCCAL INFECTION. Treatment is by antibiotic therapy (Table 20–28).

PREVENTION. Chemoprophylaxis has been shown to be effective (Table 20–29).

For more information about this subject, see *Cecil Textbook of Medicine,* 21st edition. Philadelphia, W.B. Saunders Company, 2000. Chapter 329, Meningococcal Infections, pages 1655 to 1659.

INFECTIONS CAUSED BY *HAEMOPHILUS* SPECIES

H. influenzae is the most important pathogen in this genus. It can be recovered from sites where it colonizes, such as the nasopharynx and upper respiratory tract, and from sites where it causes disease, such as blood, CSF, sputum, pleura, middle ear, female genital tract, and joints.

CLINICAL SYNDROMES. ***MENINGITIS.*** *H. influenzae* meningitis commonly occurs in children younger than age 5 and in adults with histories of skull trauma or CSF leaks.

EPIGLOTTITIS. *H. influenzae* type b is the most common cause of acute epiglottitis in both children and adults.

PNEUMONIA. *H. influenzae* is a common cause of pneumonia in both children and adults.

TRACHEOBRONCHITIS. Tracheobronchitis is a condition characterized by fever, cough, and purulent sputum that occurs in the absence of radiographic infiltrates suggestive of pneumonia. It frequently occurs in patients with known chronic lung disease.

OTITIS MEDIA. *H. influenzae* is the most frequent cause of otitis media in young children.

OBSTETRIC AND GYNECOLOGIC INFECTION. Pregnancy is associated with a significant risk for *H. influenzae* infection.

TREATMENT. Third-generation cephalosporins are currently considered to be the treatment of choice for serious *H. influenzae* infections, such as meningitis or epiglottitis. Treatment with ceftriaxone (adult dose: 1 g intravenously every 12 hours) or cefo-

Table 20–28 ■ ANTIBIOTIC MANAGEMENT OF SYSTEMIC MENINGOCOCCAL INFECTION

ANTIBIOTIC	DOSE
Penicillin G	300,000 U/kg/d IV, up to 24 million U/d
Ampicillin	150–200 mg/kg/d IV up to 12 g/d
Ceftriaxone	2 g/d IV
Chloramphenicol	For use in penicillin-allergic patients, 100 mg/kg/d IV, up to 4 g/d

taxime (adult dose: 2 g intravenously every 8 hours) should be started for patients with proven or suspected *H. influenzae* infection, and this should be continued at least until the full susceptibility data are available.

PREVENTION. The first *H. influenzae* type b vaccines were licensed for use in the United States in 1985.

For more information about this subject, see *Cecil Textbook of Medicine,* 21st edition. Philadelphia, W.B. Saunders Company, 2000. Chapter 330, Infections Caused by *Haemophilus* Species, pages 1659 to 1662.

OSTEOMYELITIS

Osteomyelitis is an infection by microorganisms that invade bone. Three pathogenetic routes of infection occur: (1) hematogenous seeding, (2) contamination accompanying surgical and nonsurgical trauma, or (3) spread from infected contiguous tissue (Table 20–30).

Table 20–29 ■ CHEMOPROPHYLAXIS AND IMMUNOPROPHYLAXIS FOR PREVENTION OF MENINGOCOCCAL INFECTION

ANTIBIOTIC	DOSE
Chemoprophylaxis	
Rifampin	Adults who are not pregnant, 600 mg PO q12h for 2 d Children >1 mo 5mg/kg PO, <1 mo 10 mg/kg PO q12h for 2 d
Ceftriaxone	Single 250-mg IM dose for adults, single 125-mg IM dose for children <15 yr
Ciprofloxacin	Adults who are not pregnant, 500 mg as a single PO dose; limited experience in children <18 and should not be used if other alternatives
Immunoprophylaxis	
Monovalent A, monovalent C, bivalent A-C or quadrivalent A, C, Y and W-135 vaccine is administered once by volume according to manufacturer. Amount of polysaccharide delivered is usually 50 μg. Vaccination should be considered an adjunct to antibiotic chemoprophylaxis for household or intimate contacts of meningococcal disease cases when appropriate serogroups are causing disease.	

Table 20–30 ■ PROMINENT PATHOGENS IN FORMS OF OSTEOMYELITIS

FORM OF OSTEOMYLELITIS	PROMINENT PATHOGENS
Hematogenous	
Childhood	*Staphylococcus aureus,* streptococci, *Haemophilus*
	Salmonella
Adult	Gram-negative bacilli, streptococci
	S. aureus
	Mycobacterium tuberculosis
	Gram-negative bacilli, staphylococci, *Candida*
	Fungi, mycobacteria
Introduced type	*S. aureus, Staphylococcus epidermidis,* gram-negative bacilli
Contiguous spread	Polymicrobial: staphylococci, streptococci, gram-negative bacilli, anaerobes
	Pasteurella
	S. aureus
	Sporothrix

DIAGNOSIS. Diagnosis requires both confirming the osseous site of involvement and identifying the etiologic microbes. Technetium diphosphonate bone scans, gallium-citrate scans, and indium-labeled leukocyte scintigraphy are far more sensitive than radiography and usually reveal increased radionuclide uptake when symptoms begin.

TREATMENT. Acute osteomyelitis is curable with adequate antimicrobial therapy and surgical débridement when necessary.

For more information about this subject, see *Cecil Textbook of Medicine,* 21st edition. Philadelphia, W.B. Saunders Company, 2000. Chapter 331, Osteomyelitis, pages 1662 to 1664.

WHOOPING COUGH (PERTUSSIS)

The etiologic agent of whooping cough is *Bordetella pertussis.* The descriptive name derives from a distressing, prolonged inspiratory effort that follows paroxysmal coughing. Whooping cough is estimated to cause 500,000 deaths yearly, primarily in infants. Lesions caused by *B. pertussis* are found principally in the bronchi and bronchioles. The incubation period lasts 7 to 14 days (rarely >2 weeks). It is customary to divide the clinical course into three stages.

20

1. *Catarrhal Stage.* Whooping cough begins with symptoms indistinguishable from those of a mild viral upper respiratory tract infection.
2. *Paroxysmal Stage.* Seven to 14 days after onset, the cough becomes more frequent, then paroxysmal. In a typical paroxysm there is a series of 5 to 20 short coughs of increasing intensity and then a deep inspiration, making the "whoop."
3. *Convalescent Stage.* Gradually the paroxysms become less

frequent and less intense. Convalescence requires 4 to 12 weeks.

COMPLICATIONS. Recurrent vomiting can lead to metabolic alkalosis or malnutrition.

For more information about this subject, see *Cecil Textbook of Medicine,* 21st edition. Philadelphia, W.B. Saunders Company, 2000. Chapter 332, Whooping Cough (Pertussis), pages 1664 to 1666.

DIPHTHERIA

Diphtheria is an acute infectious disease caused by *Corynebacterium diphtheriae.*

Diphtheria immunization protects against disease but does not prevent carriage.

CLINICAL MANIFESTATIONS. ***RESPIRATORY DIPHTHERIA.*** Infection limited to the anterior nares manifests as a chronic serosanguineous or seropurulent discharge without fever or significant toxicity. A whitish membrane may be observed on the septum. Cervical adenopathy and soft tissue edema may occur, resulting in the typical bullnecked appearance and stridor. The likelihood of toxic complications depends primarily on the interval between disease onset and administration of antitoxin. Diphtheria, at the end of the 20th century, remains a serious disease, associated with a high case fatality rate. In the United States, the diphtheria case fatality rate has remained virtually unchanged at between 5 and 10% over recent decades.

DIAGNOSIS. The decision to initiate therapy should be made on clinical grounds, because delayed treatment, especially delays in antitoxin administration, is associated with worse outcomes.

PREVENTION. The local health department must be notified. All contacts without full primary immunization and a booster dose within the preceding 5 years should receive diphtheria toxoid. Immunization with diphtheria toxoid is the only effective means of primary prevention. The primary series is four doses of diphtheria toxoid (given with tetanus toxoid and pertussis vaccine) at 2, 4, 6, and 12 to 18 months; a pre-school booster dose is given at ages 4 to 6 years. Thereafter, Td (tetanus-diphtheria toxoid, adult type) boosters should be given as part of the adolescent immunization visit (i.e., between 11 and 13 years of age), followed by doses administered every 10 years.

For more information about this subject, see *Cecil Textbook of Medicine,* 21st edition. Philadelphia, W.B. Saunders Company, 2000. Chapter 333, Diphtheria, pages 1666 to 1668.

CLOSTRIDIAL MYONECROSIS AND OTHER CLOSTRIDIAL DISEASES

The genus *Clostridium* encompasses over 60 species of gram-positive anaerobic spore-forming rods that cause a variety of infections in humans and animals by virtue of a myriad of proteinaceous exotoxins (Table 20–31)

For more information about this subject, see *Cecil Textbook of Medicine,* 21st edition. Philadelphia, W.B. Saunders Company,

Table 20–31 ■ CLINICAL DISEASES CAUSED BY CLOSTRIDIA

ORGANISM	CLINICAL DIAGNOSIS	CLINICAL FEATURES	LABORATORY FEATURES	TOXINS
Invasive Infections				
C. perfringens type a	Traumatic gas gangrene	Pain, necrotizing infection, renal impairment, shock	Renal failure ↑ CK Gas in tissues	α toxin θ toxin
C. septicum	Spontaneous gas gangrene	Pain, necrotizing infection, bowel portal	Renal failure ↑ CK Gas in tissues	α toxin
C. sordellii	Malignant edema	No pain, no fever, massive third spacing	Leukemoid reaction Hemoconcentration	?
C. tertium	Bacteremia in compromised hosts receiving antibiotics	Bacteremia, shock	Positive blood cultures	?
Gastrointestinal				
C. perfringens type a	Food poisoning	Nausea, vomiting, watery diarrhea	None	Enterotoxin
C. perfringens type c	Necrotizing enterocolitis	Bloody diarrhea, ruptured bowel	None	β toxin
C. septicum	Neutropenic enterocolitis, "typhlitis"	Right lower quadrant pain, abdominal distention	Low white blood cell count	Unknown
C. difficile	Pseudomembranous colitis	Watery, bloody diarrhea	Stools positive for organism, toxin, blood and leukocytes	Toxin A Toxin B
Neurologic				
C. tetanii	Tetanus	Spastic paralysis	None	Tetanospasmin
C. botulinum	Botulism	Flaccid paralysis	None	Botulinum toxin (A,B,E,F,G)

CK = creatine phosphokinase.

2000. Chapter 334, Clostridial Myonecrosis and other Clostridial Diseases, pages 1668 to 1670.

PSEUDOMEMBRANOUS COLITIS

Pseudomembranous colitis is a toxin-induced inflammatory process characterized by exudative plaques or pseudomembranes attached to the surface of the inflamed colonic mucosa. The disease is also referred to as "antibiotic-associated colitis" because many patients who develop the disease have no grossly visible pseudomembranes, even though biopsy may show microscopically visible pseudomembranes as well as inflammation.

Colitis associated with antimicrobial agents is almost always caused by *Clostridium difficile*. The disease results from the elaboration by this organism in the lumen of the large intestine of two exotoxins, A and B, and it is commonly referred to as *C. difficile*–associated diarrhea (CDAD).

CLINICAL MANIFESTATIONS. Diarrhea beginning more than 72 hours *after* admission to the hospital is not likely to be caused by other enteropathogens. Although the disease may begin as early as 1 day after antibiotic therapy is started, symptoms usually begin during the first week of treatment. In as many as 20% of patients, diarrhea may not begin until as long as 6 weeks *after* antimicrobials have been discontinued. Symptoms of CDAD are profuse watery diarrhea, usually without blood or mucus, and cramping abdominal pain. Most patients also have fever (although usually low grade, it may exceed 40° C [104° F]). Leukocytosis is very common, and leukemoid reactions occur with values as high as 50,000 to 100,000/mm^3 (Table 20–32).

For more information about this subject, see *Cecil Textbook of*

Table 20–32 ■ DIAGNOSING *Clostridium difficile* COLITIS

TEST
Laboratory Tests on Feces
Test for fecal leukocytes
Stool culture for *C. difficile*
Tests for the presence of fecal toxins
Cytopathic effect of toxin B in tissue cultures
Toxin A, B, or AB by ELISA
Latex agglutination for *C. difficile*
Radiologic Studies
Plain film of the abdomen
Barium enema
Computed tomography
Radionuclide scans (indium-labeled white blood cells)
Procedures
Flexible sigmoidoscopy
Colonscopy

ELISA = enzyme-linked immunosorbent assay.

Medicine, 21st edition. Philadelphia, W.B. Saunders Company, 2000. Chapter 335, Pseudomembranous Colitis, pages 1670 to 1673.

BOTULISM

Botulism is a severe neuroparalytic disease caused by botulinum toxin produced by clostridial species, usually *Clostridium botulinum.* Four categories of disease are recognized: (1) food-borne botulism, (2) infant botulism, (3) wound botulism, and (4) "other."

Food-Borne Botulism

Food-borne botulism, the most common form of botulism in the world, results from the ingestion of pre-formed toxin in inadequately prepared food. The foods most frequently implicated are home-processed (Table 20–33).

CLINICAL MANIFESTATIONS. The incubation period is usually 18 to 36 hours but may be as short as 2 hours or as long as 8 days. The bulbar musculature is usually affected first and results in diplopia, dysphonia, dysarthria, and dysphagia. Involvement of the cholinergic autonomic nervous system may result in decreased salivation with dry mouth and sore throat, ileus, or urinary retention. Mentation remains clear, patients are afebrile, and neurologic dysfunction is bilateral, but not necessarily symmetrical.

Botulism should be suspected in patients with acute flaccid paralysis, especially in the presence of bilateral sixth cranial nerve dysfunction and associated neurologic findings.

TREATMENT. Respiratory failure is the major risk and patients must be monitored carefully with liberal use of ventilatory support. Toxin may be removed from the gastrointestinal tract with gastric lavage, cathartics, and enemas early in the course of disease. The trivalent antitoxin or type-specific antitoxin for types A, B, or E is usually given to adults. The usual treatment is two vials, one given intravenously and one given intramuscularly. The antitoxin should be given as early as possible.

For more information about this subject, see *Cecil Textbook of*

Table 20–33 ■ INCIDENCE OF BOTULISM IN THE UNITED STATES, 1950–1993

DISEASE FROM	YEARS	TOXIN TYPE* A	B	E	TOTAL	CASE FATALITY
Food-borne	1950–93	436	183	196	1126	17.9%
Wound	1950–93	37	15	0	58	10.3%
Infant	1975–93	575	603	0	1190	1.1%
Other	1978–93	17	6	0	31	29.0%

*Nine cases due to type F and 323 cases with unknown toxin type.

Adapted from Hatheway C: *Clostridium botulinum. In* Gorbach SL, Bartlett JG, Blacklow NR (eds): Infectious Diseases, 2nd ed. Philadelphia, WB Saunders, 1998, pp 1919–1925.

20

Medicine, 21st edition. Philadelphia, W.B. Saunders Company, 2000. Chapter 336, Botulism pages 1673 to 1674.

TETANUS

Tetanus is a neurologic syndrome caused by a neurotoxin elaborated at the site of injury by *Clostridium tetani.* Tetanus is most common in warm climates and in highly cultivated rural areas. The greatest problem is in economically deprived countries, owing to poor immunization standards and unhygienic practices. It is estimated that the annual toll from neonatal tetanus in developing countries is 1 million. In the United States, there are 50 to 70 cases reported annually.

CLINICAL FEATURES. Forms of tetanus include generalized, localized, cephalic, and neonatal. Early features include irritability, restlessness, diaphoresis, and dysphagia with hydrophobia and drooling. Sustained trismus may result in a characteristic sardonic smile, the so-called risus sardonicus, and persistent spasm of the back musculature may cause opisthotonos. Waves of opisthotonos are highly characteristic of the disease. The diagnosis of tetanus is usually made on the basis of clinical observations. The putative agent, *C. tetani,* is infrequently recovered with cultures of the wound.

TREATMENT. Patients with tetanus require intensive care with particular attention to respiratory support, benzodiazepines, autonomic nervous system support, passive and active immunization, surgical débridement, and antibiotics directed against *C. tetani.* There may be clinical progression for about 2 weeks despite antitoxin treatment because of the time required to complete transport of toxin. Human tetanus immune globulin (TIG) should be given as

Table 20–34 ■ GUIDELINES FOR TETANUS PROPHYLAXIS IN WOUND MANAGEMENT

HISTORY OF ABSORBED TETANUS TOXOID (NO. OF DOSES)	CLEAN AND MINOR WOUNDS		OTHER WOUNDS*	
	Td†	TIG‡	Td†	TIG‡
Unknown or <3	Yes§	No	Yes†	Yes
≥3	Yes if >10 yr since last dose		Yes if >5 yr since last dose	

*Unimmunized or incompletely immunized persons (one or two doses of toxoid) should receive complete immunization with Td at time 0, 4 to 8 weeks later, and 6 to 12 months later.

†Td = tetanus and diphtheria toxoids absorbed. Children younger than 7 years old should receive DPT (diptheria and tetanus toxoids and pertussis vaccine absorbed). Too frequent booster doses of tetanus toxoid have been associated with hypersensitivity reactions.

‡TIG = tetanus immune globulin in a dose of 250 U intramuscularly. The usual prophylactic dose of equine tetanus immune globulin is 1500 to 5000 U intramuscularly. When tetanus toxoid is given concurrently there should be separate syringes and injection sites.

§Unimmunized or incompletely immunized persons should receive complete immunization with Td at time 0, 4–8 weeks later, and 6–12 months later.

soon as possible to neutralize toxin that has not entered neurons (Table 20–34).

For more information about this subject, see *Cecil Textbook of Medicine,* 21st edition. Philadelphia, W.B. Saunders Company, 2000. Chapter 337, Tetanus, pages 1675 to 1676.

DISEASES CAUSED BY NON–SPORE-FORMING ANAEROBIC BACTERIA

Anaerobic bacteria are the predominant indigenous, normal flora of the human body (Table 20–35), including the skin and oral, gastrointestinal, and vaginal mucosa (Table 20–36).

For more information about this subject, see *Cecil Textbook of Medicine,* 21st edition. Philadelphia, W.B. Saunders Company, 2000. Chapter 338, Diseases Caused by Non–Spore-Forming Anaerobic Bacteria, pages 1677 to 1680.

APPROACH TO ENTERIC INFECTIONS

Enteric infections may be approached on the basis of their epidemiologic features (Table 20–37).

TYPHOID FEVER

Typhoid fever is a bacterial disease caused by *Salmonella typhi.* It is characterized by prolonged fever, abdominal pain, diarrhea, delirium, rose spots, and splenomegaly, and complicated sometimes by intestinal bleeding and perforation. Enteric fever is synonymous with typhoid fever, which is occasionally caused also by *Salmonella enteritidis* bioserotype paratyphi A or B (Table 20–38).

TREATMENT. Chloramphenicol has remained the drug of choice since its introduction in 1948 because no other drug has been

Table 20–35 ■ OBSTETRIC-GYNECOLOGIC INFECTIONS THAT COMMONLY INVOLVE ANAEROBES

Abscesses
Pelvic
Vulvovaginal
Vaginal cuff
Tubo-ovarian
Bartholin's gland
Skene's gland
Endometritis
Myometritis
Parametritis
Pelvic cellulitis
Pelvic thrombophlebitis
Bacterial vaginosis
Salpingitis
Chorioamnionitis
IUD-associated infection
Pelvic actinomycosis
Postabortal sepsis

IUD = intrauterine device.

Table 20–36 ■ CLUES TO THE PRESENCE OF ANAEROBIC INFECTION

Infection in proximity to a mucous membrane
Foul odor to a discharge or wound
Gas or crepitus in a tissue
Infection associated with necrotic tissue or malignancy
Bacteremia with associated jaundice
Gram stain morphology consistent with anaerobes
"Sulfur" granules (actinomycosis)
Infection after human or animal bite
Dental infection
Infection after abdominal or pelvic surgery
No growth on routine bacterial culture (especially if Gram stain shows organisms)
Fistulous tracts
Any abscess
Typical clinical picture of gas gangrene or necrotizing fasciitis
Failure to respond to drugs not active against anaerobes (e.g., trimethoprim-sulfamethoxazole, aminoglycosides, older quinolones)

Adapted from Finegold SM: Anaerobic Bacteria in Human Disease. New York, Academic Press, 1977, p 42.

Table 20–37 ■ EPIDEMIOLOGIC FEATURES IMPORTANT IN DETERMINING POTENTIAL CAUSES OF ENTERIC INFECTION

EPIDEMIOLOGIC FEATURE	ETIOLOGIC AGENT TO SUSPECT
Travel to mountainous areas of North America	*Giardia lamblia*
Travel to Russia (especially St. Petersburg)	*Cryptosporidium, G. lamblia*
Travel to Nepal	*Cyclospora*
Travel to the developing tropical/semitropical world from an industrialized region	Enterotoxigenic *Escherichia coli, Shigella, Salmonella* (including *S. typhi*), other bacterial causes, *G. lamblia, Cyclospora,* and *Cryptosporidium*
Presence of associated cases (an outbreak)	Use incubation period and clinical features to determine probable cause
Antibiotic use in the last 2 wk	*Clostridium difficile*
Contact with day care centers	Any enteropathogen, often *G. lamblia, Cryptosporidium, Shigella,* or rotavirus
Homosexual male with diarrhea	Any organism spread by fecal-oral route; with proctitis, suspect *Neisseria gonorrhoeae, Chlamydia trachomatis,* herpes simplex, or *Treponema pallidium;* with AIDS, suspect any agent, especially *Cryptosporidium, Microsporidium, Cyclospora, Salmonella, Campylobacter jejuni, C. difficile, Myobacterium avium-intracellulare,* and cytomegalovirus

Table 20–38 ■ EVOLUTION OF TYPICAL SYMPTOMS AND SIGNS OF TYPHOID FEVER

DISEASE PERIOD	SYMPTOMS	SIGNS	PATHOLOGY
First week	Fever, chills gradually increasing and persisting; headache	Abdominal tenderness	Bacteremia
Second week	Rash, abdominal pain, diarrhea or constipation, delirium, prostration	Rose spots, splenomegaly, hepatomegaly	Mononuclear cell vasculitis of skin, hyperplasia of ileal Peyer's patches, typhoid nodules in spleen and liver
Third week	Complications of intestinal bleeding and perforation, shock	Melena, ileus, rigid abdomen, coma	Ulcerations over Peyer's patches, perforation with peritonitis
Fourth week and later	Resolution of symptoms, relapse, weight loss	Reappearance of acute disease, cachexia	Cholecystitis, chronic fecal carriage of bacteria

demonstrated to cause more rapid or consistent improvement of disease. Chloramphenicol is given orally in a dose of 50 to 60 mg/kg/day in four equal portions every 6 hours. After defervescence and clinical improvement the dosage can be reduced to 30 mg/kg/day to complete a 14-day course.

PREVENTION. Travelers to developing countries should avoid consuming untreated water, drinks served with ice, peeled fruits, and other food that is not served hot.

SALMONELLA INFECTIONS OTHER THAN TYPHOID FEVER

In humans, the most common clinical manifestation of *Salmonella* infection is enterocolitis, with diarrhea as the major symptom. Enteric fever produced by *S. typhi* is called typhoid fever, whereas enteric fever caused by other salmonellae is named paratyphoid fever.

Outbreaks of salmonellosis occur in institutionalized patients, who are probably more prone to develop *Salmonella* infections for three reasons. First, there are more underlying diseases that decrease host defense mechanisms; second, use of antimicrobial agents reduces the normal, protective intestinal flora; and third, institutional food prepared in bulk is more likely to be contaminated than individually prepared meals.

ENTEROCOLITIS. After an incubation period, which is usually 12 to 48 hours, the illness starts suddenly with crampy abdominal pain and diarrhea. Symptoms usually improve over a period of days, with fever lasting no more than 2 to 3 days and diarrhea no more than 5 to 7 days.

ENTERIC FEVER. Paratyphoid fever is an enteric fever syndrome identical to typhoid fever but produced by a serotype other than *S. typhi* (most often *serotypes paratyphi* A, *schottmuelleri,* or *hirschfeldii*).

BACTEREMIA. Patients with the syndrome of *Salmonella* bacteremia usually complain of fever and chills for a period of days to weeks.

Treatment

BACTEREMIA AND ENTERIC FEVER. The agents of choice to treat these disorders are the third-generation cephalosporins, such as ceftriaxone, cefotaxime, and ceftizoxime, or the fluoroquinolones, such as ciprofloxacin and ofloxacin.

SHIGELLOSIS

Shigellosis is an acute bacterial infection caused by the genus *Shigella* resulting in colitis affecting predominantly the rectosigmoid colon. “Bacillary dysentery” is synonymous with shigellosis. The disease is characterized by diarrhea, dysentery, fever, abdominal pain, and tenesmus (Table 20–39). Shigellosis is usually limited to a few days. Early treatment with antimicrobial drugs results in more rapid recovery.

TREATMENT. Appropriate antimicrobial therapy instituted early may decrease the duration of symptoms by 50% and decrease the duration of excretion of shigellae (an important epidemiologic fac-

Table 20–39 ■ EVOLUTION OF CLINICAL SYNDROMES IN SHIGELLOSIS

STAGE	TIME OF APPEARANCE AFTER ONSET OF ILLNESS	SYMPTOMS AND SIGNS	PATHOLOGY
Prodrome	Earliest	Fever, chills, myalgias, anorexia, nausea, vomiting	None or early colitis
Non-specific diarrhea	0–3 d	Abdominal cramps, loose stools, watery diarrhea	Rectosigmoid colitis with superficial ulceration, fecal leukocytes
Dysentery	1–8 d	Frequent passage of blood and mucus, tenesmus, rectal prolapse, abdominal tenderness	Colitis extending sometimes to proximal colon, crypt abscesses, inflammation in lamina propria
Complications	3–10 d	Dehydration, seizures, septicemia, leukemoid reaction, hemolytic-uremic syndrome, ileus, peritonitis	Severe colitis, terminal ileitis, endotoxemia, intravascular coagulation, toxic megacolon, colonic perforation
Post-dysenteric syndromes	1–3 wk	Arthritis, Reiter's syndrome	Reactive inflammation in HLA-B27 haplotype

Table 20–40 ■ CLINICAL PRESENTATIONS OF *Campylobacter jejuni* INFECTION

	INDUSTRIALIZED COUNTRIES	DEVELOPING COUNTRIES
Per cent of all diarrhea with *C. jejuni*	5–13	2–35
Per cent of *C. jejuni* diarrhea with:		
Fecal polymorphonuclear leukocytes	78–93	22–46
Blood in stool	60–65	5–17
Asymptomatic infection rates (%)	<2	0–39*

* Depending on age—39% if younger than 2 years old.

tor) by a far greater percentage. In adults, ciprofloxacin given orally in a dose of 500 mg twice daily for 5 days or 1 g as a single dose is the treatment of choice.

CAMPYLOBACTER ENTERITIS

Enteric infection with a member of the genus *Campylobacter* usually results in an inflammatory, occasionally bloody, diarrhea or dysentery syndrome in industrialized, temperate areas. *Campylobacter jejuni* is often the most commonly recognized cause of community-acquired inflammatory enteritis (Table 20–40).

DIAGNOSIS. History should prompt obtaining a fecal specimen in a cup if at all possible and direct microscopic examination using methylene blue or Gram stain for leukocytes or a test for fecal lactoferrin, as well as gross and/or occult blood.

THERAPY. The most important treatment for *Campylobacter* enteritis, as with all diarrheal illnesses, is adequate rehydration and maintenance fluid therapy. Indications for antibiotic treatment remain controversial. Antimotility agents should be avoided in *Campylobacter* enteritis, as with any inflammatory diarrhea.

CHOLERA

Cholera is an epidemic, acute watery diarrheal disease caused by *Vibrio cholerae.* The newly arisen *V. cholerae* O139 Bengal is now spreading globally. Large numbers of vibrios enter water sources from the voluminous liquid stools that soak clothing and linens and contaminate the environment. The setting for epidemics is often extreme poverty with lack of safe water. During interepidemic periods *V. cholerae* lurks in many brackish surface waters in an unculturable form that can be detected by specific gene amplification methods.

CLINICAL MANIFESTATIONS. Cholera can reduce a perfectly healthy, robust adult to shock and death in 4 to 6 hours. Without fluid replacement, cholera patients have signs of severe volume depletion—sunken eyes, poor skin turgor, hoarse voice, extreme thirst, faint heart sounds, weak or absent peripheral pulses, and severe muscle cramps.

TREATMENT. Early and complete replacement of fluid loss averts death and all complications. Advanced oral hydration solutions based on rice or other starchy foods hydrate efficiently and reduce diarrhea and vomiting substantially. In all except the most severe cases, oral rehydration therapy is sufficient to treat cholera, especially if started as soon as diarrhea begins.

Intravenous fluid replacement should be reserved for patients who have not received early oral replacement and are in shock and for those rapidly purging patients who exceed the capacity of oral replacement.

ENTERIC *ESCHERICHIA COLI* INFECTIONS

E. coli is the predominant aerobic, coliform species in the normal colon. However *E. coli* also can be an enteric pathogen and cause intestinal disease, usually diarrhea. Enteric *E. coli* infections are essentially acquired by the fecal-oral route, reflecting primarily a human reservoir for most recognized types of *E. coli* enteropathogens. Watery diarrhea characterizes enterotoxigenic *E. coli* infections, particularly in young children and travelers to tropical or developing areas.

The incubation period (2 to 7 days) varies with the size of the inoculum. Characteristic symptoms include malaise, abdominal cramping, anorexia, and watery diarrhea. The illness is usually self-limited to 1 to 5 days and rarely extends beyond 10 days or 2 weeks.

Hemorrhagic colitis associated with the Shiga-like toxin producing enterohemorrhagic *E. coli* (EHEC) O157:H7, O26:H11, and others is characterized by grossly bloody diarrhea often with remarkably little fever or inflammatory exudate in the stool.

DIAGNOSIS. With the exception of EHEC, which should be sought by enzyme-linked immunosorbent assay (ELISA), or other testing for the Shiga-like toxin and for sorbitol-negative EHEC O157:H7 in all patients with bloody diarrhea, definitive etiologic diagnosis of *E. coli* diarrhea requires the documentation of a specific virulence trait, such as enterotoxin, invasiveness, enteroadherence, or serotype. Except for EHEC, such tests are rarely cost-effective or clinically indicated.

THERAPY. As with all diarrheal illnesses, the primary treatment is replacement and maintenance of water and electrolytes. Because most *E. coli* diarrhea is self-limited, the role of antimicrobial agents is debated and remains of secondary importance to rehydration. In areas where the enterotoxigenic *E. coli* remains sensitive, early initiation of trimethoprim-sulfamethoxazole, tetracycline, or a quinolone antibiotic may reduce a 3- to 5-day illness to a 1- to 2-day illness if the agent is started with the first loose stool in travelers to endemic, tropical areas. On a note of caution: new data suggest antibiotic treatment increases the incidence of hemolytic uremia syndrome.

TRAVELER'S DIARRHEA

Traveler's diarrhea may be caused by various pathogens (Table 20–41) but may be prevented by using one of several drugs (Table 20–42).

Table 20-41 ■ ETIOLOGIC AGENTS OF TRAVELER'S DIARRHEA

AGENT	%
Enterotoxigenic *Escherichia coli*	30–70
Shigella	5–10
*Salmonella**	<5
*Campylobacter**	<5
Enteroaggregative *E. coli*	5–10
Rotavirus	<5
Giardia lamblia	<5
Entamoeba histolytica	<3
Cryptosporidium	<5
*Cyclospora**	<1
Others†	<1
Unknown agents	20–30

* May be higher in certain geographic areas.
† Includes Shiga's toxin–producing *E. coli, Vibrio cholerae,* non-cholera vibrios, other viruses.

EXTRAINTESTINAL INFECTIONS CAUSED BY ENTERIC BACTERIA

Bacteria constitute over half the dry weight of stool. *Bacteroides* species far outnumber other genera, at 10^{12} organisms per gram. Other anaerobes, such as fusobacteria, clostridia, and peptostreptococci, also are abundant. Among the facultative bacteria, members of the family Enterobacteriaceae predominate.

Enteric bacteria are not primary pathogens but cause disease when they escape from their usual gastrointestinal habitat.

Specific infections with enteric bacteria include peritonitis, pyelonephritis, prostatitis, meningitis (*E. coli* and *Klebsiella* are frequent causes of neonatal meningitis), pneumonia, infections from intravenous catheters, infections in neutropenia, and gram-negative bacteremia. For therapeutic purposes, the diagnosis of gram-negative

Table 20-42 ■ PREVENTION AND TREATMENT OF TRAVELER'S DIARRHEA WITH ANTIMICROBIAL AGENTS

	PREVENTION*	TREATMENT†	
ANTIMICROBIAL	Daily Dose (mg)	Dose (mg)	Duration‡ (days)
Norfloxacin	400	400 bid	3
Ciprofloxacin	500	500 bid	3
Trimethoprim-sulfamethoxazole	160:800	160:800 bid	3

* For periods up to 3 weeks.
† Loperamide given along with antimicrobial agents has given further improvement.
‡ Some studies have shown larger doses given as only a single dose to be effective.

bacteremia cannot await the results of blood cultures but must be made on clinical grounds alone.

TREATMENT. The choice of empiric antibiotics should be made on the basis of the site of the focal infection, the known antimicrobial sensitivities of previous isolates from the patient or from recent nosocomial infections in the hospital, and the patient's underlying disease.

Gram-negative bacteremia cannot be cured without eradicating the source of bacteremia.

YERSINIA INFECTIONS

Yersinia enterocolitica

Y. enterocolitica is an enteric pathogen that can cause gastroenteritis, mesenteric adenitis and ileitis ("pseudoappendicitis"), and sepsis. Infection may also trigger a variety of autoimmune phenomena, including reactive arthritis.

DIAGNOSIS. Diagnosis is based on isolation of the organism from stool, blood, or other clinical specimen.

TREATMENT. Available data do not indicate that antimicrobial therapy is efficacious in cases of uncomplicated *Y. enterocolitica* enteritis. *Y. enterocolitica* strains are susceptible in vitro to aminoglycosides, chloramphenicol, tetracycline, trimethoprim-sulfamethoxazole, third-generation cephalosporins, and quinolones. Data suggest that fluoroquinolones may be the drug of choice for extraintestinal *Y. enterocolitica* infections, in combination with a third-generation cephalosporin or an aminoglycoside in severe cases.

Yersinia pestis (Plague)

CLINICAL AND LABORATORY FEATURES. Plague presents most commonly as an acute regional lymphadenitis, or bubonic plague. In the absence of therapy, disease progresses rapidly to a septicemic phase, with marked toxicity, prostration, and shock. One of the feared complications of plague is plague pneumonia.

DIAGNOSIS. Plague can be diagnosed by isolating *Y. pestis* from blood, from an aspirate of a bubo, or from sputum.

TREATMENT AND PROGNOSIS. In the absence of therapy, plague has an estimated mortality of more than 50%; untreated primary septicemic or pneumonic plague is invariably fatal. Streptomycin was the first drug to be shown to have activity against plague, and, in the absence of controlled trials with other agents, it remains the drug of choice. Chloramphenicol and tetracycline are thought to be acceptable.

TULAREMIA

Tularemia is a rare infectious disease caused by a small gram-negative pleomorphic rod, *Francisella tularensis*. This organism is acquired from an animal reservoir. The most common form of tularemia results from *F. tularensis* penetrating the skin. Disease initiated by a tick bite is manifested by an ulcer at the site or adjacent to it. The tick defecates after feeding, and the infected feces may be scratched into the epidermis.

DIAGNOSIS. The diagnosis of ulceroglandular tularemia is made on the basis of the clinical manifestations and serologic studies.

TREATMENT. All forms of tularemia respond to the antibiotics streptomycin, gentamicin, tetracycline, and chloramphenicol. The aminoglycoside antibiotics are recommended; they produce a prompt cure of patients with the most severe form of tularemia.

DISEASES CAUSED BY PSEUDOMONADS

Pseudomonads are gram-negative aerobic bacilli that prefer moist environments and are relatively non-invasive yet can cause serious and often fatal infection when the host defense mechanism is damaged or deficient.

Pseudomonas (Burkholderia) pseudomallei causes melioidosis, which is often characterized as a glanders-like infectious disease. Patients with the acute septic form characteristically present with a short history of fever and no clinical evidence of focal infection, although skin abrasion is the presumed site of origin.

Pseudomonas aeruginosa almost never causes infection in the absence of (1) damage to a normal host defense mechanism (e.g., cancer chemotherapy–induced mucosal damage to the alimentary canal, granulocytopenia, or extensive third-degree burns); (2) deficiency or alteration in a defense mechanism (e.g., the progressive respiratory tract changes of cystic fibrosis); or (3) bypass of a normal defense mechanism.

The standard approach to suspected gram-negative sepsis, including that caused by *P. aeruginosa,* is a combination using an antipseudomonal β-lactam (penicillin or cephalosporin) with an aminoglycoside. Imipenem and perhaps the antipseudomonal quinolones—again, in combination with an aminoglycoside—are also effective.

LISTERIOSIS

Listeriosis is caused by the bacterium *Listeria monocytogenes.* The majority of afflicted patients are immunocompromised and present with meningoencephalitis. *L. monocytogenes* is distributed widely in nature throughout the world. It is recovered from water, soil, decaying vegetation, silage, sewage, insects, crustaceans, fish, birds, and wild and domestic mammals. *L. monocytogenes* is the cause of about 1% of cases of acute bacterial meningitis.

DIAGNOSIS. The microbiologic diagnosis of listeriosis is established by culture of blood, CSF, or tissue. In cases of granulomatosis infantiseptica, meconium, amniotic fluid, and lochia are cultured.

TREATMENT. Ampicillin is the antimicrobial agent of choice for listeriosis.

ACTINOMYCOSIS

Actinomycosis is a chronic bacterial infection that induces both a suppurative and a granulomatous inflammatory response. It spreads contiguously through anatomic barriers and frequently forms external sinuses, from which may extrude "sulfur granules," which are characteristic but not pathognomonic. The most common clinical forms are cervicofacial, thoracic, abdominal, and, in females, genital.

TREATMENT. Penicillin G is the drug of choice for treating an infection caused by any of the *Actinomyces.* It is given in high dosage over a prolonged period, because the infection has a tendency to recur, presumably because antibiotic penetration to areas of fibrosis and necrosis and into sulfur granules may be poor.

NOCARDIOSIS

Nocardiosis is a subacute or chronic bacterial infection that evokes a suppurative response. The most common sites of primary infection are, first, the lung and then the skin, from which bacteria may disseminate hematogenously to the CNS and other tissues. The infection often pursues a more acute and aggressive course in immunosuppressed patients.

TREATMENT. Sulfonamides are equally efficacious and are first-line agents for treatment, as is the combination of trimethoprim-sulfamethoxazole. Dosage of sulfadiazine is 6 to 10 g/day given in three to six divided doses. Dosing schedules of trimethoprim-sulfamethoxazole range from 160 mg/800 mg to 320 mg/1600 mg every 6 or 8 hours.

BRUCELLOSIS

Bacteria of the genus *Brucella* cause disease with protean manifestations (Table 20–43). Infection is transmitted to humans from

Table 20–43 ■ CLINICAL CLASSIFICATION OF HUMAN BRUCELLOSIS

	DURATION OF SYMPTOMS BEFORE DIAGNOSIS	MAJOR SYMPTOMS AND SIGNS
Subclinical		Asymptomatic
Acute and subacute	Up to 2–3 mo and 3 mo–1 yr	Malaise, chills, sweats, fatigue, headache, anorexia, arthralgias, fever, splenomegaly, lymphadenopathy, hepatomegaly
Localized	Occurs with acute or chronic untreated disease	Related to involved organs
Relapsing	2–3 mo after initial episode	Same as acute illness but may have higher fever, more fatigue, weakness, chills, and sweats
Chronic	>1 yr	Non-specific presentation but neuropsychiatric symptoms and low-grade fever most common

Table 20–44 ■ TREATMENT FOR BRUCELLOSIS

	TREATMENT
Acute	
With no endocarditis or CNS involvement	Doxycycline 200 mg/d plus rifampin 600–900 mg/d for 6 wk
	or
	Tetracycline 2 g/d for 6 wk plus streptomycin 1 g/d or gentamicin for 3 wk; alternative agents: chloramphenicol, fluoroquinolones, trimethoprim-sulfamethoxazole, imipenem
In children	Trimethoprim-sulfamethoxazole
CNS	Third-generation cephalosporin with rifampin
Localized	Surgically drain abscesses plus antimicrobial therapy for ≥6 wk
Brucella endocarditis	Bactericidal drugs; early valve replacement may be necessary

animals as a consequence of occupational exposure or ingestion of contaminated milk products. Despite the attempt to institute effective control measures, brucellosis remains a significant health and economic burden in many countries (Table 20–44).

DISEASE CAUSED BY *BARTONELLA* SPECIES

The genus *Bartonella* includes 11 species, but only 4 (*B. henselae, B. quintana, B. bacilliformis,* and *B. elizabethae*) are known to be pathogenic in humans. Three major pathologic varieties of disease are attributed to *Bartonella* infection: (1) vasculoproliferative disease, (2) endovascular disease with primary bacteremia, and (3) granulomatous disease. Examples of vasculoproliferative disease include bacillary angiomatosis and peliosis caused by *B. henselae* or *B. quintana* (formerly members of the *Rochalimaea* genus).

The state of host immune system integrity plays an important role in determining which of these disparate pathologic forms become manifest during *Bartonella* infection. For example, *B. henselae* usually causes bacillary angiomatosis in immunocompromised individuals and cat-scratch disease in immunocompetent hosts.

VASCULOPROLIFERATIVE DISEASE. Bacillary angiomatosis (epithelioid angiomatosis) was first described in 1983 in a person infected with human immunodeficiency virus (HIV). Classic bartonellosis (*B. bacilliformis* infection; Carrión's disease) is an insect-borne disorder characterized by two well-defined clinical stages: Oroya fever and verruga peruana.

BACTEREMIC DISEASE. Trench fever was described as a specific clinical entity during World War I. The agent was renamed *B. quintana.*

GRANULOMATOUS DISEASE. Cat-scratch disease affects about 22,000 persons in the United States, usually in the summer and autumn. Severe symptoms may be seen in about 2% of patients. Treatment recommendations (Table 20–45) are based on retrospective or empirical clinical observations.

Table 20–45 ■ TREATMENT SUGGESTIONS

Severe Cat-Scratch Disease*	
Doxycycline, plus	100 mg bid
rifampin	300 mg bid
or ciprofloxacin	500 mg bid
or azithromycin	500 mg qd × 1 d, then 250 mg qd × 4 d
Bacillary Angiomatosis-Peliosis or *Bartonella* Bacteremia†	
Erythromycin or	250–500 mg qid
doxycycline	100 mg bid
plus rifampin (severe disease)	300 mg bid
Azithromycin	500 mg qd × 1 d, then 250 mg/d

* Therapy with doxycycline plus rifampin or ciprofloxacin should be continued for at least 14 days.

† Treat patients with bacillary angiomatosis-peliosis for at least 3 to 4 months, patients with *Bartonella* bacteremia for 2 to 4 weeks, and patients with *Bartonella* endocarditis for at least 6 weeks.

TUBERCULOSIS

The characteristic features of tuberculosis include a generally prolonged latency period between initial infection and overt disease, prominent pulmonary disease (although other organs can be involved), and a granulomatous response associated with intense tissue inflammation and damage.

EPIDEMIOLOGY. Globally, tuberculosis is now the leading infectious cause of morbidity and mortality. The World Health Organization (WHO) estimates that approximately one third of the world's population is latently infected with *Mycobacterium tuberculosis*. From this pool, 8 to 10 million new active cases emerge per year.

PULMONARY DISEASE. Classic symptoms include the following: cough (nearly universal), variable appearance of blood streaking or gross hemoptysis, feverishness (common as the disease advances), malaise, fatigue, weight loss, non-pleuritic chest pain, and dyspnea. The chest radiograph is central to the diagnosis. Upper lung zone fibronodular shadowing involving one or both apices is seen in the majority of cases.

EXTRAPULMONARY TUBERCULOSIS. This occurs in roughly one sixth of HIV-negative adults in the United States with active disease.

TREATMENT. The CDC recommends a four-drug regimen to combat resistant strains (Table 20–46 and 20–47).

OTHER MYCOBACTERIOSES

Among the mycobacteria, *M. tuberculosis, M. bovis,* and *M. leprae* have caused most human infections. In the 1950s, however, Timpe and Runyon established that other mycobacteria could cause disease in humans and classified these organisms based on pigment production, growth rate, and colonial characteristics (Table 20–48).

Table 20–46 ■ RECOMMENDED REGIMEN OPTIONS FOR TUBERCULOSIS, UNITED STATES*

REGIMEN	MEDICATIONS	TOTAL DURATION
ATS/CDC (as modified by ACET)	INH and RIF daily for 6 mo PZA and SM or EMB daily for 2 mo	6 mo
Denver	INH, RIF, PZA, and SM daily for 2 wk; then twice weekly for 6 wk; follow with INH and RIF twice weekly for 18 wk	6 mo
Hong Kong	INH, RIF, PZA, and SM or EMB thrice weekly for 6 mo (may stop PZA, SM, or EMB after 2 mo)	6 mo
Arkansas	INH and RIF daily for 1 mo; then INH and RIF twice weekly for 8 mo	9 mo

INH = isoniazid; RIF = rifampin; PZA = pyrazinamide; SM = streptomycin; EMB = ethambutol.

* Currently, the Advisory Council for the Elimination of Tuberculosis (ACET) of the Centers for Disease Control and Prevention (CDC) advocates initial four-drug therapy for cases in communities with a background prevalence of initial drug resistance of 4% or greater. If susceptibility has been demonstrated or if resistance is deemed very unlikely, initial three-drug regimens may be used.

LEPROSY (HANSEN'S DISEASE)

Leprosy is a bacterial disease of great chronicity and low infectivity that occurs worldwide. The primary host is the human, in whom the causative agent, *Mycobacterium leprae,* accumulates largely in the skin and peripheral nerves.

CLINICAL DIAGNOSIS. Patients with leprosy are first seen and followed by dermatologists because the anesthetic cutaneous lesions are often the presenting complaint. The range in immune response

Table 20–47 ■ DOSAGE FOR ANTITUBERCULOSIS MEDICATIONS

DRUG	DAILY DOSE	USUAL ADULT DOSE THRICE/TWICE WEEKLY
Isoniazid	300 mg PO	600/900 mg
Rifampin*	600 mg PO 450 mg in persons <50 kg body weight	600/(same)
Pyrazinamide	25–30 mg/kg PO	30–35 mg/kg/(same)
Ethambutol	15 mg/kg PO	35 mg/kg/50 mg/kg
Streptomycin	12–15 mg/kg IM	15 mg/kg/(same)

* Rifampin drug interactions have been reported with anti-retroviral agents, including protease inhibitors and non-nucleoside reverse transcriptase inhibitors, oral contraceptives, anticoagulants, methadone, corticosteroids, estrogen replacement, calcium channel blockers, β-blockers, cyclosporine, antifungal agents (azols), phenytoin, theophylline, sulfonylureas, haloperidol, and others (see *Physicians' Desk Reference*).

Table 20–48 ■ NON-TUBERCULOUS MYCOBACTERIAL DISEASES AND ETIOLOGIC SPECIES

CLINICAL DISEASE	SPECIES (RUNYAN GROUP)
Pulmonary	*M. avium* complex (III) *M. kansasii* (I) *M. abscessus* (IV) *M. xenopi* (II)
Lymphadenitis	*M. avium* complex (III) *M. scrofulaceum* (II)
Cutaneous	*M. marinum* (I) *M. fortuitum* (IV) *M. chelonei* (IV) *M. abscessus* (IV) *M. ulcerans* (III)
Disseminated	*M. avium* complex (III) *M. kansasii* (I) *M. chelonei* (IV) *M. abscessus* (IV) *M. haemophilum* (III)

I = photochromogen; II = scotochromogen; III = nonpigmented; IV = rapid grower.

to *M. leprae* is reflected clinically by a wide variation of skin lesions and peripheral nerve involvement. The immunologic features of leprosy patients are shown in Table 20–49.

TREATMENT. The most commonly used drug in the therapy for leprosy is 4,4′-diaminodiphenylsulfone (dapsone, DDS). Because of the widespread emergence of dapsone-resistant strains of *M. leprae,* all patients now receive multidrug therapy.

1. *Paucibacillary disease of the polar tuberculoid and borderline tuberculoid categories.*
   a. Dapsone-sensitive *M. leprae:* dapsone is given in a dose of 100 mg/kg and rifampin in a dose of 600 mg/day for 1 year.
   b. Dapsone-resistant *M. leprae:* clofazimine at a dose of 50 to 100 mg/day is substituted for dapsone.
2. *Multibacillary disease of the borderline, borderline lepromatous, and polar lepromatous categories.*
   a. Dapsone-sensitive or dapsone-resistant *M. leprae:* dapsone is given in a dose of 100 mg/day, rifampin is given in a dose of 600 mg/day, and clofazimine is given in a dose of 50 mg/day for 2 years.

A modified schedule for Third World country control programs was issued by the WHO.

1. *Paucibacillary disease—a bacillary index of 0 at all six skin sites.* Dapsone is given in a dose of 100 mg/day, unsupervised. Rifampin is given at a dose of 600 mg once a month, supervised. Treatment is given for 6 months and is then discontinued.
2. *Multibacillary disease—a bacillary index of 1+ or more at any one of six skin sites.* Dapsone is given in a dose of 100 mg/day with clofazimine 50 mg/day, unsupervised. Rif-

Table 20–49 ■ IMMUNOLOGIC FEATURES OF LEPROSY PATIENTS

	TUBERCULOID	BORDERLINE TUBERCULOID	MID–BORDERLINE	BORDERLINE LEPROMATOUS	LEPROMATOUS
Acid-fast bacilli in skin lesions	–	–/+	+	+++	+++
Lepromin (Mitsuda) reaction	+++	+++	–	–	–
Lymphocyte transformation test	95%	40%	10%	1–2%	1–2%
Anti–*Mycobacterium leprae* antibodies	–/+	–/++	++	+++	+++
CD4+/CD8+ T-cell ratio in lesions	1.35	1.11	NT	0.48	0.20

ampin 600 mg and clofazimine 300 mg are given once monthly, supervised. This therapy is continued for 2 years.

SEXUALLY TRANSMITTED DISEASES

Sexually transmitted diseases may be caused by a number of different agents (Table 20–50) but are grouped together because of common clinical and epidemiologic features.

In males, urethritis is a common syndrome which may be gonococcal or non-gonococcal in derivation. Management of urethritis (Fig. 20–1) should include the patient and any sexual partners.

In females, vaginitis may involve yeast infection (*Candida albicans*), *Trichomonas* (*T. vaginalis*) infection, and bacterial vaginosis (Table 20–51). Bacterial vaginosis is the most common cause of vaginitis in women of childbearing age. This syndrome is probably caused by mixed infection by *Gardnerella vaginalis* and anaerobic bacteria, including the curved or common-shaped rods known as *Mobiluncus* species.

For more information about this subject, see *Cecil Textbook of Medicine,* 21st edition. Philadelphia, W.B. Saunders Company, 2000. Chapter 361, on Sexually Transmitted Diseases, pages 1738 to 1742.

Gonococcal Infections

Neisseria gonorrhoeae is a common sexually transmitted organism that causes anterior urethritis in males and endocervicitis and urethritis in females. Gonorrhea is the most common reportable infectious disease in the United States, with nearly 400,000 cases reported in 1995. The true incidence is probably twice as high.

CLINICAL PATTERNS OF DISEASE. ***GONORRHEA IN MALES.*** Gonococcal urethritis in males ("the clap" or "the strain") is characterized by a yellowish, purulent urethral discharge and dysuria. The usual incubation period is 2 to 6 days.

GONORRHEA IN FEMALES. In incidence studies, approximately one half of women infected with the gonococcus are asymptomatic or have so few symptoms that they do not seek medical care. The most commonly involved site is the endocervix (80 to 90%).

TREATMENT. Management is by antibiotic therapy (Table 20–52).

Syphilis

Syphilis is a chronic infectious disease caused by the bacterium *Treponema pallidum.* It is usually acquired by sexual contact with another infected person. Syphilis is remarkable among infectious diseases in its large variety of clinical presentations. It progresses, if untreated, through primary, secondary, and tertiary stages (Table 20–53). The early stages (primary and secondary) are infectious. Spontaneous healing of early lesions occurs, followed by a long latent period. In about 30% of untreated patients, late disease of the heart, CNS, or other organs ultimately develops.

NATURAL COURSE OF UNTREATED SYPHILIS. The incubation period from time of exposure to development of the primary lesion

Table 20–50 ■ SEXUALLY TRANSMITTED AGENTS AND THEIR SYNDROMES*

MICROORGANISM	SYNDROME
Bacteria	
Neisseria gonorrhoeae	Urethritis, cervicitis, bartholinitis, proctitis, pharyngitis, salpingitis, epididymitis, conjunctivitis, perihepatitis, arthritis, dermatitis, endocarditis, meningitis, amniotic infection syndrome
Mobiluncus spp. and *Gardnerella vaginalis*	Bacterial vaginosis
Treponema pallidum	Syphilis (multiple clinical syndromes)
Haemophilus ducreyi	Chancroid
Calymmatobacterium granulomatis	Granuloma inguinale
Shigella spp.	Enteritis in homosexual men
Campylobacter spp.	Enteritis in homosexual men
Group B *Streptococcus*	Neonatal sepsis and meningitis
Chlamydiae	
Chlamydia trachomatis	Nongonococcal urethritis, purulent hypertrophic cervicitis, epididymitis, salpingitis, conjunctivitis, trachoma, pneumonia, perihepatitis, lymphogranuloma venereum, Reiter's syndrome
Mycoplasmas	
Ureaplasma urealyticum	Nongonococcal urethritis, premature rupture of membranes and abortion
Mycoplasma hominis	Postpartum fever, pelvic inflammatory disease
Viruses	
Herpes simplex virus	Genital herpes, proctitis, meningitis, disseminated infection in neonates
Hepatitis A virus	Hepatitis in homosexual men
Hepatitis B virus	Hepatitis, periarteritis nodosa, hepatoma; especially prevalent in homosexual men
Cytomegalovirus	Congenital infection (birth defects, infant mortality, mental deficiency, hearing loss), mononucleosis syndrome
Human papillomavirus	Condyloma acuminatum, cervical and perianal
Molluscum contagiosum virus	Molluscum contagiosum
Human immunodeficiency virus	Acquired immunodeficiency syndrome and related illnesses
Protozoa	
Trichomonas vaginalis	Trichomonal vaginitis, occasional urethritis
Entamoeba histolytica	Enteritis in homosexual men
Giardia lamblia	Enteritis in homosexual men
Fungi	
Candida albicans	Vaginitis, balanitis
Ectoparasites	
Phthirus pubis	Pubic lice infestation
Sarcoptes scabiei	Scabies

* The relative importance of sexual transmission in the epidemiology of several of these agents remains to be defined; these include group B streptococci, hepatitis A virus, cytomegalovirus, *Candida albicans*, and others.

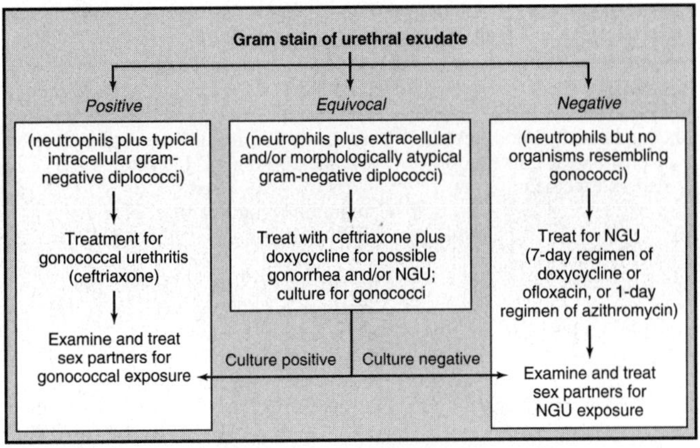

Gram stain of urethral exudate

Positive	Equivocal	Negative
(neutrophils plus typical intracellular gram-negative diplococci)	(neutrophils plus extracellular and/or morphologically atypical gram-negative diplococci)	(neutrophils but no organisms resembling gonococci)
↓	↓	↓
Treatment for gonococcal urethritis (ceftriaxone)	Treat with ceftriaxone plus doxycycline for possible gonorrhea and/or NGU; culture for gonococci	Treat for NGU (7-day regimen of doxycycline or ofloxacin, or 1-day regimen of azithromycin)
↓	Culture positive → left; Culture negative → right	↓
Examine and treat sex partners for gonococcal exposure		Examine and treat sex partners for NGU exposure

FIGURE 20–1 ■ Management of male patients with urethritis. NGU = nongonococcal urethritis.

at the place of initial inoculation of treponemes averages approximately 21 days but ranges from 10 to 90 days. A painless papule develops and soon breaks down to form a clean-based ulcer, the chancre, with raised, indurated margins. Several weeks later the patient characteristically develops a secondary stage characterized by low-grade fever, headache, malaise, generalized lymphadenopathy, and a mucocutaneous rash. The secondary lesions heal spontaneously within 2 to 6 weeks, and the infection then enters latency. About one third of untreated patients eventually develop late destructive tertiary lesions involving one or more of the eyes, CNS, heart, or other organs, including skin. These may occur at any time from a few years to as late as 25 years after infection.

TREATMENT. Management is usually by a long-term course of penicillin (Table 20–54).

LYME DISEASE

Lyme disease is a tick-borne inflammatory disorder caused by the spirochete *Borrelia burgdorferi*. Its clinical hallmark is an early

Table 20–51 ■ DIFFERENTIAL DIAGNOSIS OF VAGINITIS

CHARACTERISTICS OF VAGINAL DISCHARGE	*CANDIDA ALBICANS* VAGINITIS	*TRICHOMONAS VAGINALIS* VAGINITIS	BACTERIAL VAGINOSIS
pH	4.5	>5.0	>5.0
White curd	Usually	No	No
Odor with KOH	No	Yes	Yes
Clue cells	No	No	Usually
Motile trichomonads	No	Usually	No
Yeast cells	Yes	No	No

Table 20–52 ■ ANTIBIOTIC REGIMENS RECOMMENDED FOR GONOCOCCAL INFECTION

DIAGNOSIS	TREATMENT
Uncomplicated genital, rectal, or pharyngeal infection of men and women	Ceftriaxone 125 mg IM once, plus doxycycline 100 mg PO bid for 7 d *or* Cefixime 400 mg PO once, plus doxycycline 100 mg PO bid for 7 d *or* Ciprofloxacin 500 mg PO once, plus doxycycline 100 mg PO bid for 7 d *or* Ofloxacin 400 mg PO once, plus doxycycline 100 mg PO bid for 7 d
Gonorrhea in pregnancy	Ceftriaxone 125 mg IM once, plus erythromycin base 500 mg PO qid for 7 d *or* Spectinomycin 2 g IM, plus erythromycin (as in ceftriaxone regimen)
Salpingitis—outpatient	Cefoxitin 2 g IM, plus doxycycline 100 mg PO bid for 10–14 d *or* Ofloxacin 400 mg PO bid for 14 d, plus either clindamycin 450 mg PO qid or metronidazole, 500 mg PO bid for 14 d
Salpingitis—inpatient	Doxycycline 100 mg IV bid, plus cefoxitin 2 g IV qid until improved, followed by doxycycline 100 mg PO bid to complete 14 d of therapy; alternative regimens include clindamycin plus an aminoglycoside
Disseminated gonococcal infection	Ceftriaxone 1 g IM q24h *or* Spectinomycin 2 g IM q12h

expanding skin lesion, *erythema migrans* (Table 20–55). Lyme disease is widespread. In the United States there are three distinct foci: the Northeast, from southern Maine to Maryland; the upper Midwest; and the West in northern California. Over 90% of reported cases come from eight states: Connecticut, Maryland, Massachusetts, New Jersey, New York, Pennsylvania, Minnesota, and Wisconsin.

Table 20–53 ■ FREQUENCY OF POSITIVE SEROLOGIC TESTS IN UNTREATED SYPHILIS

STAGE	VDRL (%)	FTA-ABS (%)	MHA-TP (%)
Primary	70	85	50–60
Secondary	99	100	100
Latent or late	70	98	98

VDRL = Venereal Disease Research Laboratories; FTA-ABS = fluorescent treponemal antibody absorption (test); MHA-TP = microhemagglutination assay—*Treponema pallidum.*

Table 20–54 ■ PENICILLIN TREATMENT PRACTICE IN SYPHILIS AS RECOMMENDED BY U.S. PUBLIC HEALTH SERVICE

INDICATIONS FOR SYPHILIS THERAPY†	DOSAGE AND ADMINISTRATION*	
	Benzathine Penicillin G	**Aqueous Benzyl Penicillin G or Procaine Penicillin G**
Primary, secondary, and early latent syphilis (<1 yr); epidemiologic treatment	Total of 2.4 million U; single IM dose of 2 injections of 1.2 million U in one session	Total of 4.8 million U IM in doses of 600,000 U/d for 8 consecutive days
Late latent (>1 yr) or when CSF was not examined in "latency"; cardiovascular syphilis, late benign (cutaneous, osseous, visceral gumma)	Total of 7.2 million U IM in doses of 2.4 million U at 7-d intervals, over 21 d	Total of 9 million units IM in doses of 600,000 U/d over 15 d
Symptomatic or asymptomatic neurosyphilis	2–4 million U of aqueous (crystalline) penicillin G IV q4h for ≥10 d	2–4 million U/d procaine penicillin IM and probenecid 500 mg PO qid for 10–14 d
Congenital		
Infants	CSF normal: total of 500,000 U/kg IM in a single or divided dose at 1 session	CSF abnormal: total of 50,000 U/kg/d IM for 10 consecutive days‡
Older children	CSF normal: same as for early congenital syphilis, up to 2.4 million U	CSF abnormal: 200,000–300,000 U/kg/d IV aqueous crystalline penicillin for 10–14 d

CSF = cerebrospinal fluid
* Individual doses can be divided for injection in each buttock to minimize discomfort.
† In *pregnancy,* treatment is dependent on the stage of syphilis.
‡ For aqueous penicillin, give in two divided IV doses per day; for procaine penicillin, give as one daily dose IM.

Table 20–55 ■ EARLY SIGNS OF LYME DISEASE IN A STUDY OF 314 PATIENTS

SIGNS	NO. OF PATIENTS (%)
Erythema migrans*	314 (100)
Multiple annular lesions	150 (48)
Lymphadenopathy	
Regional	128 (41)
Generalized	63 (20)
Pain on neck flexion	52 (17)
Malar rash	41 (13)
Erythematous throat	38 (12)
Conjunctivitis	35 (11)
Right upper quadrant tenderness	24 (8)
Splenomegaly	18 (6)
Hepatomegaly	16 (5)
Muscle tenderness	12 (4)
Periorbital edema	10 (3)
Evanescent skin lesions	8 (3)
Abdominal tenderness	6 (2)
Testicular swelling	2 (1)

* Erythema migrans was required for inclusion in this study.

From Steere AC, et al: The early clinical manifestations of Lyme disease. Ann Intern Med 99:76, 1983.

The major goal of therapy in Lyme disease is to eradicate the causative organism. Like other spirochetal diseases, Lyme disease is most responsive to antibiotics early in its course (Table 20–56).

LEPTOSPIROSIS

Leptospirosis is a spirochetal infection with bacteria of the genus *Leptospira.* The severe icteric form of infection is called Weil's disease, after the investigator who in 1886 described four men with an acute but self-limited infectious illness characterized by fever, jaundice, nephritis, and hepatomegaly, and a biphasic course, with fever recurring 1 to 7 days into convalescence. The most common source of exposure in the United States is dogs, followed by livestock, rodents, and other wild animals.

Symptoms develop 7 to 12 days after exposure. Most patients have an abrupt onset of a self-limited 4- to 7-day anicteric illness characterized by the sudden onset of fever, mild to severe headache, myalgias, chills, cough, chest pain, neck stiffness, and/or prostration. Pre-tibial, raised, 1- to 5-cm erythematous lesions are seen characteristically in a form of leptospirosis called 'Fort Bragg fever.'

The diagnosis is usually made retrospectively by a four-fold rise in agglutinating antibody titer. The microscopic agglutination test (MAT) detects serum antibodies against the 21 most common serovars of *Leptospira.*

THERAPY. Doxycycline 100 mg orally twice a day for 7 days, started within 48 hours of illness, decreased the duration of illness by 2 days in one study; penicillin 2.4 to 3.6 million U/day also has been successful early treatment.

Table 20–56 ■ RECOMMENDATIONS FOR ANTIBIOTIC TREATMENT OF LYME DISEASE*

Early Lyme Disease†

Amoxicillin 500 mg tid for 21 d‡
Doxycycline 100 mg bid for 21 d
Cefuroxime axetil 500 mg bid for 21 d
Azithromycin 500 mg/d for 7 d§
(less effective than other regimens)

Neurologic Manifestations

Bell's-like palsy (no other neurologic abnormalities)
Oral regimens of doxycycline or amoxicillin for 21–28 d
Meningitis (with or without radiculoneuropathy or encephalitis)||
Ceftriaxone 2 g/d for 14–28 d
Penicillin G 20 million U d for 14–28 d
Doxycycline 100 mg bid PO or IV for 21–28 d¶

Arthritis**

Amoxicillin 500 mg tid for 30–60 d
Doxycycline 100 mg bid for 30–60 d
Ceftriaxone 2 g/d for 30 d
Penicillin G 20 million U/d for 30 d

Carditis

Ceftriaxone 2 g/d for 14–28 d
Penicillin G 20 million U/d for 14–28 d
Doxycycline 100 mg bid PO for 30 d††
Amoxicillin 500 mg tid for 30 d††

Pregnancy

Localized early disease
Amoxicillin 500 mg tid for 21 d
Any manifestation of disseminated disease
Penicillin G 20 million U/d for 14–28 d
Asymptomatic seropositivity
No treatment necessary

* These are guidelines, to be modified by new findings and to be applied always with close attention to the clinical context of individual patients.

† Without neurologic, cardiac, or joint involvement. For early Lyme disease limited to single erythema migrans lesion, 10 days may suffice.

‡ Some experts advise addition of probenecid 500 mg three times daily.

§ Experience with this agent is limited; optimal duration of therapy is unclear.

|| Optimal duration of therapy has not been established. There are no controlled trials of therapy longer than 4 weeks for any manifestation of Lyme disease.

¶ No published experience in the United States.

** An oral regimen should be selected only if there is no neurologic involvement.

†† Oral regimens have been reserved for mild carditis limited to first-degree heart block with P–R ≤ 0.30 second and normal ventricular function.

Adapted from Rahn DW, Malawista SE: Treatment of Lyme disease (special article). *In* Mandell GL, Bone RC, Cline MJ, et al (eds): 1994 Year Book of Medicine. St. Louis, Mosby–Year Book, 1994.

20

DISEASES CAUSED BY CHLAMYDIAE

Chlamydiae are among the most common of all human infectious agents and produce much disability although little mortality (Table 20–57).

In 1986, a new chlamydial pathogen was recognized—*Chlamydia pneumoniae*—which causes respiratory illness. More than 50% of adults in the United States and from other developed

Table 20–57 ■ MAJOR DISEASES CAUSED BY *Chlamydia*, AND CARDINAL EPIDEMIOLOGIC FEATURES

SPECIES	DISEASE	HOST RESERVOIR	TRANSMISSION ROUTE
C. trachomatis	Trachoma	Children	Fomites/flies
	Urethritis/cervicitis	Sexually active teenagers and adults	Direct sexual contact
	Epididymitis/salpingitis	Sexually active teenagers and adults	Direct sexual contact
	Lymphogranuloma venereum	Sexually active teenagers and adults	Direct sexual contact
	Inclusion conjunctivitis	Infected pregnant mothers	Direct perinatal contact
	Infant pneumonia		
C. psittaci	Atypical pneumonia	Birds	Aerosol
	Culture-negative endocarditis		
C. pneumoniae	Bronchitis	Humans	Respiratory droplet
	Atypical pneumonia		

countries are seropositive. Most seroconversion occurs during childhood. *C. pneumoniae* also causes bronchitis and sinusitis.

RICKETTSIAL DISEASES

Rickettsial diseases are transmitted to humans by ticks, mites, lice, fleas, or aerosols originating from animal products, or from feces of the insects noted. In general, rickettsial diseases are relatively rare, but they may be public health problems in developing countries. Clinical features of rickettsial diseases are detailed in Table 20–58.

For more information about this subject, see *Cecil Textbook of Medicine,* 21st edition. Philadelphia, W.B. Saunders Company, 2000. Chapter 371, Rickettsial Diseases, pages 1767 to 1778.

ZOONOSES

Zoonoses are most simply defined as human infections derived from animals. Approximately 200 different infectious agents, many of them rare, cause disease in humans. Highly fatal zoonoses are noted in Table 20–59. Newly characterized zoonoses are detailed in Table 20–60.

For more information about this subject, see *Cecil Textbook of Medicine,* 21st edition. Philadelphia, W.B. Saunders Company, 2000. Chapter 372, Zoonoses, pages 1778 to 1780.

VIRAL DISEASES AND ANTIVIRAL THERAPY

Viruses are among the simplest and smallest forms of life. Viruses cause cell injury and as cells are injured, disease results. Viral infection may be limited to the initial site of infection or may spread through the lymphatic, blood, or nervous systems. Viral infections may be classified according to mechanisms of pathogenesis (Table 20–61).

Advances in chemotherapy to combat viruses are increasingly common. Several antiviral agents of proven clinical value are available and for a limited number of indications (Table 20–62).

For more information about this subject, see *Cecil Textbook of Medicine,* 21st edition. Philadelphia, W.B. Saunders Company, 2000. Chapter 373, Introduction to Viral Diseases; and Chapter 374, Antiviral Therapy (Non-AIDS), pages 1780 to 1790.

VIRAL PHARYNGITIS, LARYNGITIS, CROUP, AND BRONCHITIS

Viral infections that localize to the upper and middle respiratory passages produce an acute inflammatory response and, depending on the anatomic site involved, evoke the clinical manifestations of pharyngitis, laryngitis, croup (laryngotracheobronchitis), and bronchitis (Table 20–63).

For more information about this subject, see *Cecil Textbook of Medicine,* 21st edition. Philadelphia, W.B. Saunders Company, 2000. Chapter 376, Viral Pharyngitis, Laryngitis, Croup, and Bronchitis, pages 1793 to 1794.

Table 20–58 ■ SOME CLINICAL FEATURES OF SELECTED RICKETTSIAL DISEASES

DISEASE	USUAL INCUBATION PERIOD (days)	ESCHAR	RASH			USUAL DURATION OF DISEASE (days) (RANGE)	USUAL SEVERITY*	FEVER AFTER CHEMOTHERAPY (hr)
			Onset, Day of Disease	Distribution	Type			
Typhus group								
Murine typhus	12 (8–16)	None	5–7	Trunk → extremities	Macular, maculopapular	12 (8–16)	Moderate	48–72
Epidemic typhus	12	None	5–7	Trunk → extremities	Macular, maculopapular	14 (10–18)	Severe	48–72
Brill-Zinsser disease	(10–14)	None		Trunk → extremities	Macular	7–11	Relatively mild	48–72
Spotted fever group								
Rocky Mountain spotted fever	7 (12–13)	None	3–5	Extremities → trunk, face	Macular, maculopapular, petechial	16 (10–20)	Severe†	72
Boutonneuse fever	5–7	Often present	3–4	Trunk, soles, extremities face, palms	Macular, maculopapular, petechial	10 (7–14)	Moderate	24–48
Rickettsialpox	?9–17	Often present	1–3	Trunk → face, extremities	Papulovesicular	7 (3–11)	Relatively mild	
Ehrlichiosis	7–21	None	?Rare	Unknown	Petechial	7 (3–19)	Moderate	72
Scrub typhus (tsutsugamushi disease)	1–12 (9–18)	Often present	4–6	Trunk → extremities	Macular, maculopapular	7 (3–11)	Relatively mild	
Q fever	10–19	None		None		(2–21)	Relatively mild‡	48 (occasionally slow)

* Severity can vary greatly. † Untreated disease. ‡ Occasionally subacute or chronic infections occur (e.g., hepatitis, endocarditis).

Table 20–59 ■ HIGHLY FATAL ZOONOSES

DISEASE	FATALITY RATE (%)
Creutzfeldt-Jakob disease (new variant)	100
Rabies	100
Anthrax pneumonia	100
Herpes simiae*	50–75
Ebola virus	70
Eastern equine encephalitis	50–70
Hantavirus pulmonary syndrome†	60
Yellow fever‡	20–50
Lassa fever‡	15–25
Plague*	50–80
Rocky Mountain spotted fever*	20–60
East African sleeping sickness*	20–30
Anthrax—cutaneous*	20
Tularemia	10–15
Visceral leishmaniasis*	5–25
Louse-borne relapsing fever*	5–40

* Fatality rate if untreated.
† If jaundiced.
‡ Case mortality of hospitalized patients.

INFLUENZA

Influenza is an acute febrile respiratory illness that occurs in annual outbreaks of varying severity. The causative virus infects the respiratory tract, is highly contagious, and typically produces prominent systemic symptoms early in the illness (Table 20–64). Groups with high risk of influenza complications and their immediate contacts should be immunized (Table 20–65).

RESPIRATORY COMPLICATIONS. Three kinds of pneumonic syndromes have been described: (1) primary influenza viral pneumonia, (2) secondary bacterial pneumonia, and (3) mixed viral and bacterial pneumonia.

For more information about this subject, see *Cecil Textbook of Medicine,* 21st edition. Philadelphia, W.B. Saunders Company, 2000. Chapter 379, Influenza, pages 1797 to 1800.

ADENOVIRUS DISEASES

The adenoviruses can infect and cause disease in a variety of human epithelial tissues, including those of the eye, respiratory tract, gastrointestinal tract, and urinary bladder. Most infections in immunologically competent persons are subclinical (Table 20–66).

20

For more information about this subject, see *Cecil Textbook of Medicine,* 21st edition. Philadelphia, W.B. Saunders Company, 2000. Chapter 380, Adenovirus Diseases, pages 1800 to 1802.

MEASLES

Measles is an acute, highly contagious disease characterized by fever, coryza, conjunctivitis, and both an enanthem and an exanthem. Differential diagnosis of measles includes consideration of

Text continued on page 630

Table 20–60 ▪ NEWLY CHARACTERIZED ZOONOSES

DISEASE	INFECTIOUS AGENT	CLINICAL INFORMATION	VECTOR
Ehrlichiosis, monocytic	*Ehrlichia chaffeensis*	Fever, myalgia, leukopenia	Tick bite
Ehrlichiosis, granulocytic	Human granulocytic *Ehrlichia*	Fever, myalgia, leukopenia	Tick bite
Cat-scratch disease	*Bartonella* spp.	Cervical lymphadenopathy in normal hosts and cutaneous and hepatic angiomatosis in AIDS patients	Cat scratch or bite
Hemorrhagic diarrhea	Enterohemorrhagic *Escherichia coli* O157 : H7 (other species)	Rectal bleeding, dysentery, hemolytic uremic syndrome	Contaminated, undercooked meat
Hantavirus pulmonary syndrome	Hantavirus—Sin Nombre	Adult respiratory distress syndrome	Fomites of rodents
Cryptosporidum diarrhea	*Cryptosporidium parvum* (?)	Diarrhea	Contaminated water
Dysentery	*Campylobacter jejuni*	Dysentery, Reiter's syndrome, Guillain-Barré syndrome	Contaminated chicken
Pyogenic skin ulcer	*Capnocytophaga canimorsus*	Sepsis, skin infection	Dog bites

Table 20–61 ■ VIRUSES COMMONLY ASSOCIATED WITH DIFFERENT SYNDROMES

DISEASE CATEGORY	COMMON ASSOCIATED VIRUS
Respiratory Tract	
Upper respiratory tract infection (including common cold and pharyngitis)	Rhinoviruses Coronaviruses Parainfluenza 1–3 Influenza A, B Herpes simplex Adenoviruses Echoviruses Coxsackieviruses Epstein-Barr virus Respiratory syncytial
Croup	Parainfluenza 1–3 Influenza A, B Respiratory syncytial
Bronchiolitis	Respiratory syncytial Parainfluenza 1–3
Pneumonia (adults)	Influenza A
Pneumonia (children)	Respiratory syncytial Parainfluenza 1–3 Influenza A
Central Nervous System	
Aseptic meningitis	Mumps Coxsackievirus B1–5 Coxsackievirus A9 Echovirus 4, 6, 9, 11, 14, 18, 30, 31
Paralysis	Poliovirus 1–3
Encephalitis	Human immunodeficiency virus 1 Alphaviruses Flaviviruses Bunyaviruses Herpes simplex 1 Enterovirus 71 Mumps
Genitourinary Tract	
Vulvovaginitis, cervicitis	Herpes simplex 2
Penile and vulvar lesions	Herpes simplex 2 Molluscum contagiosum Human papillomavirus 6, 10, 11, 40–45, 51
Acute hemorrhagic cystitis	Adenovirus 11
Ocular	
Conjunctivitis	Adenovirus 3, 4, 7, 8, 19 Herpes simplex Varicella-zoster Measles
Acute hemorrhagic conjunctivitis	Enterovirus 70 Coxsackievirus A24
Immune System	
Acquired immunodeficiency syndrome	Human immunodeficiency virus 1

Table continued on following page

20

Table 20–61 ■ VIRUSES COMMONLY ASSOCIATED WITH DIFFERENT SYNDROMES *Continued*

DISEASE CATEGORY	COMMON ASSOCIATED VIRUS
Gastrointestinal Tract	
Gastroenteritis	Rotavirus Norwalk-like agents Adenovirus
Hepatitis	Hepatitis A Hepatitis B Hepatitis C Hepatitis D Hepatitis E Epstein-Barr virus Cytomegalovirus
Skin	
Maculopapular rash	Measles Rubella Parvovirus B19 Echoviruses Coxsackievirus A16 Enterovirus 71
Hemorrhagic rash	Herpesvirus G Alphavirus Bunyavirus Flaviviruses
Localized lesions	Herpes simplex Human papillomavirus 1, 2, 4, 41 Molluscum contagiosum
Neonatal	
Teratogenic effects	Rubella Cytomegalovirus
Disseminated disease	Coxsackievirus B1–5 Echoviruses Hepatitis B Parvovirus B19 Cytomegalovirus Herpes simplex
Lower respiratory disease	Respiratory syncytial Influenza
Enteritis	Rotavirus
Other	
Arthritis	Rubella Parvovirus B19 Hepatitis B
Myositis	Togaviruses Influenza B
Carditis	Coxsackievirus B
Parotitis, pancreatitis, and orchitis	Mumps

Modified from Manegus MA, Douglas RG Jr: Viruses, rickettsiae, chlamydiae, and mycoplasmas. *In* Mandell GL, Douglas RG Jr, Bennett JE (eds): Principles and Practice of Infectious Diseases, 3rd ed. New York, Churchill Livingstone, 1990.

Table 20–62 ■ INDICATIONS FOR THE USE OF AVAILABLE ANTIVIRAL AGENTS

INDICATION	ANTIVIRAL AGENT	ROUTE	DOSE	COMMENTS
Respiratory syncytial virus infection (infants)	Ribavirin	Aerosol	Diluted in sterile water to a concentration of 20 mg/mL, then delivered via aerosol for 12–18 hr/d for 3–7 d	Only for infants at high risk
Life- or sight-threatening cytomegalovirus (CMV) infections in immunocompromised hosts	Ganciclovir	IV	5.0 mg/kg q12h × 14 d	Maintenance therapy of 5.0 mg/kg/d recommended for AIDS patients; leukopenia is a frequent complication; in bone marrow transplant patients with CMV pneumonia, CMV immune globulin may be a useful adjunct
	Foscarnet	IV		
	Cidofovir	IV	5 mg once weekly × 3	Induction therapy
		IV	5 mg biweekly	Maintenance
Condyloma acuminatum	Interferon alfa	Intralesional	1.0 million U injected into the base of each lesion, up to 3 times per week for 3 wk	Flu-type symptoms may occur with administrations
Influenza A infection	Amantadine	Oral	Adults: 100–200 mg/d for 5–7 d Children ≤ 9 yr: 4.4–8.8 mg/kg/d for 5–7 d not to exceed 150 mg/d	Normal person >65 yr should receive 100 mg/d
Prophylaxis against influenza A virus infection	Amantadine	Oral	Adults: 100–200 mg/d Children ≤ 9 yr: 4.4–8.8 mg/kg/d (not to exceed 150 mg/d)	Continued for the duration of the epidemic or for 2 wks in conjunction with influenza vaccination (until vaccine-induced immunity develops); normal persons >65 yrs should receive 100 mg/d
	Rimantadine	Oral	100 mg PO bid × season	
Herpes simplex virus (HSV) encephalitis	Acyclovir	IV	10 mg/kg (1-hr infusion) q8h for 10–14 d	Morbidity and mortality are significantly lower in patients treated with acyclovir than with vidarabine
Neonatal herpes	Acyclovir	IV	10 mg/kg (1-hr infustion) q8h for 10 d	Efficacy of vidarabine is established; vidarabine and acyclovir show equal efficacy

Table continued on following page

Table 20–62 ■ INDICATIONS FOR THE USE OF AVAILABLE ANTIVIRAL AGENTS *Continued*

INDICATION	ANTIVIRAL AGENT	ROUTE	DOSE	COMMENTS
Mucocutaneous HSV in immunocompromised hosts	Acyclovir	IV	5.0 mg/kg (1-hr infusion) q8h for 7 d	Choice of topical, PO, or IV preparation depends on clinical severity and setting; topical acyclovir is appropriate only when it can be applied to all lesions; it does not affect untreated lesions or systemic symptoms
	or			
	Acyclovir	Oral	400 mg 3–5 times/d for 10 d	
	Valaciclovir		500 mg bid PO	10 d
	Famciclovir	Oral	500 mg tid	10 d
Prophylaxis against mucocutaneous HSV during intense immunosuppression	Acyclovir	Oral	200 mg 3–4 times/d	Oral therapy most convenient; lesions recur when therapy stops
	or			
	Acyclovir	IV	5 mg/kg/q8h	Lesions recur when therapy stops
Treatment of initial genital HSV infections	Acyclovir	Oral	200 mg 5 times/d for 10 d or 400 mg tid × 10 d	Drug of choice in most clinical settings; treatment has no effect on subsequent recurrence rates
	or			
	Acyclovir	IV	5 mg/kg (1-hr infusion) q8h for 5–7 d	For patients requiring hospitalization or with neurologic or other visceral complications
	Valaciclovir	Oral	1 g bid	5–10 d
	Famciclovir	Oral	250 mg tid	5–10 d
Recurrent genital herpes	Acyclovir	Oral	400 mg tid for 5 d	No effect on subsequent reucrrence rates; efficacy greater if used early in attack
	Valaciclovir	Oral	500 mg bid or 1 g qd	5–7 d
	Famciclovir	Oral	250 mg tid	5–7 d

Prophylaxis against frequently recurring genital herpes	Acyclovir	Oral	200 mg 3–5 times/d	Occasional "breaking through" attacks and/or asymptomatic virus shedding during treatment; re-evaluation every 6 mo recommended
	Valaciclovir	Oral	500 mg bid or 1 g/d	
	Famciclovir	Oral	250 mg tid	
Treatment of HSV keratitis	Trifluorothymidine	Topical	1 drop of 0.1% ophthalmic solution q2h while awake (up to 9 drops/d)	3% acyclovir ointment (ophthalmic) is equal or superior to idoxuridine, vidarabine, and trifluridine for treatment of HSV keratitis but is not available in United States
	or			
	Vidarabine	Topical	One-half-inch ribbon of 3% ophthalmic ointment 5 times/d	
	or			
	Idoxuridine	Topical	One-half-inch ribbon of 0.5% ophthalmic ointment 5 times/d	
Localized herpes zoster in immunocompetent hosts	Acyclovir	Oral	800 mg 5 times/d for 7–10 d	Shortens time to lesion healing, but not shown to decrease the incidence of post-herpetic neuralgia
	or			
	Famiclovir		250 mg tid × 5–7 d	
	or			
	Valaciclovir		1 g tid × 5–7 d	
Chickenpox in immunocompromised hosts	Acyclovir	IV	500 mg/m² (1-hr infusion) q8h for 7 d	In the absence of comparative data, acyclovir is preferred because of its ease of administration and lower toxicity
Treatment of severe localized or disseminated herpes zoster in immunocompromised hosts	Acyclovir	IV	500 mg/m² or 12.4 mg/kg (1-hr infusion) q8h for 5–7 d	Comparative trials in severe localized and disseminated herpes zoster are underway; pending results, acyclovir is preferred because of its ease of administration and lower toxicity
	or			
	Valaciclovir	Oral	1 g tid	7–10 d
	Famciclovir	Oral	500 mg tid	7–10 d
Chronic hepatitis B	Interferon alfa	SC	10×10^6 U 3 times a week for 16 wk or 5×10^6 U/d for 16 wk	Patients must have compensated liver disease
Chronic hepatitis C	Interferon alfa	SC	3×10^6 U 3 times a week for 24 wk	Must have compensated liver disease
	+ ribavirin	Oral	500–600 mg bid	Reduce dose if hemoglobin falls below 10 g/dL

Table 20–63 ■ RELATIVE IMPORTANCE OF VIRUSES CAUSING PHARYNGITIS, LARYNGITIS, CROUP, AND BRONCHITIS

	OCCURRENCE IN INDICATED ILLNESS*			
VIRUS	Pharyngitis	Laryngitis	Croup	Bronchitis
Influenza				
A	++++	++++	+	++++
B	++	++		++
Parainfluenza				
1	++	++	++++	++
2	+	+	+++	+
3	++	++	++++	++
Respiratory syncytial	+		+	+++
Adenovirus	++++	++		++
Coronavirus	+	+		+++
Rhinovirus	+	+		+
Enterovirus	+			
Herpes simplex	+		+	+

* Graded from minimal (+) to major (++++) importance; blank means unlikely occurrence.

rubella, scarlet fever, infectious mononucleosis, secondary syphilis, drug eruptions, toxic shock syndrome, and Kawasaki syndrome (Table 20–67).

For more information about this subject, see *Cecil Textbook of Medicine,* 21st edition. Philadelphia, W.B. Saunders Company, 2000. Chapter 381, Measles, pages 1802 to 1805.

Table 20–64 ■ AGE-SPECIFIC RATES FOR ILLNESS AND MORTALITY DURING URBAN INFLUENZA EPIDEMICS

AGE (yr)	PHYSICIAN VISITS PER 100	ARD HOSPITALIZATIONS PER 10,000	P + I MORTALITY PER 100,000
<5	28	43	3
5–14	14	5	1
15–44	10	8	1
45–54	9	13	10
55–64	10	21	10
≥65	—	73	104

ARD = acute respiratory disease; P + I = pneumonia and influenza; — = not stated.

Adapted from Glezen WP: Anatomy of an urban influenza epidemic. *In* Hannoun C, Kendal AP, Klenk HD, et al (eds): Options for the Control of Influenza II. Amsterdam, Elsevier Science, 1993, p 12.

Table 20–65 ▪ TARGET GROUPS FOR INFLUENZA IMMUNIZATION

Groups at Increased Risk of Complications

Persons aged ≥65 yr
Residents of nursing homes and other chronic care facilities
Patients with chronic pulmonary (including asthma) or cardiac disorder
Patients with chronic metabolic disease (including diabetes), renal dysfunction, hemoglobinopathies, or immunosuppression
Children and teens receiving long-term aspirin
Pregnant women who will be in second or third trimester during influenza season

Groups in Contact with High-Risk Persons

Physicians, nurses, and other health care providers
Employees of nursing homes and chronic care facilities
Providers of home care to high-risk persons
Household members (including children) of high-risk persons

Other Groups

Providers of essential community services (e.g., police, fire)
International travelers
Students, dormitory residents
Anyone wishing to reduce risk of influenza

Adapted from Advisory Committee on Immunization Practices, Centers for Disease Control and Prevention. MMWR 47(No. RR-6):1–26, 1998.

Table 20–66 ▪ ADENOVIRUS SEROTYPES AND ASSOCIATED SYNDROMES

HOST AND DISEASE CATEGORY	EPIDEMIOLOGIC FEATURES	ASSOCIATED ADENOVIRUS SEROTYPES
Immunocompetent Hosts		
Pharyngoconjunctival fever	Epidemics in schools, families, and the military, associated with swimming pools	3, 7
Epidemic keratoconjunctivitis	Sporadic epidemics in schools, families, and industrial sites; may cause nosocomial outbreaks; more common in fall and winter	8, 19, 37
Endemic upper respiratory disease	Seen predominantly in children, in families, and day care settings	1, 2, 5
Acute respiratory disease of military recruits		3, 4, 7, 14, 21
Acute hemorrhagic cystitis	Male predominance	7, 11, 21, 35
Gastroenteritis	Predominant in children <2 yr	40, 41
Immunocompromised Hosts		
Transplantation		7, 11, 31, 34, 35
Acquired immunodeficiency syndrome		Multiple, 35, 42–47

20

Table 20–67 ■ A GUIDE TO THE DIFFERENTIAL DIAGNOSIS OF MEASLES

	CONJUNCTIVITIS	RHINITIS	SORE THROAT	ENANTHEM	LEUKOCYTOSIS	SPECIFIC LABORATORY TESTS AVAILABLE
Measles	++	++	0	+	0	+
Rubella	0	±	±	0	0	+
Exanthem subitum	0	±	0	0	0	+
Enterovirus infection	0	±	±	0	0	+
Adenovirus infection	+	+	+	0	0	+
Scarlet fever	±	±	++	0	+	+
Infectious mononucleosis	0	0	++	±	±	+
Drug rash	0	0	0	0	0	0

0 = not usually present or no test available; ± = variable in occurrence; + = present or test available (virus or bacterial culture, serology); ++ = present and severe.

MUMPS

Mumps is an acute systemic viral infection that occurs most commonly in children, is usually self-limited, and is clinically characterized by non-suppurative parotitis.

The diagnosis of mumps is usually made on the basis of clinical findings in a child who presents with fever and parotitis, particularly if the individual is known to be susceptible and has been exposed to mumps during the preceding 2 to 3 weeks.

PREVENTION. In the United States, mumps vaccine is administered in combination with the measles and rubella vaccines (MMR) to children at age 12 to 15 months and produces protective antibody levels in more than 95% of recipients. A second dose of MMR is recommended for children at age 4 to 6 years. The mumps vaccine is also indicated for susceptible adults.

For more information about this subject, see *Cecil Textbook of Medicine,* 21st edition. Philadelphia, W.B. Saunders Company, 2000. Chapter 384, Mumps, pages 1808 to 1810.

HERPES SIMPLEX VIRUS INFECTIONS

The word *herpes* means "to creep or crawl," in reference to the spreading nature of the observed skin lesions. More recently, infection has been defined by the spectrum of illnesses caused by herpes simplex virus (HSV). A unique characteristic of the herpesviruses is their ability to establish latent infection, persist in an apparently inactive state for varying amounts of time, and then be reactivated (Fig. 20–2).

Clinical manifestations include the mucocutaneous infections gingivostomatitis, genital herpes, and herpetic keratitis; neonatal HSV

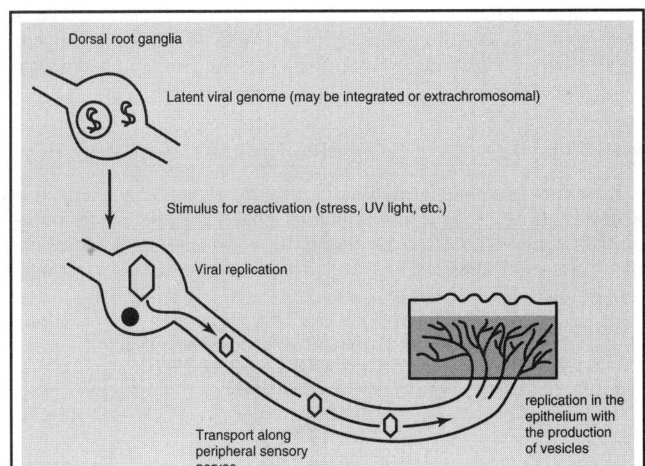

FIGURE 20–2 ■ Schematic diagram of herpes simplex virus latency and reactivation.

20

infection; and herpes simplex encephalitis. HSV infections also afflict the immunocompromised host.

For more information about this subject, see *Cecil Textbook of Medicine,* 21st edition. Philadelphia, W.B. Saunders Company, 2000. Chapter 385, Herpes Simplex Virus Infections, pages 1810 to 1814.

INFECTIONS ASSOCIATED WITH HUMAN CYTOMEGALOVIRUS

Host immunity is thought to be protective, because clinical evidence of infection rarely develops in the immunocompetent host. Abnormalities in immune responses caused by immunosuppressive drugs after allotransplantation, retroviral infections in patients with HIV, or developmental immune dysfunction in the fetus predispose these unique populations to human cytomegalovirus (HCMV)–induced disease.

Although infection in the immunocompetent host rarely results in clinically apparent disease, infrequently normal hosts will exhibit a mononucleosis-like syndrome. Approximately 8% of cases of infectious mononucleosis may be caused by HCMV. Clinically, this infection is indistinguishable from mononucleosis caused by Epstein-Barr virus, with the exception that it is heterophile negative. Non-specific constitutional symptoms predominate. Laboratory abnormalities include atypical lymphocytosis, chemical hepatitis and cholestasis, and, less frequently, thrombocytopenia.

THERAPY. Two agents, ganciclovir and foscarnet, have been shown to be virostatic in vitro and in vivo. Clinical trials have documented efficacy of these agents in treating invasive HCMV disease in both transplant and AIDS patients. Both have significant toxicity. Local therapy for HCMV retinitis has included intraocular injection of cidofovir and antisense oligonucleotides. Both therapies are well tolerated and lack systemic toxicity.

For more information about this subject, see *Cecil Textbook of Medicine,* 21st edition. Philadelphia, W.B. Saunders Company, 2000. Chapter 386, Infections Associated with Human Cytomegalovirus, pages 1814 to 1816.

INFECTIOUS MONONUCLEOSIS: EPSTEIN-BARR VIRUS INFECTION

Infectious mononucleosis is a clinical syndrome characterized by malaise, headache, fever, pharyngitis, pharyngeal lymphatic hyperplasia, lymphadenopathy, atypical lymphocytosis, heterophile antibody, and mild transient hepatitis. The syndrome occurs most com-

Table 20–68 ■ CLINICAL MANIFESTATIONS OF INFECTIOUS MONONUCLEOSIS

Splenomegaly (50%)
Vomiting (20%)
Hepatitis (20–50%)
Jaundice (5%)
Palatal petechiae
Rash (4%)
Albuminuria (10%)

monly in adolescents and young adults (Table 20–68). Primary Epstein-Barr virus (EBV) infection is the cause of almost all typical infectious mononucleosis syndromes. EBV is a herpesvirus.

Latent EBV infection is also associated with B-cell lymphomas in immunosuppressed patients, with Burkitt-type lymphoma in African children, with some of the sporadic Burkitt-type lymphomas that occur in developed societies, with about 50% of cases of Hodgkin's disease, with some T-cell lymphomas in adolescents or young adults, and with anaplastic nasopharyngeal carcinoma.

ENTEROVIRUSES

Enteroviruses, so named because they generally infect the alimentary tract and are shed in the feces, cause a variety of diseases (Table 20–69).

ASEPTIC MENINGITIS. Aseptic meningitis is the most common significant illness caused by non-polio enteroviruses (Table 20–70), and these viruses are responsible for more than 80% of the cases of aseptic meningitis in which an etiologic agent is identified.

Treatment and Prevention

Specific antiviral chemotherapy and chemoprophylaxis are not yet available for enterovirus infections. Treatment is symptomatic and, in severe disease, supportive. Corticosteroids should not be administered during acute enterovirus infections. Strenuous exercise and intramuscular injections should also be avoided during the acute, presumably viremic, phase of symptomatic enterovirus infections.

Table 20–69 ■ CLASSIFICATION OF HUMAN ENTEROVIRUSES*

ENTEROVIRUS GROUP	NO. OF SEROTYPES	NUMERICAL DESIGNATION	GROWTH IN PRIMATE CELL CULTURE
Poliovirus	3	1–3	+
Coxsackievirus, group A	23	A1–22, A24†	+/–‡
Coxsackievirus, group B	6	B1–6	+
Echovirus	31	1–9, 11–27, 29–34§	+
Enterovirus	4	68–71‖	+

* Many enterovirus strains have been isolated that do not conform to these criteria.

† Coxsackievirus A23 has been reclassified as echovirus 9.

‡ Except for a few serotypes (e.g., A7, A9, A16), primary isolates of group A coxsackieviruses grow poorly or not at all in cell culture; virus isolation requires inoculation of suckling mice.

§ Echovirus 10 has been reclassified as reovirus type 1; echovirus 28 has been reclassified as rhinovirus 1A.

‖ Hepatitis A virus, formally classified as human enterovirus 72, is now classified as heparnavirus in the picornavirus family.

20

Table 20–70 ■ CLINICAL MANIFESTATIONS OF NON-POLIO ENTEROVIRUS INFECTIONS

Asymptomatic infection
Undifferentiated febrile illness ("summer grippe") with or without respiratory symptoms
Aseptic meningitis
Encephalitis
Paralytic disease (poliomyelitis-like)
Myopericarditis
Pleurodynia
Herpangina
Hand-foot-and-mouth disease
Exanthem
Common cold
Lower respiratory tract infections (broncheolitis, pneumonia)
Acute hemorrhagic conjunctivitis*
Generalized disease of the newborn

* Conjunctivitis without hemorrhage is frequently seen in association with other manifestations in patients infected with many group A and group B coxsackieviruses and echoviruses, especially coxsackieviruses A9, A16, and B1–5 and echoviruses 2, 7, 9, 11, 16, and 30.

VIRAL GASTROENTERITIS

Viral gastroenteritis (acute infectious nonbacterial gastroenteritis, epidemic diarrhea, winter vomiting disease, sporadic infantile gastroenteritis) is a common acute infectious disease of all age groups, characterized by vomiting or watery diarrhea, or both, that may be accompanied by fever, nausea, anorexia, and malaise. It ranges from a mild, self-limited illness of short duration to life-threatening dehydration, especially in infants and young children.

Rotaviruses are the major known etiologic agents of severe diarrhea in infants and young children in most areas of the world and are usually associated with sporadic or endemic infantile gastroenteritis.

HEMORRHAGIC FEVER VIRUSES

The viral hemorrhagic fevers encompass syndromes that vary from febrile hemorrhagic disease with capillary fragility to acute severe shock leading rapidly to death. The causative agents include arthropod-borne and rodent-associated viruses. The rodent-associated viruses do not require an arthropod vector but are transmitted directly to vertebrates by aerosol spread or contact with infected excreta or body secretions of the rodent. The reservoir and natural mode of transmission for the African hemorrhagic fever viruses Marburg and Ebola are not known. At least 18 viruses cause human hemorrhagic fevers. All contain RNA, and nearly all are zoonoses. (Table 20–71)

OTHER ARTHROPOD-BORNE VIRUSES

There are nearly 500 arthropod-borne viruses, and at least 100 of these infect humans. They cause fever, rash, or polyarthritis (Table 20–72) or CNS infection and encephalitis (Table 20–73).

Text continues on page 641

Table 20–71 ■ CLINICAL PARAMETERS OF VIRAL HEMORRHAGIC FEVERS

DISEASE	VIRAL AGENT	INCUBATION PERIOD (days)	CLINICAL SYNDROMES				ARDS	CASE FATALITY RATE (%)
			Hemorrhage	Hepatitis	Encephalitis	Nephropathy		
Yellow fever	Yellow fever	3–6	Major	Major	Absent	Moderate	Absent	2–20
Dengue hemorrhagic fever	Dengue 1–4	5–8	Moderate	Moderate	Absent	Absent	Absent	2–10
Rift Valley fever	Rift Valley fever	3–6	Major	Major	Moderate	Absent	Absent	0.2–10
Crimean-Congo hemorrhagic fever	Crimean-Congo hemorrhagic fever	2–9	Major	Major	Minor	Absent	Absent	30–50
Kyasanur Forest disease	Kyasanur Forest disease	3–8	Minor	Minor	Moderate	Absent	Absent	5–10
Omsk hemorrhagic fever	Omsk hemorrhagic fever	3–8	Minor	Minor	Moderate	Absent	Absent	0.4–2.5
Hemorrhagic fever with renal syndrome	Hantaan, Puumala, Dobrava, Seoul	2–42	Moderate	Rare	Minor	Major	Absent	2–5
Hantavirus pulmonary syndrome	Sin Nombre	12–16	Minor	Minor	Absent	Minor	Major	40–50
Venezuelan hemorrhagic fever	Guanarito	7–14	Moderate	Rare	Rare	Minor	Absent	33
Brazilian hemorrhagic fever	Sabiá	8–12	Major	Minor	Minor	Minor	Absent	33
Argentine hemorrhagic fever	Junin	10–14	Minor	Rare	Moderate	Minor	Absent	10–20
Bolivian hemorrhagic fever	Machupo	7–14	Moderate	Rare	Moderate	Minor	Absent	15–30
Lassa fever	Lassa	3–16	Minor	Major	Minor	Minor	Absent	15
African hemorrhagic fever	Marburg	3–9	Major	Major	Minor	Absent	Absent	20–30
	Ebola	3–18	Major	Major	Minor	Absent	Absent	53–88

ARDS = adult respiratory distress syndrome.

Table 20–72 ■ ARTHROPOD-BORNE VIRUSES THAT CAUSE FEVER, RASH, OR POLYARTHRITIS

FAMILY (GENUS)*	HUMAN DISEASE	DISTRIBUTION	VECTOR
Togaviridae (*Alphavirus*)			
Mayaro	Fever, arthritis, rash	South America	Mosquito
Ross River	Arthritis, rash, sometimes fever	Australia, South Pacific	Mosquito
Chikungunya	Fever, arthritis, hemorrhagic fever	Africa, Asia, Philippines	Mosquito
O'nyong-nyong	Fever, arthritis, rash	Africa	Mosquito
Sindbis	Arthritis, rash, sometimes fever	Africa, Europe, Australia	Mosquito
Flaviviridae (*Flavivirus*)			
Dengue (4 types)	Fever, rash, hemorrhagic fever	Worldwide (tropics)	Mosquito
Yellow fever	Fever, hemorrhagic fever	Tropical Americas, Africa	Mosquito
West Nile	Fever, rash, hepatitis, encephalitis	Asia, Europe, Africa	Mosquito
Bunyaviridae (*Bunyavirus*)			
Oxopouche	Fever	Brazil, Panama	Midge
Bunyaviridae (*Phlebovirus*)			
Sandfly fever viruses	Fever	Asia, Africa, tropical Americas	Sandfly, mosquito
Rift Valley fever	Fever, hemorrhagic fever, encephalitis, retinitis	Africa	Mosquito
Bunyaviridae (*Hantavirus*)			
Sin Nombre, others	Pulmonary disease	Americas	Rodent
Reoviridae (*Coltivirus*)			
Colorado tick fever	Fever	Western United States	Tick

* Shown are the most important of more than 100 arboviruses that infect humans.

Table 20–73 ■ ARTHROPOD-BORNE VIRUSES THAT CAUSE ACUTE CENTRAL NERVOUS SYSTEM INFECTION AND ENCEPHALITIS

VIRUS BY GROUP	MODE OF TRANSMISSION	GEOGRAPHIC DISTRIBUTION
Viruses Principally Associated with the Encephalitis Syndrome; Epidemic and Endemic		
Togaviridae (*Alphavirus*)		
Eastern equine encephalitis	Mosquito	Eastern North America, Caribbean, South America
Western equine encephalitis	Mosquito	Western North America, South America
Venezuelan equine encephalitis	Mosquito, possibly other	Florida, Central and South America
Flaviviridae (*Flavivirus*)		
St. Louis encephalitis	Mosquito	North America, Caribbean, Central and South America
Japanese encephalitis	Mosquito	East and Southeast Asia, India
Rocio encephalitis	Mosquito	Brazil
Murray Valley encephalitis	Mosquito	Australia
Tick-borne encephalitides		
Russian spring-summer and Central European encephalitis	Tick, ingestion of milk	Europe, former U.S.S.R.
Louping ill	Tick	British Isles
Powassan	Tick	North America
Bunyaviridae, California subgroup		
California encephalitis, LaCrosse, Jamestown Canyon, snowshoe hare	Mosquito	North America, China, former U.S.S.R.

Table continued on following page

Table 20–73 ■ ARTHROPOD-BORNE VIRUSES THAT CAUSE ACUTE CENTRAL NERVOUS SYSTEM INFECTION AND ENCEPHALITIS *Continued*

VIRUS BY GROUP	MODE OF TRANSMISSION	GEOGRAPHIC DISTRIBUTION
Viruses Principally Associated with Other Syndromes, but Occasionally Causing Encephalitis; Epidemic and Endemic		
Togaviridae (*Alphavirus*)		
Sinbis (febrile illness with rash)	Mosquito	Africa, Europe
Semliki Forest (febrile illness)	Mosquito	Africa, Southeast Asia
Flaviviridae (*Flavivirus*)		
West Nile (febrile illness with rash)	Mosquito	Africa, Middle East
Kyasanur Forest disease*	Tick	India
Omsk hemorrhagic fever*	Tick	Central Asia
Bunyaviridae (*Phlebovirus*)		
Rift Valley fever (febrile illness, hemorrhagic fever, retinitis)	Mosquito, direct contact	Africa
Crimean hemorrhagic fever*—Congo	Tick	Eastern Europe, former U.S.S.R., Africa
Reoviridae, orbivirus		
Colorado tick fever (febrile illness)	Tick	Western North America
Rare and Sporadic Infections Associated with Encephalitis		
Flaviviridae (*Flavivirus*)		
Ilheus†	Mosquito	South America
Negishi	Tick	Japan, China
Langat*	Tick	Asia
Orthomyxovirus		
Thogoto	Tick	Africa

* Tick-borne hemorrhagic fevers.

† Encephalitis recorded in laboratory infections or experimental infections of cancer patients only; significance in naturally acquired infections unknown.

Table 20–74 ■ COMMON SYSTEMIC MYCOSES

DISEASE	CAUSATIVE FUNGUS
Aspergillosis	*Aspergillus* spp.
Zygomycosis (mucormycosis)	*Mucor* and *Rhizopus* spp.
Candidiasis	*Candida* spp.
Cryptococcosis	*Cryptococcus neoformans*
Blastomycosis	*Blastomyces dermatitidis*
Coccidioidomycosis	*Coccidioides immitis*
Histoplasmosis	*Histoplasma capsulatum*
Paracoccidioidomycosis	*Paracoccidioides brasiliensis*
Sporotrichosis	*Sporothrix schenckii*

THE MYCOSES

The terms *fungal diseases* and *mycoses* are used interchangeably. Fungal infections that involve only the skin and its appendages are referred to as cutaneous or superficial mycoses. Those fungal infections acquired primarily by inhalation and involving organs such as the lungs, skin, liver, spleen, and CNS are considered systemic mycoses (Table 20–74).

Although amphotercin B remains the standard of therapy for many systemic fungal diseases, it does have some disadvantages in that it must be administered intravenously and it is associated with a high toxicity profile. Several other classes of antifungal drugs are also available (Table 20–75).

Brief profiles of several important mycotic disorders are given here.

For more information about this subject, see *Cecil Textbook of Medicine,* 21st edition. Philadelphia, W.B. Saunders Company, 2000. Chapter 393, Introduction to the Mycoses, pages 1858 to 1860.

Table 20–75 ■ CURRENTLY AVAILABLE DRUGS FOR THERAPY OF SYSTEMIC MYCOSES BY CLASS AND MECHANISM OF ACTION

CLASS OF ANTIFUNGAL DRUG WITH EXAMPLES	MECHANISM OF ACTION
Polyene Nystatin Amphotercin B	Binds irreversibly to ergosterol, resulting in increased permeability of cell membrane with leakage of intracellular contents
Azole Clotrimazole Miconazole Ketoconazole Fluconazole Itraconazole	Blocks synthesis of ergosterol via inhibition of cytochrome P-450–dependent enzyme, 14α-demethylase
Substituted pyrimidine Flucytosine	Inhibits both DNA and protein synthesis

Histoplasmosis

Causative fungus	*Histoplasma capsulatum*
Primary geographic distribution	Worldwide; endemic in northern and south central United States
Primary route of acquisition	Respiratory (inhalation of spores)
Principal sites of disease	Lungs, lymph nodes, liver, spleen, bone marrow, adrenal glands, gastrointestinal tract
Opportunistic infection in compromised hosts	Frequent, especially in AIDS patients
Drug of choice for most patients	Itraconazole
Alternative therapy	Amphotericin B, ketoconazole, or fluconazole

For more information about this subject, see *Cecil Textbook of Medicine,* 21st edition. Philadelphia, W.B. Saunders Company, 2000. Chapter 394, Histoplasmosis, pages 1860 to 1862.

Coccidioidomycosis

Causative fungus	*Coccidioides immitis*
Primary geographic distribution	Lower Sonoran deserts of the Western Hemisphere including parts of Arizona, California, New Mexico, west Texas, and parts of Central and South America
Primary route of acquisition	Respiratory (inhalation of arthroconidia)
Principal site of disease	Lungs most common; spread to skin, bones, meninges, and other viscera uncommon but serious
Opportunistic infection in compromised hosts	Diffuse pneumonia and widespread infections common in patients with T-lymphocyte defects or during high-dose corticosteriod therapy
Drug of choice for most patients	No antifungal is required for uncomplicated pneumonia; fluconazole or itraconazole for progressive forms of infection
Alternative therapy	Amphotericin B (especially with diffuse pneumonia or rapidly progressive infections); ketoconazole

For more information about this subject, see *Cecil Textbook of Medicine,* 21st edition. Philadelphia, W.B. Saunders Company, 2000. Chapter 395, Coccidioidomycosis, pages 1863 to 1864.

Blastomycosis

Causative fungus	*Blastomyces dermatitidis*
Primary geographic distribution	Endemic in northern and south central United States

Primary route of acquisition	Respiratory (inhalation of spores)
Principal sites of disease	Lungs, skin, bone, joints, prostate
Opportunistic infection in compromised hosts	Infrequent
Drug of choice for most patients	Itraconazole
Alternative therapy	Amphotericin B, ketoconazole, or fluconazole

For more information about this subject, see *Cecil Textbook of Medicine,* 21st edition. Philadelphia, W.B. Saunders Company, 2000. Chapter 396, Blastomycosis, pages 1865 to 1866.

Paracoccidioidomycosis

Causative fungus	*Paracoccidioides brasiliensis*
Primary geographic distribution	Endemic in Mexico, Central America, and parts of South America
Primary route of acquisition	Respiratory (inhalation of spores)
Principal sites of disease	Lungs, mucous membranes, skin, lymph nodes, liver, and spleen
Opportunistic infection in compromised hosts	Infrequent
Drug of choice for most patients	Itraconazole
Alternative therapy	Sulfonamide, amphotericin B, or ketoconazole

For more information about this subject, see *Cecil Textbook of Medicine,* 21st edition. Philadelphia, W.B. Saunders Company, 2000. Chapter 397, Paracoccidioidomycosis, pages 1866 to 1867.

Cryptococcosis

Causative fungus	*Cryptococcus neoformans*
Primary geographic distribution	Worldwide
Primary route of acquisition	Respiratory (inhalation of spores)
Principal sites of disease	Lungs, CNS, blood, skin, bone, joints, prostate
Opportunistic infection in compromised hosts	Frequent, especially in corticosteroid-treated and AIDS patients
Drug of choice in most patients	Amphotericin B (with or without flucytosine) or fluconazole
Alternative therapy	Itraconazole

For more information about this subject, see *Cecil Textbook of Medicine,* 21st edition. Philadelphia, W.B. Saunders Company, 2000. Chapter 398, Cryptococcosis, pages 1867 to 1870.

Sporotrichosis

Causative fungus	*Sporothrix schenckii*
Primary geographic distribution	Worldwide, mainly in temperate and tropical areas
Primary route of acquisition	Cutaneous inoculation
Principal sites of disease	Skin, lymphatics; less commonly, lungs and joints

Opportunistic infection in compromised hosts	Infrequent
Drug of choice for most patients	Itraconazole
Alternative therapy	Cutaneous disease: saturated solution of potassium iodide, fluconazole, or surgery Extracutaneous disease: amphotericin B

For more information about this subject, see *Cecil Textbook of Medicine,* 21st edition. Philadelphia, W.B. Saunders Company, 2000. Chapter 399, Sporotrichosis, pages 1870 to 1871.

Candidiasis

Causative fungus	*Candida* species (*C. albicans* most common)
Primary geographic distribution	Worldwide; part of normal flora of humans and in environment
Primary route of acquisition	Endogenous; person-to-person
Principal sites of disease	Mucous membranes (oropharynx, vagina), skin, esophagus, blood, liver, spleen, kidneys, eyes, heart
Opportunistic infection in compromised hosts	Frequent; e.g., mucosal disease in patients with AIDS and deep-organ disease in patients with granulocytopenia
Drug(s) of choice for most patients	Mucosal disease: topical or oral azole drug (clotrimazole or fluconazole) Deep-organ disease: amphotericin B or fluconazole
Alternative therapy for deep-organ disease	Amphotericin B plus flucytosine

For more information about this subject, see *Cecil Textbook of Medicine,* 21st edition. Philadelphia, W.B. Saunders Company, 2000. Chapter 400, Candidiasis, pages 1871 to 1875.

Aspergillosis

Causative fungus	*Aspergillus* species: *A. fumigatus, A. flavus, A. niger, A. terreus*
Primary geographic distribution	Ubiquitous: human habitat, soil, water, air
Primary route of acquisition	Inhaling spores
Principal site of disease	Lung
Opportunistic infection in compromised hosts	Invasive form, pulmonary
Drug of choice for most patients	Amphotericin, itraconazole
Alternative therapy	None

For more information about this subject, see *Cecil Textbook of Medicine,* 21st edition. Philadelphia, W.B. Saunders Company, 2000. Chapter 401, Aspergillosis, pages 1875 to 1877.

Pneumocystis carinii PNEUMONIA

Pneumocystis carinii pneumonia (PCP) remains the most frequent case-defining infection in acquired immunodeficiency syndrome (AIDS), despite an almost 50% decrease in the number of first episodes. A large number of second or third episodes also occur annually in AIDS patients, although these are less well reported.

CLINICAL MANIFESTATIONS. Early recognition and treatment are imperative. The onset of PCP in AIDS patients is usually insidious. The cardinal manifestation is a hacking, typically nonproductive cough that may have been present for weeks. Pneumothoraces that may be associated with refractory bronchopleural fistulas and chronic lung cavitation are an increasingly frequent presentation. In some AIDS patients, PCP may present as an occult febrile illness, with few or no respiratory symptoms. Infection with *P. carinii* may occur outside the lung in 0.5 to 3.0% of patients with PCP. Clinical presentations have included external auditory polyps, mastoiditis, choroiditis, cutaneous lesions or digital necrosis secondary to vasculitis, small bowel obstruction, ascites with gross nodules in the stomach and duodenum, hepatic or splenic infiltration, hilar or mediastinal lymphadenopathy, thyroiditis, thymic involvement, and cytopenia due to bone marrow infection. Hypoxemia is the most useful marker of PCP and is highly predictive of outcome.

RADIOGRAPHY. Routine chest radiographs typically show interstitial infiltrates, beginning in perihilar areas and spreading to the lower and finally upper lung fields in a butterfly pattern.

DIAGNOSIS. Bronchoalveolar lavage (BAL) is the cornerstone of diagnosis and consistently has a sensitivity of 86 to 96%.

TREATMENT. Therapeutic regimens for PCP are shown in Table 20–76.

ADJUNCTIVE CORTICOSTEROIDS. The major breakthrough in the search for more effective therapies for PCP has been the irrefutable evidence that mortality for severe episodes can be reduced nearly two-fold by use of corticosteroids within 72 hours after beginning specific anti-*Pneumocystis* therapy (Table 20–77).

For more information about this subject, see *Cecil Textbook of Medicine,* 21st edition. Philadelphia, W.B. Saunders Company, 2000. Chapter 402, *Pneumocystis carinii* Pneumonia, pages 1877 to 1883.

Table 20–76 ■ ESTABLISHED THERAPIES FOR INITIAL TREATMENT OF *Pneumocystis carinii* PNEUMONIA

Intravenous Therapy	
Trimethoprim-sulfamethoxazole	5 mg/kg of trimethoprim component q6–8h
Pentamidine*	4 mg/kg once daily
Trimetrexate plus leucovorin	For patients <50 kg: 1.5 mg/kg trimetrexate once daily plus leucovorin 0.5 mg/kg IV or PO q6h For patients 50–80 kg: 1.2 mg/kg trimetrexate daily plus leucovorin 0.5/kg IV or PO q6h For patients >80 kg: 1.0 mg/kg trimetrexate daily plus leucovorin 0.8 mg/kg IV or PO q6h Continue leucovorin for 72 hr after last dose of trimetrexate
Clindamycin plus primaquine base (oral)†	600–900 mg q8h plus 15–30mg PO once daily
Oral Therapy	
Trimethoprim-sulfamethoxazole	2 double-strength tablets tid
Trimethoprim plus dapsone	4–5 mg/kg tid plus 100 mg once daily
Clindamycin plus primaquine base†	450–600 mg tid or qid plus 15–30 mg once daily
Atovaquone‡	750 mg tid
Aerosol Therapy	
Pentamidine	600 mg daily via Respirgard II§

* Intramuscular therapy may cause sterile abscesses and should be avoided.

† The combination is not advisable in situations in which absorption may be impaired (severe hypoxemia, vomiting, diarrhea, ileus, malabsorption) because clindamycin alone has no activity against *P. carinii*.

‡ Must be given with fatty food because serum concentrations are 2- or 3-fold lower when drug is administered on an empty stomach.

§ Administered at 50 psi and 8 L/minute of oxygen.

Table 20–77 ■ ADJUNCTIVE CORTICOSTEROIDS* FOR PATIENTS WITH *Pneumocystis carinii* PNEUMONIA AND (A − a)$DO_2 \geq 35$ mm Hg *or* $PaO_2 \leq 70$ mm Hg

DRUG	DOSE	TREATMENT DAYS
Oral		
Prednisone	40 mg bid	1–5
	40 mg once daily	6–10
	20 mg once daily	11–21
Intravenous		
Methylprednisolone	30 mg bid	1–5
	30 mg once daily	6–10
	15 mg once daily	11–21

* Efficacy established only when adjunctive corticosteroids are initiated within 72 hours of starting specific treatment for *P. carinii* infection.

CHAPTER 21

THE HUMAN IMMUNODEFICIENCY VIRUS AND ACQUIRED IMMUNODEFICIENCY SYNDROME

BIOLOGY OF HUMAN IMMUNODEFICIENCY VIRUSES

The selective loss of CD4+ helper T lymphocytes in patients with AIDS implicated an agent with T-lymphocyte cell tropism. As expected for an etiologic agent, HIV-1 was shown to be uniformly present in subjects with AIDS and to reproduce the hallmark of the disease, destruction of T lymphocytes, in tissue culture (Fig. 21–1).

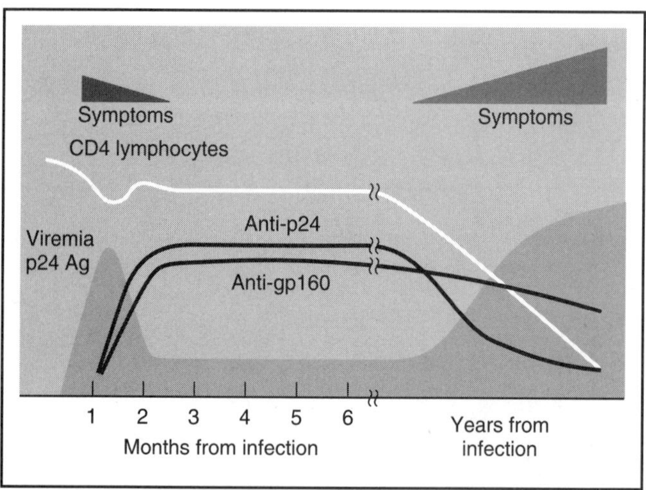

FIGURE 21–1 ■ Natural history model for HIV-1 infection. Viremia denotes cell-free infectious virus in plasma, p24 Ag denotes circulating viral p24 antigen in plasma, and anti-p24 and anti-gp 160 correspond to antibodies to viral core and envelope proteins.

For more information about this subject, see *Cecil Textbook of Medicine,* 21st edition. Philadelphia, W.B. Saunders Company, 2000. Part XXIII: HIV and the Acquired Immunodeficiency Syndrome, pages 1889 to 1945.

PREVENTION OF HIV INFECTION

Prevention of HIV infection requires an understanding of the modes of viral transmission, the populations at risk, and the established guidelines to avoid high-risk exposures (Table 21–1). HIV has been identified in virtually every body fluid and tissue.

NEUROLOGIC COMPLICATIONS OF HIV-1 INFECTION

The neurologic complications of HIV-1 infection are both common and varied. Only rarely do the central (CNS) and peripheral nervous systems of HIV-infected patients remain unaffected through the course of untreated disease (Table 21–2). The focal brain disorders seen with HIV infection are cerebral toxoplasmosis,

Table 21–1 ■ DEFINITIONS OF EXPOSURES TO BLOOD AND BODY FLUIDS FROM HIV-INFECTED PATIENTS

	CHEMOPROPHYLAXIS*
Massive parenteral exposure	
Transfusion of blood	Recommended
High-inoculum injection of blood (>1 mL) or laboratory materials containing high viral titers	
Definite parenteral exposure	
Deep intramuscular injury with a needle contaminated with blood or a body fluid	Recommended
Small-volume injection of blood or body fluid (<1 mL)	
Laceration caused by an instrument contaminated with blood or body fluids	
Laceration inoculated with blood, body fluids, or virus samples (research materials)	
Possible parenteral exposure	
Subcutaneous or superficial injury with an instrument or needle contaminated with blood or body fluids	Available
Injury with a contaminated instrument or needle which does not cause visible bleeding	
Previous wound or skin lesion contaminated with blood or body fluids	
Mucous membrane exposure to blood or body fluids	
Doubtful parenteral exposure	
Subcutaneous injury by instrument or needle contaminated with noninfectious fluids†	Discouraged
Contamination of a wound, previous skin lesion, or mucous membrane with noninfectious fluids	
Intact skin visibly contaminated with blood	

* Dual nucleoside therapy (e.g., zidovudine plus lamivudine), usually with a potent protease inhibitor or non-nucleoside reverse transcriptase inhibitor (NNRTI).

† Body fluids considered to be potentially infectious include blood, blood products, cerebrospinal fluid, amniotic fluid, menstrual discharge, inflammatory exudate, pleural fluid, peritoneal fluid, pericardial fluid, and any fluid visibly contaminated with blood. All other fluids are considered non-infectious.

Table 21–2 ■ PATHOPHYSIOLOGIC CLASSIFICATION OF SOME COMMON NEUROLOGIC COMPLICATIONS OF LATE HIV-1 INFECTION

UNDERLYING PROCESS	EXAMPLES
Opportunistic infections	Cerebral toxoplasmosis Cryptococcal meningitis Progressive multifocal leukoencephalopathy Cytomegalovirus encephalitis, polyradiculitis
Opportunistic neoplasms	Primary CNS lymphoma Metastatic lymphoma
Conditions possibly related to HIV-1 itself	AIDS demential complex Aseptic meningitis Predominantly sensory polyneuropathy
Metabolic and vascular complications of systemic disease	Hypoxic, sepsis-related encephalopathies Stroke (nonbacterial thrombotic endocarditis, coagulopathies)
Toxic reactions	Dideoxyinosine, dideoxycytidine neuropathies AZT myopathy
Functional (psychiatric) disorders	Anxiety disorders Psychotic depression

AZT = zidovudine.

progressive multifocal leukoencephalopathy, and primary CNS lymphoma. Although the three all have a subacute onset and may be clinically indistinguishable, they tend to have somewhat different temporal profiles (Table 21–3).

PULMONARY MANIFESTATIONS OF HIV INFECTION

Lung disease, specifically *Pneumocystis carinii* pneumonia (PCP), was the first recognized mode of expression of infection with HIV (Fig. 21–2). Although the differential diagnosis of lung disease in a person with HIV infection is quite broad, the probabilities of the various diagnoses can be reduced in a given patient by knowing the patient's symptoms, HIV transmission category, and

Table 21–3 ■ COMPARATIVE CLINICAL FEATURES OF CEREBRAL TOXOPLASMOSIS, PRIMARY CNS LYMPHOMA, AND PROGRESSIVE MULTIFOCAL LEUKOENCEPHALOPATHY

	TEMPORAL PROFILE	LEVEL OF ALERTNESS	FEVER
Cerebral toxoplasmosis	Days	Reduced	Common
Primary CNS lymphoma	Days to weeks	Variable	Absent
Progressive multifocal leukoencephalopathy	Weeks	Preserved	Absent

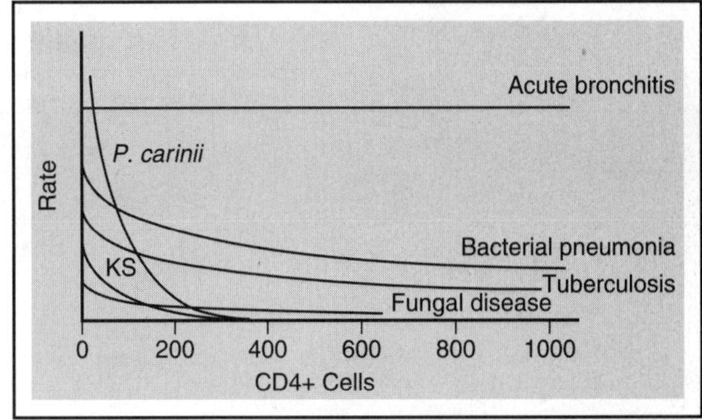

FIGURE 21–2 ■ The relative frequency and spectrum of lung diseases change as the CD4+ lymphocyte count declines. This graph presents a conceptual depiction of these changes. The x-axis could also be equated with time following acquisition of HIV infection.

CD4+ lymphocyte count and further refined by the findings on the chest film (Fig. 21–3).

Much of the improved survival for patients with HIV infection in recent years owes to the prevention of PCP. Hence, the use of antipneumocystis agents such as trimethoprim-sulfamethoxazole, dapsone, pentamidine aerosol, and atovaquone for persons with HIV infection and CD4+ lymphocyte counts of less than 200 cells per microliter is a high-priority intervention.

GASTROINTESTINAL MANIFESTATIONS OF AIDS

The gastrointestinal tract is an especially common site for clinical expression of HIV infection (Table 21–4) and is an important factor in morbidity from opportunistic infections in late-stage disease, as well as gastrointestinal complications from antiretroviral agents or other drugs (Table 21–5). Nearly all opportunistic infections occur when the CD4+ count is less than 200/mm^3, and almost all seem to respond well to immune reconstitution when achieved with antiretroviral therapy. Oral candidiasis (thrush) is encountered at some time in 80 to 90% of all patients with advanced stages of HIV infections.

AIDS ENTEROPATHY. Endoscopy in patients with advanced AIDS often shows morphologic changes in the small bowel in the absence of evidence of a superimposed opportunistic infection.

21

MALNUTRITION AND WASTING. The average patient with late-stage AIDS loses 15 to 20% of baseline weight. Protein-calorie malnutrition is a common and important sequela that may accelerate progressive immunosuppression

HEPATOBILIARY DISEASE. The prevalence of markers for hepatitis B (hepatitis B surface antigen [HbsAg], antibody to HbsAg, or antibody to hepatitis B core antigen) is 35 to 80% in AIDS patients.

CONDITIONS NECESSITATING ABDOMINAL SURGERY. The most common clinical syndromes in persons with HIV infection

HIV infection (known or suspected), CD4+ count ≤ 300, cough, dyspnea ± fever
Chest film
Normal
Abnormal
Purulent sputum
Diffuse infiltrate
Focal infiltrate
Yes
No
DLCO < 75%
No
Yes
Purulent sputum
No
Yes
Symptomatic Rx ± antimicrobials
Induced sputum for AFB, *P. carinii*, mycobacterial culture
Sputum Gram stain, culture, blood culture
Antimicrobial Rx based on results
P. carinii, or AFB absent
P. carinii, or AFB present
Bronchoscopy with BAL
Treat
No diagnosis
P. carinii, AFB, fungi
KS
Repeat BAL, Tb Bx
Treat
? Treat

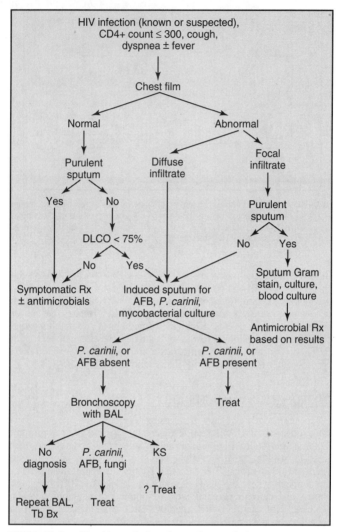

FIGURE 21–3 ■ Algorithm of the diagnostic approach to patients who are known or suspected of having HIV infection resulting in significant immunocompromise: ≤300 CD4+ lymphocytes per microliter. DLCO = pulmonary diffusing capacity for carbon monoxide; AFB = acid-fast bacilli; BAL = bronchoalveolar lavage; Tb Bx = transbronchial lung biopsy; KS = Kaposi's sarcoma.

that require abdominal surgery are peritonitis associated with perforation secondary to cytomegalovirus (CMV) infection, lymphoma of the gut (most frequently manifested as involvement of the terminal ileum by obstruction or bleeding), Kaposi's sarcoma, and *Mycobacterium avium-intracellulare* infection involving the retroperitoneal lymph nodes or spleen.

Table 21–4 ■ ESOPHAGEAL COMPLICATIONS OF HIV INFECTION

AGENT	FREQUENCY* (%)	CD4 COUNT (mm^3)	CLINICAL FEATURES	DIAGNOSIS	TREATMENT
Candida	50–70	<200	Odynophagia, thrush, diffuse pain, usually afebrile	Usually treated empirically Endoscopy shows plaques	Fluconazole
Cytomegalovirus (CMV)	10–20	<50	Odynophagia, focal pain, usually febrile	Biopsy of ulcer to show CMV inclusions	Ganciclovir
Herpes simplex virus (HSV)	2–5	<200	Odynophagia, oral HSV lesions common, usually afebrile	Biopsy of ulcer to show HSV inclusions	Acyclovir
Idiopathic	10–20	<300	Odynophagia, focal pain, usually afebrile	Negative biopsy of ulcer	Prednisone or thalidomide

* Approximate frequency in HIV-infected patients with odynophagia.

21

Table 21–5 ■ AGENTS OF ACUTE AND CHRONIC DIARRHEA

AGENT	FREQUENCY* (%)	CD4 COUNT (mm^3)	CLINICAL FEATURES	DIAGNOSIS	TREATMENT
Acute Diarrhea					
Salmonella	5–15	Any	Watery diarrhea, fever	Stool and blood culture	Fluoroquinolone
Clostridium difficile	10–15	Any	Cramps, watery diarrhea, fever	Stool toxin assay	Metronidazole
Enteric viruses	15–30	Any	Watery diarrhea, usually afebrile	None	Symptomatic
Idiopathic	25–40	Any	Variable	Negative culture, O&P exam, and *C. difficile* toxin	Symptomatic
Chronic Diarrhea					
Cryptosporidium	10–30	<100	Watery diarrhea, fever variable, may be devastating fluid losses	Stool O&P with AFB	Paromomycin ± azithromycin
Microsporidia	15–30	<100	Watery diarrhea, afebrile	Stool trichrome stain	Albendazole (*Enterocytozoon intestinalis*)
Isospora	1–3	<100	Watery diarrhea	Stool O&P	TMP-SMX
Mycobacterium avium	10–20	<50	Watery diarrhea, fever, wasting	Blood culture	Clarithromycin + ethambutol
Cytomegalovirus	15–40	<50	Watery or bloody diarrhea; fever, fecal WBCs	Colon biopsy	Ganciclovir
Idiopathic	20–30	Any	Watery diarrhea	Negative culture, O&P, *C. difficile* toxin, endoscopy	Symptomatic

O&P = ova and parasites; AFB = acid-fast bacillus; TMP-SMX = trimethoprim-sulfamethoxazole; WBCs = white blood cells.
* Frequency among HIV-infected patients with acute or chronic diarrhea.

CUTANEOUS SIGNS OF AIDS

Infection by HIV may produce a transient macular roseola-like eruption. As HIV infection progresses, infectious processes and neoplastic disease are most often seen. Patients also may have symptoms such as pruritus without visible skin lesions. Superficial infections such as dermatophytosis, candidiasis, and scabies may be extensive and have altered appearances. Human papillomavirus–induced lesions may occur, ranging from persistent verrucae to severe anogenital condylomas. Chronic herpetic lesions may not have the characteristic morphologic characteristics of acute lesions in immunocompetent individuals. Mycobacterial infections produced by *Mycobacterium tuberculosis, M. avium-intracellulare, M. haemophilum,* and others affect the skin in patients with AIDS. Bacillary angiomatosis, caused by *Bartonella henselae* or *Bartonella quintana,* produces vascular proliferations in the skin as well as in other sites. Reiter's syndrome, with typical cutaneous findings, is being found with increased frequency in patients with AIDS. Mucous membranes are commonly affected by infectious processes. The most common neoplasm in the context of AIDS is Kaposi's sarcoma. A number of poorly classified eruptions occur in AIDS patients. Best known is seborrheic dermatitis, which occurs in the usual locations but can be persistent and difficult to treat.

OPHTHALMOLOGIC MANIFESTATIONS OF AIDS

Infectious or noninfectious ocular disorders, some of which may lead to severe visual impairment, have been reported in 40 to 90% of patients with AIDS (Table 21–6).

HEMATOLOGY AND ONCOLOGY IN AIDS

A signature abnormality of HIV infection is the decline in the number of CD4+ lymphocytes over time. However, other cytopenias also are seen in advanced disease, with anemia reported in 60%, thrombocytopenia in 40%, and neutropenia in 50% of patients.

Kaposi's Sarcoma

Kaposi's sarcoma (KS) is the most frequent neoplastic manifestation of HIV infection and is one of the Centers for Disease Control and Prevention (CDC) criteria that define an HIV-infected individual as having AIDS. KS is often a cutaneous non-blanching red macule. As lesions increase in size, they often have surrounding ecchymoses and acquire more of a violet hue. At times, the lesions may become nodular and, with advanced disease, the lesions may become confluent with large plaques developing, particularly on the legs. Chemotherapy may provide symptomatic relief (Table 21–7).

Non-Hodgkin's Lymphoma

B-cell lymphoma frequently occurs in immunosuppressed individuals. HIV infection provides a permissive environment for the development of lymphoma. Lymphoma in this setting may be regarded as an opportunistic neoplasm and is considered an AIDS-defining illness. Genetic evidence of Epstein-Barr virus is found in

Table 21–6 ■ DIAGNOSTIC FEATURES OF IMPORTANT CAUSES OF HIV-ASSOCIATED RETINITIS

FEATURE	CYTOMEGALOVIRUS	ACUTE RETINAL NECROSIS (VZV, HSV)	TOXOPLASMOSIS	SYPHILIS
Ocular symptoms	Floaters, visual field defect or decreased visual acuity	Same	Same	Same
	Painless	Pain common	± Photophobia	± Photophobia
Associated clinical findings	AIDS	Orolabial herpes, trigeminal zoster	AIDS, encephalitis	Rash, hearing loss
Typical retinal lesion	Cottage-cheese exudate with hemorrhage	Confluent, gray or pale retina	White or yellow exudate	Variable
Typical retinal location	Adjacent to major vessel	Peripheral	Multifocal	Focal or posterior
Risk of retinal detachment	+++	++++	++	+
Serology, culture	Not helpful	Viral culture of skin lesion	*Toxoplasma gondii* IgG titer	VDRL, FTA-ABS

VZV = varicella-zoster virus; HSV = herpes simplex virus; FTA-ABS = fluorescent treponemal antibody absorption (test).
Modified from Culbertson WW: Infection of the retina in AIDS. Int Ophthalmol Clin 29:108, 1989.

Table 21–7 ■ TREATMENT OF KAPOSI'S SARCOMA

Chemotherapy, single-agent	Liposomal doxorubicin	20 mg/m² IV every 3 wk
	Liposomal daunorubicin	40 mg/m² IV every 2 wk
	Paclitaxel	100 mg/m² IV every 2 wk
Combined therapy	Bleomycin/vincristine	Bleomycin 15 U IV Vincristine 2 mg IV every 2–3 wk
	Doxorubicin-bleomycin-vincristine	Doxorubicin 20 mg/m² Bleomycin 15 μm² IV Vincristine 2 mg IV every 3 wk

about one half of B-cell lymphomas in AIDS patients and virtually all primary CNS lymphomas in AIDS.

Other Malignancies

The incidence of Hodgkin's disease has been estimated to be up to 18-fold greater in HIV-infected patients compared to the HIV-seronegative population. In patients with HIV infection and Hodgkin's disease, the clinical presentation usually includes B symptoms (fever, night sweats, anorexia, and weight loss).

Anal cancer and, to a lesser extent, cervical cancer occur with a higher incidence in HIV-infected patients. This is due to the high prevalence of papillomavirus infection in groups at risk for HIV and the dysplasia associated with it.

RENAL, CARDIAC, ENDOCRINE, AND RHEUMATOLOGIC MANIFESTATIONS OF HIV INFECTION

Infection with the human immunodeficiency virus type 1 (HIV-1) is a multisystem disease. HIV-related renal, cardiac, endocrine, and rheumatologic diseases are more insidious in presentation. As overall survival of HIV-infected patients continues to improve and therapeutic regimens become more sophisticated, clinicians will undoubtedly encounter disorders of these organ systems with increasing frequency.

RENAL DISEASE. Renal disease associated with HIV infection may present as fluid-electrolyte and acid-base abnormalities, acute renal failure, coincidental renal disorders, or a glomerulopathy directly related to the underlying HIV infection. Renal dysfunction may be a complication in management of HIV-infected patients (Table 21–8).

CARDIAC DISEASE. A wide variety of cardiac abnormalities have been reported in HIV-infected patients, including ventricular dysfunction, myocarditis, pericarditis, endocarditis, and arrhythmias. Most often, cardiac involvement is clinically silent and is noted as an incidental finding at autopsy.

ENDOCRINE DISORDERS. Endocrine dysfunction has not been prominent in HIV infection. Nonetheless, all glands of the endocrine system may be infiltrated with opportunistic infections or malignancies or may be affected by drugs used to treat HIV-related

Table 21–8 ■ DRUGS WITH NEPHROTOXIC POTENTIAL COMMONLY USED IN THE TREATMENT OF HIV-RELATED DISEASE

Acyclovir	Non-steroidal anti-inflammatory agents
Aminoglycosides	Penicillins
Amphotericin B	Pentamidine
Aspirin	Phenytoin
Cephalosporins	Rifabutin
Cimetidine	Rifampin
Cisplatin	Spiramycin
Dapsone	Sulfonamides
Ethambutol	Tetracyclines
Foscarnet	Thiazides
Ganciclovir	Trimethoprim

Table 21–9 ■ RHEUMATOLOGIC DISEASES ASSOCIATED WITH HIV INFECTION

- Autoimmune phenomena
  - Anticardiolipin antibodies
  - Antigranulocyte antibodies
  - Antilymphocyte antibodies
  - Antinuclear antiodies
  - Antiplatelet antibodies
  - Circulating immune complexes
  - Cryoglobulins
  - Rheumatoid factor
- Dermatologic
  - Dermatomyositis
  - Malar flush
  - Psoriasis
- Joint disease
  - Arthralgias
  - Arthritis
  - Enthesopathies
  - HIV-associated arthritis
  - "Painful articular syndrome"
  - Psoriatic arthritis
  - Reactive arthropathy
  - Reiter's disease
  - Septic arthritis
  - Systemic lupus erythematosus (lupus-like syndrome)
- Myopathies
  - Infectious (septic) myositis
  - Myalgias
    - Idiopathic
    - Zidovudine-associated
  - Necrotizing, noninflammatory myopathy
  - Nemaline rod polymyositis
  - Polymyositis
  - Pyomyositis
- Sjögren's syndrome
  - Sicca complex
- Vasculitis
  - Central nervous system angiitis
  - Eosinophilic vasculitis
  - Henoch-Schönlein purpura
  - Hypersensitivity (drug-induced)
  - Leukocytoclastic vasculitis
  - Polyarteritis nodosa
  - Unspecified vasculitis

Table 21–10 ■ NAMES AND USUAL ADULT ORAL DOSES OF ANTI-HIV DRUGS

DRUG	DOSAGE
Nucleoside Reverse Transcriptase Inhibitors	
Zidovudine (AZT)	200 mg tid or 300 mg bid*
Didanosine (ddI)	>60 kg: 200 mg bid (tablets) between meals†
	<60 kg: 125 mg bid (tablets) between meals†
Zalcitabine (ddC)	0.75 mg tid
Stavudine (d4T)	>60 kg: 40 mg bid
	<60 mg: 30 mg bid
Lamivudine (3TC)	>50 kg: 150 mg bid*
	<50 kg: 2 mg/kg bid
Abacavir	300 mg bid
Non-Nucleoside Reverse Transcriptase Inhibitors	
Nevirapine	200 mg/d for 14 d, then 200 mg bid
Delavirdine	400 mg tid (in water as slurry)
Efavirenz	600 mg once daily at nighttime
Protease Inhibitors	
Indinavir	800 mg q8h between meals or with low-fat meal
Ritonavir	600 mg q12h with food if possible
Saquinavir	
Hard-gel capsule	600 mg tid with large meal
Soft-gel capsule	1200 mg tid with large meal
Nelfinavir	750 mg tid with food or light snack

* Zudovudine is also available in a combined capsule with lamivudine.

† For the buffered powder formulation of didanosine, the doses are 250 mg twice daily for patients > 60 kg and 167 mg twice daily for patients < 60 kg.

disorders. More recently, hyperlipidemia and lipodystrophy have been associated with the use of highly active antiretroviral therapy, especially with certain protease inhibitors. The specific cause of these disorder remains unclear. The subtle presentations of endocrine diseases create difficult diagnostic challenges. The most common abnormality of endocrine function noted clinically is hypogonadism.

RHEUMATOLOGIC DISEASE. Rheumatologic manifestations of HIV disease are being recognized with increased frequency. Musculoskeletal complains are reported in 33 to 75% of HIV-infected patients and may present as a variety of rheumatologic disorders. (Table 21–9).

TREATMENT

Recent developments have increased the complexity of therapy (Table 21–10). It is now generally accepted that a goal of anti-HIV therapy should be to completely inhibit HIV replication in a patient to the extent possible. HIV has an extremely high mutation rate (approximately one mutation for every one to three genomes copied), and resistant strains can emerge to any of the available drugs. (Table 21–11).

Table 21-11 ■ PREFERRED ANTIRETROVIRAL COMBINATION REGIMENS FOR INITIAL THERAPY IN PATIENTS WITH ESTABLISHED HIV INFECTION*

Preferred regimens include one drug or combination from the top column plus one of the nucleoside reverse transcriptase inhibitor combinations in the bottom column. Listings in each column are in random order, not priority order.

NON-NRTI
- Indinavir
- Nelfinavir
- Ritonavir
- Saquinavir–soft gel
- Ritonavir plus saquinavir (soft or hard gel)
- Efavirenz

plus

NRTI COMBINATIONS
- Zidovudine plus didanosine
- Stavudine plus didanosine
- Zidovudine plus zalcitabine
- Zidovudine plus lamivudine
- Stavudine plus lamivudine

NRTI = nucleoside reverse transcriptase inhibitor.

* Based on recommendations of the panel convened by the Department of Health and Human Services and the Henry J. Kaiser Family Foundation.

CHAPTER 22

DISEASES OF PROTOZOA AND METAZOA

The magnitude of parasitic infections worldwide is staggering. One billion people are infected with ascariasis or trichuriasis, and 600 million are infected with malaria and either schistosomiasis or filariasis.

Probably nowhere else in clinical medicine is the question "Where have you been?" more important than in the diagnosis of parasitic and helminthic disease.

There are a limited number of effective agents for protozoal and helminthic infections. Fortunately, most parasites remain susceptible to the limited armamentarium of available agents. The situation is decidedly different with malaria, where chloroquine resistance is now worldwide.

MALARIA

Malaria is characterized by recurrent fever and chills associated with the synchronous lysis of parasitized red blood cells. Malaria is produced by intraerythrocytic parasites of the genus *Plasmodium.* Four plasmodia produce malaria in humans: *P. falciparum, P. vivax, P. ovale,* and *P. malariae.* The severity and characteristic manifestations of malaria are governed by the infecting species, the magnitude of the parasitemia, the metabolic effects of the parasite, and the cytokines released as a result of the infection.

DIAGNOSIS. The most direct way to diagnose malaria is to examine Giemsa-stained thick or thin smears using oil immersion magnification (×1000). Identification of the parasite is key to management of the disease (Table 22–1).

TREATMENT. Successful treatment of patients with malaria depends primarilly on effective antimalarial drugs (Table 22–2).

AFRICAN TRYPANOSOMIASIS (SLEEPING SICKNESS)

Known widely as sleeping sickness, African trypanosomiasis is an acute and chronic disease caused by *Trypanosoma brucei.* The parasites are transmitted to humans through the bite of tsetse flies located in 36 countries of Africa. In humans, there are two distinct forms of the disease, East African trypanosomiasis caused by *T. brucei rhodesiense* and West African trypanosomiasis caused by *T. brucei gambiense.* Although there is some clinical overlap, East African trypanosomiasis primarily causes an acute febrile illness

For more information about this subject, see in *Cecil Textbook of Medicine,* 21st edition. Philadelphia, W.B. Saunders Company, 2000. Part XXIV: Diseases of Protozoa and Metazoa, pages 1946 to 2006.

Table 22–1 ■ MALARIA PARASITES THAT INFECT HUMANS

PLASMODIUM SPECIES	PARASITEMIA (μL bd)	COMPLICATIONS	
P. falciparum	$\geq 10^6$	Coma (cerebral malaria) Hypoglycemia Pulmonary edema, renal failure Anemia	
P. vivax	$\leq$25,000	Late (2–3 mo) splenic rupture	
P. ovale	$\leq$25,000	—	
P. malariae	$\leq$10,000	Immune complex nephrotic syndrome	
	MORPHOLOGY		
	Red Blood Cell (RBC) Size	**Schüffner's Dots**	**Stages**
P. falciparum	No RBC enlargement	Absent	Rings, occasionally gametocytes
P. vivax	Enlarged host RBC	Present	All forms
P. ovale	Enlarged host RBC	Present	All forms
P. malariae	No RBC enlargement	Absent	All forms
	RELAPSE FROM HYPNOZOITES	**ANTIMALARIAL RESISTANCE**	
P. falciparum	No	Chloroquine, meftoquine, pyrimethamine-sulfadoxine, plus partial resistance to quinine and quinidine	
P. vivax	Yes	Chloroquine	
P. ovale	Yes	None known	
P. malariae	No	None known	

Table 22–2 ■ CHEMOPROPHYLAXIS OF MALARIA*

For Areas without Chloroquine-Resistant *Plasmodium falciparum*	
Chloroquine phosphate (Aralen)	500 mg/wk (300 mg chloroquine base) during exposure and for 4 wk after leaving the endemic area
For Areas with Chloroquine-Resistant *Plasmodium falciparum*	
Mefloquine (Lariam)	250 mg/wk during exposure and for 4 wk after leaving the endemic area
Doxycycline	100 mg/d during exposure and for 4 wk after leaving the endemic area

Alternatives for areas with chloroquine-resistant *P. falciparum* include proguanil 200 mg/day plus weekly chloroquine, although this regimen has not been approved by the FDA and breakthroughs occur with some frequency in areas with chloroquine-resistant *P. falciparum*. Updated information on malaria chemoprophylaxis may be obtained from the CDC hot line and websites at 404-223-4559, 404-332-4565, and www.cdc.gov, respectively.

with myocarditis and meningoencephalitis that is rapidly fatal if not treated, whereas West African trypanosomiasis is characterized as a chronic debilitating disease with mental deterioration and physical wasting.

TREATMENT. Suramin* is the drug of choice for the early hemolymphatic stage of both *T. b. gambiense* **and** *T. b. rhodesiense* infections before central nervous system (CNS) invasion has occurred. Suramin does not cross the blood-brain barrier in increased amounts, and it does not cure the disease once CNS invasion has occurred. The dose is 20 mg/kg of body weight given intravenously up to a maximum single dose of 1 g. Suramin is a toxic drug that may result in idiosyncratic reactions in some patients (1 in 20,000). The drug is excreted entirely by the kidneys. Pentamidine isethionate* is an alternative drug for treating early hemolymphatic African trypanosomiasis, but it is much less active against *T. b. rhodesiense* than is suramin. The arsenical melarsoprol* (Mel B) is the treatment of choice for both Gambian and Rhodesian sleeping sickness once involvement of the CNS has occurred. Untreated African sleeping sickness is almost invariably fatal.

AMERICAN TRYPANOSOMIASIS (CHAGAS' DISEASE)

Chagas' disease results from infection with the protozoan parasite *Trypanosoma cruzi*. *T. cruzi* is usually transmitted as a zoonosis. Various species of blood-sucking reduviid bugs become infected when they take a blood meal from animals or humans who have circulating parasites, trypomastigotes, in the blood.

T. cruzi and its arthropod vectors are widely distributed from the southern United States through Mexico and Central America into South America down to central Argentina and Chile. The parasite is restricted to the Western Hemisphere. In endemic areas, first exposure to *T. cruzi* generally is subclinical and unnoticed. When those initially exposed do have clinical manifestations, the disease is an acute systemic infection. Chronic Chagas' disease, in contrast, evolves as a later sequela with specific organ involvement and no systemic features.

Myocarditis, accompanied by tachycardia and non-specific ECG changes, can occur in the acute stage. Cardiac signs and symptoms are the most common manifestations of chronic disease and are likely to begin with palpitations, dizziness, precordial discomfort, and even syncope. These reflect a variety of arrhythmias. Sudden death due to ventricular tachycardia in an otherwise healthy young adult in not unusual.

The *diagnosis of chronic Chagas' disease* requires demonstration of antibodies to *T. cruzi* in the presence of the characteristic cardiac abnormalities and/or megadisease.

TREATMENT. Two drugs with reasonable antitrypanosomal activity are currently in use for treating Chagas' disease. One of these is a nitrofuran derivative, nifurtimox,* which has been extensively

*Available from the Centers for Disease Control and Prevention (CDC), Atlanta, GA. Drug Service (404-639-3670).

Table 22–3 ■ CLINICAL SYNDROMES OF LEISHMANIASIS

Visceral leishmaniasis
Kala-azar (spleen, bone marrow, liver, etc.)
Old World cutaneous leishmaniasis
Single or limited number of skin lesions
Diffuse cutaneous leishmaniasis
New World cutaneous leishmaniasis
Single or limited number of skin lesions
Diffuse cutaneous leishmaniasis
Mucosal leishmaniasis

evaluated. Nifurtimox* is the only drug available in the United States for treating Chagas' disease; it is used in a dose of 8 to 10 mg/kg/day.

LEISHMANIASIS

Leishmaniasis comprises a spectrum of clinical disease produced by *Leishmania* species. An estimated 350 million people worldwide live in areas where there is a risk of infection (Table 22–3).

TREATMENT. ***VISCERAL LEISHMANIASIS.*** Pentavalent antimonials and meglumine antimoniate have been the mainstays of therapy for visceral leishmaniasis. They are still used in many countries, but therapeutic failures are increasingly recognized in some areas. Amphotericin B and pentamidine have been effective. Liposome-encapsulated amphotericin B recently became the first drug licensed for the treatment of visceral leishmaniasis in the United States. It is likely to emerge as the treatment of choice. Stibogluconate sodium is available in the United States through the CDC Drug Service.

CUTANEOUS LEISHMANIASIS. Pentavalent antimonials, stibogluconate sodium, and meglumine antimoniate effectively treat cutaneous leishmaniasis in many situations.

TOXOPLASMOSIS

Toxoplasma gondii is a protozoan parasite. The *acute acquired* infection in humans is usually asymptomatic. However, clinical and/or pathologic evidence of disease (toxoplasmosis) may occur, particularly in the immunocompromised patient, the congenitally infected fetus and child, and those in whom chorioretinitis develops during the acute acquired infection.

CLINICAL MANIFESTATIONS. ***ACUTE INFECTION IN IMMUNOCOMPETENT PATIENTS.*** *T. gondii* infection is symptomatic in only approximately 10% of immunocompetent patients. In these patients, toxoplasmosis most often presents as lymphadenopathy.

OCULAR TOXOPLASMOSIS IN IMMUNOCOMPETENT PATIENTS. *T. gondii* infection has been reported to be responsible for approximately 35% of retinochoroiditis in older children and adults in the United States.

TOXOPLASMOSIS IN IMMUNOCOMPROMISED PATIENTS. Toxoplasmosis in the immunocompromised patient in most cases is the

---

*Must be obtained from CDC, Atlanta, GA (404-639-3670).

result of reactivation of latent infection. Numerous conditions that compromise the immune system have been associated with toxoplasmosis, with the highest frequencies in patients with acquired immunodeficiency syndrome (AIDS), Hodgkin's disease or other lymphoma, and in other patients who are on high-dose corticosteroids and/or other immunosuppressive agents for treatment of malignancies. Toxoplasmosis can be diagnosed by isolation of the organism, polymerase chain reaction (PCR), demonstration of tachyzoites in tissues or body fluids by histologic or cytologic analysis, and serologic testing.

TREATMENT. The need for and duration of therapy depend on the clinical manifestations of toxoplasmosis and the immune status of the patient (Tables 22–4 and 22–5).

CRYPTOSPORIDIOSIS

Cryptosporidiosis is a leading cause of endemic and epidemic diarrheal disease worldwide. Diarrhea is the predominant symptom in all groups. In otherwise healthy adults, the incubation period is 2 to 14 days, followed by the onset of non-inflammatory (watery and non-bloody) diarrhea. *Corynebacterium parvum* infection is diagnosed by stool examination.

THERAPY. The cornerstone of therapy is fluid replacement, and in immunocompromised patients, an attempt to reverse the immunodeficiency. *Mycobacterium avium-intracellulare* chemoprophylaxis with rifampin and the macrolide clarithromycin in AIDS patients is protective against the development of cryptosporidiosis. There is no clearly demonstrated successful drug therapy once infection is established.

GIARDIASIS

Giardia lamblia is the most common human protozoan enteric pathogen worldwide and causes both endemic and epidemic diarrheal illnesses. The parasite is also often carried asymptomatically by humans.

CLINICAL DISEASE. Giardiasis presents in one of three clinical forms: (1) asymptomatic carrier state; (2) acute, self-limited diarrheal illnesses; (3) chronic diarrhea associated with malabsorption.

DIAGNOSIS. Giardiasis is diagnosed by demonstration of the cysts or, more rarely, trophozoites of *G. lamblia* in fecal specimens.

THERAPY. The nitroimidazoles, metronidazole and tinidazole (not available in the United States) are most often the drugs of choice and are more than 90% efficacious.

AMEBIASIS

The parasite *Entamoeba histolytica* infects 1% of the world's population, with the disease burden highest in poor, developing areas. Disease syndromes caused by *E. histolytica* are summarized in Table 22–6. Evaluation of amebic colitis and liver abscess is seen in Figure 22–1. Treatment regimens for amebiasis are summarized in Table 22–7.

Table 22–4 ■ GUIDELINES FOR ACUTE AND MAINTENANCE THERAPY OF TOXOPLASMIC ENCEPHALITIS IN AIDS PATIENTS

	ACUTE THERAPY	MAINTENANCE THERAPY*
Suggested Regimens		
Pyrimethamine plus	200 mg loading dose PO, then 50–75 mg qd	25–50 mg qd
Folinic acid (leucovorin) plus one of the following:	10–20 mg PO, IV, or IM qd (up to 50 mg qd)	10–20 mg qd
Sulfadiazine *or*	1.0–1.5 g PO q6h	0.5–1.0 g PO qid
Clindamycin	600 mg PO or IV q6h (up to IV 1200 mg q6h)	450–600 mg q6h
Pyrimethamine-sulfadoxine (Fansidar)	No adequate data	1 tablet biweekly
Alternative Regimens†		
Trimethoprim-sulfamethoxazole	5 mg PO or IV (trimethoprim component)/kg q6h	No adequate data
Pyrimethamine plus	No adequate data	50 mg qd
Folinic acid		10–20 mg qd
Pyrimethamine and folinic acid plus one of the following:	As in suggested regimens	As in suggested regimens
Clarithromycin *or*	1 g q12h PO	1 g q12h
Azithromycin *or*	1200–1500 mg PO qd	1200–1500 mg qd
Atovaquone *or*	750 mg PO q6h	750 mg q6h
Dapsone	100 mg PO qd	100 mg biweekly

* Drugs administered orally.
† Data inadequate for definitive recommendation.
Adapted from Liesenfeld O, Wong SY, Remington JS: Toxoplasmosis in the setting of AIDS. *In* Merigan TC Jr, Bartlett JG, Bolognesi D (eds): Textbook of AIDS Medicine. Baltimore, Williams & Wilkins, 1999, pp 225–259.

Table 22–5 ■ PRIMARY PROPHYLAXIS FOR TOXOPLASMOSIS IN AIDS PATIENTS*

For the *Toxoplasma gondii*–seropositive HIV-infected patient†	
Trimethoprim-sulfamethoxazole	1 DS tablet qd
	2 DS tablet biweekly
Pyrimethamine-dapsone	Pyrimethamine 50 mg once a week, plus dapsone, 50 mg qd
	Pyrimethamine 25 mg biweekly, plus dapsone 100 mg biweekly
	Pyrimethamine 75 mg once a week, plus dapsone 200 mg once a week
Pyrimethamine-sulfadoxine	3 tablets every 2 wk
(Fansidar)	1 tablet biweekly
For prevention of congenital transmission of *T. gondii* in seropositive, HIV-infected pregnant women‡	
Spiramycin	1 g q8h

AIDS = acquired immunodeficiency syndrome; HIV = human immunodeficiency syndrome; DS = double strength.

* Drugs are administered orally.

† These regimens have been reported to be effective for primary prophylaxis of toxoplasmic encephalitis in AIDS patients.

‡ Although at present no data are available on the efficacy of prophylaxis against congential transmission in this group of patients, we consider it prudent to recommend spiramycin because preliminary studies suggest that the transmission rate for congenital toxoplasmosis in these women is remarkably and significantly higher than in non–HIV-infected *T. gondii*–seropositive women.

Adapted from Liesenfeld O, Wong SY, Remington JS: Toxoplasmosis in the setting of AIDS. *In* Merigan TC Jr, Bartlett JG, Bolognesi D (eds): Textbook of AIDS Medicine. Baltimore, Williams & Wilkins, 1999, pp 225–259.

Table 22–6 ■ CLINICAL SYNDROMES ASSOCIATED WITH *ENTAMOEBA HISTOLYTICA* INFECTION

Intestinal Disease

Asymptomatic infection
Acute rectocolitis (dysentery)
Fulminant colitis with perforation
Toxic megacolon
Chronic nondysenteric colitis
Ameboma

Extraintestinal Disease

Liver abscess
Liver abscess complicated by:
  Peritonitis
  Empyema
  Pericarditis
Lung abscess
Brain abscess
Genitourinary disease

From Mandell GL, Douglas RG Jr, Bennett JE (eds): Principles and Practices of Infectious Diseases, 3rd ed. New York, Churchill Livingstone, 1989.

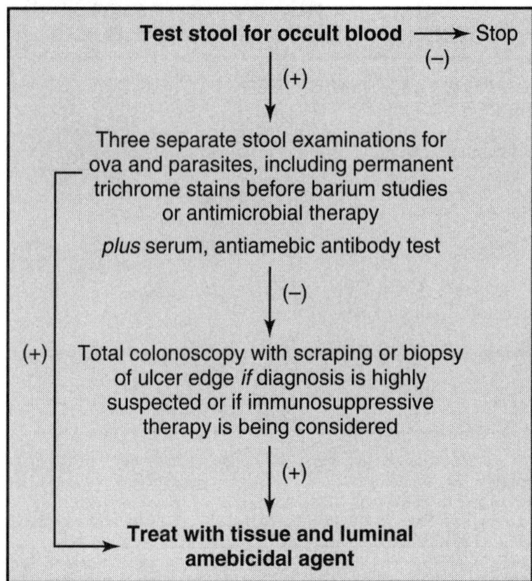

FIGURE 22–1 ■ Diagnostic evaluation for acute amebic rectocolitis in a patient with suggestive epidemiology and clinical manifestations. (From Kass EH, Platt R [eds]: Current Therapy in Infectious Disease—3. Philadelphia, BC Decker, 1990.)

Table 22–7 ■ THERAPEUTIC REGIMENS FOR TREATMENT OF AMEBIASIS*

Cyst Passers
Diloxanide furoate 500 mg bid × 10 d, *or*
Paromomycin 30 mg/kg/d in three divided doses × 5–10 d, *or*
Tetracycline 250 mg four times a day × 10 d, then diiodohydroxyquin 650 tid × 20 d
Invasive Rectocolitis
Metronidazole 750 mg tid × 5–10 d *or*
2.4 g/d × 2–3 d *or*
50 mg/kg × 1 dose
plus diloxanide furoate or paromomycin *or* if metronidazole not tolerated
Dehydroemetine, 1.01–1.5 mg/kg/d × 5 d plus diloxanide furoate or paromomycin
Liver Abscess
Metronidazole 750 mg tid × 5–10 d or 2.4 g/d × 1–2 d plus diloxanide furoate or paromomycin or if metronidazole not tolerated
Dehydroemetine 1.0–1.5 mg/kg/d × 5 d plus diloxanide furoate or paromomycin

* All dosages are for oral administration except dehydroemetine, which is given intramuscularly; metronidazole can be used intravenously.

Adapted with permission from Mandell GL, Douglas RG Jr, Bennett JE (eds): Principles and Practices of Infectious Diseases, 3rd ed. New York, Churchill Livingstone, 1989.

CESTODE INFECTIONS

Although the cestodes are often referred to collectively as "tapeworms," not all cestode parasites develop into tapeworms in the human host (Table 22–8).

SCHISTOSOMIASIS (BILHARZIASIS)

Schistosomiasis is one of the most important parasitic diseases of humans. It is estimated that over 200 million people are currently infected worldwide. There are five major species of *Schistosomia* affecting humans. The endemicity of schistosomiasis depends on the urban disposal of urine (*S. haematobium*) and feces (*S. mansoni, S. japonicum, S. intercalatum, S. mekongi*), the presence of suitable snail hosts, and human exposure to cercariae.

Clinical manifestations of schistosomiasis are divided into schistosome dermatitis, acute schistosomiasis, and chronic schistosomiasis. Acute disease is more frequently observed in people living outside the endemic areas of schistosomiasis. The disease is characterized by fever, chills, hepatosplenomegaly, lymphadenopathy, weight loss, headache, and cough.

In chronic schistosomiasis, tissue injury is mediated by egg-induced granulomas and subsequent appearance of fibrosis. Because the habitat of *S. mansoni, S. japonicum, S. mekongi,* and *S. intercalatum* worms is the mesenteric blood vessels, the intestines are involved primarily and egg embolism results in secondary involvement of the liver. Hepatosplenic involvement is the most important cause of morbidity in *S. mansoni* and *S. japonicum* infections.

A definitive diagnosis of schistosomiasis can be made only by finding schistosome eggs in feces, urine, or a biopsy specimen, usually from the rectum.

MANAGEMENT. Chemotherapy is by far the major tool for the control and cure of schistosomiasis. Three compounds are currently in use—metrifonate, oxamniquine, and praziquantel—and all three are included in the World Health Organization's list of essential drugs.

LIVER, INTESTINAL, AND LUNG FLUKE INFECTIONS

Approximately 50 million people are infected worldwide with liver, intestinal, or lung flukes (Table 22–9).

TREATMENT. Chemotherapy for fluke infections has become a more effective management strategy with the introduction of praziquantel. This orally administered 1-day anthelmintic results in cure rates of 70 to 90%. The recommended dose of praziquantel is 75 mg/kg body weight divided into three doses and given in 1 day. A 2-day course of praziquantel is necessary for treatment of paragonimiasis.

NEMATODE INFECTIONS

Nematodes, or roundworms, include a vast number of species of free-living and parasitic helminths. Mebendazole is the treatment of choice (Table 22–10).

Table 22–8 ■ COMMON HUMAN CESTODE INFECTIONS

SPECIES	STAGE FOUND IN HUMANS	COMMON NAME	PATHOLOGY	THERAPY
Diphyllobothrium latum	Adult	Fish tapeworm	Pernicious anemia	Niclosamide Praziquantel
Hymenolepis nana	Adult	Dwarf tapeworm	Rarely symptomatic	Niclosamide Praziquantel
Taenia saginata	Adult	Beef tapeworm	Rarely symptomatic	
Taenia solium	Adult	Pork tapeworm	Rarely symptomatic	Niclosamide Praziquantel
	Larva	Cysticercosis	Brain and tissue cysts	Albendazole Praziquantel Surgery
Echinococcus granulosus	Larva	Hydatid cyst disease	Solitary tissue cysts	Surgery Albendazole
Echinococcus multilocularis	Larva	Alveolar cyst disease	Multilocular cysts	Surgery Albendazole
Taenia multiceps	Larva	Bladderworm, coenurosis	Brain and eye cysts	Surgery
Spirometra mansonoides	Larva	Sparganosis	Subcutaneous larvae	Surgery

Table 22–9 ■ MAJOR LIVER, INTESTINAL, AND LUNG FLUKE INFECTIONS IN HUMANS

INFECTION (GENUS)	CAUSATIVE ORGANISMS	SECOND INTERMEDIATE HOST
Opisthorchiasis (*Opisthorcis*)	*O. viverrini* *O. felineus*	Cyprinoid fish
Clonorchiasis (*Clonorchis*)	*C. sinensis*	Carp fish
Fascioliasis (*Fasciola*)	*F. hepatica* *F. gigantica*	Aquatic vegetation or water
Fasciolopsiasis (*Fasciolopsis*)	*F. buski*	Aquatic plants
Paragonimiasis (*Paragonimus*)	*P. westermani*	Freshwater and brackish water crabs

FILARIASIS

The filariases are a group of arthropod-borne parasitic diseases of humans caused by threadlike nematodes that in their mature adult stage reside in the lymphatics or in connective tissue (Table 22–11).

Table 22–10 ■ TREATMENT FOR INTESTINAL NEMATODES

NEMATODE	TREATMENT
Hookworm	Mebendazole 100 mg PO bid for 3 d; do not give to pregnant women; iron supplementation (if warranted by anemia and complicating illnesses)
Ascaris	Mebendazole 100 mg PO bid for 3 d; children with heavy infections, biliary tract obstruction: piperazine 50–75 mg/kg body weight for 2 d
Enterobius	Pyrantel pamoate 11 mg/kg once, with a repeated dose 2 wk later; maximum single dose, 1 g; several treatments may be required (every 3–4 mo) if exposure continues (i.e., in institutional setting)
Trichuris	Mebendazole, at same dosage as for ascariasis
Other animal nematodes	
Trichostrongylus	Pyrantel pamoate 11 mg/kg once; maximum dose of 1 g
Anisakis	Thiabendazole 25 mg/kg bid for 3 d if surgery is not required
Capillaria	Mebendazole 200 mg bid for 20 d; alternative: albendazole, 400 mg/d for 10 d; supportive care: replacement of fluid and electrolytes, high-protein diet
Gnathostoma	For subcutaneous lesions: surgical removal; for CNS infection: albendazole 400 mg bid for 21 d

Table 22–11 ■ THE COMMON FILARIAL PARASITES OF HUMANS

SPECIES	DISTRIBUTION	VECTOR	PRIMARY PATHOLOGY	MICROFILARIAE		
				Primary Location	Periodicity	Presence of Sheath
Wuchereria bancrofti	Tropics worldwide	Mosquitoes	Lymphatic, pulmonary	Blood, hydrocele fluid	Nocturnal, subperiodic	+
Brugia malayi	Southeast Asia, West Pacific	Mosquitoes	Lymphatic, pulmonary	Blood	Nocturnal, subperiodic	+
Brugia timori	Indonesia	Mosquitoes	Lymphatic	Blood	Nocturnal	+
Onchocerca volvulus	Africa, Central and South America	Black fly	Skin, eye, lymphatic	Skin, eye	None or minimal	–
Loa loa	Africa	Deer fly	Allergic	Blood	Diurnal	+
Mansonella perstans	Africa, South America	Midge	? Allergic	Blood	None	–
Mansonella streptocerca	Africa	Midge	Skin	Skin	None	–
Mansonella ozzardi	Central and South America	Midge	Vague	Blood	None	–

CHAPTER 23

NEUROLOGY

APPROACH TO THE PATIENT

The neurologic history is the most important component of neurologic diagnosis. Symptoms of acute onset suggest a vascular cause or seizure; symptoms that are subacute in onset suggest a mass lesion such as a tumor or abscess; symptoms that have a waxing and waning course with exacerbations and remissions suggest a demyelinating cause; symptoms that are chronic and progressive suggest a degenerative disorder. Principles of evaluation include the following:

1. Carefully identify the chief complaint or major problem. Establishing a diagnosis that does not incorporate the chief complaint frequently focuses attention on a coincidental process irrelevant to the patient's concerns.
2. Listen carefully to the patient for as long as is necessary. During this time, the examiner can also assess mental status, including speech, language, fund of knowledge, and affect, and observe the patient for facial asymmetry, abnormalities of ocular movements, and an increase or a paucity of spontaneous movements, as seen with movement disorders.
3. Steer the patient away from discussions of previous diagnostic test results.
4. Take a careful history. Many neurologic illnesses are complications of underlying medical disorders or are due to adverse effects of drugs. A large number of neurologic disorders are hereditary. Absence of a family history of a disease is seldom an argument against considering that the patient may have a hereditary condition. Two specific features of neurologic disorders are important to consider in obtaining a family pedigree. *Anticipation,* the worsening of a disease with successive generations, is a feature of the trinucleotide repeat diseases. Many *mitochondrial* genetic diseases are transmitted only from mothers to their male and female offspring. Occupation plays a major role in various neurologic disorders such as carpal tunnel syndrome.
5. Interview surrogate historians. A family member may provide key details.
6. Summarize the history for the patient to ensure that all details were covered sufficiently to make a tentative diagnosis.
7. End by asking the patient what he or she thinks is wrong to evaluate the patient's concerns about and insight into the condition.

For more information about this subject, see in *Cecil Textbook of Medicine,* 21st edition. Philadelphia, W.B. Saunders Company, 2000. Part XXV: Neurology, pages 2007 to 2223.

Clinical Diagnosis

Ask yourself, Can one disease account for all of the symptoms and signs? Formulate a diagnostic opinion in anatomic terms. Is the history suggestive of a single (e.g., stroke or tumor) *focus* or of multiple sites of nervous system involvement (e.g., multiple sclerosis)? Or is the process a disease of *a system:* vitamin B_{12} deficiency, myopathy, or polyneuropathy?

Traumatic injury inflicted by family members or other close contact with patients is usually difficult to detect by medical history and examination. A host of neurologic disorders can be the result of the intentional ingestion of toxins. Patients do not usually give an accurate account of their use of these agents.

Neurologic Examination

Head circumference should be measured in patients with central nervous system (CNS) or spinal cord disease (normally 55 ±5 cm in adults). Head enlargement should suggest a long-standing anomaly of the brain or spinal cord. The skin should be inspected for cafe au lait maculas, adenoma sebaceum, vascular malformations, lipomas, neurofibromas, and other lesions. Neck range of motion, straight leg raising, and spinal curvature (scoliosis) should be assessed. Carotid auscultation for bruits is indicated. Limitation of joint range of motion or painless swelling of joints is often a sign of an unsuspected neurologic lesion.

The mental status must be assessed for level of consciousness, orientation, memory, language function, affect, and judgment. Cranial nerve function includes visual acuity (with and without correction); optic fundi; visual fields; pupils (size and reactivity to direct and consensual light); ocular motility; jaw, facial, palatal, neck, and tongue movement; and hearing.

Motor system examination includes muscle tone (flaccid, spastic, or rigid), muscle size (atrophy or hypertrophy), and muscle strength. Gait, stance, and coordination are assessed. The patient should be observed for tremor, fasciculations, and other abnormal movements.

Sensory testing need not be detailed unless there are sensory symptoms. However, vibration perception in the toes, as well as the normality of perception of pain, temperature, and light touch in the hands and feet, should be assessed.

Muscle stretch reflexes and plantar responses should always be assessed, evaluating right-left symmetry and disparity between proximal or distal reflexes or arm versus leg reflexes. Biceps, triceps, brachioradialis, quadriceps, and ankle reflexes should be quantitated on a scale of 1 to 4 (4 = clonus; 3 = spread; 2 = brisk; 1 = hypoactive).

The rapid examination required for a patient with an altered state of consciousness is much different from that of an alert, aware individual. Attention should focus on the examination of (1) level of consciousness, (2) respiratory pattern, (3) eyelid position and eye movements, (4) pupils, (5) corneal reflexes, (6) optic fundi, (7) motor responses.

Neurologic Diagnostic Procedures

Sampling of *cerebrospinal fluid* (CSF) via lumbar puncture often provides an important clue as to the pathologic process involved (Table 23–1). A lumbar puncture should not be performed in patients who have obstructive, non-communicating hydrocephalus or a focal CNS mass lesion causing raised intracranial pressure (ICP).

Electroencephalography (EEG) is performed by securing 20 electrodes to the scalp at predetermined locations. The major usefulness of EEG is for diagnosis and categorization of a seizure disorder, but EEGs are neither highly sensitive nor completely specific for diagnosing seizures. In fact, only about 50% of patients with seizures show epileptiform activity on the first EEG. Repeating the EEG with provocative maneuvers, such as sleep deprivation, hyperventilation, and photic stimulation, may increase this percentage to 90%. Conversely, about 1% of adults who are neurologically normal and who never had a seizure will have epileptiform activity on an EEG. In herpes simplex encephalitis, periodic lateralizing epileptiform discharges emanating from the temporal lobes are frequently present. Triphasic slow waves are the hallmark of hepatic encephalopathy. The EEG is also helpful in confirming brain death.

A *nerve conduction study* (NCS) (Table 23–2) is helpful in documenting the existence of a neuropathy, quantifying its severity, and noting its distribution (i.e., whether it is distal, proximal, or diffuse). The NCS can give clues about whether the underlying pathologic process is axonal or demyelinating. An NCS is also helpful in diagnosing compressive neuropathies, such as carpal tunnel syndrome. F waves are helpful in diagnosing Guillain-Barré syndrome.

The *repetitive stimulation study* is a method of measuring electrical conduction properties at the neuromuscular junction. In myasthenia gravis, the amplitudes of the evoked potentials become progressively smaller with repetitive stimulation. In the myasthenic syndrome (Lambert-Eaton syndrome), an increment is seen in the amplitudes of the evoked potentials with repetitive electrical stimulation.

Electromyography (EMG) studies the electrical activity of muscle in four settings: (1) insertional activity (occurring within the first second of needle insertion); (2) spontaneous activity (electrical activity at rest); (3) voluntary activity (electrical activity with muscle contraction); and (4) recruitment pattern (change in electrical activity with maximal contraction) (Table 23–3). The EMG can help to determine whether weakness is due to anterior horn cell disease, nerve root disease, peripheral neuropathy, or an intrinsic disease of muscle itself (myopathy). The EMG can differentiate acute denervation from chronic denervation. In addition, based on which muscles have an abnormal EMG pattern, it is possible to determine whether the neuropathy is due to a lesion of a nerve root (radiculopathy), the brachial or lumbosacral plexus (plexopathy), an individual peripheral nerve (mononeuropathy), or multiple peripheral nerves (polyneuropathy). The EMG is also helpful in differentiating active (inflammatory) myopathies from chronic myopathies. The active myopathies include dermatomyositis, polymyositis, inclusion

Table 23–1 ■ CHARACTERISTIC CEREBROSPINAL FLUID FORMULAS

	TURBIDITY AND COLOR	OPENING PRESSURE	WBC COUNT (mm^3)	DIFFERENTIAL	RBC COUNT	PROTEIN	GLUCOSE
Normal	Clear, colorless	70–180 mm H_2O	0–5	Mononuclear	0	$<$60 mg/dL	$>$2/3 serum
Bacterial meningitis	Cloudy, straw-colored	↑	↑↑	PMNs	0	↑↑	↓
Viral meningitis	Clear or cloudy, colorless	↑	↑	Lymphocytes	0	↑	Normal
Fungal and tuberculous meningitis	Cloudy, straw-colored	↑	↑	Lymphocytes	0	↑↑	↓↓
Viral encephalitis	Clear or cloudy, straw-colored	Normal to ↑	↑	Lymphocytes	0 (herpes ↑)	Normal to ↑	Normal
Subarachnoid hemorrhage	Cloudy, pink	↑	↑	PMNs and lymphocytes	↑↑	↑	Normal (early) ↓ (late)
Guillain-Barré syndrome	Clear, yellow	Normal to ↑	0–5	Mononuclear	0	↑	Normal

WBC = white blood cell; RBC = red blood cell; PMNs = polymorphonuclear leukocytes.

Table 23–2 ■ NERVE CONDUCTION STUDY ABNORMALITIES

ABNORMALITY	CLINICAL CORRELATE
Reduced amplitude of CMAP	Axonal neuropathy
Prolonged terminal latency	Demyelinating neuropathy Distal compressive neuropathy
Conduction block	Severe focal compressive neuropathy Severe demyelinating neuropathy
Slowed conduction velocity	Demyelinating neuropathy

CMAP = compound muscle action potential.

body myositis, and some forms of muscular dystrophy, such as Duchenne's dystrophy. It may take several weeks for a muscle to develop EMG signs of acute denervation following nerve transection.

The pattern reversal *visual evoked response* (PVER) measures conduction velocities for central visual pathways, in particular the optic nerves. PVER testing is helpful when multiple sclerosis is suspected clinically.

The *brain stem auditory evoked response* (BAER) measures conduction velocities for central auditory pathways in the brain stem. BAER testing is helpful in diagnosing acoustic schwannoma.

Table 23–3 ■ ELECTROMYOGRAPHIC (EMG) ABNORMALITIES

ABNORMALITY	CLINICAL CORRELATE
Insertional Activity	
Prolonged	Acute denervation Active (usually inflammatory) myopathy
Spontaneous Activity	
Fibrillations and positive waves	Acute denervation Active (usually inflammatory) myopathy
Fasciculations	Chronic neuropathies Motor neuron disease (rare fasciculations may be normal)
Myotonic discharges	Myotonic disorders Acid maltase deficiency
Voluntary Activity	
Neuropathic potentials: large-amplitude, long-duration, polyphasic potentials	Chronic neuropathies and anterior horn cell diseases
Myopathic potentials: small-amplitude, short-duration, polyphasic potentials	Chronic myopathies Neuromuscular junction disorders
Recruitment	
Reduced	Chronic neuropathies
Rapid	Chronic myopathies

The *somatosensory evoked response* (SER) measures conduction velocities for central somatosensory pathways in the posterior columns of the spinal cord, brain stem, thalamus, and primary sensory cortex in the parietal lobes. SER testing, like PVER, is helpful when multiple sclerosis is suspected clinically.

Electronystagmography accurately records eye movements and nystagmus following certain proactive maneuvers. Spontaneous nystagmus suggests a vestibular lesion, as does an imbalance in the nystagmus evoked by these maneuvers in the right and left ears.

Imaging Studies

Magnetic resonance imaging (MRI) is at present the most commonly used imaging modality for the CNS (Table 23–4). MRI is generally the best modality for imaging the spinal cord and the spaces surrounding it. The exceptions to MRI as a first study are discussed below. Plain skull films are rarely, if ever, indicated.

To rule out subarachnoid hemorrhage, non-contrast *computed tomography* (CT) is the fastest, most sensitive, and most specific imaging modality. The next study following a positive CT is an angiogram. CT is more sensitive and specific with respect to calcification. CT, with or without contrast depending on the goals (Table 23–5), is also the first study in other clinical situations, including acute head trauma or facial trauma, sinusitis, temporal bone problems such as inflammatory or congenital lesions, and the immediate postoperative craniotomy patient.

Magnetic resonance angiography (MRA) is rapidly replacing conventional angiography. MRA is the best non-invasive technique for evaluating the extracranial vasculature for the presence of a hemodynamically significant lesion of the carotid arteries, dissection of the vertebral and carotid arteries, extracranial traumatic fistula, extracranial vasculitis such as giant cell arteritis, or congenital abnormalities of the vessels such as fibromuscular disease. The limitations of extracranial MRA include a tendency to overestimate stenosis.

For more information about this subject, see *Cecil Textbook of Medicine,* 21st edition. Philadelphia, W.B. Saunders Company, 2000. Chapter 442, Neurologic Diagnostic Procedures; and Chapter 443, Radiologic Imaging Procedures, pages 2009 to 2023.

COMA AND DISORDERS OF AROUSAL

Coma is a sleeplike state from which the patient cannot be aroused. Consciousness requires an intact and functioning brain stem reticular activating system and its cortical projections. The reticular formation begins in the midpons and ascends through the dorsal midbrain to synapse in the thalamus for its thalamocortical connections. A brain stem or bihemispheric dysfunction must satisfy these anatomic requirements or it is not the cause of the patient's unconsciousness. In addition to structural lesions, meningeal inflammation, metabolic encephalopathy, or seizure satisfies the anatomic requirements and completes the differential diagnosis of the patient in coma.

Meningeal irritation caused by infection or blood in the subarachnoid space is among the most important early considerations in coma evaluation as it is treatable and (especially with purulent

Table 23–4 ■ IMAGING METHODOLOGIES FOR NEUROLOGIC PROBLEMS

NEUROLOGIC PROBLEM/DISORDER	IMAGING METHODOLOGY	COMMENT
Vague symptoms	MRI without and with contrast	Once a physician decides that an imaging study is warranted, MRI is the most sensitive modality for the initial imaging evaluation
Headache not secondary to subarachnoid hemorrhage	MRI without and with contrast	Best method to triage this particular group of headache patients
Rule out subarachnoid hemorrhage	CT without contrast	Best imaging method to detect subarachnoid hemorrhage
Rule out intracranial aneurysm (high probability, e.g., acute third nerve palsy)	Conventional angiography	Definitive
Familial history of aneurysm or predisposing condition, e.g., polycystic kidney disease	MRA	Nonvasive and excellent at detecting aneurysms
Rule out stroke	CT	CT is fast and can detect whether or not there is an intraparenchymal hemorrhage or ischemic infarction
	Diffusion-weighted MRI	Fast and extremely sensitive for the diagnosis of acute stroke
Rule out neoplasm	MRI without and with contrast	Most sensitive imaging test
Rule out multiple sclerosis	MRI without and with contrast	Most sensitive imaging test
Rule out infection/inflammation	MRI without and with contrast	Most sensitive imaging test
Dementia work-up	MRI without contrast (rarely is contrast helpful)	The first test should be MRI to detect any lesion such as a frontal meningioma that might be responsible for dementia syndrome; normal-pressure hydrocephalus and multi-infarct dementia can also be easily demonstrated; PET and SPECT scanning may also be helpful
Seizures/epilepsy	MRI without and with contrast	The first test should be MRI to detect any lesion that is the seizure source; other useful techniques may be SPECT, PET, and MRS
Head trauma	Acute—CT; MRI is additionally useful as well as for follow-up	CT is the fastest method to assess head trauma; MRI is more sensitive and specific for detecting diffuse axonal injury
Intrinsic spinal cord lesion	MRI without and with contrast	Most sensitive imaging modality for detecting of spinal cord disease
Extradural spinal process	MRI without and with contrast and CT myelogram	For nonneoplastic disease, MRI without contrast is all that is required; CT myelogram is particularly useful for cervical spine degenerative disease

MRI = magnetic resonance imaging; CT = computed tomography; MRA = magnetic resonance angiography; PET = positron emission tomography; SPECT = single photon emission computed tomography; MRS = magnetic resonance spectroscopy.

Table 23-5 ■ INDICATIONS FOR UNENHANCED AND ENHANCED IMAGING (CT/MRI) IN DISEASES OF THE BRAIN AND SPINE

UNENHANCED IMAGES	ENHANCED
Hemorrhagic event	Infection
Ischemic event	Inflammation
Congenital anomaly	Neoplasia—either primary or metastatic
Head trauma	Process thought to involve the leptomeninges, nerve roots
Neurodegenerative disease	Seizures
Degenerative disease of the spine (not operated on)	Intrinsic spinal cord lesions or suspected lesions in the subarachnoid space
Spinal cord trauma	Extradural spinal cord lesions from primary neoplastic or metastatic lesions
	Postoperative spine to separate scar from recurrent disk

CT = computed tomography; MRI = magnetic resonance imaging.

meningitis) may not be diagnosed by CT scan (Table 23–6). Metabolic abnormalities result in diffuse dysfunction of the nervous system without localized signs.

Hemispheric mass lesions result in coma either by expanding across the midline laterally to compromise both cerebral hemispheres or by impinging on the brain stem to compress the rostral reticular formation. These processes have been referred to as *lateral herniation* (lateral movement of the brain) and *transtentorial herniation* (vertical movement of hemispheric content across the cerebellar tentorium, which separates the hemispheric compartment from the brain stem and posterior fossa). Brain stem mass lesions produce coma by directly compromising the reticular formation.

A premonitory headache supports a diagnosis of meningitis, encephalitis, or intracerebral or subarachnoid hemorrhage. The sudden apoplectic onset of coma is particularly suggestive of ischemic or hemorrhagic stroke affecting the brain stem or of subarachnoid hemorrhage or intracerebral hemorrhage with intraventricular rupture. Lateralized symptoms of hemiparesis or aphasia prior to coma occur with hemispheric masses.

The physical examination is critical, quickly accomplished, and diagnostic. The issues are three: (1) Does the patient have meningitis? (2) Are there signs of a mass lesion? (3) Is this a diffuse syndrome of exogenous or endogenous metabolic cause?

Passive neck flexion should be carried out in all comatose patients unless head trauma is likely to have occurred. When the neck is passively flexed, attempting to bring the chin within a few fingerbreadths of the chest, patients with irritated meninges will reflexively flex one or both knees. This sign (Brudzinski's reflex) is usually asymmetrical and not dramatic. In the absence of lateralized signs (such as hemiparesis) indicating a superimposed mass lesion, a lumbar puncture should be performed immediately. The time required for CT scanning may cause a fatal therapeutic delay. An alternative approach is to obtain blood cultures and immediately initiate antibiotic therapy with subsequent lumbar puncture. Despite a short period of antibiotic treatment, the CSF cell count, glucose

Table 23–6 ■ CAUSES OF COMA WITH NORMAL COMPUTED TOMOGRAPHIC SCAN RESULT

- Meningeal
  - Subarachnoid hemorrhage (uncommon)
  - Bacterial meningitis
  - Encephalitis
  - Subdural empyema
- Exogenous toxins
  - Sedative drugs/barbiturates
  - Anesthetics/γ-hydroxybutyrate*
  - Alcohol
  - Stimulants
    - Phencyclidine†
    - Cocaine/amphetamine‡
  - Psychotropic drugs
    - Cyclic antidepressants
    - Phenothiazines
    - Lithium
  - Anticonvulsants
    - Opioids
    - Clonidine§
    - Penicillins
    - Salicylates
    - Anticholinergics
    - Carbon monoxide/cyanide/methemoglobinemia
- Endogenous toxins/deficiencies/derangements
  - Hypoxia/ischemia
  - Hypoglycemia
  - Hypercalcemia
  - Osmolar
    - Hyperglycemia
    - Hyponatremia
    - Hypernatremia
  - Organ system failure
    - Hepatic encephalopathy
    - Uremic encephalopathy
    - Pulmonary insufficiency (CO_2 narcosis)
- Seizures
  - Prolonged post-ictal state
  - Spike wave stupor
- Hypo-/hyperthermia
- Multifocal disorders presenting as metabolic coma
  - Disseminated intravascular coagulopathy (DIC)
  - Sepsis
  - Pancreatitis
  - Vasculitis
  - Thrombotic thrombocytopenic purpura (TTP)
  - Fat emboli
  - Hypertensive encephalopathy
  - Diffuse micrometastases
- Brain stem ischemia
  - Basilar artery stroke
  - Brain stem or cerebellar hemorrhage
- Conversion/malingering

* General anesthetic, similar to γ-aminobutyric acid; recreational drug and body building aid characterized by rapid onset, rapid recovery, often with myoclonic jerking and confusion; deep coma (2–3 hours; Glasgow coma scale = 3) with maintenance of vital signs.

† Coma associated with cholinergic signs: lacrimation, salivation, bronchorrhea, and hyperthermia.

‡ Coma after seizures or status, i.e., a prolonged post-ictal state.

§ An antihypertensive agent active through the opiate receptor system; overdose frequent when used to treat narcotic withdrawal.

level, and protein content are unchanged, and the Gram stain and culture often produce positive findings.

Structural and metabolic causes of coma can be distinguished by neurologic examination. This task is accomplished by focusing on three features of neurologic examination: (1) the motor response to a painful stimulus, (2) pupillary function, and (3) reflex eye movements.

Expanding hemispheric masses at their early stage (early diencephalic, i.e., compromising the brain above the thalamus) will produce appropriate movement of one upper extremity toward the painful stimulus (see Fig. 23–1). The contralateral arm will reflect a hemiparesis. As the mass expands to involve the thalamus (late diencephalic), the response to pain is now reflex arm flexion associated with extension and internal rotation of the legs (decorticate posturing); asymmetry of the response in the upper extremities will be seen. With further brain compromise at the midbrain level, the reflex posturing now changes in the arms so that both arms and legs respond by extension (decerebrate posturing); at this level the asymmetry tends to be lost. With further compromise to the level of the pons, the most frequent finding is no response to painful stimulation, although spinal movements of leg flexion may occur.

Metabolic lesions do not compromise the brain in the progressive level-by-level manner seen with hemispheric masses and rarely produce the asymmetrical motor signs typical of masses. Reflex posturing may be seen, but it lacks the asymmetry of decortication.

If the pupils constrict to a bright light, the midbrain is intact; if they do not, the midbrain has been compromised. In mass lesions, the loss of pupillary reactivity from a hemispheric mass is asymmetrical, with the pupil homolateral to the mass losing reactivity before its contralateral fellow.

In metabolic coma, one feature is central to the examination: pupillary reactivity is present. The reaction is lost only when coma is so deep the patient requires ventilatory and blood pressure support.

Reflex eye movements are brought about by passive head rotation to stimulate the semicircular canal input to the vestibular system (doll's eye maneuver), or by inhibition of function of one semicircular canal by infusion of ice water against the tympanic membrane (caloric testing). In metabolic coma, reflex eye movements may be lost or retained. Caloric testing is not useful in drug-induced coma.

Brain stem mass lesions are most commonly vascular. Reflex lateral eye movements, the pathways for which traverse the pons and midbrain, are particularly affected, and the reflex postures of decortication and decerebration typical of brain stem injury are common findings.

Prolonged alteration in consciousness after an unwitnessed seizure may produce diagnostic confusion. In a post-ictal state, the examination will detect reactive pupils and inducible eye movements (in the absence of overtreatment with anticonvulsants) and may detect upgoing toes; if the onset of the seizure was in a focal motor area of the cortex, there may be a prolonged hemiparesis (Todd's paresis).

Emergency management of the patient with a decreased level of consciousness includes assurance of airway adequacy and support

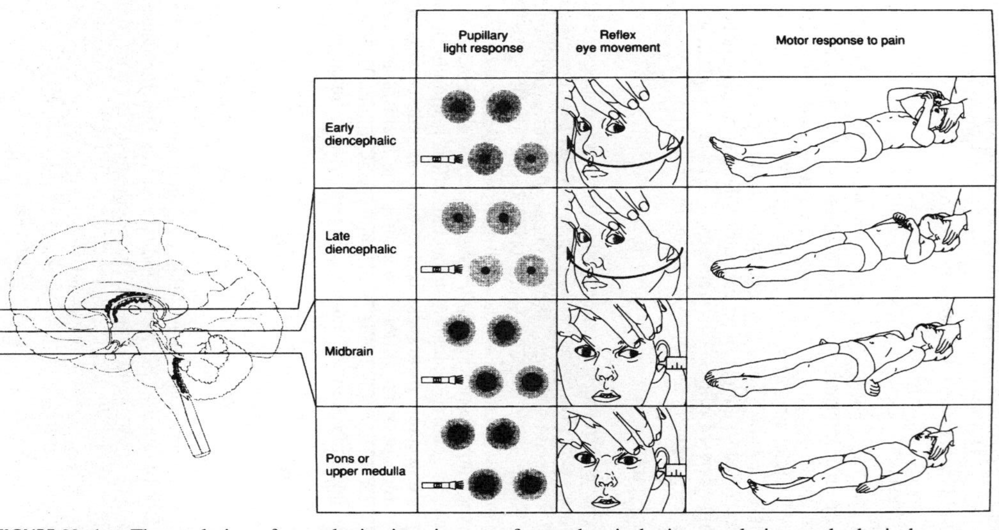

FIGURE 23–1 ■ The evolution of neurologic signs in coma from a hemispheric mass lesion as the brain becomes functionally impaired in a rostral-caudal manner. Early and late diencephalic levels are levels of dysfunction just above (early) and just below (late) the thalamus. (From Aminoff MJ, Greenberg DA, Simon RP: Clinical Neurology. Norwalk, CT, Appleton & Lange, 1996.)

of ventilation and of circulation. Assessment of serum glucose and electrolyte levels, hepatic and renal function, prothrombin and partial thromboplastin times, complete blood count, and drug screen should be done. The patient should be given dextrose 25 g intravenously (IV) (typically 50 mL of 50% dextrose) to treat possible hypoglycemic coma. As administration of dextrose alone can precipitate or worsen Wernicke's encephalopathy in thiamine-deficient patients, thiamine 100 mg must be given IV. A possible opiate overdose should be treated with naloxone 0.4 to 1.0 to 1.2 mg IV.

Coma-Like States

Locked-in syndrome patients are those in whom a lesion (usually hemorrhage or an infarct) transects the brain stem at a point below the reticular formation (therefore sparing consciousness) but above the ventilatory nuclei of the medulla (therefore, precluding death). Such patients are awake. Voluntary eye movement, especially vertical, is preserved, and patients open and close their eyes or produce appropriate numbers of blinking movements in answer to questions. *Psychogenic unresponsiveness* is a diagnosis of exclusion.

Vegetative States

Whereas coma represents a state lacking both wakefulness and awareness, in a vegetative state patients have awakened from coma but have not regained awareness. Wakefulness is manifested by eye opening and sleep-wake cycles. Acute brain injury resulting in a vegetative state first produces coma, with the patient later awakening into the vegetative condition. Brain stem reflexes are intact.

A persistent vegetative state is suspected after 1 month in a patient without detectable awareness of the environment. A vegetative state is termed *persistent* after 3 months if the brain injury was medical and after 12 months if the brain injury was traumatic. Rare patients show late improvement but none regain normal function.

Brain Death

A diagnosis of brain death depends upon documentation of irreversible cessation of all brain functions, including those of the brain stem. The absence of hemispheric function is documented by unreceptivity and unresponsiveness. Purely spinal reflexes may be maintained. Documentation of irreversibility requires that the cause of the coma be known and that it be adequate to explain the clinical findings of brain death. An isoelectric EEG is frequently useful. However, deep coma from sedative drugs or hypothermia below 20° C can produce EEG flattening. In addition, patients clinically brain dead may have residual EEG activity.

Syncope

Syncope is loss of consciousness associated with loss of postural tone (Table 23–7). The episode is caused by global impairment of blood flow to the brain. Syncope must be differentiated from seizures.

Each syncopal episode should be reviewed with attention to events and symptoms preceding the spell, what happened during

Table 23-7 ■ CAUSES OF EPISODIC LOSS OF CONSCIOUSNESS

	PATIENTS IN EACH CATEGORY (%)
Reflex-mediated	
Vasovagal	18
Carotid sinus sensitivity	1
Situational	
Micturition, defecation, cough	5
Orthostatic hypotension	8
Medication-induced	3
Psychiatric/hyperventilation	2
Neurologic (seizures, TIAs, subclavian steal)	10
Cardiac	
Organic heart disease*	4
Arrhythmias†	14
Unknown‡	34

TIAs = transient ischemic attacks.

* Aortic stenosis, hypertrophic cardiomyopathy, pulmonary embolism, myxoma, myocardial infarction, coronary spasm, tamponade, aortic dissection.

† Sinus node disease, second- and third-degree heart block, pacemaker failure, drug-induced bradyarrhythmias, ventricular tachycardia, torsades de pointes, supraventricular tachycardia.

‡ Half would have neurocardiogenic syncope by tilt table testing.

Data from Linzer M, Yang E, Estes NA, et al., Ann Intern Med 126:989–996, 1997 and 127:76–86, 1997. Also compiled from studies published 1980–1997 (prior to tilt table testing).

the spell of unconsciousness, and the time course of regaining orientation once consciousness is regained.

Loss of consciousness so rapid that a prodrome is absent may occur with seizures and with some cardiac arrhythmias such as asystole. Palpitations during the prodrome occur with tachyarrhythmias but may also introduce vasovagal events. Extreme exertion (cardiac), an emotional or painful stimulus (vasovagal), a rapid change in posture (orthostatic), and straining at urination (situational) help in identifying the cause.

Body stiffening and limb jerking occur with generalized seizures, but also from other causes of cerebral hypoperfusion. Such muscle jerking is often multifocal and can be synchronous or asynchronous. In contrast to epileptic seizures, which generally produce tonic-clonic activity for at least 1 to 2 minutes, muscle jerking in syncope rarely persists longer than 30 seconds. Urinary incontinence during the spell is frequently used to support or refute a diagnosis of epilepsy; however, fainting with a full bladder can result in incontinence, whereas seizures with an empty bladder will not. Tongue biting favors seizures. Recovery of orientation and consciousness following vasovagal or reflex-mediated syncope occurs simultaneously. Recovery of orientation following syncope of cardiac origin is proportional to the duration of the unconsciousness but is usually rapid (0 to 10 seconds); with periods of malignant arrhythmia producing unconsciousness of 2 minutes, confusion on waking is less than 30 seconds. Following seizures, however, the period of confusion, often with agitation, continues for 2 to 20 minutes following recovery of consciousness.

REFLEX MEDIATED SYNCOPE. Vasovagal spells, or simple faints, are the most common cause of syncope. Precipitating factors include pain, trauma, fatigue, blood loss, or prolonged motionless standing. Vagally mediated situational syncope can be induced by micturition, defecation, or swallowing, or during episodes of glossopharyngeal neuralgia. Vagally mediated hypotension and bradycardia combine to produce cerebral hypoperfusion, with a resultant prodrome of lightheadedness, nausea, tinnitus, diaphoresis, salivation, pallor, and dimming of vision. The patient loses consciousness and postural tone and falls with either flaccid or stiff limbs; eyes are open, often with an upward gaze. The patient is pale and diaphoretic and has dilated pupils.

Carotid sinus syncope results from vagal stimulation from the carotid sinus producing hypotension or bradycardia. Carotid sinus massage may be diagnostic and can be performed only in the absence of carotid bruits. Induction of asystole greater than or equal to 3 seconds, hypotension, or both constitute a positive test. False-positive results are common.

A non-vagally mediated situational syncope occurs with coughing (cough syncope). Coughing increases intrathoracic venous pressure, which is transmitted to the intracranial veins; the resultant transient increase in ICP impairs blood flow.

The term "neurocardiogenic syncope" has come into use to describe spells of cerebral hypoperfusion in the absence of a demonstrable cardiac cause or recognized vasovagal precipitants or situational triggers. Half of all patients with syncope of unknown cause may fall into this category. The patient's typical symptoms may be reproduced during head-up tilt table testing.

CEREBROVASCULAR SYNCOPE. Loss of consciousness can be a component of a basilar artery transient ischemic attack (TIA), but unconsciousness alone is virtually never the initial sign. Vertigo, diplopia or visual field disturbances, and dysarthria or ataxia are common. Recovery of consciousness may require 30 to 60 minutes. Neuropsychiatric syncope is a diagnosis of exclusion.

CARDIOGENIC SYNCOPE. Syncope that occurs during exercise or is associated with palpitations is particularly suggestive of a cardiac cause of syncope (pages 74 to 75). Premonitory symptoms may be those of cerebral hypoperfusion (faintness, tinnitus, and dimming of vision), but these symptoms may be absent with asystole because of the rapid fall in cardiac output and precipitous decline in cerebral blood flow resulting in abrupt loss of consciousness. Evaluation for arrhythmias should begin with a rhythm strip (with a 5% yield), followed by Holter monitoring for 24 hours (symptoms occur during the monitoring in approximately 20% of patients). With recurrent events, long-term ambulatory loop electrocardiography (ECG) is useful. Intracardiac electrodiagnostic testing is useful in selected patients with syncope.

ORTHOSTATIC HYPOTENSION. Postural hypotension can result in syncope that may be recurrent. The diagnosis is supported by noting a fall of 30 mm Hg or greater in systolic pressure or a fall of 10 mm Hg or greater in diastolic pressure between testing in the recumbent versus the upright posture.

SYNCOPE IN THE ELDERLY. The elderly often have multiple factors contributing to syncope. Orthostatic syncope is particularly likely to occur 15 to 75 minutes after a meal or following rapid change of posture.

For more information about this subject, see *Cecil Textbook of Medicine,* 21st edition. Philadelphia, W.B. Saunders Company, 2000. Chapter 444, Coma and Disorders of Arousal; Chapter 445, Persistent Vegetative State; Chapter 446, Brain Death; and Chapter 447, Syncope, pages 2023 to 2030.

DISORDERS OF SLEEP

Sleep stages are defined electroencephalographically and behaviorally (Table 23–8). *Insomnia* is the perception of inadequate sleep, either in amount or quality, usually not associated with daytime sleepiness. Treatment of depression, elimination of stimulant drugs, and providing an optimal sleep environment are general principles of sleep hygiene. For sleep onset, triazolam (Halcion) or zolpidem (Ambien) are rapidly acting, short half-life compounds. For sleep maintenance, longer-acting drugs, such as flurazepam (Dalmane) or quazepam (Doral), are more effective.

Narcolepsy is a disorder of excessive daytime sleepiness associated with abnormalities in rapid eye movement (REM) sleep. When fully expressed, the quartet of narcolepsy, cataplexy, hypnagogic hallucinations, and sleep paralysis occurs. Narcoleptic hypersomnia occurs most often in settings of sedentary activity and with boredom. However, narcoleptic sleep attacks may also occur during conversation, meals, and while driving. The diagnosis is made on the basis of a typical and persistent history of excessive daytime sleepiness in the absence of underlying nocturnal sleep disorders producing daytime somnolence and is confirmed by the documentation of sleep-onset REM (latency <15 minutes) and an abnormal multiple sleep latency test.

Treatment should begin with planned 15- to 20-minute naps throughout the day. Pharmacologic therapy has traditionally relied on stimulants (methylphenidate 5 to 60 mg or dextroamphetamine 5 to 50 mg daily). Modafinil (α-adrenergic agonist) 100 or 200 mg at morning and noon was effective in a recent controlled trial.

Cataplexy is associated with narcolepsy in about 70% of cases. The cataplectic phenomenon is that of emotion-induced, reflex muscular atonia, which spares respiratory muscles. Laughter is the most common inducer. Most attacks last less than a minute. Cataplectic attacks can be attenuated in most patients by clomipramine 10 to 150 mg/day.

Sleep paralysis is a frightening event with awareness of paralysis of all but the ventilatory and extraocular muscles. Hypnogogic and hypnopompic hallucinations may be associated. Serotonin (5-hydroxytryptamine, 5-HT), reuptake inhibitors that suppress REM sleep (clomipramine), or fluoxetine 10 to 40 mg/day have been prescribed.

Obstructive sleep apnea occurs in 2 to 5% of the adult American population (see pages 174 to 175). 23

For more information about this subject, see *Cecil Textbook of Medicine,* 21st edition. Philadelphia, W.B. Saunders Company, 2000. Chapter 448, Disorders of Sleep and Arousal, pages 2030 to 2033.

Table 23–8 ■ STAGES OF SLEEP

SLEEP STAGE	EEG	EYE MOVEMENTS	EMG ACTIVITY	IMAGERY
Wakefulness	Alpha and beta activity (low voltage fast)	Random, rapid	Active, spontaneous	Vivid, external
NREM sleep				
Stage I (drowsiness)	Theta activity	Slow, rolling	Attenuated, episodic	Dulled
Stage II (light sleep)	Sleep spindles, K complexes	Slow/absent	Attenuated	Non-vivid
Stages III and IV (slow wave sleep)	Delta activity	Absent	Attenuated	
REM sleep	Low amplitude, irregular	Abrupt, rapid	Absent	Vivid, bizarre

NREM = non-rapid eye movement; REM = rapid eye movement.

DISORDERS OF COGNITION

Regional Cerebral Dysfunction

Many neurologic disorders affect the cerebral hemispheres in a regionally specific, or focal, fashion.

FRONTAL LOBES. Lesions in Broca's area cause a predictable language disturbance, or *aphasia,* characterized by loss of the orderly execution of language. In this non-fluent or motor aphasia, the patient's verbal output is sparse with short agrammatic phrases, word-finding abnormalities, and impaired repetition. Comprehension is relatively preserved. *Apraxia* is loss of the ability to perform organized motor acts despite relative preservation of strength, sensation, and comprehension.

Damage to the dorsolateral pre-frontal cortex on the convexity of the frontal lobe is characterized by a memory retrieval deficit, reduced fluency of output, and an inability to think abstractly. Lesions cause reduced verbal fluency, and patients with right-sided lesions have a reduced ability to produce varied figures.

Damage to the lateral orbitofrontal cortex is frequently manifested as disturbed social behavior, including disinhibited, impulsive, and tactless responses. Idiopathic obsessive-compulsive disorder is associated with increased metabolism of the orbitofrontal cortex and the caudate nuclei. Acquired obsessive-compulsive behavior and occasionally mania may arise after damage to the orbitofrontal circuit. This area is prone to damage by closed head trauma.

The medial frontal portion of the frontal lobe mediates analysis of the emotional relevance of stimuli, and damage to it results in an apathetic state with reduced interest. The most profound form of this state is *akinetic mutism.*

PARIETAL LOBES. Lesions of the primary somatosensory area cause loss of tactile sensation on the contralateral side of the body. With unilateral lesions, these deficits are most profound on the contralateral side of the body. The most common aura associated with seizures originating from the parietal lobe is contralateral numbness and tingling. Lesions of the left parietal lobe produce deficits in varied aspects of communication. Comprehension and semantics (word meaning) are typically most affected.

Alexia, or the inability to read, is often accompanied by *agraphia,* the inability to write. In cases of alexia with agraphia, the lesion typically involves the angular gyrus of the left parietal lobe. *Apraxias,* in which subjects pantomime poorly or are unable to perform gestures on command, occur with lesions of the left inferior parietal lobule, left pre-motor cortex, and corpus callosum.

Lesions of the right parietal lobe are frequently characterized by *hemispatial neglect.* In this condition, the subjects do not attend to stimuli in the neglected sphere contralateral to the lesion. They may ignore the left half of the visual field, the left half of their body, auditory stimuli from the left hemispace, or anything in the left hemiuniverse. A milder form of neglect called extinction has been described; in extinction, subjects are capable of attending to contralateral stimuli but when presented with stimuli simultaneously on both sides respond only to the ipsilateral side. Anosognosia, or the lack of knowledge of one's deficit, often accompanies hemispatial neglect arising from right parietal lesions.

OCCIPTIAL LOBES. In complete cortical blindness, or blindness caused by bilateral destruction of the occipital lobes or their afferents, retention of pupillary responses reflects intact visual input to the brain stem. Denial of blindness, or *Anton's syndrome,* frequently occurs in association with damage to the visual cortex.

When the occipitoparietal areas are damaged bilaterally, *simultagnosia* may occur. In this condition the subject is unable to attend to more than a small part of the visual field at once and consequently has difficulty understanding whole scenes.

Infarction in the distribution of the posterior cerebral arteries is a frequent cause of occipital lobe damage; head injury, tumors, and many other processes can affect the occipital lobes as well. Hallucinations can occur as a result of occipital lobe injury.

TEMPORAL LOBES. Complete destruction of the primary auditory area unilaterally does not result in appreciable hearing deficits. A condition termed *pure word deafness,* in which patients are unable to understand spoken language but do not have a more general auditory agnosia or aphasia, occasionally occurs.

Lesions in the posterosuperior temporal lobe of the left hemisphere cause Wernicke's aphasia, in which fluent paraphasic output and impairment in language comprehension are the predominant features. Focal seizures arising from the temporal lobe may give rise to changes in ongoing language function and to sensory, emotional, or psychic phenomena.

LIMBIC LOBE. Situated between the neocortex and brain stem structures, the limbic system plays a role in mediating the experience of emotions, visceral responses, and storage of memories. Lesions of the limbic lobe can also produce profound deficits in memory.

Characteristic visceral and psychic phenomena occur with epileptic activity arising from limbic structures. Olfactory sensations are classically associated with involvement of the uncus in the medial temporal lobe. Psychic sensations of déjà vu, jamais vu, dreamlike states, and depersonalization may occur along with associated impairment in consciousness. Profound acute depression, fear, or extreme pleasure is sometimes seen.

Amnesia and Aphasia

AMNESIA. Short-term memory involves holding information for a minute or less. Long-term memory involves holding information for longer than a minute. Two types of long-term memory are distinguished: recent memory (new learning) and remote memory (the retrieval of old established information). Amnesia refers to difficulty learning new information and is primarily concerned with recent memory (Table 23–9).

A common way to assess verbal memory is a word list learning task. For the screening examination, a list of 3 or 4 words may suffice; however, for a more extended examination, a list of 10 or 16 words with multiple repetitions is preferable. In the 3- to 4-word tests, the examiner repeats the word list until the patients are able to repeat the words on their own; subsequently, the examiner asks them to recall the words after a 5-minute delay.

Table 23–9 ■ CAUSES OF AMNESIA

Alzheimer's disease and other dementias
Cerebrovascular
Posterior cerebral artery and other strokes involving the hippocampi
Infarction in the medial thalamic nuclei
Ruptured anterior communicating artery aneurysms
Anoxic/ischemic encephalopathy or hypoglycemia
Head trauma
Encephalitides
Herpes simplex and other infections
Limbic and other paraneoplastic syndromes
Mass lesions involving the limbic system
Thiamine deficiency or Wernicke-Korsakoff syndrome
Epileptic seizures
Electroconvulsive therapy
Temporal lobe surgery
Transient global amnesia
Psychogenic amnesia

"Memory loss" may result from deficits in attention or other cognitive process rather than from amnesia. An initial step in the differential diagnosis of a memory complaint is to exclude the presence of delirium or an acute confusional state.

Clinicians need to distinguish neurologically based amnesia from the syndrome of "psychogenic amnesia." The most common amnesic syndrome is dementia.

Anoxia and ischemia are common causes of residual memory impairment. Traumatic brain injury is another common cause. The extent of post-traumatic (anterograde) amnesia is a good gauge of the severity of the head injury. Herpes simplex encephalitis, complex partial and generalized seizures, as well as electroconvulsive therapy, can cause amnesia. The Wernicke-Korsakoff syndrome and rupture of an anterior communicating aneurysm can also cause amnesia.

APHASIA. Aphasia is the loss or impairment of language caused by brain dysfunction. The most common causes of focal aphasias are strokes. Neurodegenerative processes such as Alzheimer's disease also commonly produce aphasia.

Aphasia can result from any lesion in the language areas of the brain. In almost all right-handed persons, the left hemisphere is dominant for language. Most left-handed and ambidextrous persons are also left hemisphere language dominant.

The different language disorders or aphasias have different patterns of impaired language skills (Table 23–10). Non-fluent verbal output characterizes Broca's aphasia. Spontaneous speech is sparse, effortful, dysarthric, dysprosodic, short in phrase length, and agrammatic. Most patients with Broca's aphasia have right-sided weakness. The most striking abnormality of Wernicke's aphasia is a disturbance in comprehension. Treatment of aphasic patients includes speech and language therapy.

Alzheimer's Disease and Related Dementias

Evaluation of dementia starts with a detailed history of the initial problem not only from the patient but from family members or

Table 23–10 ■ APHASIA SYNDROMES

SYNDROME	SPONTANEOUS SPEECH	REPETITION	COMPREHENSION	NAMING	READING	WRITING	HEMIPARESIS	HEMISENSORY DEFECT	VISUAL FIELD DEFECT	NEUROPATHOLOGY IN LEFT HEMISPHERE
Broca's	Non-fluent	Poor	Good	Poor	Poor	Poor	Common	Rare	Rare	Posterior inferior frontal lobe
Wernicke's	Fluent, paraphasic	Poor	Poor	Poor	Poor	Poor	Rare	Variable	Variable	Posterior superior temporal lobe
Conduction	Fluent, paraphasic	Poor	Good	Variable	Good	Variable	Rare	Variable	Rare	Arcuate fasciculus region
Global	Non-fluent	Poor	Poor	Poor	Poor	Poor	Common	Common	Common	Combinations of the above three
Transcortical										
Motor	Non-fluent	Good	Good	Poor	Good	Poor	Common	Rare	Rare	Frontal, beyond Broca's area
Sensory	Fluent	Good	Poor	Poor	Poor	Poor	Rare	Common	Common	Parietal-temporal junction
Mixed	Non-fluent	Good	Poor	Poor	Poor	Poor	Common	Common	Common	Combination of the above two
Anomic	Fluent	Good	Good	Poor	Variable	Variable	Variable	Variable	Rare	Multiple sites
Subcortical										
Anterior	Non-fluent, paraphasic	Good	Good	Poor	Poor	Poor	Common	Rare	Rare	Putamen, globus pallidus
Posterior	Fluent, paraphasic	Good	Poor	Poor	Poor	Poor	Rare	Common	Variable	Thalamus

caregivers of the patient as well. Baseline intellectual and emotional functions should be determined. The mental status examination begins with observations of the patient's appearance and behavior during the evaluation. Screening tests such as the Mini-Mental Status Examination (Table 23–11) can be used to determine a numerical cognitive baseline value.

The presence of focal neurologic deficits leads one to consider non-Alzheimer disease dementias. Rigidity and other extrapyramidal signs suggest Parkinson's disease, dementia with Lewy bodies, or vascular dementia. Gait abnormalities occur with normal-pressure hydrocephalus. Most of the many causes of dementia are rare and may be excluded with a thorough history and evaluation (Table 23–12). The term *pseudodementia* has been used to describe dementia associated with a psychiatric illness

Neuroimaging is helpful to detect tumors, subdural hematomas, and strokes. Scans may also show focal atrophy in specific locations, such as frontotemporal atrophy in the frontotemporal dementias. A lumbar puncture is indicated if the serum VDRL is positive or in cases of suspected CNS infections or demyelination.

ALZHEIMER'S DISEASE. Alzheimer's disease is the most common cause of degenerative dementia. Nearly 10% of the population older than 65 years is affected.

Four genes have been linked to Alzheimer's disease. Chromosome 21 carries the gene coding for the precursor of β-amyloid,

Table 23–11 ■ THE MINI-MENTAL STATUS EXAMINATION

	SCORE
Orientation: What is the month, day, year, season? Where are you, what floor, city, county, and state? (Score 1 point for each item correct.)	10
Registration: State 3 items (ball, flag, tree). (Score 1 point for each item that the patient registers *without* you having to repeat the words. You may repeat the words until the patient is able to register the words but do not give him/her credit. You must also tell the patient that he/she should memorize those words and that you will ask him/her to recall those words later.)	3
Attention: Can you spell the word WORLD forwards, then backward? Can you subtract 7 from 100, and keep subtracting 7? (100-93-86-79-72, etc.) (Do both items but give credit for best of the two performances.)	5
Memory: Can you remember those 3 words I asked you to memorize? (Do not give clues or multiple choice.)	3
Languages	
Naming: Can you name (show) a pen and a watch?	2
Repetition: Can you repeat "No if's, and's or but's?"	1
Comprehension: Can you take this piece of paper in your right hand, fold it in half, then put it on the floor? (Score 1 point for each item done correctly.)	3
Reading: Read and obey, "CLOSE YOUR EYES."	1
Writing: Can you write a sentence?	1
Visuospatial: Have the patient copy intersecting pentagons	1
Total	30

Table 23–12 ■ MAJOR CAUSES OF DEMENTIA

Major causes of dementia
Degenerative disorders
Alzheimer's disease
Frontotemporal dementia
Dementia with Lewy bodies
Corticobasal ganglionic degeneration
Parkinson's disease
Huntington's disease
Progressive supranuclear palsy
Conditions associated with anoxia
Cardiac disease
Pulmonary insufficiency
Post-anoxia dementia
Chronic renal failure
Uremic encephalopathy
Dialysis dementia
Hepatic diseases
Portal-systemic encephalopathy
Electrolyte abnormalities
Hypernatremia
Hyponatremia
Hypercalcemia
Vascular dementia
Head trauma
Dementia pugilistica
Multiple contusions
Subdural hematoma
Myelin disorders
Multiple sclerosis
Adult-onset leukodystrophies
CNS infections
Prion diseases (Creutzfeldt-Jakob, Gerstmann-Straussler-Shenker, fatal familial insomnia)
Encephalitis/chronic meningitis
AIDS and AIDS-related infections
Neurosyphilis
CNS tumors
Cerebral effects of systemic malignancies
Hydrocephalus
Vitamin deficiency states
Thiamine (B_1)
Cobalamin (B_{12})
Endocrinopathies
Thyroid disturbances
Adrenal disease
Intoxication/toxicity
Medications
Alcohol
Other toxins
Inflammatory disorders

amyloid precursor protein. One gene, presenilin 1 (*PS1*), is on chromosome 14; another, presenilin 2 (*PS2*), is on chromosome 1. Apolipoprotein E (apo E) is a plasma protein involved in cholesterol transport and is encoded by a gene on chromosome 19; the E4 allele has been identified as a risk factor.

Memory disturbance occurs early in the disease; patients have difficulty learning and remembering new material. Aphasia, apraxia, and acalculia develop as the disease progresses, and apathy or paranoia may occur. Patients may wander, pace, and repeat the same questions. Sleep-wake cycle abnormalities may become evident. Activities of daily living decline throughout the illness. Other causes of dementia should be excluded by history, examination, and the laboratory studies described above.

Acetylcholinesterase inhibitors, tacrine and donepezil, are efficacious not only in improving cognition, as shown by a modest increase, but also improving the neuropsychiatric disturbances. In general, they should be used early in the course of Alzheimer's disease. Vitamin E has been shown to slow progression of Alzheimer's disease. Randomized trials have shown no benefit from estrogen replacement therapy. Trials are in progress to study anti-inflammatory agents.

Controlling the environment may help patients. Ancillary help is imperative as the caregiver burden increases.

FRONTOTEMPORAL DEMENTIA. Frontotemporal dementia may account for as many as 20% of patients with pre-senile dementia secondary to primary cerebral degeneration. The onset is usually insidious and may be manifested by subtle personality and affective changes. The pathologic process starts in the frontal and temporal lobes, and patients subsequently have clinical symptoms of depression, anxiety, and disinhibited behavior. Cholinesterase inhibitors are not useful in frontotemporal dementia.

DEMENTIA WITH LEWY BODIES. Dementia with Lewy bodies accounts for 15 to 25% of all degenerative dementias; it shares clinical and pathologic features with Alzheimer's disease and is regarded by some as an Alzheimer disease variant. The clinical features include fluctuations in cognition, visual hallucinations, and parkinsonian motor signs. The cholinergic deficit appears to be more severe than that of Alzheimer's disease. Cholinesterase inhibitors (tacrine and donepezil) may be beneficial.

VASCULAR DEMENTIA. Vascular dementia is the second most common dementia of the elderly in the United States. Vascular dementia may result from strategically placed single infarcts, multiple infarcts, small vessel disease, hypoperfusion, amyloid angiopathy, and brain hemorrhage.

When compared with Alzheimer's disease, patients with vascular dementia tend to have an earlier age of onset, and the duration of survival after the onset of mental status changes is shorter. Historically, cognitive dysfunction may develop abruptly, and patients may experience stepwise deterioration. Clinically, patients may have focal signs. Features of pseudobulbar palsy, including emotional lability, dysarthria, and dysphagia, are often present.

The diagnosis is facilitated by brain imaging demonstrating moderate to severe ischemic white matter changes subcortically or focal cortical infarctions. Vascular dementia is treated by stroke prevention.

Subcortical Degenarative Diseases

The reported prevalence of dementia in patients with *Parkinson's disease* varies widely but is thought to be in the range of 35 to 55%. The principal features include slowing of cognition, failure to initiate activities spontaneously, poor word list generation, a retrieval deficit–type memory disturbance, and executive dysfunction.

Therapies improve the motor symptoms of the disease but afford little or no cognitive benefit. Cholinesterase inhibitors may be useful.

Early signs of *Huntington's disease* include personality changes of irritability, apathy, and untidiness, which usually begin in midlife. Depression is common and leads to suicide in up to 8% of males and 6% of females.

In *progressive supranuclear palsy,* cognitive decline tends to be mild until late in the disease, when characteristic features of a subcortical dementia develop.

For more information about this subject, see *Cecil Textbook of Medicine,* 21st edition. Philadelphia, W.B. Saunders Company, 2000. Chapter 449, Disorders of Cognition, pages 2033 to 2047.

PSYCHIATRIC DISORDERS

Depression and Suicidality

The core clinical features of the depressive disorders are included in the diagnostic criteria for a major depressive episode and for dysthymia (Table 23–13). These disorders tend to recur.

Major depressive episodes clearly cluster in families. Lifetime

Table 23–13 ■ DIAGNOSTIC CRITERIA FOR DEPRESSIVE DISORDERS

Major Depressive Episode

1. At least 5 of the following symptoms have been present during the same 2-wk period and represent a change from previous functioning; at least one of the symptoms is either depressed mood or loss of interest or pleasure
   a. Depressed mood most of the day, nearly every day
   b. Markedly diminished interest or pleasure in all, or almost all, activities most of the day, nearly every day
   c. Significant weight loss or weight gain when not dieting, or decrease or increase in appetite nearly every day
   d. Insomnia or hypersomnia nearly every day
   e. Psychomotor agitation or retardation nearly every day; observable by others
   f. Fatigue or loss of energy nearly every day
   g. Feelings of worthlessness or excessive or inappropriate guilt (which may be delusional) nearly every day
   h. Diminished ability to think or concentrate, or indecisiveness, nearly every day
   i. Recurrent thoughts of death, recurrent suicidal ideation without a specific plan, or a suicide attempt or a specific plan for committing suicide
2. a. It cannot be established that an organic factor initiated and maintained the disturbance
   b. The disturbance is not a normal reaction to the death of a loved one.
3. At no time during the disturbance have there been delusions or hallucinations for as long as 2 wk in the absence of prominent mood symptoms (i.e., before the mood symptoms developed or after they have remitted)
4. Not superimposed on schizophrenia, schizophreniform disorder, delusional disorder, or psychotic disorder; no other specific diagnosis

Dysthymia

1. Depressed mood for most of the day for at least 2 yr
2. Presence, while depressed, of 2 or more of the following:
   a. Poor appetite
   b. Insomnia or hypersomnia
   c. Low energy or fatigue
   d. Low self-esteem
   e. Poor concentration or difficulty making decisions
   f. Feelings of hopelessness
3. During the 2-yr period, the person has never been without the symptoms for more than 2 mo at a time
4. No major depressive episode has been present during the first 2 yr of the disturbance
5. There has not been an intermixed manic episode
6. The disturbance does not occur during the course of a psychotic disorder
7. The symptoms are not caused by the physiologic effects of a substance
8. The symptoms cause significant distress or functional impairment

prevalence rates for major depressive disorders are 15 to 20%. Completed suicides are common in the United States, accounting for some 30,000 deaths each year.

The symptoms of depression are variable for each individual and sometimes are difficult to recognize. The treatment plan must be individualized.

The selective serotonin reuptake inhibitors (SSRIs) are the initial therapy. For sertraline, the dose is 50 mg once daily for almost all patients. The dosage can be increased to 100 mg/day after 3 weeks if there is no evidence of symptom improvement. As an alternative, paroxetine can be started at 20 mg once daily and increased at similar intervals to 50 mg.

The tricyclic antidepressants have the disadvantage that they affect neurochemical systems not thought to be essential for antidepressant efficacy. Tricyclic antidepressants have a wide range of side effects, including postural hypotension, cardiac tachyarrhythmias, urinary retention, and constipation. These drugs are considered second-line agents for the treatment of depression.

The monoamine oxidase (MAO) inhibitors are limited by their potentially dangerous interactions with dietary tyramine or other agents with sympathomimetic or serotonergic properties. Use of these drugs should generally be initiated by psychiatrists.

Trazodone and nefazodone inhibit the reuptake of 5-HT at the synapse. Trazodone has some sedating properties, which makes it useful in agitated patients with disturbed sleep, particularly elderly persons. Bupropion is a novel monocyclic compound in that it inhibits the reuptake of dopamine but has little effect on other adrenergic systems.

Bipolar Disorders

Bipolar disorders are marked swings in mood from major depressive episodes to major manic episodes. At times it is difficult to distinguish an excited schizophrenic patient from a manic one (Table 23–14). The average age at onset is about 30 years, but about 20% of patients have an onset before the age of 20. The lifetime risk for development of bipolar illness ranges from 0.6 to 0.9%. There is a 72% concordance in monozygotic twins.

The treatment has three distinct aspects: (1) the manic episode, (2) the major depressive episode, and (3) long-term maintenance therapy. The treatment of the acute manic phase is usually undertaken in the hospital. Lithium is not useful for the acute management of mania, but benzodiazepines, particularly lorazepam, can effectively control most acute manic states.

Lithium effectively prevents relapses in most bipolar illnesses. Before lithium therapy is begun, a complete blood cell count, urinalysis, electrolytes, creatinine level, blood urea nitrogen level, thyroid studies, and a baseline ECG and EEG should be obtained. The starting dose of lithium carbonate in acute mania is generally 300 mg three or four times per day. Lithium has a half-life of 24 to 36 hours, and it takes at least 4 days to achieve a steady state. Its specific therapeutic effectiveness is not evident until at least 4 to 10 days after institution of therapy. Lithium does not work immediately for acutely agitated or manic patients but should nonetheless be started early in anticipation of maintenance use. It is necessary

Table 23–14 ■ MAJOR DIAGNOSTIC CRITERIA FOR A MANIC EPISODE

A distinct period of abnormally and persistently elevated, expansive, or irritable mood, lasting at least 1 wk (or any duration if hospitalization is necessary)

During the period of mood disturbance, at least 3 of the following symptoms have persisted (4 if the mood is only irritable) and have been present to a significant degree:

1. Inflated self-esteem or grandiosity
2. Decreased need for sleep (e.g., feels rested after only 3 hr of sleep)
3. More talkative than usual or feels pressure to keep talking
4. Flight of ideas or subjective experiences that thoughts are racing
5. Distractibility (i.e., attention too easily drawn to unimportant or irrelevant external stimuli)
6. Increase in goal-directed activity (either socially, at work or school, or sexually) or psychomotor agitation
7. Excessive involvement in pleasurable activities that have a high potential for painful consequences (e.g., engaging in unrestrained buying sprees, sexual indiscretions, or foolish business investments)

The mood disturbance is sufficiently severe to cause marked impairment in occupational functioning or in usual social activities or relationships with others to necessitate hospitalization to prevent harm to self or others

The symptoms are not due to the direct effects of a substance (e.g., drugs of abuse, medications) or a general medical condition (e.g., hyperthyroidism)

---

to monitor the serum level of lithium; adequate levels for acute illness are in the range of 0.8 to 1.4 mEq/L. For maintenance therapy, satisfactory responses accompany blood levels of 0.4 mEq/L. Elevation of serum lithium levels to more than 2 mEq/L is toxic and represents a medical emergency requiring immediate hospitalization and possibly hemodialysis.

Antiepileptic drugs have increasingly been used as alternative or adjunctive therapy. Antimania doses of carbamazepine are similar to those used for epilepsy and range from 600 to 1600 mg/day on a thrice-daily schedule, aiming for a serum level of 6 to 12 μg/mL. Valproic acid is also effective in doses from 800 to 1800 mg/day, also on a thrice-daily schedule aiming for a serum level above 50 μg/mL.

Anxiety Disorders

It is useful clinically to consider the anxiety disorders in two different patterns: (1) chronic, generalized anxiety, and (2) episodic, panic-like anxiety. Lifetime prevalence rates for DSM (*Diagnostic and Statistical Manual of Mental Disorders*) diagnosable anxiety disorders are as high as 30% for women and 19% for men (Table 23–15).

Sustained use of benzodiazepines and tricyclic antidepressants is equally effective in patients with panic disorder. A representative initial dosing regimen is imipramine 10 mg thrice daily, or alprazolam 0.5 mg twice daily. The MAO inhibitors and the SSRIs have also been demonstrated to have efficacy in panic disorder.

Antihistamines such as diphenhydramine 25 mg three times a

Table 23–15 ■ DIAGNOSTIC CRITERIA FOR PANIC DISORDERS

One or more panic attacks (discrete periods of intense fear or discomfort) have occurred that (1) were unexpected (i.e., did not occur immediately before or on exposure to a situation that almost always caused anxiety) and (2) were not triggered by situations in which the person was the focus of others' attention.

Either 4 attacks have occurred within a 4-week period or 1 or more attacks have been followed by a period of at least 1 month of persistent fear of having another attack.

At least 4 of the following symptoms developed during at least 1 of the attacks:

Shortness of breath (dyspnea) or smothering sensations
Dizziness, unsteady feelings, or faintness
Palpitations or accelerated heart rate (tachycardia)
Trembling
Sweating
Choking
Nausea or abdominal distress
Depersonalization or derealization
Numbness or tingling sensations (paresthesias)
Flashes (hot flashes) or chills
Chest pain or discomfort
Fear of dying
Fear of "going crazy" or of doing something uncontrolled

During at least some of these attacks, at least 4 of the symptoms developed suddenly and increased in intensity within 10 min of the beginning of the first symptom noticed in the attack.

---

day can be tried for some patients. Buspirone is a non-benzodiazepine antianxiety agent which sometimes provides relief at doses of 5 mg twice a day initially. All the benzodiazepines are effective in many patients. Lorazepam is often the first used, since it is relatively short-acting (half-life of 10 to 15 hours) and easier to titrate in elderly or medically ill patients. Because its half-life is shorter than drugs such as diazepam, lorazepam must be taken at least twice and often three times per day. A dosage of 0.5 mg twice daily is the initial regimen for most patients. The dose should be increased by 0.5 mg/day at 3-day intervals until target symptoms resolve or sedative side effects supervene.

The Somatoform Disorders

The long-term goal of treatment for the somatoform disorders (Table 23–16) is to enable the patient to convert from a medical to a psychiatric patient.

Character Disorders

The goal of management of character disorders (Table 23–17) is to help the patient to increase his or her awareness of the dysfunctional interpersonal traits.

Schizophrenic Disorders

Seventy per cent of persons with schizophrenia (Table 23–18) become ill between the ages of 15 and 35 years. Ten to 15 per cent

Table 23–16 ■ THE SOMATOFORM DISORDERS

DISORDER	FEATURES
Somatization disorder	Chronic, multisystem disorder characterized by complaints of pain, gastrointestinal and sexual dysfunction, and pseudoneurologic symptoms; onset is usually early in life, and psychosocial and vocational achievements are limited
Conversion disorder	Syndrome of symptoms or deficits mimicking neurologic or medical illness in which psychological factors are judged to be of etiologic importance
Pain disorder	Clinical syndrome characterized predominantly by pain in which psychological factors are judged to be of etiologic importance
Hypochondriasis	Chronic preoccupation with the idea of having a serious disease; the preoccupation is usually poorly amenable to reassurance
Body dysmorphic disorder	Preoccupation with an imagined or exaggerated defect in physical appearance
Somatoform-like Disorders	
Factitious disorder	Intentional production or feigning of physical or psychological signs when external reinforcers (e.g., avoidance of responsibility, financial gain) are not clearly present
Malingering	Intentional production or feigning of physical or psychological signs when external reinforcers (e.g., avoidance of responsibility, financial gain) are present
Dissociative disorders	Disruptions of consciousness, memory, identity, or perception judged to be due to psychological factors

Table 23–17 ■ CHARACTER DISORDERS

PERSONALITY TYPE	CHARACTERISTIC BEHAVIOR PATTERNS
Paranoid	Distrust and suspiciousness
Schizoid	Detachment from social relationships, with a restricted range of emotional expression
Schizotypal	Eccentricities in behavior and cognitive distortions; acute discomfort in close relationships
Antisocial	Disregard for rights of others; a defect in the experience of compunction or remorse for harming others
Borderline	Instability in interpersonal relationships, self-image, and affective regulation
Histrionic	Emotional overreactivity, theatrical behaviors, and seductiveness
Narcissistic	Persisting grandiosity, need for admiration, and lack of empathy for others
Avoidant	Social inhibition, feelings of inadequacy, and hypersensitivity to negative evaluation
Dependent	Submissive and clinging behaviors
Obsessive-compulsive	Rigid, detail-oriented behaviors, often associated with compulsions to perform tasks repetitively and unnecessarily

Table 23–18 ■ SCHIZOPHRENIA AND OTHER PSYCHOTIC DISORDERS

Characteristic Symptoms

At least 2 of the following, each present for a major portion of time during a 1-mo period (or less if successfully treated):

1. Delusions
2. Hallucinations
3. Disorganized speech (e.g., frequent derailment, jumping from one topic to another or incoherence)
4. Grossly disorganized or catatonic behavior
5. Negative symptoms (i.e., affective flattening, alogia, or avolition)

(*Note:* only 1 characteristic symptom is required if delusions are bizarre or hallucinations consist of a voice keeping up a running commentary on the person's behavior or thoughts, or involve 2 or more voices conversing with each other.)

Social/Occupational Dysfunction

For a significant portion of the time since the onset of the disturbance, 1 or more major areas of functioning (e.g., work, interpersonal relations, or self-care) are markedly below the level achieved before the onset (or when the onset is in childhood or adolescence, failure to achieve expected level of interpersonal, academic, or occupational achievement).

Duration

Continuous signs of the disturbance persist for at least 6 mos. This 6-mo period must include at least 1 mo of characteristic symptoms as described above (i.e., active-phase symptoms) and may include periods of prodromal or residual symptoms. During these prodromal or residual periods, the signs of the disturbance may be manifested by only negative symptoms or 2 or more of the characteristic symptoms present in an attenuated form (e.g., odd beliefs, unusual perceptual experiences).

Schizoaffective and Mood Disorder Exclusion

Schizoaffective disorder and mood disorder with psychotic features have been ruled out because either (1) no major depressive or manic episodes have occurred concurrently with the active-phase symptoms, or (2) if mood episodes have occurred during active phase symptoms, their total duration has been brief in relation to the duration of the active and residual periods.

Substance/General Medical Condition Exclusion

The disturbance is not due to the direct effects of a substance (e.g., drugs of abuse, medication) or a general medical condition.

---

of the offspring of schizophrenic parents have the disease. During a 25- to 30-year period, about one third of patients show some recovery or remission.

Typical initial treatment regimens include risperidone 2 mg twice daily, increasing to 6 to 10 mg/day total dose after 1 week if tolerated. An alternative is olanzapine, starting at 5 mg/day and increasing by 5-mg increments at weekly intervals to the 15- to 20-mg range. An important risk in the use of antipsychotic drugs is the development of tardive dyskinesia, a syndrome of involuntary movements, usually choreoathetoid, that can affect the mouth, lips, tongue, extremities, or trunk.

For more information about this subject, see *Cecil Textbook of Medicine,* 21st edition. Philadelphia, W.B. Saunders Company,

2000. Chapter 450, Psychiatric Disorders in Medical Practice, pages 2047 to 2056.

AUTONOMIC DISORDERS AND THEIR MANAGEMENT

The peripheral autonomic nervous system consists of three main divisions: (1) the *parasympathetic* division, which includes the outflow from the cranial nerves and the low lumbar and sacral spinal cord; (2) the *sympathetic* division, which comprises the autonomic outflow from the thoracic and high lumbar segments of the spinal cord; and (3) the *enteric* nervous system, which includes neurons that are intrinsic to the wall of the gut.

Systemic Dysautonomia

Widespread failure of the autonomic nervous system may evolve acutely or subacutely as part of a *parainfectious inflammatory polyneuropathy* (of the Guillain-Barré syndrome type). Wide swings in blood pressure and heart rate occur. Cardiac arrhythmias of all types may occur, presumably as a result of the instability of autonomic innervation of the cardiac conducting system. A similar subacute pandysautonomia is also seen in severe cases of *tetanus.*

Amyloid neuropathy often includes a major autonomic component which may be manifested as a gastrointestinal motility disorder or orthostatic hypotension. Similarly, *diabetic neuropathy,* although it is often dominated by sensory or motor complaints, may cause widespread autonomic failure. The neuropathy of *acute intermittent porphyria* or certain toxic agents such as *Vacor* (a rat poison) may have a prominent autonomic component. Acute poisoning with *organophosphate insecticides* that block acetylcholinesterase results in a hypercholinergic state, including miosis and cardiac slowing, which lasts for several days. Other peripheral neuropathies that may have an autonomic component are renal failure, toxic neuropathies (vinca alkaloids, perhexiline maleate, thallium, arsenic, mercury, organic solvents, acrylamide), vasculitis (systemic lupus erythematosus, rheumatoid arthritis, mixed connective tissue disease), thiamine deficiency, leprosy, Charcot-Marie-Tooth disease, and Fabry's disease.

Autonomic failure may be associated with *Parkinson's disease.* The Shy-Drager syndrome is part of a spectrum of *multiple systems atrophy* characterized by degeneration of central autonomic control nuclei in which evidence of cerebellar and extrapyramidal involvement is generally present but not evidence of peripheral autonomic degeneration on formal testing. *Pure autonomic failure* may also develop as a chronic degenerative condition in middle age or late adult life as a result of loss of neurons in the autonomic ganglia.

TREATMENT. Orthostatic hypotension is generally the most disabling aspect of autonomic degeneration. Treatment with elastic stockings or even entire lower body suits can improve standing blood pressure. Treatment with fludrocortisone (0.1 mg once to three times a day) expands intravascular blood volume and causes an elevation in blood pressure in all positions. Midodrine is the pro-drug of a direct sympathetic agonist; a starting dose of 10 mg three times a day may increase blood pressure. L-Dihydroxyphenylserine is a promising new drug that is a synthetic precursor of norepinephrine; it has shown encouraging results in some, but not all, trials.

Regional Dysautonomia

The most common cause of regional dysautonomia is injury to the cranial sympathetic innervation arising from the superior cervical ganglion, or *Horner's syndrome.* Miosis, ptosis, and anhidrosis may occur. The most common cause of Horner's syndrome is atherosclerotic disease affecting the vasa nervorum originating in the carotid artery. However, Horner's syndrome may also be seen when an intrathoracic or cervical tumor involves the sympathetic chain. *Paraspinal tumors* at lower levels along the sympathetic chain may cause loss of sweating over the involved dermatomes.

Following injury to peripheral nerves, aberrant regeneration may result in a severe pain syndrome known as *causalgia.* Normally innocuous sensory stimulation, such as covering the affected limb with a sheet or with clothing, may cause excruciating burning pain associated with variable autonomic changes. Atrophic changes in the skin and bone may reflect abnormal sympathetic innervation or disuse. One theory holds that the chronic pain may be due to *reflex sympathetic dystrophy.*

MOTOR SYMPTOMS

Fatigue can be a sign of upper motor neuron disease (corticospinal pathways) and is a common complaint of established multiple sclerosis and other multifocal CNS diseases. Similarly, any process that produces bilateral corticospinal tract or extrapyramidal disease can produce fatigue.

Muscle tremors, jerks, twitches, cramps, and spasms that occur in an entire limb or in more than one muscle group concurrently are caused by CNS disease. The intense muscle contractions of *tetany* are often painful. Usually a reflection of hypocalcemia, tetany can occasionally be seen without demonstrable electrolyte disturbance. Similarly, in the syndrome of *tetanus* produced by a clostridial toxin, intensely painful, life-threatening muscle contractions arise from hyperexcitable peripheral nerves.

SENSORY SYMPTOMS

Cutaneous sensation is observed by at least two distinct systems. Pain and temperature appreciation and aspects of tactile sensation are subserved by one system. The sensory receptors consist of naked nerve endings, from which impulses are conducted in the dorsal root ganglia, and impulses pass along the central processes of these neurons to the spinal cord, where they synapse in the dorsal horn.

A second sensory system subserves crude and light touch, position sense, and tactile localization or discrimination. The afferent pathways consist of large myelinated fibers that pass to the spinal cord via the dorsal root ganglia and ascend in the ipsilateral posterior and, to a lesser extent, the posterolateral columns of the cord to reach the posterior column. 23

Paresthesias may include a feeling of tingling, crawling, itching, compression, tightness, cold, or heat, and are sometimes associated with a feeling of heaviness. The term *dysesthesia* refers to abnormal sensations, often tingling, painful, or uncomfortable, that occur after innocuous stimuli. *Hypesthesia* and *hypalgesia* denote a loss or impairment of touch or pain sensibility, respectively, and *hyperesthesia* and *hyperalgesia* indicate a lowered threshold to tactile or painful stimuli, respectively.

Disorders of *peripheral nerves* commonly lead to sensory disturbances that depend upon the population of affected nerve fibers. Examination reveals that vibration, position, and movement sensations are impaired, and movement becomes clumsy and ataxic. Pain and temperature appreciation are relatively preserved. The tendon reflexes are lost early. Examples include diabetes. Most sensory neuropathies are characterized by a distal distribution of sensory loss.

Sensory changes in a *radiculopathy* will conform to a root territory. In cauda equina syndromes, sensory deficits involve multiple roots and may lead to saddle anesthesia and loss of the normal sensation associated with the passage of urine or feces.

Lesions of the *posterolateral columns* of the cord, as occur in multiple sclerosis, vitamin B_{12} deficiency, and cervical spondylosis, lead often to a feeling of compression in the affected region and to Lhermitte's sign (paresthesias radiating down the extremities on neck flexion). Conversely, lesions of the *anterolateral region* of the cord (as by cordotomy) or *central lesions* interrupting fibers crossing to join the spinothalamic pathways (as in syringomyelia) lead to an impairment of pain and temperature appreciation with relative preservation of vibration, joint position sense, and light touch.

Lateral hemisection of the cord (*Brown-Séquard syndrome*) leads to ipsilateral pain, hyperesthesia, and impaired vibration and joint position sense below the level of the lesion, and to contralateral impairment of pain and temperature appreciation. Patients with a central cord lesion that interrupts fibers crossing in the cord develop a *syringomyelic syndrome* affecting the involved segments, with impairment of pain and temperature appreciation but preservation of vibration and joint position senses and the ability to localize touch. In patients with a severe transverse myelitis or complete cord transection, all sensation is lost below the level of the lesion, although spinal reflex activity is preserved except in the acute stage of spinal shock.

Motor deficits may also be present and help to localize the lesion. Upper motor neuron dysfunction from cervical lesions leads to quadriplegia, whereas more caudal lesions lead to paraplegia. Lesions below the level of the first lumbar vertebra may simply compress the cauda equina, leading to lower motor neuron deficits from a polyradiculopathy and to impairment of sphincter and sexual functions.

Lateral medullary lesions (Wallenberg's syndrome) typically lead to a crossed sensory deficit, with loss of pain and temperature appreciation on the ipsilateral face. With lesions at the level of the *thalamus* or more rostrally, all sensory modalities are lost on the side opposite the lesions. Spontaneous pain is common, and diverse cutaneous stimuli may cause unpleasant painful sensations.

For more information about this subject, see *Cecil Textbook of*

Medicine, 21st edition. Philadelphia, W.B. Saunders Company, 2000. Chapter 451, Autonomic Disorders and Their Management; Chapter 452, Disorders of Motor Function; and Chapter 453, Major Sensory Symptoms, pages 2057 to 2066.

HEADACHES AND OTHER HEAD PAIN

Over 90% of the population experience headache of one type or another at least once during life. Fortunately, most patients with recurrent or chronic headaches suffer from a primary headache disorder for which no ominous underlying source can be found. A headache signifies activation of the primary afferent fibers that innervate cephalic blood vessels, chiefly meningeal or cerebral blood vessels.

Primary Headache Disorders

MIGRAINE HEADACHES. Migraine is the second most common primary headache disorder and has a prevalence of about 12%. Migraine falls into two categories: (1) migraine without an aura (previously called common migraine), which occurs in about 85% of patients, and (2) migraine with an aura (previously called classic migraine), which occurs in about 15% of patients. Migraine patients may report prodromal symptoms, including hyperactivity, mild euphoria, lethargy, depression, craving for certain foods, fluid retention, and frequent yawning. Prodromal symptoms should not be confused with the migraine aura that consists of transient episodes of focal neurologic dysfunction appearing 1 to 2 hours before the onset of a migraine headache and resolving within 60 minutes. Typical aura symptoms include (1) homonymous (rarely monocular) visual disturbance, classically an expanding scotoma with a scintillating margin; (2) unilateral paresthesias and/or numbness; (3) unilateral weakness; and (4) dysphasia or other language disturbances.

The headache phase is similar with or without an aura. It typically consists of 4 to 72 hours of unilateral throbbing head pain of moderate to severe intensity that is worsened by routine physical exertion and associated with nausea, photophobia, and phonophobia. *Complicated migraine* refers to attacks associated with aura symptoms lasting for more than 1 hour. Migraine attacks that persist for longer than 72 hours despite treatment are classified as *status migrainosus.*

Non-pharmacologic treatment includes behavior modification techniques such as the avoidance of triggering factors, biofeedback, relaxation training, rational motive therapy, self-hypnosis, and meditation. *Pharmacologic treatment of migraine* includes abortive therapy given to shorten the attack or reduce headache severity. If migraines cause disability more than 3 days per month, daily prophylactic treatment may be taken.

Mild attacks may be treated with simple analgesics such as acetaminophen (suggested dose, 650 to 1000 mg) or non-steroidal anti-inflammatory drugs (NSAIDs: aspirin 900 to 1000 mg, ibuprofen 1000 to 1200 mg, naproxen 500 to 825 mg, or ketoprofen 100 to 200 mg). *Moderate headaches* may respond to the combination of acetaminophen, isometheptene mucate, and dichloralphenazone. Infrequent headaches of moderate-to-severe intensity may be treated with butalbital, a barbiturate, combined with caffeine, aspirin, and/or acetaminophen. Ergotamine, 2 mg sublingually or 1 to 2 mg orally (PO), is typically most effective if given early in the migraine attack.

Moderate-to-severe attacks may be treated outside the hospital with oral or intranasal formulations of a serotonin 5-HT receptor agonist like sumatriptan at 25 or 50 mg PO, 20 mg intranasally, or 6 mg subcutaneously (SC); dihydroergotamine 1 to 2 mg intranasally; and, more recently, new second-generation sumatriptan-like drugs such as naratriptan, zolmitriptan, and rizatriptan.

Very severe attacks sometimes require the administration of IV or intramuscular (IM) agents in the emergency department. Dihydroergotamine may be administered SC or IV. Meperidine, an opioid analgesic, is frequently administered IM, but parenteral opioids should be limited to patients with infrequent, severe attacks for whom other treatments are contraindicated. Chlorpromazine 10 mg IV may be used.

In general, preventive treatment is recommended (1) if headaches limit work or normal daily activity 3 or more days per month, (2) if the symptoms accompanying headache are severe or prolonged, and (3) if previous migraine was associated with a complication (e.g., cerebral infarction). The prophylactic agents fall into seven groups and include:

1. β-Adrenergic blockers: propranolol 40 to 240 mg, atenolol 50 to 150 mg, nadolol 20 to 80 mg, timolol 20 to 60 mg, and metoprolol 50 to 300 mg
2. NSAIDs: aspirin 1000 to 1300 mg, naproxen 480 to 1100 mg, ketoprofen 150 to 300 mg
3. Tricyclic antidepressants: amitriptyline 10 to 120 mg, nortriptyline 10 to 75 mg
4. Calcium channel antagonists: verapamil 120 to 480 mg, flunarizine 5 to 10 mg
5. Anticonvulsants: divalproex sodium 750 to 1000 mg, gabapentin 900 to 1800 mg
6. Serotoninergic drugs: methysergide 4 to 8 mg, cyproheptadine 8 to 20 mg
7. MAO inhibitor: phenelzine 30 to 60 mg

CLUSTER HEADACHES. Cluster headaches consist of recurrent episodes of unilateral, orbital, supraorbital, or temporal head pain usually accompanied by ipsilateral autonomic signs, including conjunctival injection, lacrimation, rhinorrhea, nasal congestion, ptosis, miosis, eyelid edema, and facial sweating. The attacks last from 15 minutes to 3 hours.

Oxygen inhalation (100%) delivered at a rate of 8 L/minute for 15 minutes through a loose-fitting face mask is a safe and effective treatment. Ergotamine tartrate is effective and well tolerated. Sumatriptan 6 mg SC is usually successful and reduces both pain and conjunctival injection within 15 minutes. Verapamil and ergotamine tartrate are effective and well-tolerated prophylactic agents. Lithium carbonate may also be beneficial in the episodic form of the disease; the usual therapeutic range is 0.3 to 0.8 mmol/L. Prednisone is frequently used in dosages of 60 to 80 mg/day for 1 week, followed by a taper in dosage over a period of 2 to 4 weeks.

TENSION-TYPE HEADACHE. Tension-type headache is the most common of the primary headache disorders, with a lifetime prevalence between 30 and 78%. Tension-type headache occurs in episodic and chronic forms. Episodic headache consists of recurrent attacks of tight, pressing (bandlike), bilateral, mild-to-moderate head pain that lasts from minutes to days. Tension-type headaches do not worsen with routine physical exertion and are not associated with nausea, although photophobia or phonophobia may be present. Episodic tension-type headaches usually respond to simple analgesics such as acetaminophen 650 to 1000 mg or to NSAIDs such as aspirin 900 to 1000 mg, ketoprofen 12.5 to 50 mg, ibuprofen 200 to 800 mg, or naproxen 250 to 500 mg. Tricyclic antidepressants decrease both the frequency and the severity of attacks.

EXERTIONAL AND ORGASMIC HEADACHE. In some individuals, exertion or various types of exercise may trigger bilateral throbbing or pressure-like headaches that persist for several minutes up to 48 hours. In rare cases, coital headache may be associated with unruptured cerebral aneurysms; the possibility of aneurysm should be excluded. Exertional headache can sometimes be prevented by ingestion of ergotamine or indomethacin before the planned exertion.

Secondary Headache Disorders

Headache may be the initial complaint in a host of CNS and systemic abnormalities (see Table 23–19).

GIANT CELL ARTERITIS. Giant cell arteritis most often affects people older than 60 years and can result in rapid and permanent loss of vision. Features suggestive of temporal arteritis include (1) orbital or frontotemporal head pain described as dull and constant with superimposed jabbing sensations; (2) aggravation of pain by cold temperatures; (3) pain in the jaw or tongue upon chewing (jaw claudication); (4) accompanying constitutional symptoms such as weight loss, anemia, polymyalgia rheumatica, mononeuropathy, and elevated liver enzymes; and (5) decreased visual acuity. The erythrocyte sedimentation rate (ESR) is elevated in 95% of cases.

In patients with an elevated ESR, methylprednisolone 500 to 1000 mg IV every 12 hours for 48 hours should be followed by oral prednisone 80 to 100 mg/day for 14 to 21 days, with a gradual taper over 12 to 24 months.

SUBSTANCE-INDUCED HEADACHES. Headaches may occur with acute exposure or as a result of withdrawal from many types of substances (Table 23–20).

HEADACHES ASSOCIATED WITH INCREASED INTRACRANIAL PRESSURE. Headaches in brain tumor patients are usually dull and bifrontal, although they tend to be worse on the side of the tumor. They are more often qualitatively similar to tension-type headache than to migraine and tend to be intermittent and of moderate intensity. They are accompanied by nausea about half the time and are usually resistant to common analgesics. Factors that should increase suspicion of an intracranial tumor include papilledema, new neurologic deficits, initial attack of prolonged head-

Table 23–19 ■ SECONDARY HEADACHE DISORDERS

Headaches Associated with Cranial Vascular Abnormalities
Subarachnoid hemorrhage
Intracerebral, epidural, and subdural hematoma
Unruptured vascular malformation
Arteriovenous malformation
Saccular aneurysm
Carotid or vertebral artery dissection
Carotidynia
Cerebral intra-arterial occlusion
Venous thrombosis
Arterial hypertension
Headaches Associated with Non-Vascular Intracranial Disorders
Intracranial neoplasms
High- and low-pressure headaches
Inflammatory disorders
Temporal (giant cell) arteritis
Tolosa-Hunt syndrome
Intracranial sarcoidosis
Intracranial infection
Acute meningitis
Meningoencephalitis
Brain abscess
Headaches Associated with Systemic Abnormalities
Systemic infection, viral, bacterial, treponemal, etc.
Substance-induced headaches, exposure and withdrawal
Metabolic disturbance
Hypoxia, altitude sickness, sleep apnea
Hypercapnia
Hypoglycemia
Dialysis
Head and Facial Pain Associated with Disorders of Cranial Nerves
Neuralgias
Trigeminal neuralgia
Glossopharyngeal neuralgia
Occipital neuralgia
Herpes zoster
Head and Facial Pain Associated with Disorders of Other Cranial Structures
Glaucoma
Sinusitis
Temporomandibular joint disease
Dental pain
Neck abnormalities

ache occurring after the age of 45, previous malignancy, cognitive abnormality, or altered mental status.

Idiopathic intracranial hypertension (pseudotumor cerebri) is a syndrome composed of headache, papilledema, and transient visual symptoms that occur in the absence of CSF abnormalities, except for elevated ICP. The diagnosis is made by lumbar puncture (CSF pressure >250 mm Hg; normal CSF composition) after excluding a mass lesion by neuroimaging. Weight reduction should be attempted. Furosemide, a potent loop diuretic, must be given with

Table 23–20 ■ SUBSTANCES INDUCING HEADACHE

After Acute Exposure	
Alcohol	Indomethacin
Amphotericin B	Monosodium glutamate
Azithromycin	Nifedipine
Carbon monoxide	Nitrates/nitrites
Cimetidine	Ondansetron
Cocaine/crack	Phenylethylamine
Danazol	Ranitidine
Diclofenac	Reserpine
Dipyridamole	Tyramine
Estrogen/birth control pills	Timolol ophthalmic drops
Fluconazole	Verapamil
Following Withdrawal after Chronic Use	
Alcohol	
Barbiturates	
Caffeine	
Ergotamine	
Opiate analgesics	

potassium supplementation and may cause hypotension. If drug treatment is ineffective, repeated lumbar punctures may sometimes be useful.

HEADACHE ASSOCIATED WITH DECREASED INTRACRANIAL PRESSURE. Decreased ICP (<50 to 90 mm H_2O) (usually caused by a decrease in CSF volume) is commonly associated with dull, throbbing, sometimes severe headaches that are probably caused by reduced brain buoyancy. Low-pressure headaches often become more intense upon standing or sitting upright and may be relieved by lying down. Headaches most commonly follow lumbar puncture, intracranial surgery, ventricular shunting, trauma, and various systemic medical conditions such as severe dehydration, postdialysis status, diabetic coma, uremia, or hyperpnea. If the headache is prolonged, the possibility of a persistent CSF leak may be investigated by radioisotope cisternography or CT myelography. Treatment strategies include corticosteroids, oral fluid or salt intake, IV fluids, CO_2 inhalation, methylxanthines such as theophylline 300 mg three times per day, caffeine 500 mg IV, or intrathecal autologous blood patch.

Head and Facial Pain Associated with Disorders of Cranial Nerves

TRIGEMINAL NEURALGIA. Trigeminal neuralgia, also known as *tic douloureux,* is a sharp, often electric shock–like pain that occurs in a rapid series of jabs (lasting seconds to minutes) in one or more division of the trigeminal nerve. When trigeminal neuralgia occurs in persons younger than 40 years, a specific cause can often be found, such as demyelination (multiple sclerosis, especially when bilateral) and compression by vascular abnormalities or tumors (myeloma, metastatic carcinoma, cholesteatoma, chordoma, acoustic neuroma, trigeminal neuroma). The initial work-up should include MRI studies, which detail the cerebellopontine angle and the entry foramen. In the absence of a structural cause, treatment usually consists of administering drugs such as carbamazepine 400 to 1200 mg, valproate 500 to 1500 mg, phenytoin 200 to 500 mg, baclofen 40 to 80 mg, or clonazepam 2 to 6 mg.

GLOSSOPHARYNGEAL NEURALGIA. Glossopharyngeal neuralgia is characterized by paroxysmal pain within the distribution of the vagus and glossopharyngeal nerves. The pain is most often felt in or around the ear, tongue, jaw, or larynx and can be triggered by swallowing, talking, chewing, clearing the throat, yawning, or tasting spicy food or cold liquids. The usual cause of glossopharyngeal neuralgia appears to be microvascular compression, although abscess and tumor are sometimes associated. Medical treatment is similar to that for trigeminal neuralgia and includes slow introduction of carbamazepine 400 to 1200 mg or baclofen 40 to 80 mg.

POST-HERPETIC NEURALGIA. A useful definition of *post-herpetic neuralgia* requires persistence of pain for 3 months after skin healing because pain resolves slowly in many patients as inflammation subsides. Patients describe three components: (1) a constant, deep, aching, bruised, or burning sensation; (2) a spontaneous, recurrent, lancinating, shooting, or electric shock–like pain; and (3) an allodynic (pain from a usually non-painful stimulus), superficial, sharp, radiating, burning, tender, dysesthetic, or "itch"-like sensation evoked by wearing clothing or by gentle touch. Double-blind controlled trials have provided evidence of efficacy for topical agents in the form of capsaicin cream and local anesthetic patches, oral opioids, tricyclic antidepressants, and the anticonvulsant medication gabapentin.

COMPLEX REGIONAL PAIN SYNDROME (CRPS; REFLEX SYMPATHETIC DYSTROPHY AND CAUSALGIA). CRPS has two forms, CRPS I and CRPS II. CRPS I replaces the term *reflex sympathetic dystrophy* and describes a pain syndrome that usually develops after an initiating noxious event, is not limited to the distribution of a single peripheral nerve, and is apparently disproportional to the inciting event. CRPS I is associated at some point with evidence of edema, changes in skin blood flow, abnormal sweating (sudomotor activity) in the region of the pain, and (or) allodynia or hyperalgesia.

CRPS II (formerly causalgia) is the same syndrome in patients with demonstrable peripheral nerve injury. Not all patients have dystrophy, and a few have dystrophy but no pain.

Symptoms of CRPS may begin gradually in the days or weeks after an injury or may be manifested within a few hours. The "acute" stage, is heralded by pain that seems more severe than that usually caused by the initial injury, has a prominent burning or aching component, and is increased by dependency of the affected part, any physical contact, or emotional upset. The "dystrophic" stage is notable for a change from edema to induration, cool hyperhidrotic skin, and livedo reticularis or cyanosis. Hair loss and ridged, cracked, or brittle nails may be apparent. MRI demonstrates bone marrow abnormalities consistent with CRPS. The "atrophic" stage is associated with proximal spread of pain and irreversible tissue damage. The skin is thin and shiny, digits are wasted, and flexion or Dupuytren's contractures may occur. Radiographs are invariably abnormal, often with ankylosis.

Treatment outcomes are disappointing. A conservative approach combines physical therapy, medication management, individual and group counseling and education, and judicious use of local anesthetic nerve blocks. Surgical sympathectomy and other destructive procedures are seldom of benefit.

FIBROMYALGIA SYNDROME. The diagnosis of fibromyalgia syndrome requires widespread pain on both sides of the body and pain both above and below the waist. More than 75% of patients also complain of symptoms such as morning stiffness, chronic fatigue, and sleep disturbance. Current therapy includes non-pharmacologic approaches such as exercise-based programs and cognitive behavioral therapies. Both tricyclic and SSRI-type antidepressants have proved beneficial in clinical trials.

For more information about this subject, see *Cecil Textbook of Medicine,* 21st edition. Philadelphia, W.B. Saunders Company, 2000. Chapter 454, Headaches and Other Head Pain; and Chapter 455, Other Specific Pain Syndromes, pages 2066 to 2073.

NEUROCUTANEOUS SYNDROMES

Neurofibromatosis

Neurofibromatosis encompasses a wide spectrum of syndromes with neurocutaneous lesions. Although at least eight variants have been described, only two are well-recognized, genetically distinct entities: NF-1 and NF-2.

NF-1 corresponds to the classic disorder described by von Recklinghausen. The NF-1 gene is located on chromosome 17q and expresses a protein designated as neurofibromin. Clinical criteria for the diagnosis include (1) six or more cafe au lait macules larger than 5 mm in pre-pubescent patients and more than 15 mm in post-pubescent individuals, (2) two or more neurofibromas of any type or one plexiform neurofibroma, (3) axillary or inguinal freckling, (4) sphenoid bone dysplasia, (5) optic glioma, (6) Lisch nodules (iris hamartomas), and (7) a family history of NF-1. The diagnosis is made when at least two or more of the above criteria are present. Subcutaneous neurofibromas may be painful or disfiguring and can be excised surgically. Intraspinal and intracranial tumors are approached surgically. Optic nerve gliomas may be treated with radiation. Genetic counseling is important.

NF-2, or central neurofibromatosis, is an autosomal dominant syndrome. The classic pathologic abnormality in NF-2 is bilateral eighth cranial nerve schwannomas. The NF-2 gene is located on chromosome 22q. The gene product (merlin) is a cytoskeletal protein. Although skin lesions may be present in up to 30% of patients with NF-2, the diagnosis is based on the presence of the following criteria: (1) bilateral eighth nerve tumors detected by MRI; (2) a family member with either NF-2 or unilateral eighth nerve lesions that may include neurofibromas, meningiomas, or schwannomas; and (3) juvenile posterior subcapsular lenticular opacities. Surgical treatment may be indicated in patients with intramedullary spinal tumors.

Tuberous Sclerosis

The classic clinical criteria for diagnosis of tuberous sclerosis include mental subnormality, epilepsy, and skin lesions. Diagnosis is usually clinical and is confirmed by calcified or uncalcified hamartomas on imaging studies. Neurologic manifestations in most patients are seizures and mental retardation.

Sturge-Weber Syndrome

Sturge-Weber syndrome is characterized by the presence of facial vascular nevi (port-wine stain), epilepsy, cognitive deficits, and less frequently, hemiparesis or hemiplegia, hemianopia, or glaucoma. Treatment is aimed at the epilepsy.

Von Hippel-Lindau Disease

Von Hippel-Lindau disease (CNS angiomatosis) is an autosomal dominant disorder caused by a defective tumor suppressor gene at chromosome 3p25-p26 and characterized by retinal angiomas, brain and spinal cord hemangioblastomas, renal cell carcinomas, endolymphatic sac tumors, pheochromocytomas, papillary cystadenomas of the epididymis, angiomas of the liver and kidney, and cysts of the pancreas, kidney, liver, and epididymis. Symptoms typically begin during the third or fourth decade. Retinal inflammation with exudate, hemorrhage, and retinal detachment from the retinal angiomas typically antedates the cerebellar complaints. Headache, vertigo, and vomiting result from the cerebellar tumor. Other cerebellar findings are common. Treatment is symptomatic.

Syringohydromyelia

Syringohydromyelia is a condition in which the central canal of the spinal cord (hydromyelia), the substance of the spinal cord (syringomyelia), or the brain stem (syringobulbia) is expanded by the presence of fluid under pressure. Symptoms most commonly begin in late adolescence or early adulthood. Classically, patients have asymmetrical segmental weakness and atrophy of the hands and arms, loss of upper limb deep tendon reflexes, and dissociated sensory loss (with impaired perception of pain and temperature but preservation of light touch and proprioception) in the neck, arms, and upper part of the trunk. In the legs, muscle tone is increased and the reflexes are hyperactive. Extension into the medulla may cause nystagmus or lower cranial neuropathies. The diagnosis is made by MRI.

In patients with Chiari II malformations, adequate shunting of the lateral ventricles may result in collapsing the syrinx. Syringohydromyelia in patients with spinal tumors is treated by surgery. Patients with narrowing of the craniocervical junction are treated by bony foramen magnum decompression. Patients with arachnoidal scarring are typically treated by insertion of a syringopleural or syringoperitoneal shunt.

For more information about this subject, see *Cecil Textbook of Medicine,* 21st edition. Philadelphia, W.B. Saunders Company, 2000. Chapter 456, Neurocutaneous Syndromes, pages 2074 to 2075.

THE EXTRAPYRAMIDAL DISORDERS, INCLUDING PARKINSONISM

The term *extrapyramidal* refers to the anatomic and functional characteristics that distinguish the basal ganglia–regulated motor system from the pyramidal (corticospinal) and cerebellar systems. Extrapyramidal movement disorders are *hypokinesias,* characterized by poverty and slowness of movement; *hyperkinesias,* manifested by abnormal involuntary movements; and miscellaneous motor disturbances (Table 23–21).

The six paired nuclei that constitute the basal ganglia include the caudate nucleus, putamen, globus pallidus (or pallidum), nucleus accumbens, subthalamic nucleus, and substantia nigra. The caudate nucleus and putamen are often referred to as the *corpus striatum.* The term *lenticular nucleus* refers to the putamen and globus pallidus combined.

Parkinsonism

Parkinsonism is a clinical syndrome dominated by four cardinal signs: tremor at rest, bradykinesia, rigidity, and postural instability. Less prominent manifestations concern the mood and intellect, autonomic function, and the sensory system. The average age at onset is 55 years, with about 1% of persons 60 years or older having the disease. One subtype is characterized by tremor as the dominant parkinsonian feature. The postular instability–gait difficulty subtype shows more bradykinesia and dementia, as well as a more rapidly progressive course.

Bradykinesia is clinically manifested by slowness of automatic and spontaneous movements and an impaired ability to initiate voluntary movements (akinesia). This symptom presumably results from loss of the inhibitory dopamine input to the striatum and hypoactivity of the neurons in the external segment of the globus pallidus. Rigidity, another cardinal sign of parkinsonism, is demonstrated clinically by increased resistance against passive movement of a body part, usually associated with the cogwheel phenomenon. Postural instability resulting from loss of righting reflexes can cause propulsion (tendency to fall forward) and retropulsion (tendency to fall backward).

Bradykinesia accounts for general slowing in movements and activities of daily living, lack of facial expression (hypomimia or masked facies), staring expression resulting from a decreased frequency of blinking, impaired swallowing causing drooling (sialorrhea), hypokinetic and hypophonic dysarthria, monotonous speech,

Table 23–21 ■ MOVEMENT DISORDERS

HYPOKINESIAS	HYPERKINESIAS	MISCELLANEOUS
Parkinsonism	Tremor	Ataxia
Hypomimia	Dystonia	Gait disorders
Dysarthria	Chorea	Hyperexplexia
Sialorrhea	Athetosis	Hemifacial spasm
Micrographia	Ballism	Myokymia
Shuffling gait	Tics	Stiff-person syndrome
Other signs of bradykinesia and rigidity	Myoclonus	Psychogenic
	Sterotypy	
	Akathisia	
	Restless legs	
	Paroxysmal dyskinesias	

small handwriting (micrographia), difficulty in arising from a chair, shuffling gait with short steps, decreased automatic movements, and start hesitation and freezing.

Parkinson's Disease

The typical pathologic features of Parkinson's disease are neuronal loss with depigmentation of the substantia nigra and Lewy bodies, which are eosinophilic cytoplasmic inclusions in neurons. Motor symptoms result chiefly from degeneration of the nigrostriatal pathway, which causes a deficiency of dopamine in the putamen and, to a lesser degree, the caudate nucleus. The cognitive deficits and some neurobehavioral symptoms have been attributed to degeneration of the dopaminergic mesocortical and mesolimbic pathways. Two mutations have been identified in the gene coding for α-synuclein on chromosome 4q in families with autosomal dominant Parkinson's disease.

TREATMENT. Many neurologists favor the use of a combination of deprenyl, anticholinergics, and amantadine until they no longer provide satisfactory control of parkinsonian symptoms. At that point, many authorities believe that dopamine agonists should be used. Improvement may be sufficient to delay the introduction of levodopa by several months or years and thus delay the onset of levodopa-related complications. Dopamine agonists also smooth out the motor fluctuations associated with chronic levodopa therapy. Dopamine agonists include cabergoline, pramipexole, ropinirole, bromocriptine, and pergolide.

When patients continue to be troubled by their parkinsonian symptoms despite deprenyl, anticholinergics, amantadine, and a dopamine agonist, levodopa combined with carbidopa, a peripheral dopa decarboxylase inhibitor, is added to the antiparkinsonian regimen. The starting dosage of carbidopa-levodopa is 25:100 mg (controlled release) twice daily, to be gradually increased to three times per day.

Slow-release preparations of carbidopa-levodopa (e.g., Sinemet CR, Madopar CR) prolong the plasma (and presumably brain) levels and may be useful in treating or preventing motor fluctuations. Another strategy designed to prolong levodopa response takes advantage of the inhibition of catechol *o*-methyltransferase by drugs such as tolcapone and entacapone. The most common central side effects of levodopa include psychiatric problems, dyskinesias, and clinical fluctuations. Patients will lose their response to levodopa because of natural progression of the disease and development of complications.

Stereotactic thalamotomy is still occasionally used in an attempt to ameliorate disabling tremor. Both the ablative and stimulating pallidotomy and high-frequency deep brain stimulation have been found to be particularly effective in smoothing out motor fluctuations and eliminating levodopa-induced dyskinesias. Surgical transplantation of fetal substantia nigra into the striatum remains under investigation.

Secondary Parkinsonism

In general, post-encephalitic parkinsonism has a slower progression and is more sensitive to levodopa therapy. Cerebrovascular disease accounts for a small proportion of parkinsonism. Drugs that block dopamine receptors, such as antipsychotic and antiemetic agents, can cause a parkinsonian syndrome clinically indistinguishable from idiopathic parkinsonism.

Approximately 10 to 15% of all patients with parkinsonian findings have a more widespread disorder classified clinically as "parkinsonism-plus syndrome." Such patients suffer from supranuclear ophthalmoparesis (progressive supranuclear palsy), dysautonomia (Shy-Drager syndrome), ataxia (olivopontocerebellar atrophy), laryngeal stridor, apraxia, dementia, and a combination of dementia and motor neuron disease.

For more information about this subject, see *Cecil Textbook of Medicine,* 21st edition. Philadelphia, W.B. Saunders Company, 2000. Chapter 459, Introduction to the Extrapyramidal Disorders; and Chapter 460, Parkinsonism, pages 2077 to 2083.

OTHER MOVEMENT DISORDERS

Tremors

Tremor is a rhythmic oscillatory movement produced by alternating or synchronous contractions of opposing muscle groups. Tremors are divided into rest or action tremors; the latter are further subdivided into postural or contraction tremors. *Rest tremor,* usually asymmetrical at onset, is the typical tremor of Parkinson's disease. *Postural tremor,* with a frequency ranging between 4 and 12 Hz, is most typically seen in patients with essential tremor. *Kinetic (intention) tremors* are slow and more irregular movements with a rate of 1.5 to 3.0 Hz. Kinetic tremors usually indicate an abnormality of the cerebellum or its outflow pathways.

Essential tremor is the most common type of tremor. The tremor is inherited in an autosomal dominant pattern with high penetrance. Affected patients lack the hypokinetic features and rigidity of Parkinson's disease. Essential tremor also frequently involves the head and voice. Some forms occur during a specific activity, such as writing.

β-Adrenergic blocking drugs (e.g., propranolol 20 to 240 mg/day) are the most effective agents. Other occasionally useful drugs include primidone, lorazepam, and alprazolam.

Dystonias

Dystonia is a syndrome dominated by involuntary, sustained (tonic) or spasmodic (rapid or clonic), patterned, and repetitive muscle contractions frequently causing twisting (e.g., torticollis), flexing or extending (e.g., writer's cramp, retrocollis), and squeezing (e.g., blepharospasm) movements or abnormal postures. Dystonia can fluctuate in intensity and is exacerbated by stress, fatigue, activity, or a change in posture. It subsides during sleep, relaxation, and hypnosis. The most common form is *cervical dystonia.*

Occasionally, a specific and potentially treatable cause of dystonia can be identified. One of the most important examples is *Wilson's disease.* Tardive dystonia is a persistent form of dystonia caused by exposure to dopamine receptor blocking drugs such as major tranquilizers (e.g., chlorpromazine, thioridazine, fluphenazine, thiothixene, haloperidol, loxapine, amoxapine) and certain antiemetics (e.g., prochlorperazine, metoclopramide).

Treatment consists of supportive therapy (e.g., relaxation techniques, prostheses), medications, botulinum toxin injections, and surgery. Anticholinergic drugs are sometimes beneficial.

Choreas

Chorea consists of continuous, abrupt, rapid, brief, flowing, unsustained, irregular, and random jerklike movements. A characteristic feature of chorea is the inability to maintain voluntary sustained contraction.

Huntington's disease is an autosomal dominant disorder with complete penetrance. Dementia and various emotional and psychiatric disturbances are prominent. Neuropsychological symptoms may precede motor changes. Cognitive changes are loss of recent memory and impaired judgment. The duration of illness from onset to death is about 15 years.

The mutation responsible for the disease consists of an unstable enlargement of the CAG repeat sequence in the 5′ end of a large (210 kb) gene, *IT15*. This gene, located at 4p16.3, encodes a protein called *huntingtin*. Treatment is symptomatic.

Athetosis and Ballism

Athetosis is a slow form of chorea characterized by twisting, writhing movements. Athetosis usually does not respond to pharmacologic therapy.

Ballism is a form of forceful, flinging, high-amplitude, coarse chorea. Because the involuntary movement usually affects only one side of the body, the term *hemiballism* is used. The condition is often preceded by hemiparesis associated with a hemorrhagic or ischemic stroke. Dopamine-blocking and -depleting drugs benefit most patients with hemiballism, but the disorder usually subsides spontaneously within several weeks.

Tics

Tics are involuntary, abrupt, sudden, isolated, brief movements (*motor tics*); sounds produced by the nose, mouth, or throat (*vocal-phonic tics*); or sensations (*sensory tics*). The most common cause of tics is the *Gilles de la Tourette syndrome,* a genetic disorder. The following criteria are diagnostic:

1. Both multiple motor and one or more phonic tics must be present, although not necessarily concurrently.
2. The tics occur many times, nearly every day, or intermittently over a period of more than a year.
3. The anatomic location, number, frequency, complexity, type, and severity of tics change over time
4. Onset is before age 21 years.
5. Involuntary movements and noises cannot be explained by other medical conditions.

Many affected patients suffer from obsessive-compulsive disorder. Judicious use of dopamine receptor blocking drugs, such as fluphenazine, pimozide, and haloperidol, may reduce the frequency and severity of tics and ameliorate impulsive and aggressive behavior.

Myoclonus

Myoclonus is a jerklike movement produced by a sudden, rapid, and brief contraction (positive myoclonus) or a muscle inhibition (negative myoclonus). Two forms of myoclonus are associated with sleep: physiologic sleep myoclonus, occurring normally during the initial phases of sleep, and nocturnal myoclonus, now called periodic movements of sleep, often associated with restless legs syndrome as well as with abnormal involuntary movements while the person is awake. Causes of generalized myoclonus include acute and prolonged hypoxia and ischemia; various metabolic, infectious, and toxic factors; and exposure to neuroleptic drugs (tardive myoclonus). Clonazepam, lorazepam, valproate, carbamazepine, and 5-hydroxytryptophan (5-HTP) have been reported to have antimyoclonic activity.

For more information about this subject, see *Cecil Textbook of Medicine,* 21st edition. Philadelphia, W.B. Saunders Company, 2000. Chapter 461, Tremors; Chapter 462, Dystonias; Chapter 463, Choreas, Athetosis, and Ballism; and Chapter 464, Tics, Myoclonus, and Stereotypes, pages 2083 to 2087.

DEGENERATIVE DISEASES OF THE NERVOUS SYSTEM

An important common mutation mechanism in single-gene disorders involves the expansion of the normal genome by runs of three DNA bases, known as trinucleotide repeats. Individuals in successive generations are often more severely affected at a younger age. This phenomenon, known as anticipation, occurs as the unstable trinucleotide repeats expand between parents and offspring. Trinucleotide repeat disorders, in which genomic expansion occurs in the coding region, appear to represent adult-onset, gain-of-function disorders. These include the spinocerebellar ataxias. In contrast, if the repeat is located in a non-coding region, the disorder frequently occurs at a younger age, represents a loss of function, and involves multiple organs. Friedreich's ataxia is an example of a trinucleotide repeat occurring in a non-coding region.

Friedreich's Ataxia

The clinical diagnosis of Friedreich's ataxia is made when patients meet the following criteria: (1) usual onset during puberty; (2) progressive ataxia with loss of lower extremity deep tendon reflexes; (3) presence of Babinski's sign (extensor plantar responses); and (4) 5 or more years of disease and a family history compatible with autosomal recessive inheritance. Other common clinical features include nystagmus, dysarthria, stocking-glove neuropathy, and pes cavus with weakness in the lower extremities. Diagnosis is made by positive genetic testing. No treatment, other than supportive measures, is currently available.

Spinocerebellar Ataxia

The predominant clinical feature of spinocerebellar ataxia types 1 to 7 and Machado-Joseph disease is ataxia, followed by dysarthria and ophthalmoplegia. Additional clinical signs include dementia, optic atrophy, retinal pigmentary degeneration, deafness, dysphagia, extrapyramidal and pyramidal findings, and peripheral neuropathy. Diagnosis is made by positive genetic testing in a patient with appropriate clinical signs and symptoms. No specific therapy is currently available for the spinocerebellar ataxias.

Hereditary Spastic Paraplegia

Pure hereditary spastic paraplegia, also known as Strümpell's disease, is usually an autosomal dominant disorder. Patients have progressive gait disturbance, spasticity of lower extremities, and hyperreflexia, frequently grade 4, with Babinski's sign. The differential diagnosis includes other genetic conditions, spinal cord disease from structural lesions, multiple sclerosis, and vitamin deficiencies or retroviral infections. No specific treatment is currently available.

For more information about this subject, see *Cecil Textbook of Medicine,* 21st edition. Philadelphia, W.B. Saunders Company, 2000. Chapter 465, Introduction to Degenerative Diseases of the Nervous System; Chapter 466, Hereditary Cerebellar Ataxias and Related Disorders; and Chapter 467, Hereditary Spastic Paraplegias, pages 2087 to 2089.

MOTOR NEURON DISEASES

Motor neuron diseases are a heterogeneous group of disorders that selectively affect upper or lower motor neurons or both (Table 23–22).

Sporadic amyotrophic lateral sclerosis (ALS) accounts for approximately 80% of all cases of acquired motor neuron disease, whereas the remaining 20% of patients have either only lower motor neuron signs or a familial form of ALS. The 80% of patients who have sporadic ALS present with spasticity, hyperreflexia, and Babinski's sign in the setting of progressive muscle wasting and weakness (lower motor neuron signs). Patients with ALS have brain stem and spinal cord atrophy with loss of motor neurons and associated extensive gliosis.

Painless, progressive weakness is the usual presenting sign and symptom of ALS. Usually focal in onset, weakness then spreads to contiguous muscle groups. Weakness is accompanied by muscle atrophy. Patients frequently experience muscle cramps because of

Table 23–22 ■ THE MAJOR ACQUIRED MOTOR NEURON DISEASES

Acute: anterior poliomyelitis
Chronic
- Sporadic amyotrophic lateral sclerosis (ALS)
- Postpoliomyelitis syndrome, motor neuron loss associated with spinocerebellar degeneration, multisystem atrophy, Creutzfeldt-Jakob disease

ALS-like syndromes
- Motor neuron disease with gammopathy or paraproteinemia, heavy metal intoxication, hexoseaminidase A deficiency, paraneoplastic motor neuronopathy

Primary lateral sclerosis (rare)

fasciculations. Spasticity is common, and patients may complain of spontaneous clonus.

ALS can present with bulbar dysfunction. Patients experience dysarthria. Dysphagia with choking is common. The absence of spontaneous swallowing results in sialorrhea, or drooling. Early in ALS, patients complain of dyspnea with exertion and frequently sigh at rest.

Several aspects of neurologic function are usually spared in ALS. These include mentation, extraocular movements, bowel and bladder function, and sensation.

The diagnosis of definite ALS is made when upper and lower motor neuron signs are present in the bulbar region and two other spinal regions or in three spinal regions. Nerve conduction studies with repetitive stimulation and EMG confirm lower motor neuron degeneration and exclude disorders of the neuromuscular junction, such as myasthenia gravis, and disorders of peripheral nerve and muscle. The EMG, neuroimaging, and clinical laboratory tests exclude the most common ALS-related disorders: polyradiculopathy with myelopathy, post-polio syndrome, multifocal motor neuropathy, motor neuron disease with paraproteinemia, heavy metal intoxication, hexoseaminidase A deficiency, paraneoplastic motor neuronopathy, and syringomyelia and syringobulbia.

The only drug currently available is riluzole. The average 5-year survival is 25%.

For more information about this subject, see *Cecil Textbook of Medicine,* 21st edition. Philadelphia, W.B. Saunders Company, 2000. Chapter 468, Motor Neuron Diseases, pages 2089 to 2092.

CEREBROVASCULAR DISEASES

Approximately 80% of strokes are caused by too little blood flow (ischemic stroke), and the remaining 20% are nearly equally divided between hemorrhage into brain tissue (parenchymatous hemorrhage) and hemorrhage into the surrounding subarachnoid space (subarachnoid hemorrhage). Stroke incidence has stabilized at approximately 0.5 to 1.0 per 1000 population. Stroke remains the third leading cause of medically related deaths and the second most frequent cause of neurologic morbidity in developed countries.

Cerebrovascular Anatomy

The brain is supplied by the left and right internal carotid and vertebral arteries (Fig. 23–2). Each common carotid artery bifurcates into an internal and external artery, in most persons just below the angle of the jaw. The *internal carotid artery* divides into the *anterior* and *middle cerebral arteries.* The internal carotid artery gives off the *ophthalmic, posterior communicating,* and *anterior choroidal arteries.* Branches of the external carotid artery include the *facial artery* and the *superficial temporal artery.*

The vertebral arteries usually arise from the subclavian arteries. The vertebral arteries ascend through the transverse foramina and exit at C1. The vertebral arteries unite at the medullopontine junction to form the *basilar artery.* The basilar artery bifurcates at the pontomesencephalic junction into the *posterior cerebral arteries.*

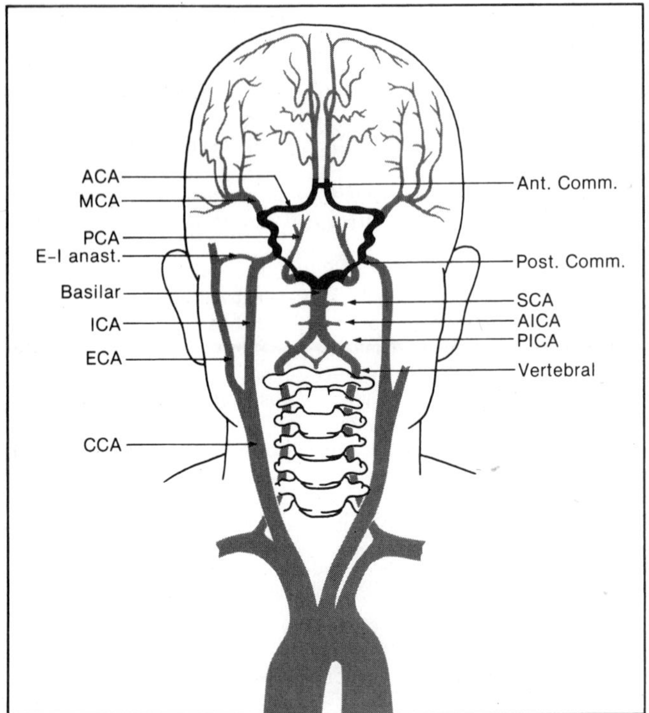

FIGURE 23–2 ■ Extracranial and intracranial arterial supply to the brain. Abbreviations for intracranial and extracranial arteries are as follows: ACA = anterior cerebral artery; MCA = middle cerebral artery; PCA = posterior cerebral artery; E-I anast. = extracranial-intracranial anastomosis; ICA = internal carotid artery; ECA = external carotid artery; CCA = common carotid artery; Ant. Comm. = anterior communicating artery; Post. Comm. = posterior communicating artery; SCA = superior cerebellar artery; AICA = anterior inferior cerebellar artery; PICA = posterior inferior cerebellar artery. (Modified from Lord R: Surgery of Occlusive Cerebrovascular Disease. St Louis, CV Mosby Company, 1986; with permission.)

Intracranial branches of the vertebral arteries include the *anterior spinal artery* and the *posterior inferior cerebellar arteries.*

The *circle of Willis* is formed by the union at the base of the brain of both anterior cerebral arteries via the *anterior communicating artery* and the middle cerebral arteries with the posterior cerebral arteries on each side via the *posterior communicating arteries.*

The *anterior cerebral arteries* supply the frontal poles, the superior surfaces of the cerebral hemispheres, and all of the medial surfaces of both cerebral hemispheres with the exception of the calcarine cortex. The *anterior choroidal artery* supplies the anterior hippocampus, uncus, amygdala, globus pallidus, tail of the caudate nucleus, lateral thalamus, geniculate body, and a large portion of the most inferoposterior limb of the internal capsule.

The *middle cerebral artery* is the vessel most frequently involved in ischemic stroke. The territory of the middle cerebral artery includes the major motor and sensory areas of the cortex, the areas for contraversive eye and head movement, the optic radiations, auditory sensory cortex, and, in the dominant hemisphere, the motor and sensory areas for language.

Posterior cerebral arteries supply the inferior surface of the temporal lobe and the occipital lobe. The brain stem is supplied by the *posterior inferior cerebellar* arteries, and by the *anterior inferior* and *superior cerebellar* arteries.

The veins in the brain, unlike those in many other parts of the body, do not accompany the arteries. Cortical veins drain into the superior sagittal sinus. Deeper structures drain into the inferior sagittal sinus and great cerebral vein (of Galen), which join at the straight sinus. The straight sinus joins the superior sagittal sinus. Each cavernous sinus communicates with its contralateral twin and surrounds the ipsilateral carotid artery; both drain posteriorly into the petrosal sinuses, which in turn drain into the sigmoid sinus.

Physiology

Unlike muscle or other tissues, the brain stores few glucose, glycogen, or other high-energy phosphate reserves but instead relies on a sizable and well-regulated blood flow to satisfy its immediate needs for energy. Cerebral blood flow (CBF) averages 60 mL/100 g of brain per minute.

Mechanical hyperventilation to a $PaCO_2$ of 20 to 25 mm Hg reduces CBF by approximately 40 to 45% and normal adult cerebral blood volume from 50 mL to approximately 35 mL. This 15-mL reduction often suffices to retard the progression of cerebral herniation.

At mean arterial pressures above 150 mm Hg, blood flow increases and capillary pressure rises, while at mean arterial pressures below 50 mm Hg, CBF falls. In patients with chronic hypertension, the upper and lower autoregulatory limits are shifted toward higher systemic pressures. Consequently, too rapid therapeutic reduction of blood pressure to apparently normal levels carries the risk of further lowering CBF in hypertensive patients with ongoing cerebral ischemia. Chronic treatment with antihypertensive agents readjusts the autoregulatory curve toward more normal values.

The blood-brain barrier protects the brain against the fluctuating composition of blood and minimizes the entry of potentially toxic compounds. Lipid-soluble compounds rapidly diffuse across, whereas polar compounds must be transported on special carrier molecules.

Pathophysiology and Pathology of Cerebral Ischemia

Cerebral hypoxia-ischemia can be divided into focal or multifocal ischemia from vascular occlusion, global ischemia from complete failure of cardiovascular pumping, and diffuse hypoperfusion hypoxia caused by respiratory disease or reduced perfusion pressure. Focal cerebral ischemia, resulting most frequently from embolic or thrombotic occlusion of extracranial or intracranial blood vessels, variably reduces blood flow within the involved vascular territory.

Focal cerebral ischemia sufficient to cause clinical signs or symptoms and lasting only 15 to 30 minutes causes irreversible injury to specific, highly vulnerable neurons. If the ischemia lasts an hour or longer, infarction of part or all of the involved vascular territory is inevitable.

Global cerebral ischemia, typically caused by cardiac asystole or ventricular fibrillation, reduces blood flow to zero throughout all of the brain. Global ischemia lasting more than 5 to 10 minutes is usually incompatible with recovery of consciousness in normothermic humans.

Diffuse cerebral hypoxia, uncomplicated by cerebral ischemia, is limited to conditions of mild to moderate hypoxemia. Pure cerebral hypoxia causes cerebral dysfunction but not irreversible brain injury. Persons with pure cerebral hypoxia from altitude sickness, pulmonary disease, or severe anemia present with confusion, cognitive impairment, and lethargy.

For more information about this subject, see *Cecil Textbook of Medicine,* 21st edition. Philadelphia, W.B. Saunders Company, 2000. Chapter 469, Cerebrovascular Diseases—Principles, pages 2092 to 2099.

ISCHEMIC CEREBROVASCULAR DISEASE

Stroke is defined as a neurologic deficit lasting more than 24 hours caused by reduced blood flow in a particular artery supplying the brain. The usual pathologic outcome is infarction. *Unstable strokes* are those in which symptoms and signs either improve or deteriorate after the onset. A *transient ischemic attack,* by contrast, is defined arbitrarily as a similar neurologic deficit lasting less than 24 hours. Nevertheless, most TIAs resolve within an hour. The relevant clinical distinction is whether the ischemia has caused brain damage.

The identification of patients with worsening signs and symptoms, frequently referred to as *progressing stroke* or *stroke in evolution,* is particularly important, since if the cause can be identified, treatment to limit brain damage may be possible. Progression of cerebral edema, which usually maximizes by 3 or 4 days, contributes to neurologic deterioration with large strokes but not with smaller ones. Bleeding into the infarct affects as many as 40% of patients but seldom causes new symptoms.

An important distinction is between a *complete* and an *incomplete stroke.* The terms refer to whether the affected vascular territory has been completely involved; if not, more brain remains at risk of additional focal ischemia, making treatment an urgent matter.

Clinical Manifestations and Vascular Syndromes (Table 23–23)

The carotid artery bifurcation and origin of the internal carotid artery provide the most frequent sites for atherothrombosis of cerebral blood vessels. Flow through the ophthalmic artery is often affected sufficiently to produce *transient monocular blindness* (also called amaurosis fugax).

Most ischemic strokes involve part or all of the territory of the middle cerebral artery, usually caused by emboli from the heart or extracranial carotid arteries. Emboli may occlude the main stem of

Table 23–23 ■ CLINICAL MANIFESTATIONS OF ISCHEMIC STROKE

OCCLUDED BLOOD VESSEL	CLINICAL MANIFESTATIONS
ICA	Ipsilateral blindness (variable) MCA syndrome (see below)
MCA	Contralateral hemiparesis, sensory loss (arm, face worst) Expressive aphasia (dominant) or anosognosia and spatial disorientation (non-dominant) Contralateral inferior quadrantanopsia
ACA	Contralateral hemiparesis, sensory loss (worst in leg)
PCA	Contralateral homonymous hemianopsia or superior quadrantanopsia Memory impairment
Basilar apex	Bilateral blindness Amnesia
Basilar artery	Contralateral hemiparesis, sensory loss Ipsilateral bulbar or cerebellar signs
Vertebral artery or PICA	Ipsilateral loss of facial sensation, ataxia, contralateral hemiparesis, sensory loss
Superior cerebellar artery	Gait ataxia, nausea, dizziness, headache progressing to ipsilateral hemiataxia, dysarthria, gaze paresis, contralateral hemiparesis, somnolence

ICA = internal carotid artery; MCA = middle cerebral artery; ACA = anterior cerebral artery; PCA = posterior cerebral artery; PICA = posterior inferior cerebellar artery.

the middle cerebral artery but more frequently produce distal occlusions of either the superior or inferior branch.

The superior cerebellar artery supplies most of the cerebellar cortex. Occlusion of this vessel is the most common cause of *cerebellar infarction,* characterized initially by gait ataxia, headache, nausea, vomiting, dizziness, ipsilateral clumsiness, and dysarthria.

Vertebrobasilar ischemia often produces multifocal lesions, scattered on both sides and along a considerable longitudinal extent of the brain stem. Basilar artery occlusion produces massive brain stem dysfunction. The *locked-in state* is one possible consequence; in this condition, paralysis of the limbs and most of the bulbar muscles means that the patient can communicate only by moving the eyes or eyelids to command.

Diagnosis

The history should emphasize the precise onset of the clinical deficit and the course since onset (stable or unstable). Preceding TIAs are more likely to be associated with an ischemic than a hemorrhagic stroke. Headache more often occurs with hemorrhage and embolus than with atherothrombotic ischemic stroke. The initial evaluation should include a thorough search for vascular disease risk factors.

The neurologic examination serves to localize the lesion site, but the general medical examination more frequently provides clues to pathogenesis. The arterial blood pressure in both arms, cardiac rhythm, and other cardiac abnormalities, such as murmurs or opening snaps, should be carefully recorded. The vascular examination should include gentle palpation of the carotid arteries and auscultation of their course in the neck. Ophthalmoscopy can detect retinal cholesterol or platelet-fibrin emboli, as well as evidence of chronic hypertensive or diabetic disease.

Hematologic tests include complete blood and platelet counts (to evaluate for polycythemia, thrombocytosis, bacterial endocarditis, and severe anemia). Blood should be taken to evaluate glucose, prothrombin time, partial thromboplastin time, and a lipid profile. In the elderly, determination of the ESR should be performed urgently to exclude giant cell arteritis. In the young, the presence of antiphospholipid antibodies helps to identify immune-related disease processes predisposing to stroke. Other blood tests (e.g., protein C, protein S, measurements of viscosity or platelet function, and tests for collagen-vascular diseases) may be indicated in younger patients who lack obvious causes for their strokes.

All stroke patients require a standard 12-lead ECG and a rhythm strip. Transthoratic echocardiography or, preferably, transesophageal echocardiography is useful in patients with focal stroke who (1) are young, (2) have no detectable atherothrombosis of the appropriate extracranial vessel, regardless of age; or (3) have no detectable risk factors. CT scanning cannot always detect cerebral infarction. Only about 5% of strokes are visible on CT scan within the first 12 hours. Detection increases to approximately 50% between 24 and 48 hours and approximately 90% by the end of 1 week.

Contrast-enhancing agents carry a small risk of neurotoxicity, and they may normalize the CT density of an otherwise small hypodense infarct, making the infarct less visible. Accordingly, one should use contrast-enhancing agents during the acute phase of the ischemic stroke only to seek out a mass lesion and only after a non-contrast scan has been obtained.

MRI is more sensitive than CT. If the diagnosis remains in doubt, MRI may be used after the acute phase to verify infarction.

Direct examination of the common, internal, and external carotid arteries is best achieved with duplex ultrasonography. Limitations include (1) access to only the portion of the carotid circulation that lies between the clavicles and mandible; (2) absorption of sound waves within a mural plaque, which may "shadow" and obscure a plaque on a distal vessel wall; and (3) echolucency of acute thrombi, which can be indistinguishable from flowing blood.

The direction and velocity of blood flow in the intracranial blood vessels originating from the circle of Willis can be examined with low-frequency pulsed transcranial Doppler. The intracranial blood vessels also can be examined on reconstructed CT or MRI images. An evolving technique involves the imaging of flowing blood using MRA.

Intracranial and extracranial cerebral angiography of elderly patients prone to ischemic stroke carries a 1 to 4% risk of producing a reversible neurologic deficit and a 0.5 to 1.0% risk of permanent neurologic deficits or death. Accordingly, angiography should be reserved for specific indications in which it may reveal abnormalities amenable to therapy. Digital subtraction arteriography permits use of smaller amounts of intravascular contrast material and may thus be of lower risk.

Differential Diagnosis

Deficits that evolve over weeks are usually caused by a brain mass, either a primary or metastatic brain tumor or brain abscess. Subdural hematoma should be distinguishable from stroke by the hematoma's more prolonged course and its combination of diffuse and focal dysfunction.

TIAs may be confused with classic or complicated migraine. Hemorrhagic stroke often enters the differential diagnosis for ischemic stroke, making the CT scan necessary. Other illnesses included in the differential diagnosis of vertebrobasilar ischemia include nonspecific dizziness, Meniere's disease, or peripheral vestibulopathy.

Causes and Pathogenesis

Atherosclerosis accounts for approximately two thirds of all ischemic strokes and an even greater proportion of those affecting patients over the age of 60 years (Table 23–24). Atherosclerosis causes strokes either by in situ stenosis or occlusion or by embolization of plaque thrombus material to distal cerebral vessels.

Cerebral emboli of a cardiac source may account for up to one third of all ischemic strokes. Mural ventricular thrombi, atrial thrombi, vegetations from acute or subacute infective endocarditis, nonbacterial endocarditis (in association with cancer), Libman-Sacks endocarditis (associated with systemic lupus erythematosus), and prosthetic heart valves carry a high risk of systemic (including cerebral) embolism. Cardiac myxomas embolize from either overlying thrombus or the tumor itself.

Atrial fibrillation, with or without valvular disease, strongly increases the risk of embolic ischemic stroke. The risk is highest shortly after development of atrial fibrillation. Embolism can also accompany therapeutic cardioversion.

Emboli of venous origin have long been known to cross a patent foramen ovale into the systemic circulation. Studies using bubble echocardiography have found that 40% of stroke patients under age 55 with a normal cardiac evaluation by history, physical examination, and ECG have a patent foramen ovale detected by bubble echocardiography.

CNS vasculitis, although a rare cause of stroke, is itself not uncommon and should enter the differential diagnosis whenever a young patient presents with a stroke or a patient of any age presents with a diffuse unexplained encephalopathy. Symptoms of CNS vasculitis include cognitive disturbances, headache, and seizures (encephalopathy). The diagnosis depends on the angiographic appearance of a "beadlike" segmental narrowing of cerebral blood vessels and/or the finding of characteristic inflammatory histopathology. Cerebral angiograms may appear normal in 20 to 30% of histologically positive cases. The diagnosis of CNS vasculitis is aided by the presence or absence of peripheral nervous system or systemic organ involvement and by identifying the underlying cause of the inflammation.

Table 23–24 ■ CAUSES OF ISCHEMIC STROKE

ATHEROSCLEROSIS

EMBOLI OF CARDIAC ORIGIN

Mural thrombus
- Myocardial infarction
- Cardiomyopathy

Valvular heart disease
- Rheumatic heart disease
- Bacterial endocarditis
- Nonbacterial endocarditis (carcinoma, Libman-Sacks disease)
- Mitral valve prolapse
- Prosthetic valve

Arrhythmia (atrial fibrillation)
Cardiac myxoma
Paradoxical emboli

VASCULITIDES

Primary central nervous system vasculitis
Systemic necrotizing vasculitis (polyarteritis nodosa, allergic angiitis)
Hypersensitivity vasculitis (serum sickness, drug-induced, cutaneous vasculitis)
Collagen-vascular diseases (rheumatoid arthritis, scleroderma, Sjögren's disease)
Giant cell arteritis (temporal arteritis, Takayasu's arteritis)
Wegener's granulomatosis
Lymphomatoid granulomatosis
Behçet's disease
Infectious vasculitis (neurovascular syphilis, Lyme disease, baterial and fungal meningitis, tuberculosis, acquired immunodeficiency syndrome, ophthalmic zoster, hepatitis B)

HEMATOLOGIC DISORDERS

Hemoglobinopathies (sickle cell, Hb SC)
Antiphospholipid antibodies (lupus anticoagulant, anticardiolipin antibody)
Hyperviscosity syndromes (polycythemia, thrombocytosis, leukocytosis, macroglobulinemia, multiple myeloma)
Secondary hypercoagulable states (carcinoma, pregnancy, puerperium)
Primary hypercoagulable states (Table 11–31)

DRUG-RELATED

Street drugs (cocaine, crack, amphetamines, lysergic acid diethylamide, phencyclidine, methylphenidate, sympathomimetics, heroin, pentazocine)
Alcohol
Oral contraceptives

OTHER

Fibromuscular dysplasia
Arterial dissection (trauma, spontaneous, Marfan syndrome)
Migraine
Subarachnoid hemorrhage or vasospasm
Other emboli (fat, bone marrow, air)
Moyamoya

Primary arteritis of the CNS, also called granulomatous arteritis of the CNS, causes headache and encephalopathy-like symptoms in young or middle-aged individuals. Temporal arteritis and Takayasu's arteritis are characterized by a granulomatous vasculitis of medium-sized and large arteries. Temporal arteritis affects predominantly patients over the age of 60, causing constitutional symptoms such as fever, malaise, weight loss, and headache. Biopsy of the superficial temporal artery provides the definitive diagnosis. Takayasu's arteritis primarily affects young women and mainly involves the aortic arch, the large brachiocephalic arteries derived from the arch, and the abdominal aorta.

Bacterial, fungal, and viral infections can induce CNS vasculitis and cerebral ischemia. Neurosyphilis and its meningovascular complications have increased considerably in recent years.

Among the hemoglobinopathies, sickle cell disease is by far the most common cause of stroke. Ischemic stroke occurs in approximately 15% of patients with Hb SS and in a much smaller percentage of those with sickle cell trait (Hb SA) or Hb SC.

Cellular hyperviscosity, associated with polycythemia, thrombocytosis, or leukocytosis of any cause, can reduce blood flow below threshold levels for cerebral dysfunction and injury. Hematocrits above 50%, white blood cell counts above 150,000/μL, and platelet counts in excess of 1 million/μL increase the risk of stroke.

Cancer, particularly the adenocarcinomas, pregnancy, and the puerperium have all been associated with a hypercoagulable state that predisposes to arterial and venous thrombosis. Approximately 25% of patients with macroglobulinemia experience some form of cerebral ischemia.

Disorders of proteins C and S are associated with ischemic vascular disease. Because of incomplete penetrance, the occurrence of thrombosis and stroke in the adult is extremely rare.

A strong epidemiologic association links a group of antiphospholipid antibodies to cerebral ischemia manifested clinically as atypical migraine, TIA, recurrent strokes, or ischemic encephalopathy. The syndrome usually affects patients younger than 50 years. The risk of ischemic and hemorrhagic stroke is increased from 4- to 13-fold among users of high-dose estrogen contraceptives. An extensive list of street drugs has also been associated with stroke.

Fibromuscular dysplasia affects the carotid and vertebral arteries, usually at the level of C2. It produces ischemic stroke both by the hemodynamic effects of stenosis and by thromboembolism. The condition is also associated with aneurysm formation and with arterial dissection. A dissecting aortic aneurysm can occlude major branches of the aorta supplying the cranial circulation and produce ischemic strokes.

Carotid artery dissections can sometimes be recognized clinically by intense ipsilateral pain. Angiography may be needed for diagnosis, but MRI is sometimes sufficient.

Reactive vascular narrowing (vasospasm) causes ischemic strokes in two settings. Vasospasm causes substantial disability in patients with subarachnoid hemorrhage. Vasospasm also presumably explains the ischemic strokes seen in a small number of patients with migraine headaches.

Fat emboli typically occur several days after trauma that includes fracture of long bones. Although focal ischemic strokes may occur, more typically the condition manifests with seizures and a diffuse encephalopathy consistent with disseminated embolization. Associated findings include petechiae and fat emboli visible on funduscopic examination.

Air emboli can occur with open heart surgery, in patients with pneumothorax, or in divers who ascend too rapidly to the surface. Air emoli cause altered mental status and seizures.

Moyamoya is a rare condition. Diagnosis requires demonstration of bilateral terminal internal carotid artery occlusion that involves the origins of the middle and anterior cerebral arteries. An abnormal vascular network develops at the base of the brain and is believed to provide collateral circulation. The abnormal collateral channels appear as a "smoky haze," hence the Japanese term *moyamoya*.

Prevention and Treatment of Stroke and Transient Ischemic Attacks

Patients clinically diagnosed as having acute cerebral ischemia should be admitted to the hospital unless the deficit has existed for several days and is stable (Table 23–25). Admission is also advised for patients with new-onset TIAs or those in whom TIAs are occurring with markedly increasing frequency or severity (crescendo TIAs).

ACUTE PHARMACOTHERAPY. Patients who present within 3 hours of onset of ischemic stroke and who meet specific inclusion and exclusion criteria (Table 23–26) should be considered for tissue plasminogen activator (tPA) in a dose of 0.9 mg/kg IV (maximum dose 90 mg), 10% as a bolus and the remaining 90% by infusion over 60 minutes. Anticoagulants and aspirin are contraindicated for the first 24 hours after tPA therapy. Despite a significant increase in intracerebral hemorrhage, mortality is unchanged and neurologic outcome is significantly improved at 3 months when such patients are treated with tPA.

For patients who present within 24 hours of symptom onset and who have signs of unstable or progressing atherothrombotic stroke, one approach is to give IV heparin. IV heparin is maintained for 3 to 7 days while a decision is made about long-term prophylactic therapy with either antiplatelet drugs or warfarin. Patients with stable, complete strokes or those admitted with new-onset or crescendo TIAs are often placed on aspirin therapy prophylactically at admission.

PREVENTION OF STROKE. The reduction of stroke risk factors, through therapy for hypertension, diabetes mellitus, smoking cessation, atherosclerosis, and cardiac arrhythmias (Table 23–27), is largely responsible for the marked decline in the incidence of stroke during the past 30 to 40 years. Strong evidence derived from meta-analyses supports the use of prophylactic aspirin to protect against strokes in patients with prior strokes or TIAs. Similarly, prophylactic antiplatelet therapy with ticlopidine or clopidogrel has also been shown to protect against such secondary events.

Endarterectomy significantly reduces ipsilateral stroke in patients with recent stroke or TIA and angiographically proven 70 to 99% ipsilateral carotid artery stenosis provided the rate of perioperative morbidity and mortality is less than 5 to 10%. Selected patients with symptomatic stenosis of 50 to 69% may benefit marginally

Table 23–25 ▪ EVALUATION OF ACUTE FOCAL NEUROLOGIC DYSFUNCTION

STABILIZE VITAL SIGNS

↓
- Establish and maintain airway
- Nasal O_2
- Repeat vital signs every 15 min
- Treat temperatures $>$ 100° F
- Record but do not treat BP $<$ 220/120
- Blood lab (CBC with differential and platelet count, electrolytes, glucose, BUN, PT, PTT, ESR)
- ECG with rhythm strip

RECORD HISTORY

↓
- Time of symptom onset and course?
- Anatomic localization?
- Headache or meningeal symptoms?
- Vascular risk factors?
- Medications or illicit drug use?

MEDICAL EXAMINATION

↓
- Cardiovascular examination (BP in both arms, cardiac murmurs and rhythm, auscultate neck for bruits, palpate peripheral pulses)
- Hematologic (examine integument for coagulopathies)
- General examination

NEUROLOGIC EXAMINATION

↓
- Anatomic localization
- Examine for head trauma, meningeal signs
- Ophthalmoscopy for retinal emboli, hypertension, papilledema

HEAD CT SCAN WITHOUT CONTRAST

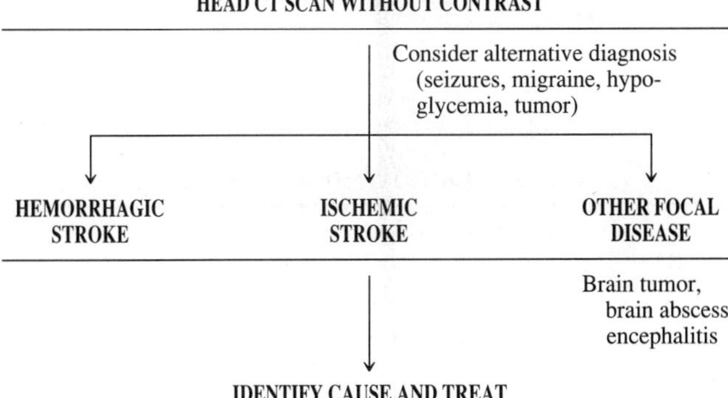

IDENTIFY CAUSE AND TREAT

(see Table 23–26).

BP = blood pressure; BUN = blood urea nitrogen; PT = prothrombin time; PTT = partial thromboplastin time; ESR = erythrocyte sedimentation rate; ECG = electrocardiogram; CT = computed tomography; CBC = complete blood count.

Table 23–26 ■ INCLUSION AND EXCLUSION CRITERIA FOR USE OF INTRAVENOUS TISSUE PLASMINOGEN ACTIVATOR IN STROKE

Inclusion Criteria

≥18 yrs of age
Clinical diagnosis of ischemic stroke
Persistent neurologic deficit
Baseline CT scan showing no evidence of intracranial hemorrhage
Initiation of tPA therapy within 3 hr of symptom onset

Exclusion Criteria

Rapidly improving or minor symptoms such as isolated ataxia or sensory symptoms
CT scan showing possible intracranial hemorrhage or large infarct (sulcal effacement, mass effect, edema)
History of seizure at stroke onset
Stroke or serious head trauma within 3 mo
History of intracranial hemorrhage, arteriovenous malformation, or aneurysm
Symptoms consistent with subarachnoid hemorrhage
Major surgery or serious trauma within 2 wk
Gastrointestinal or urinary tract hemorrhage within 3 wk
Systolic BP > 185 mm Hg; diastolic BP > 110 mm Hg; aggressive treatment required to lower BP below specified limits prior to tPA therapy
Glucose <50 mg/dL or >400 mg/dL
Arterial puncture at noncompressible site or lumbar puncture within 1 wk
Platelet count <100,000/mm^3
Heparin within 48 hr and associated with elevated aPTT
Oral anticoagulants associated with elevated PT > 15 sec or INR > 1.5
Pregnancy

tPA = tissue plasminogen activator; CT = computed tomography; BP = blood pressure; aPTT = activated partial thromboplastin time; PT = prothrombin time; INR = international normalized ratio.

Table 23–27 ■ PREVENTION OF STROKE

Treatment of hypertension and diabetes mellitus
Smoking cessation
Limited alcohol intake
Control of diet and obesity
Thoughtful use of oral contraceptives
Antiplatelet drugs or anticoagulants for atrial fibrillation and selected acute myocardial infarctions
Antiplatelet drugs for symptomatic carotid or vertebrobasilar atherosclerosis
Endarterectomy for symptomatic carotid artery stenosis of 70–99% in selected patients with perioperative morbidity or mortality risk of <5–10%
Endarterectomy for symptomatic carotid artery stenosis of 50–69% in selected patients with perioperative morbidity or mortality risk of <6%
Endarterectomy for asymptomatic carotid artery stenosis of >60% in selected patients with perioperative morbidity or mortality risk of <3%

from endarterectomy if the perioperative morbidity rate is below 6%. Patients with less than 50% stenosis are best treated medically. Endarterectomy significantly reduces ipsilateral stroke in patients with asymptomatic carotid artery stenosis of 60% or higher if perioperative morbidity and mortality rates are less than 3%.

Venous Stroke

The most dangerous form of venous disease arises when the superior sagittal sinus is occluded, but obstruction of a transverse sinus or one of the major veins over the cerebral convexity also can produce significant damage. Venous occlusions occur most commonly in association with coagulopathies, often in the puerperal period or in patients with disseminated cancer, and sometimes as a result of contiguous disease, such as infection or cancer. Superior sagittal sinus obstruction can result in bilateral weakness and sensory changes in the legs. The differential diagnosis of venous obstruction can include traditional arterial strokes but more often extends to diffuse processes such as herpes simplex encephalitis and meningitis. Management relies on heparin.

Diffuse Ischemia

Brief diffuse cerebral ischemia causes syncope without permanent sequelae. By contrast, prolonged diffuse ischemia has devastating consequences. The most common cause is cardiac asystole or other forms of overwhelming cardiopulmonary failure. Other than prompt and aggressive efforts to restore cardiovascular circulation, no treatments have been found to help patients who are comatose after cardiac arrest.

For more information about this subject, see *Cecil Textbook of Medicine,* 21st edition. Philadelphia, W.B. Saunders Company, 2000. Chapter 470, Ischemic Cerebrovascular Disease, pages 2099 to 2109.

HEMORRHAGIC CEREBROVASCULAR DISEASE

Approximately 20% of all strokes consist of intracranial hemorrhages, half into the subarachnoid space and half within the brain itself. The acute rise in ICP from arterial rupture causes loss of consciousness in about half of patients, and many of these die of cerebral herniation. However, patients who survive often show remarkable recovery.

Subarachnoid hemorrhage (SAH) is caused by rupture of surface arteries (aneurysms, vascular malformations, head trauma), with blood usually limited to the CSF space (Table 23–28). Intracerebral hemorrhage is most frequently caused by the rupture of arteries lying deep within the brain substance (hypertensive hemorrhage, vascular malformations, head trauma). Blood within the cerebral ventricles results either from reflux of subarachnoid blood through the fourth ventricular foramena or by extension from a site of intraparenchymal hemorrhage.

Rupture of a saccular or berry aneurysm causes approximately 80% of all SAHs; 5% are caused by mycotic aneurysm rupture, and an even smaller percentage reflects bleeding from atherosclerotic, neoplastic, or dissecting cerebral aneurysms. The patho-

Table 23–28 ■ CAUSES OF SPONTANEOUS INTRACRANIAL HEMORRHAGE

Arterial aneurysms
Berry aneurysm
Fusiform aneurysm
Mycotic aneurysm
Aneurysm with vasculitis
Cerebrovascular malformations
Hypertensive-atherosclerotic hemorrhage
Hemorrhage into brain tumor
Systemic bleeding diatheses
Hemorrhage with vasculopathies
Hemorrhage with intracranial venous infarction

genesis of saccular aneurysms reflects a combination of congenital, acquired, and hereditary factors. Microaneurysmal dilations (<2 mm) of the circle of Willis arteries occur in 15 to 20% of the population. Larger (>5 mm) aneurysms are found in 5% of the population, characteristically distributed at the arterial bifurcations. Fusiform or ectatic aneurysms develop most frequently in the basilar artery but also may affect the internal, middle, and anterior cerebral arteries. They rarely rupture and are difficult to treat when they do because their shape and stiff walls preclude easy surgical clipping. Mycotic cerebral aneurysms are caused by septic degeneration of arterial wall muscle and elastic tissue. They form in distal cerebral arteries at the point where small septic cardiogenic emboli lodge. They are frequently multiple.

Clinical Presentation

Focal headaches occasionally signal compression of pain-sensitive structures from an expanding aneurysm. "Sentinel" leaks cause sudden, focal head pain and may be accompanied by nausea or vomiting or may cause meningeal irritation.

Compression syndromes from cerebral aneurysms include compression of the oculomotor nerve, amnesia combined with varying degrees of third cranial nerve paresis, and quadriparesis from large, strategically placed, basilar-tip aneurysms. Giant aneurysms cause unilateral ophthalmoplegia and orbital pain.

Rupture of saccular aneurysms into the subarachnoid space seldom is associated with focal signs or symptoms. Nearly half of patients so affected lose consciousness, at least transiently, as ICP exceeds cerebral perfusion pressure. Patients commonly recall the sudden onset as producing the "most excruciating headache" of their life.

SAH causes meningeal irritation, nuchal rigidity, and photophobia. Subhyaloid retinal hemorrhages occur in 20 to 30% of patients. Blood pressure is frequently elevated, and body temperature usually rises.

CT scans reveal subarachnoid blood within the basal cisterns in about three fourths of patients within 48 hours of bleeding. A contrast-enhanced CT scan may aid in the identification of an arteriovenous malformation.

If the CT scan fails to show blood, a lumbar puncture is diagnostic. A traumatic lumbar puncture usually can be distinguished from SAH by the failure of the latter to show a decrease in the red blood cell count between the first and last tubes of the CSF. The CSF pressure is usually elevated and may remain so for many days.

Cerebral angiography remains the definitive study to detect the source of SAH. Because as many as 33% of patients with aneurysmal SAHs harbor multiple cerebral aneurysms, both carotid and vertebral arteries should be examined. Cerebral angiography fails to detect the source of bleeding in 10 to 20% of cases. Such patients are thought to have a better prognosis. Cerebral angiography is recommended immediately in patients who have septic endocarditis and SAHs to search for possible mycotic aneurysms. The presence of back pain or spinal cord symptoms at onset should prompt a search for a spinal source of hemorrhage. Repeat cerebral angiography is indicated 3 to 4 weeks later when the initial angiogram is negative and no other clues to the bleeding site can be found.

The medical complications of SAH include cardiac myonecrosis and arrhythmias attributed to abnormal levels of circulating epinephrine. Symptomatic hyponatremia may also develop from secretion of atrial natriuretic factor by the heart leading to salt and water wasting.

Late neurologic complications include rebleeding from the same aneurysm, cerebral vasospasm and its ischemic consequences, hydrocephalus caused by blockage of CSF outflow pathways, and occasionally seizures. Approximately 30% of patients with aneurysmal SAH rebleed during the first month.

Cerebral vasospasm as diagnosed by cerebral angiography has been reported in up to 75% of patients with SAH, 50% of whom have strokelike neurologic signs and symptoms. The peak onset for vasospasm is between days 3 and 14. Communicating hydrocephalus may develop as early as the first or second week after SAH.

Treatment

The definitive therapy for a ruptured saccular aneurysm consists of surgical clipping of the aneurysm to prevent rebleeding. Medical therapy aims to reduce the risk of rebleeding and cerebral vasospasm and to prevent other medical complications before and after surgical intervention. Hypertension should be treated, but not aggressively. Systolic pressures of 160 to 170 mm Hg and diastolic pressures of 90 to 100 mm Hg are acceptable. Nimodipine should be given in a dosage of 60 mg PO every 4 hours for 21 days. Although it does not reduce the frequency of vasospasm, nimodipine lowers by one third the incidence of cerebral infarction in patients suffering SAH and cerebral vasospasm.

Because the incidence of aneurysmal rebleeding is highest during the first 2 weeks after SAH and the mortality rate associated with each hemorrhage approaches 40 to 50%, the aneurysm should be clipped as soon as possible. Nevertheless, undertaking aneurysmal surgery in the presence of active vasospasm has consistently been associated with poor neurologic outcomes. As a result, most surgeons avoid operating during days 3 to 10, when maximal cerebral vasospasm is likely.

Unruptured mycotic aneurysms should be treated with antibiotics appropriate for the infecting organism and followed angiographically. Single aneurysms and those in surgically accessible areas should be considered for prompt surgical clipping.

Unruptured cerebral aneurysms detected incidentally during cerebral angiography bleed at a yearly rate of 1 to 3%. Saccular aneurysms less than 5 mm should be followed carefully, aneurysms between 5 and 10 mm can be considered for surgical clipping, and those larger than 10 mm should be clipped at the earliest convenience.

Hemorrhage from Vascular Malformations

ARTERIOVENOUS MALFORMATIONS. The most common symptomatic vascular anomaly is the arteriovenous malformation (AVM). AVMs can be located anywhere in the brain and can produce headaches, seizures, focal neurologic deficits, and intracranial hemorrhage. Most AVMs manifest with intracranial hemorrhage, while a lower proportion cause seizures or progressive neurologic disability. The initial hemorrhage tends to occur during the second through fourth decades, with the risk of rebleeding averaging approximately 6 to 7% the first year, 2% after 5 years, and 1 to 2% thereafter. AVMs can bleed into the subarachnoid space, into the brain parenchyma, or into the ventricular system.

Approximately 30% of patients who harbor an AVM have seizures, of which about 50% have a focal onset. Focal neurologic deficits independent of seizures also develop, resulting from vascular thrombosis and brain tissue hypoperfusion caused by either vascular compression or a steal syndrome. AVM-associated headaches closely resemble migraine.

CT scanning with contrast is diagnostic in approximately 85% of patients. MRI is equally, if not more, effective in diagnosis. Angiography remains the definitive test. Because approximately 10% of AVMs are associated with saccular aneurysms, four-vessel angiography is indicated even if the AVM is defined by unilateral carotid injection.

Large cerebral hemorrhages usually produce catastrophic, acute syndromes. The onset is often associated with physical (or emotional) activity. Common early features include alterations in consciousness, headache, nausea, and vomiting. Hemorrhages also can produce less severe dysfunction which may be indistinguishable clinically from ischemic stroke. Clinical evolution over hours is common and is usually attributed to secondary brain swelling.

Patients with massive hemorrhages of the putamen become lethargic or comatose within minutes to hours of onset and concurrently experience contralateral weakness (including that of the face) and a contralateral hemianopsia and gaze paresis (with eyes deviated toward the hemorrhage). Some patients with thalamic hemorrhages lose consciousness early in the clinical course, but those who are awake often experience hemiparesis, sensory changes, and homonymous hemianopsia.

Pontine hemorrhage usually causes coma. In a coma, small reactive pupils are common, oculovestibular responses are lost early, and vomiting often occurs at onset. Patients usually have quadriplegia and bilateral extensor posturing.

Cerebellar hemorrhage initially spares the brain stem, so consciousness is usually preserved in the early stages. Occipital headache is usually the first symptom, followed by unsteady gait, clumsiness, nausea, and vomiting, which may be severe and repetitive. Motor weakness is seldom prominent at onset. Deterioration can result from extension into or compression of the brain stem, herniation of cerebellar tissue, or hydrocephalus.

Non-contrast CT scans demonstrate areas of hemorrhage as zones of increased density. One advantage of MRI is its ability to detect small hemorrhages, especially in the brain stem. Hypertension should be controlled. AVMs that manifest with either seizure or headache may be treated conservatively. In other cases, interventional therapeutic options include surgical resection of the AVM, embolization of the feeding arteries, and radiation-induced thrombosis.

OTHER VASCULAR MALFORMATIONS. *Venous angiomas,* the most common cerebrovascular malformations, are composed entirely of veins and usually lie close to the brain's surface. Hemorrhage from a venous angioma is uncommon and rarely fatal.

Telangiectasias are uncommon vascular anomalies usually located deep in the brain and rarely producing symptoms. Hemorrhage from these small vessels can occasionally be fatal.

Cavernous angiomas are large sinusoidal channels served by large feeding arteries and veins. Many of the channels thrombose. They are readily detected by CT scan and rarely bleed, but they can cause headaches and seizures.

Focal Cerebral Hemorrhage

Focal hemorrhage occurs spontaneously in three common settings: hypertension, ruptured AVMs, and amyloid angiopathy. Additional contributing causes are excessive anticoagulation, systemic bleeding diatheses, and trauma.

Hypertension can produce hemorrhages throughout the brain, but hemorrhage usually occurs in four central locations: external capsule–putamen, internal capsule–thalamus, central pons, and cerebellum. Bleeding producing central hemorrhages is believed to result from rupture of microaneurysms in small, intracerebral arteries (50 to 150 μm in diameter).

Amyloid angiopathy is a pathologic diagnosis increasingly encountered in the elderly. Unrelated to generalized amyloidosis and occasionally hereditary, the condition often appears in the brains of patients with Alzheimer's disease and has been associated with non-hypertensive hemorrhages.

Anticoagulation, fibrinolysis, and other hematologic abnormalities can be associated with intracerebral hemorrhages. Warfarin anticoagulation has been implicated in about 10% of primary intracerebral hemorrhages. Cerebral hemorrhages occur in leukemia, polycythemia, hemophilia, and other clotting abnormalities, and they also occur in patients using amphetamines and cocaine. Trauma also causes intracerebral (as well as subarachnoid) hemorrhage.

Management is supportive, but vigilance for transtentorial or foramen magnum herniation must be exercised. Blood pressure should not be lowered precipitously. Direct surgical evaluation seldom is justified. With the cerebellum, lateral ventricular shunting appears to produce results as good as or better (fewer neurologic residua) than surgical removal of hematomas, although lesions more than 3 cm in diameter that continue to compress the brain stem after the shunt is placed occasionally benefit from evacuation.

The prognosis with intraparenchymal hemorrhage is surprisingly good in patients who survive the acute illness, but about 20% of patients who survive hemorrhage require institutionalization. Epidemiologic data strongly suggest that control of hypertension reduces the risk of hypertensive intraparenchymal hemorrhage.

For more information about this subject, see *Cecil Textbook of Medicine,* 21st edition. Philadelphia, W.B. Saunders Company, 2000. Chapter 471, Hemorrhagic Cerebrovascular Disease, pages 2109 to 2115.

INFECTIONS AND INFLAMMATORY DISORDERS OF THE NERVOUS SYSTEM

Parameningeal Infections

Parameningeal CNS infections include those that affect brain parenchyma directly (brain abscess), those that produce suppuration in potential spaces covering the brain and spinal cord (epidural abscess and subdural empyema), those that produce occlusion of the contiguous venous sinuses and cerebral veins (cerebral venous sinus thrombosis), and remote infectious processes (bacterial endocarditis and sepsis) that result in diffuse, multifactorial involvement of the CNS.

Brain Abscess

Brain abscess is an uncommon disorder, accounting for only 2% of intracranial mass lesions (Table 23–29). The most commonly isolated pathogens are aerobic and microaerobic streptococci and gram-negative anaerobes such as *Bacteroides* and *Prevotella* spe-

Table 23–29 ■ BRAIN ABSCESS: PRESENTING FEATURES IN 43 CASES

Headache	72%
Lethargy	71%
Fever	60%
Nuchal rigidity	49%
Nausea, vomiting	35%
Seizures	35%
Ocular palsy	27%
Confusion	26%
Visual disturbance	21%
Weakness	21%
Dysarthria	12%
Stupor	12%
Papilledema	10%
Dysphasia	9%
Hemiparesis	9%
Dizziness	7%

From Chan CH, Johnson JD, Hofstetter M, et al: Brain abscess: A study of 45 consecutive cases. Medicine (Baltimore) 65:415, 1986. © 1986, The Williams & Wilkins Company, Baltimore.

cies. Less commonly, gram-negative aerobes and *Staphylococcus* spp. are isolated.

CSF examination is not useful in diagnosis because the findings range from normal to those of purulent meningitis, depending on the walling off of the brain abscess or its closeness to CSF compartments.

Pyogenic brain abscesses are treated with antibiotics combined with surgical aspiration or excision. Aspiration offers the advantage of identifying the infecting organism and may be performed stereotactically with CT guidance while the patient is under local anesthesia.

Spinal Epidural Abscess

Infection within the epidural space about the spinal cord is an uncommon but readily diagnosable and treatable potential cause of paralysis and death.

Patients are usually systemically ill with fever (to 38° to 39° C). The initial feature is acute or subacute neck or back pain, with focal percussion tenderness a prominent sign in the great majority; stiff neck and headache are common. As the infection progresses over hours, days, or weeks, radicular pain occurs.

The differential diagnosis includes compressive and inflammatory processes involving the spinal cord (transverse myelitis, intervertebral disk herniation, epidural hemorrhage, metastatic tumor).

Venous Sinus Thrombosis Secondary to Infection

SEPTIC CAVERNOUS SINUS THROMBOSIS. Presenting symptoms are headache or lateralized facial pain, followed in a few days to weeks by fever, and involvement of the orbit, producing proptosis and chemosis secondary to obstruction of the ophthalmic vein.

LATERAL SINUS THROMBOSIS. The symptoms consist of ear pain followed by headache, nausea, vomiting, and vertigo, evolving over several weeks. On examination, most patients are febrile. Mastoid swelling may be seen. Sixth cranial nerve palsies can occur.

SEPTIC SAGITTAL SINUS THROMBOSIS. This uncommon condition occurs as a consequence of purulent meningitis, infections of the ethmoidal or maxillary sinuses spreading via venous channels, compound infected skull fractures, or rarely, neurosurgical wound infections. Symptoms include manifestations of elevated ICP (headache, nausea, and vomiting) that evolve rapidly to stupor and coma. Neurologic complications of infectious endocarditis occur in one third of patients with bacterial endocarditis and triple the general mortality rate of the disease.

SUBDURAL EMPYEMA. Subdural empyema is responsible for one fifth of localized intracranial infections and results from direct or indirect extension from infected paranasal sinuses. Symptoms initially reflect those of chronic otitis or sinusitis, as well as lateralized headache (a universal feature), fever, and obtundation.

CRANIAL EPIDURAL ABSCESS. Infections of the epidural space coexist most often with subdural empyema and less frequently with chronic sinusitis or otitis alone. The diagnosis is made with MRI or contrast-enhanced CT scan.

Neurosyphilis

CLINICAL SYNDROMES. The clinical manifestations of neurosyphilis are divided into acute syphilitic meningitis, cerebrovascular syphilis, syphilitic dementia (general paresis), and tabes dorsalis. These entities may overlap clinically, however, and two syndromes may coexist, as in taboparesis. These clinical subtypes of neurosyphilis each develop in a predictable time frame after the primary infection (Fig. 23–3).

CEREBROSPINAL FLUID EXAMINATION. A chronic inflammatory response in the CSF (Table 23–30) accompanies each of the clinical syndromes of neurosyphilis; this leukocytosis, in conjunction with a positive syphilis serologic result on the CSF, both establishes the diagnosis of active neurosyphilis and monitors the response to therapy.

Acute Viral Meningitis and Encephalitis

The term *viral meningitis* refers to infection of the leptomeninges, *viral encephalitis* refers to infection of the brain parenchyma, and *viral meningoencephalitis* is sometimes used when both meninges and brain parenchyma appear to be infected, although viral encephalitis is almost always accompanied by meningeal inflammation.

Many viruses can cause acute encephalitis or meningitis; others may result in subacute or chronic encephalitis. Enteroviruses are the most common cause of aseptic meningitis.

Viral meningitis and encephalitis are relatively common disorders. In one study in Rochester, Minnesota, for example, the incidence of aseptic meningitis was nearly 11 per 100,000 person-years, and that of viral encephalitis was more than 7 per 100,000 person-years.

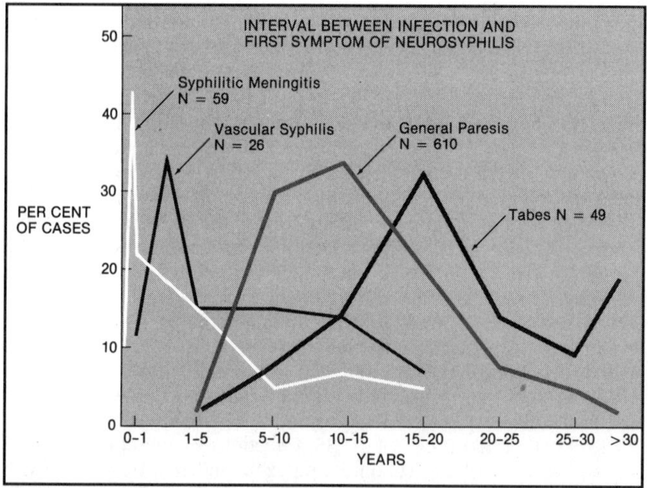

FIGURE 23–3 ■ Interval between primary and symptomatic neurosyphilis by type (meningeal, vascular, paretic, tabetic), abstracted from the literature and presented as percentage of total cases within type. (From Simon RP: Neurosyphilis, Arch Neurol 42:606, 1985. Copyright 1985, American Medical Association.)

Table 23–30 ■ CEREBROSPINAL FLUID (CSF) FINDINGS IN VARIOUS NEUROSYPHILITIC SYNDROMES

SYNDROME	OPENING PRESSURE (mm H_2O)	WBC COUNT (mm^3)	GLUCOSE (mg/dL)	PROTEIN (mg/dL)	GAMMA GLOBULIN*	VDRL	
						Blood	CSF
Meningitis	170	154 (94% L)	29	95		1:64	1:4
Cerebrovascular	192	58 (87% L)	41	119	IgG index 0.93	1:512	1:16
Paresis		220	49	305	IgG index 1.99	1:128	1:8
Tabes dorsalis (active)		62		140		1:15	1:28
Tabes dorsalis (inactive)		2	76	43		1:16	1:2

*Normal IgG index = 0.23 to 0.64.

WBC = white blood cell; VDRL = Veneral Disease Research Laboratory; L = lymphocytes; IgG = immunoglobulin G.

From Simon RP, Bayne LL: Neurosyphilis. *In* Martin J, Tyler K (eds): Infections of the Central Nervous System (Contemporary Neurology Series, Vol. 41). Philadelphia, FA Davis, 1993, pp. 237–256.

Poliomyelitis

Poliomyelitis selectively destroys the motor neurons of the spinal cord and brain stem, resulting in flaccid asymmetrical weakness. Until recently one of the most feared of all human infectious diseases, poliomyelitis is now almost entirely preventable by vaccination.

Acute poliomyelitis is separated into two distinct phases: "minor illness" and "major illness." The minor illness coincides with viremia and consists of fever, headache, and sore throat, which resolve within 1 to 2 days. In some patients, this is followed by the major illness, which is characterized by abrupt onset of fever, headache, vomiting, and meningismus. CSF pleocytosis is present at this stage. The symptoms of aseptic meningitis resolve within 5 to 10 days. Asymmetrical muscle weakness is the hallmark of the illness. It is typically preceded by intense myalgia. About 50% of patients develop acute urinary retention. The motor deficit rarely progresses for more than 3 to 5 days.

Rabies

Rabies is a viral infection with nearly worldwide distribution that affects principally wild and domestic animals; however, it also involves humans, in which case it results in devastating, almost invariably fatal encephalitis.

After an incubation period averaging 1 to 2 months, clinical rabies usually begins with a prodromal phase of nonspecific symptoms of malaise, fever, and headache, but more specific local symptoms are present at the site of the original bite. These include itching, paresthesia, or other sensations that begin in the area of the healed wound and then spread to a wider region, reflecting ganglioneuritis.

Within a few days, the full-blown illness begins, taking one of two forms: encephalitic (*furious*) or paralytic (*dumb*) rabies, perhaps depending on the source and strain of the infecting virus. In its initial phase, encephalitic rabies is often distinguished from other viral infections by irritability and hyperactivity of a number of automatic reflexes. Hydrophobia, with reflexive intense contraction of the diaphragm and accessory respiratory and other muscles, is induced on attempts to drink, or even by the mere sight of water.

Rabies is usually suspected on the basis of a history of animal bite or other exposure. But in as many as one third of cases, no such history is obtained. Definitive antemortem diagnosis is established by immunohistochemical identification of rabies virus antigen in hair follicle nerve endings of biopsied skin, usually obtained from the nape of the neck.

TREATMENT AND PREVENTION. Established CNS disease cannot be cured. The first step in management is to administer prompt local wound care, thoroughly washing the wound with soap and water, then applying iodine or 70% ethanol. In the absence of previous vaccination, both passive (rabies immune globulin of human origin) and active (diploid cell vaccines) immunizations are administered. Rabies immune globulin should be injected in and around the wound and should not be administered into the same limb in which the vaccine is given.

PROGRESSIVE MULTIFOCAL LEUKOENCEPHALOPATHY

Progressive multifocal leukoencephalopathy (PML) was demonstrated to be associated with infection of oligodendrocytes by JC virus, a papovavirus widely distributed among humans. JC virus exhibits a neurotropism exclusive to glial cells. PML was the first demyelinating disease to be unequivocally associated with a viral infection.

The clinical hallmark of PML is the presence of focal neurologic symptoms and signs associated with radiographic evidence of white matter disease in the absence of mass effect. The most common initial symptoms include weakness, speech abnormalities, and cognitive disturbances, each seen in approximately 40% of patients. Gait disturbances, sensory loss, and visual impairment occur in approximately 20 to 30%. Seizures and brain stem symptoms are less common.

The diagnosis of PML may be strongly suggested by the clinical manifestations and the radiographic imaging result. When the former are coupled with a positive JC viral polymerase chain reaction (PCR) finding in the CSF, the diagnosis of PML is virtually certain. However, unequivocal confirmation requires brain biopsy.

PML usually progresses to death with a mean survival of 6 months.

PRION DISEASES

Several human diseases have been attributed to a unique infectious protein referred to as the *prion.* The prototypical human illness is Creutzfeldt-Jakob disease (CJD), subacute spongiform encephalopathy. Other prion illnesses of humans include kuru, Gerstmann-Straussler-Scheinker syndrome, and familial fatal insomnia. Prion-related illnesses are unique in that they may be hereditary, may occur spontaneously, or may be acquired by contamination by the agent.

The clinical manifestations of CJD are protean. Prodromal symptoms are reported in as many as one fourth of patients. These symptoms include altered sleep patterns and appetite, weight loss, changes in sexual drive, and complaints of impaired memory and concentration. Typically, the patient has a rapidly progressive dementia associated with myoclonus. The dementia is generally global in nature. Myoclonus occurs in approximately 90% of patients. Visual abnormalities, cerebellar ataxia, and pyramidal and extrapyramidal manifestations are observed.

The clinical tetrad supporting the diagnosis of CJD consists of a subacute progressive dementia, myoclonus, typical periodic complexes indicated on EEG, and a normal CSF result.

The result of gross pathologic examination shows brain atrophy. The pathologic hallmarks are generally maximal in the cortex but are also seen in basal ganglia, thalamus, and cerebellum.

Although the illness is not communicable in the conventional sense, there is a risk of handling materials contaminated with the prion protein.

REYE'S SYNDROME

Reye's syndrome is a form of hepatic encephalopathy with fatty infiltration of the liver, markedly raised ICP, and brain edema. The illness follows one of several common viruses or hepatotoxicity from commonly used drugs.

Reye's syndrome appears to be due to an abnormality of mitochondrial fatty acid metabolism. Reye's syndrome usually follows a viral infection. The syndrome most commonly follows influenza A, influenza B, or varicella-zoster. Epidemiologic studies strongly support a link between the use of aspirin and Reye's syndrome.

Reye's syndrome is a biphasic disorder. As symptoms of the initial viral illness begin to improve, intractable vomiting appears in association with lethargy or delirium. Signs of CNS deterioration include the development of generalized seizures, deepening obtundation, and transtentorial herniation. The CSF is under increased pressure but is acellular, with otherwise normal constituents.

TREATMENT. Hypoglycemia and electrolyte abnormalities must be corrected. Appropriate measures should be taken to monitor ICP continuously in more severely affected patients, as judicious control of intracranial hypertension contributes to a favorable outcome. Mortality is about 10%.

For more information about this subject, see *Cecil Textbook of Medicine,* 21st edition. Philadelphia, W.B. Saunders Company, 2000. Chapter 472, Infections and Inflammatory Disorders of the Nervous System, pages 2116 to 2141.

THE DEMYELINATING DISEASES

Multiple Sclerosis and Related Conditions

Multiple Sclerosis

Multiple sclerosis (MS) is a disorder of unknown cause, defined clinically by typical symptoms, signs, and disease progression, and characterized pathologically by scattered areas of inflammation, demyelination, and axonal injury affecting the brain, optic nerves, and spinal cord.

CEREBROSPINAL FLUID. Immune activation within the CNS is a cardinal feature of MS. Increased CSF immunoglobulin levels, reflecting the presence of intrathecal humoral immune activation, appear in 80 to 90% of MS patients. CSF gamma-globulin normally represents less than 13% of total CSF protein, but in MS patients the proportion often rises much higher. Discrete "oligoclonal" bands can be detected in 70 to 80% of patients.

In the presence of slight mononuclear pleocytosis and normal protein levels, the presence of oligoclonal bands, selectively increased IgG levels, and free κ light chains provide strong support for the diagnosis of MS.

IMAGING PROCEDURES. CT brain scans sometimes reveal hypodense regions in white matter, but the imaging modality is relatively insensitive. Head MRI scans show abnormalities in more than 85% of patients with clinically definite MS. Typical lesions are multifocal, appear hyperintense on intermediate and T2-weighted MRI, and occur predominantly in the periventricular cere-

Table 23–31 ■ CONDITIONS COMMONLY MISTAKEN FOR MULTIPLE SCLEROSIS

Vascular diseases
Small vessel cerebrovascular disease
Vasculitis
Structural lesions
Craniocervical junction tumor, malformation of base of skull
Anomaly
Posterior fossa tumor or arteriovenous malformation
Spinal cord tumor or cervical spondylosis
Degenerative diseases
Motor system disease
Spinocerebellar degeneration
Infections
HTLV-1 infection
HIV myelopathy or HIV-related cerebritis
Lyme disease
Other conditions
Vitamin B_{12} deficiency
Sjögren's syndrome
Sarcoidosis
Nonspecific MRI abnormalities

HTLV-1 = human T-cell lymphotropic virus type 1; HIV = human immunodeficiency virus; MRI = magnetic resonance imaging.

bral white matter, corpus callosum, cerebellum, cerebellar peduncles, brain stem, and spinal cord.

CLINICAL MANIFESTATIONS. Clinical errors confound the diagnosis of MS. Most commonly this occurs in a patient with clear neurologic disease who has an alternative diagnosis (Table 23–31).

TREATMENT. For major clinical exacerbations, methylprednisolone, 500 or 1000 mg/day IV for 3 days, can be administered safely in an outpatient setting, followed by prednisone 60 mg in a single morning dose for 3 days, tapering off over 12 days.

IMMUNOMODULATORY THERAPY. Two forms of recombinant interferon (IFN-β), interferon β-1a (Avonex) and interferon β-1b (Betaseron), have been approved for use in relapsing remitting MS patients. Betaseron is administered at a dose of 8 million IU SC every other day, whereas Avonex is administered at a dose of 6 million IU/week IM.

CENTRAL NERVOUS SYSTEM COMPLICATIONS OF VIRAL INFECTIONS AND VACCINES

Several reasonably distinct patterns of CNS complications of viral infections and vaccines have been delineated. Two of these, *acute disseminated encephalomyelitis* (Table 23–32) and *acute necrotizing hemorrhagic encephalopathy,* appear to be mediated by immune mechanisms and have a peripheral nervous system counterpart, acute inflammatory polyneuropathy, or the Guillain-Barré syndrome. The third includes Reye's syndrome, acute toxic en-

Table 23–32 ■ CARDINAL FEATURES OF ACUTE DISSEMINATED ENCEPHALOMYELITIS

Preceding event, usually viral illness
Latent period followed by acute onset of multifocal or diffuse CNS signs
Potential for full recovery
Pathologic features of perivascular inflammation and demyelination; vessel damage and hemorrhage variable

cephalopathy, and acute cerebellar ataxia of childhood, which are likely to be toxic in origin.

For more information about this subject, see *Cecil Textbook of Medicine,* 21st edition. Philadelphia, W.B. Saunders Company, 2000. Chapter 482, Multiple Sclerosis and Related Conditions; and Chapter 483, Central Nervous Systems Complications of Viral Infections and Vaccines, pages 2141 to 2151.

THE EPILEPSIES

Epilepsy is a term applied to a group of chronic conditions whose major clinical manifestation is the occurrence of epileptic seizures—sudden and usually unprovoked attacks of subjective experiential phenomena, altered awareness, involuntary movements, or convulsions.

Although a diagnosis of epilepsy requires the presence of seizures, not all seizures imply epilepsy (Table 23–33).

About 70% of adults and 40% of children with new-onset epilepsy have partial (focal) seizures. In most of these, it is not possible to identify a specific cause, although the focal nature of the seizures generally implies a cerebral injury or lesion (so-called cryptogenic epilepsy).

Seizures are classified by their clinical manifestations (semiology) supplemented by EEG data (Table 23–34). *Complex* partial seizures impair consciousness and produce unresponsiveness. *Psychomotor, temporal lobe,* and *limbic* seizures are terms that have been used in the past to describe ictal behaviors now classified as complex partial seizures. Automatisms (the "psychomotor" element) are not uniformly present in complex partial seizures.

GENERALIZED SEIZURES. Generalized seizures begin diffusely and involve both cerebral hemispheres simultaneously from the outset. They lack clinical and EEG features that indicate a localized cerebral origin.

Generalized tonic-clonic seizures (*grand mal convulsions*) are characterized by abrupt loss of consciousness with bilateral tonic extension of the trunk and limbs (*tonic phase*).

Absence seizures (*petit mal seizures*) occur mainly in children and are characterized by sudden, momentary lapses in awareness (the absence attack), staring, rhythmic blinking, and, often, a few small clonic jerks of arms or hands. Behavior and awareness return immediately to normal. There is no postictal period.

Myoclonic seizures manifest as rapid, recurrent, brief muscle jerks that can occur bilaterally, synchronously or asynchronously, or unilaterally without loss of consciousness.

Table 23–33 ■ POTENTIAL CAUSES OF ACUTE SYMPTOMATIC SEIZURES

Medical Conditions

- Metabolic derangements
  - Hyponatremia (<120 mEq/L)—especially acute
  - Hypernatremia (>150–155 mEq/L)—especially acute
  - Hypoglycemia (<40 mg/dL)
  - Hyperglycemia (>400 mg/dL)
  - Hyperosmolality (>320 mOsm/L)
  - Hypocalcemia (<7 mg/dL)
  - Respiratory alkalosis—acute
- Drug-induced seizures
  - Isoniazid, penicillins
  - Theophylline, aminophylline
  - Lidocaine
  - Meperidine
  - Ketamine, halothane, enflurane, methohexital
  - Amitriptyline, maprotiline, imipramine, doxepin, fluoxetine
  - Haloperidol, trifluoperazine, chlorpromazine
  - Ephedrine, phenylpropanolamine, terbutaline
  - Methotrexate, BCNU, asparaginase
  - Cyclosporine
  - Cocaine (crack), phencyclidine, amphetamines
  - Alcohol (withdrawal)
- Illnesses
  - Eclampsia
  - Hypertensive encephalopathy
  - Liver failure
  - Polyarteritis nodosa
  - Porphyria
  - Renal failure
  - Sickle cell disease
  - Syphilis
  - Systemic lupus erythematosus
  - Thrombotic thrombocytopenic purpura
  - Whipple's disease

Neurologic Conditions

- Angiitis of the nervous system
- Meningitis
- Encephalitis
- Acute head trauma (impact seizures)
- Stroke
- Brain abscess
- Brain tumor

Atomic seizures ("drop attacks") occur most often in children with diffuse encephalopathies and are characterized by sudden loss of muscle tone.

DIAGNOSIS. A clear history should describe the patients's seizures, neurologic status between attacks, and relevant risk factors for epilepsy (Table 23–35). 23

ELECTROENCEPHALOGRAPHY. EEG is the most important diagnostic test for epilepsy.

DIFFERENTIAL DIAGNOSIS. Not every paroxysmal event is a seizure, and misidentification of other conditions as epilepsy leads

Table 23–34 ■ INTERNATIONAL LEAGUE AGAINST EPILEPSY CLASSIFICATION OF EPILEPTIC SEIZURES AND SYNDROMES

Classification of Seizures

I. Partial (focal) seizures
  A. Simple partial seizures (consciousness not impaired)
    1. With motor signs (including jacksonian, versive, and postural)
    2. With sensory symptoms (including visual, somatosensory, auditory, olfactory)
    3. With psychic symptoms (including dysphasia, hallucinatory, and affective changes)
    4. With autonomic symptoms
  B. Complex partial seizures (consciousness is impaired)
    1. Simple partial onset followed by impaired consciousness
    2. With impairment of consciousness at onset
    3. With automatisms
  C. Partial seizures evolving to secondarily generalized seizures
II. Generalized seizures of nonfocal origin
  A. Absence seizures
  B. Myoclonic seizures; myoclonic jerks (single or multiple)
  C. Tonic-clonic seizures
  D. Tonic seizures
  E. Atonic seizures
III. Unclassified epileptic seizures

Classification of Epileptic Syndromes

I. Idiopathic epilepsy syndromes (focal or generalized)
  A. Benign neonatal convulsions
  B. Benign partial epilepsy of childhood
  C. Childhood absence epilepsy
  D. Juvenile myoclonic epilepsy
  E. Idiopathic epilepsy, otherwise unspecified
II. Cryptogenic or symptomatic epilepsy syndromes (focal or generalized)
  A. West's syndrome (infantile spasms)
  B. Lennox-Gastaut syndrome
  C. Epilepsia partialis continua
  D. Temporal lobe epilepsy
  E. Frontal lobe epilepsy
  F. Post-traumatic epilepsy
  G. Other symptomatic epilepsies, otherwise unspecified
III. Other epilepsy syndromes of uncertain or mixed classification
  A. Neonatal seizures
  B. Febrile seizures
  C. Reflex epilepsy
  D. Adult non-convulsive status epilepticus
  E. Other unspecified

to ineffective, unnecessary, and potentially harmful treatment (Table 23–36).

TREATMENT. Drugs used to treat seizures are listed in Table 23–37. Surgical intervention should be considered when seizures fail to respond to antiepileptic drugs and when they continue to disrupt the patient's quality of life.

Status Epilepticus

Status epilepticus can take either convulsive or nonconvulsive forms. Convulsive status epilepticus is a medical emergency that

Table 23–35 ■ ESSENTIAL FEATURES OF THE SEIZURE HISTORY

Date and circumstances of first attack
First consistent event in the seizure: Is there an aura? Are initial symptoms and signs focal or lateralizing?
Subsequent evolution of the seizure, in sequence
Postictal manifestations (e.g., Todd's paralysis)
Is there more than one seizure type?
Average rate of occurrence; longest seizure-free interval since onset
Seizure precipitants (alcohol, sleep deprivation, particular stimuli, stress)
Is there a pattern to seizure occurrence (circadian, catamenial)?
Has there been a change in characteristics of the seizure?
Symptoms of neurologic or systemic disease between seizures: Are these static, intermittent, or progressive?
Risk factor for epilepsy (e.g., family history, cerebral injury)

requires timely and appropriate treatment to minimize serious systemic and neurologic morbidity. Non-convulsive status presents as a new-onset sustained confusional state. Treatment protocols are designed to eliminate seizure activity and to identify and treat any underlying medical or neurologic disorder (Table 23–38).

For more information about this subject, see *Cecil Textbook of Medicine,* 21st edition. Philadelphia, W.B. Saunders Company, 2000. Chapter 484, The Epilepsies, pages 2151 to 2163.

Table 23–36 ■ NONEPILEPTIC EPISODIC DISORDERS IN ADOLESCENTS AND ADULTS

- Movement disorders
  - Myoclonus
  - Paroxysmal choreoathetosis
  - Episodic ataxias
  - Hyperexplexia (startle disease)
- Migraine
  - Confusional
  - Vertebrobasilar
- Syncope and cardiac arrhythmias*
- Behavioral and psychiatric disorders
  - Psychogenic seizures*
  - Hyperventilation syndrome*
  - Panic disorder*
  - Dissociative states ("fugue states")
  - Episodic dyscontrol
- Narcolepsy and sleep apnea
  - Automatic behavior syndrome
  - Partial cataplexy
- Transient ischemic attacks
- Transient global amnesia*
- Acute confusional states
- Alcoholic blackouts*
- Hypoglycemic attacks

*Most commonly encountered.

Table 23–37 ■ DRUGS USED IN TREATING DIFFERENT TYPES OF SEIZURES

TYPE OF SEIZURE	DRUGS
Simple and complex partial	Carbamazepine, phenytoin, valproate, gabapentin, lamotrigine, tiagabine, topiramate
Secondarily generalized	Carbamazepine, phenytoin, valproate, gabapentin, lamotrigine, tiagabine, topiramate
Primary generalized seizures	
Tonic-clonic	Valproate, carbamazepine, phenytoin, lamotrigine
Absence	Ethosuximide, valproate, lamotrigine
Myoclonic	Valproate, clonazepam
Tonic	Valproate, felbamate, clonazepam

INTRACRANIAL AND SPINAL TUMORS

More than 18,000 new cases of primary brain tumors are treated each year in the United States. Metastases are even more frequent and contribute considerably to suffering and death from systemic cancer. The classification of brain tumors is confusing but can be simplified into metastatic, primary extra-axial, and primary intra-axial (Table 23–39).

IMAGING AND OTHER DIAGNOSTIC PROCEDURES. Brain imaging by MRI or CT scans is an indispensable component of modern diagnosis of the presence, but not the type, of brain tumor (Table 23–40). MRI is almost always superior to CT scanning in diagnosing intracranial mass lesions.

TREATMENT. In almost every instance in which a brain tumor is suspected on the basis of the combined results of history, physical findings, and imaging studies, the *first consideration is its surgical resectability.*

RADIATION THERAPY. All forms of external beam radiation, whether gamma photons emitted from cobalt-60 sources or x-rays generated from linear accelerators, act similarly. Other non-operative radiosurgical techniques include the gamma knife and linear accelerators adapted to provide focused therapeutic beams. Efficacy has been shown for metastases but not for gliomas.

CHEMOTHERAPY. Chemotherapy for brain tumors may be effective, but has had a disappointing record.

For more information about this subject, see *Cecil Textbook of Medicine,* 21st edition. Philadelphia, W.B. Saunders Company, 2000. Chapter 485, Intracranial Tumors, pages 2164 to 2168.

SPINAL TUMORS

Tumors that cause nerve root or spinal cord compression can be paravertebral, extradural, intradural, or intramedullary. Most of those causing spinal cord compression are extradural and metastatic. Intramedullary neoplasms cause symptoms both by invading and compressing spinal structures; the tumors may be either benign or malignant.

Table 23–38 ■ PROTOCOL FOR TREATING STATUS EPILEPTICUS

TIME (min)*	ACTION
0–5	Diagnose status epilepticus by observing continued seizure activity or 1 additional seizure.
	Give oxygen by nasal cannula or mask; position patient's head for optimal airway patency; consider intubation if respiratory assistance is needed.
	Obtain and record vital signs at onset and periodically thereafter; control any abnormalities as necessary; initiate ECG monitoring.
	Establish an IV in one or both arms using catheter; draw venous blood samples for glucose level, serum chemistries, hematology studies, toxicology screens, and determinations of antiepileptic drug levels.
	Assess oxygenation with oximetry or periodic arterial blood gas determinations.
6–9	If hypoglycemia is established or a blood glucose determination is unavailable, administer glucose; in adults, give 100 mg of thiamine first, followed by 50 mL of 50% glucose by direct push into the IV; in children, the dose of glucose is 2 mL/kg of 25% glucose.
10–20	Administer either 0.1 mg/kg of lorazepam at 2 mg/min or 0.2 mg/kg of diazepam at 5 mg/min by IV. If diazepam is given, it can be repeated if seizures do not stop after 5 min; if diazepam is used to stop the status, phenytoin should be administered immediately to prevent recurrent status.
21–60	If status persists, administer 15–20 mg/kg of phenytoin by IV no faster than 50 mg/min in adults and 1 mg/kg/min in children. Monitor ECG and blood pressure during the infusion. Phenytoin is incompatible with glucose-containing solutions: the IV should be purged with normal saline before the phenytoin infusion.
>60	If status does not stop after 20 mg/kg of phenytoin administration, give additional doses of 5 mg/kg to a maximal dose of 30 mg/kg.
	If status persists, give 20 mg/kg of phenobarbital by IV at 100 mg/min. When phenobarbital is given after a benzodiazepine, the risk of apnea or hypopnea is great, and assisted ventilation is usually required.
	If status persists, give anesthetic doses of drugs such as pentobarbital. Ventilatory assistance and vasopressors are virtually always necessary.

ECG = electrocardiogram; IV = intravenous line.

*Time starts at seizure onset.

From Dodson WE, DeLorenzo RJ, Pedley TA, et al: Treatment of convulsive status epilepticus: Recommendations of the Epilepsy Foundation of America's working group on status epilepticus. JAMA 270:854, 1993.

Table 23–39 ■ COMMON BRAIN TUMORS IN ADULTS WITH PERCENTAGE INCIDENCE BY CATEGORY*

METASTATIC	PRIMARY EXTRA-AXIAL	PRIMARY INTRA-AXIAL
Lung (37)	Meningioma (80)	Glioblastoma (47)
Breast (19)	Acoustic neuroma (10)	Anaplastic astrocytoma (24)
Melanoma (16)	Pituitary adenoma (7)	Astrocytoma (15)
Colorectum (9)	Other (3)	Oligodendroglioma (5)
Kidney (8)		Lymphoma (2)
Other (11)		Other (7)

*These figures, given in parentheses, can be extremely variable from one center to another, depending on referral pattern. They are given here as general estimates based upon many published series.

The differential diagnosis of paravertebral tumor includes disorders that cause paravertebral pain with or without compression of nerve roots. *Myofascial pain syndrome* causes low back or neck paravertebral pain with referred pain into arms or legs.

The differential diagnosis of extradural neoplasms includes inflammatory disease of bone and epidural abscess (e.g., vertebral tuberculosis, bacterial osteomyelitis), acute or subacute epidural hematomas, herniated intervertebral disks, spondylosis, and, very rarely, extramedullary hematopoiesis (in patients with severe and chronic anemia). MRI often distinguishes these from tumor, but sometimes a definitive diagnosis requires biopsy of the lesion either via decompressive laminectomy or by percutaneous needle biopsy.

INTRADURAL EXTRAMEDULLARY TUMORS. Most intradural tumors are benign. Meningiomas and neurofibromas are by far the most common.

INTRAMEDULLARY TUMORS. The most common intramedullary spinal tumors are astrocytomas (usually low-grade) and ependymomas.

For more information about this subject, see *Cecil Textbook of Medicine,* 21st edition. Philadelphia, W.B. Saunders Company, 2000. Chapter 487, Spinal Tumors, pages 2171 to 2172.

INTRACRANIAL HYPERTENSION

CSF pressure in excess of 250 mm H_2O is usually a manifestation of serious neurologic disease and is most often associated with

Table 23–40 ■ THE MAIN DIFFERENTIAL DIAGNOSES OF BRAIN TUMORS

Hematomas, especially in tumors that have a tendency to bleed, such as melanoma
Abscesses, including fungal
Granulomas
Parasitic infections, such as cysticercosis
Vascular malformations, especially those without arteriovenous shunts
Solitary large plaques of multiple sclerosis
Progressive strokes (rare)

Table 23–41 ■ SYMPTOMS AND SIGNS OF INTRACRANIAL HYPERTENSION

Common

Headache
Tinnitus
Vomiting (with or without nausea)
Visual obscurations, visual loss, photopsias
Papilledema
Diplopia
Lethargy and increased sleep
Psychomotor retardation
Pain on eye movement

Less Common

Hearing distortion or loss
Vertigo
Facial weakness
Shoulder or arm pain
Neck pain or rigidity
Ataxia
Paresthesias of extremities
Anosmia
Trigeminal neuralgia

rapidly expanding mass lesions (Table 23–41). The initial treatment of any patient with increased ICP whose neurologic status is deteriorating is aimed at reducing the volume of the intracranial contents in an attempt to prevent brain damage (Table 23–42).

BENIGN INTRACRANIAL HYPERTENSION. Benign intracranial hypertension is a syndrome of increased ICP unaccompanied by localizing neurologic signs, intracranial mass lesion, or CSF outflow obstruction in an alert, otherwise healthy-looking patient. Such patients are almost always obese and more often are women. Benign intracranial hypertension (also called pseudotumor cerebri or idiopathic intracranial hypertension) can be associated with a variety of systemic and iatrogenic disorders (Table 23–43).

HYDROCEPHALUS. Hydrocephalus refers to the net accumulation of CSF within the cerebral ventricles and their consequent

Table 23–42 ■ EMERGENCY TREATMENT OF IMPENDING HERNIATION IN ACUTELY DECOMPENSATING PATIENTS

THERAPY	DOSAGE OR PROCEDURE	ONSET (DURATION OF ACTION)
Hyperventilation	Lower $Pa{CO_2}$ to 25–30 mm Hg	Seconds (minutes)
Osmotherapy	Mannitol 0.5–2.0 g/kg IV over 15 min followed by 25 g as needed	Minutes (hours)
Corticosteroids	Dexamethasone 50 mg IV push, followed by 50 mg/day in divided doses	Hours (days)

23

Table 23–43 ■ SYSTEMIC AND IATROGENIC DISORDERS ASSOCIATED WITH BENIGN INTRACRANIAL HYPERTENSION

Commonly Prescribed Drugs
Nalidixic acid
Nitrofurantoin
Phenytoin
Sulfonamides
Tetracycline
Vitamin A
Endocrine and Metabolic Disorders
Addison's disease
Cushing's syndrome
Hypoparathyroidism
Menarche, pregnancy, oral contraceptives
Obesity and irregular menses
Steroid therapy or withdrawal
Hematologic Disorders
Cryoglobulinemia
Iron deficiency anemia
Miscellaneous Disorders
Dural venous sinus obstruction or thrombosis
Head trauma
Internal jugular vein ligation
Systemic lupus erythematosus
Middle ear disease

enlargement. Although acute obstructive hydrocephalus usually produces a sudden increase in intraventricular pressure. CSF pressure is frequently normal (or low) in patients with chronic hydrocephalus (Table 23–44).

Table 23–44 ■ CAUSES OF HYDROCEPHALUS

Acute
Cerebellar hemorrhage/infarction
Colloid cyst of the 3rd ventricle
Exudative meningitis
Head trauma
Intracranial tumor or hematoma
Spontaneous subarachnoid hemorrhage
Viral encephalitis
Chronic
Aqueductal stenosis
Ectasia and elongation of the basilar artery (rare)
Granulomatous meningitis
Head trauma
Hindbrain malformations
Meningeal carcinomatosis
Brain and spinal cord tumors
Spontaneous subarachnoid hemorrhage
Syringomyelia

For more information about this subject, see *Cecil Textbook of Medicine,* 21st edition. Philadelphia, W.B. Saunders Company, 2000. Chapter 488, Intracranial Hypertension and Hypotension, pages 2172 to 2175.

HEAD INJURY

Primary Damage

Primary traumatic damage to the brain can be separated into several basic processes: diffuse axonal injury, intracranial hematoma and contusion, and subarachnoid hemorrhage (Table 23–45).

Intracranial Hematomas

Epidural hematomas often result from moderate-impact injuries. The early detection of epidural hemorrhage is of utmost importance because most affected patients do not initially have irreversible brain damage. Thus, prompt surgical evacuation can be associated with a favorable outcome.

Subdural hematomas are divided into two subgroups—acute and chronic—based on timing of presentation; these manifest as distinct syndromes. An *acute subdural hematoma* almost always signifies severe brain injury. Most such patients are unconscious from impact, and half die.

Chronic subdural hematomas usually become symptomatic between 1 and 6 weeks following injury and are not infrequently located bilaterally. They often follow trivial injuries, such as striking the head on a door with no associated loss of consciousness. A few of these resolve spontaneously, and for the remainder, treatment is relatively straightforward.

Intraparenchymal hemorrhage or *contusion* can occur anywhere throughout the brain, yet most frequently it is identified in characteristic regions of the frontal and temporal poles, where the brain overlies the bony ridges of the skull base. Contusions vary in size and act as mass lesions.

For more information about this subject, see *Cecil Textbook of Medicine,* 21st edition. Philadelphia, W.B. Saunders Company, 2000. Chapter 490, Head Injury, pages 2178 to 2181.

SPINE AND SPINAL CORD INJURY

Spinal cord injury is a devastating problem that disproportionately affects young males.

Nature of the Injury

About half of all serious spinal injuries affect the cervical level of the spine, with nearly 50% of such patients rendered quadriplegic as a result.

Spinal cord injuries can be categorized as complete or incomplete on the basis of the quantity of residual neurologic function. Acute, complete injuries most often produce *spinal shock,* with loss of all sensorimotor functions, including flaccidity and loss of reflexes at and below the level of injury. Less severe injuries can produce a *central cord syndrome* resulting from ischemia or hematomas.

Table 23–45 ■ SIGNS OF POTENTIAL INTRACRANIAL CATASTROPHE AND WHAT THEY MAY SIGNIFY

SIGNS	CHANGES	POTENTIAL MEANING
Respiration	Rate > 20/min	Pulmonary edema or pneumonitis
Pulse	Change > 10/min or heart rate < 60/min	Each may indicate elevated ICP with transtentorial herniation
Blood pressure	Change in systolic > 15 mm Hg or widening pulse pressure	Each may indicate elevated ICP with transtentorial herniation
Headache*	Is it increasing?	Often indicates increased ICP
Pupils	Enlargement Asymmetry Irregular shape (oval) Decrease in reactivity Change from preresuscitation	Increased mass effect New hemorrhage Recurrent hemorrhage
Motor	Decrease of 1 point on GCS New focal deficit	Increased mass effect New hemorrhage Recurrent hemorrhage
Level of consciousness	Abrupt decrease	Increased ICP Seizures Hypotension
	Transient	Seizures Hypoxia
	Progressive decrease	Re-hemorrhage Brain stem involvement Septicemia Electrolyte imbalance Vasospasm Hydrocephalus

GCS = Glasgow coma scale; ICP = intracranial pressure.
* All changes except headache may occur in both awake and unconscious patients.

In the presence of one spinal axis injury, the incidence of a second non-contiguous fracture is 15%. It is imperative to search for this possibility and to document the integrity of the spinal column from occiput to sacrum.

Emergency Management

At the accident site, three major concerns are paramount: (1) maintenance of ventilation, (2) protection against shock, and (3) neck immobilization to prevent further spinal cord damage.

Hospital Care

There is no treatment that reverses the devastation of acute spinal cord injury. Treatment is focused on preventing secondary injury by (1) appropriate immobilization, and (2) maintenance of spinal cord perfusion (mean arterial blood pressure should be maintained above 80 to 85 mm Hg with volume resuscitation, cautiously supplemented with pharmacologic pressors).

Autonomic dysfunction complicates the convalescence of more than half of the patients who suffer severe spinal cord injuries above the midthoracic level.

For more information about this subject, see *Cecil Textbook of Medicine,* 21st edition. Philadelphia, W.B. Saunders Company, 2000. Chapter 491, Spine and Spinal Cord Injury, pages 2181 to 2183.

MECHANICAL LESIONS OF NERVE ROOTS AND SPINAL CORD

Neck and Back Pain

Neck or back pain is usually short-lived and responds to symptomatic measures (Table 23–46). Examination commonly reveals spasm of the paraspinal muscles and limitation of spinal movements. Local tenderness may also be present. Spinal compression should be suspected when neck flexion leads to pain in the thoracic or lumbar region or when Lhermitte's sign is positive. Focal tenderness over a spinous process suggests vertebral involvement by tumor or infection.

MANAGEMENT. If a cervical fracture is suspected following trauma, the neck is immobilized and radiographed. Acute hemorrhage may require evacuation, and infection requires antimicrobial therapy. Many patients with chronic neck or back pain have no surgically remedial lesion, and a multidisciplinary approach is necessary to ensure that symptoms resolve. This may include the use of analgesics, NSAIDs, or tricyclic antidepressants.

For more information about this subject, see *Cecil Textbook of Medicine,* 21st edition. Philadelphia, W.B. Saunders Company, 2000. Chapter 493, Neck and Back Pain, pages 2185 to 2187.

INTERVERTEBRAL DISK

The intervertebral disk that is interposed between two adjacent intervertebral bodies consists of a soft, gelatinous, inner nucleus pulposus (a remnant of the notochord) that serves as a shock absorber. With advancing years, the nucleus becomes harder, less

Table 23–46 ■ CAUSES OF BACK PAIN

	COMMON	LESS COMMON
Mechanical		
Degenerative	Disk protrusion Osteoarthritis Facet syndrome Spinal stenosis	
Congenital	Spinal stenosis	Spondylolisthesis Spondylolysis Transitional vertebra Other structural anomalies
Deformity	Scoliosis	
Muscle	Myofascial syndrome Spasm	
Metabolic	Osteoporosis	Paget's disease Gout
Trauma	Compression fracture Lumbosacral/sacroiliac strain Subluxation Muscle injury	
Tumors	Metastatic disease Multiple myeloma	Benign bone/neural tumors (e.g., meningioma, osteoid osteoma, hemangioma) Osteosarcoma
Inflammatory disease	Ankylosing spondylitis Arachnoiditis Rheumatoid arthritis	Enteropathic arthropathy Psoriatic arthropathy
Infections	Herpes zoster	Disk infections Epi- or subdural abscess Meningitis
Referred pain		Aortic aneurysm Cardiac/pericardial disease Pelvic/retroperitoneal disease Pulmonary/pleural disease Visceral disease
Non-organic disease	Anxiety Conversion reaction Psychosis Litigation-related Malingering Chronic pain syndrome Substance abuse	

resilient, and more susceptible to trauma. Consequently, tears tend to develop in the annulus, through which a portion of the nucleus pulposus may herniate.

LUMBOSACRAL DISK DISEASE. Protrusion of an intervertebral disk may lead to a radiculopathy. With involvement of sacral fibers, disturbances of bladder and bowel function are important complications (Table 23–47).

CERVICAL DISK DISEASE. Cervical roots may be compressed by a protruded intervertebral disk or by an abnormality involving the facet joint or joints of Luschka. Disk herniation is the most

Table 23–47 ■ DIAGNOSIS OF LOWER LUMBAR AND SACRAL RADICULOPATHY

	PAIN	WEAKNESS (SELECTED MUSCLES)	SENSORY LOSS	REFLEX LOSS
L4	Across thigh and medial leg to medial malleolus	Quadriceps Thigh adductors Tibialis anterior	Medial leg	Knee
L5	Posterior thigh and lateral calf, dorsum of foot	Extensor digitorum brevis and longus Peronei	Dorsum of foot	
S1	Buttock and posterior thigh, calf, and lateral foot	Extensor digitorum brevis Peronei Gastrocnemius Soleus	Sole or lateral border of foot	Ankle
S2–4	Posterior thigh, buttocks, and genitalia	Gastrocnemius Soleus Abductor hallucis Abductor digiti quinti pedis Sphincter muscles	Buttocks, anal region, and genitalia	Bulbocavernosus Anal

Table 23–48 ■ DIAGNOSIS OF CERVICAL RADICULOPATHY

	PAIN	WEAKNESS (SELECTED MUSCLES)	SENSORY LOSS	REFLEX LOSS
C5	Neck, shoulder, and interscapular region; lateral arm	Deltoid Spinati Rhomboids	Lateral border of shoulder and upper arm	Biceps (brachioradialis)
C6	Shoulder; lateral forearm and first 2 digits	Biceps Brachioradialis Extensor carpi radialis	Lateral forearm and first 2 digits	Brachioradialis (biceps)
C7	Interscapular region, posterior arm, mid-forearm	Triceps Extensor carpi and digitorum Flexor carpi radialis	Midforearm and middle digit	Triceps
C8	Medial forearm and hand	Extensor carpi and digitorum Flexor digitorum sublimis and profundus Flexor carpi ulnaris	Medial forearm and hand, and 5th digit	Finger flexors (triceps)
T1	Medial arm to elbow	Intrinsic hand muscles	Medial arm to elbow	

common cause (Table 23–48). Cervical pain, which is often attributed to compression, angulation, or stretch of the nerve roots, generally subsides with time, even though the anatomic abnormality may persist and the root remains distorted.

For more information about this subject, see *Cecil Textbook of Medicine,* 21st edition. Philadelphia, W.B. Saunders Company, 2000. Chapter 494, Intervertebral Disk Disease, pages 2187 to 2189.

VASCULAR DISORDERS INVOLVING THE SPINAL CORD

The spinal cord is supplied by the anterior and paired posterior spinal arteries, which are fed by segmental vessels at different levels.

Ischemic Myelopathies

Ischemia may contribute to the neurologic deficit that occurs in patients with space-occupying lesions, and those with post-traumatic or post-irradiation myelopathies. Disease of the abdominal aorta may cause an ischemic myelopathy. Severe hypotension from any cause has been associated with an ischemic myelopathy. When acute ischemia leads to a transverse myelopathy, patients present with the sudden onset of a flaccid areflexic paraplegia or quadriplegia, analgesia and anesthesia below the level of the lesion, and retention of urine and feces.

Venous infarction of the cord occurs most commonly in association with an arteriovenous malformation but occasionally in association with sepsis, malignant disease, or vertebral disorders.

Neurogenic Intermittent Claudication

The development of pain or a neurologic deficit after exercise or with certain postures that extend the lumbar spine, and their relief by rest or change in posture (leaning forward), has been designated *neurogenic intermittent claudication.*

Hemorrhage

Hematomyelia (hemorrhage into the spinal cord) or spinal subarachnoid hemorrhage may occur from trauma, spinal vascular malformations, intradural spinal neoplasms, coarctation of the aorta, or ruptured spinal aneurysms. It may be associated with connective tissue diseases, blood dyscrasias, or anticoagulant therapy.

For more information about this subject, see *Cecil Textbook of Medicine,* 21st edition. Philadelphia, W.B. Saunders Company, 2000. Chapter 496, Vascular Disorders Involving the Spinal Cord, pages 2190 to 2192.

DISEASES OF THE PERIPHERAL NERVOUS SYSTEM

Pathophysiology of Peripheral Neuropathies

Normal function of myelinated nerve fibers depends on the integrity of both the axon and its myelin sheath. Nerve action potentials jump from one node of Ranvier to the next. This rapid saltatory conduction depends on the insulating properties of the myelin sheaths. The simplest type of nerve injury is transection of the axon. The axon distal to the site of transection degenerates while that proximal to the injury survives and has the potential for regeneration. This pattern of *distal axonal degeneration* or *"dying back"* of nerve fibers results from a wide variety of metabolic, toxic, and heritable causes.

Demyelination of a peripheral nerve at even a single site can block conduction, resulting in a functional deficit identical to that seen after axonal degeneration.

For more information about this subject, see *Cecil Textbook of Medicine,* 21st edition. Philadelphia, W.B. Saunders Company, 2000. Chapter 498, Pathophysiology of Peripheral Neuropathies, page 2193.

Immune-Mediated Neuropathies

The Guillain-Barré syndrome is usually characterized by weakness or paralysis affecting more than one limb, usually symmetrically, associated with loss of tendon reflexes and with increased spinal fluid protein without pleocytosis. Since the advent of polio vaccination, Guillain-Barré syndrome has become the most frequent cause of acute flaccid paralysis throughout the world. Guillain-Barré syndrome is virtually synonymous with *acute inflammatory demyelinating polyneuropathy* (Table 23–49).

CLINICAL MANIFESTATIONS. The initial symptoms often consist of tingling and "pins-and-needles sensations" in the feet and may be associated with dull low back pain. By the time of presentation, which usually occurs within hours up to 10 days after the first symptoms, weakness has usually developed. Progression can be alarmingly rapid, so that critical functions such as respiration can be lost within a few days or even a few hours.

CHRONIC INFLAMMATORY DEMYELINATING NEUROPATHY. Chronic inflammatory demyelinating neuropathy (CIDP) differs from Guillain-Barré syndrome primarily in the time course and in the absence of identifiable antecedent events. Blinded trials showed that, unlike Guillain-Barré syndrome, most cases of CIDP respond to corticosteroids alone. Some patients with CIDP respond to plasmapheresis and with IV gamma globulin.

NEUROPATHIES ASSOCIATED WITH MONOCLONAL GAMMOPATHIES. Monoclonal proteins of IgM, IgG, and IgA types are all associated with neuropathy. In some instances the monoclonal protein has been shown to cause the neuropathy.

IMMUNE-MEDIATED ATAXIC NEUROPATHIES. In this category there are three disorders: *carcinomatous sensory neuropathy, sensory ganglionitis associated with features of Sjögren's syndrome,* and *idiopathic sensory ganglionitis.* All three are characterized clinically by subacute or slowly developing proprioceptive sensory loss leading to gait ataxia and inability to localize arms and/or legs.

VASCULITIC NEUROPATHIES. Peripheral nerves have extensive collateral circulation and are relatively invulnerable to occlusion of large peripheral arteries. By contrast, they are susceptible to focal interruption of circulation within the individual nerve fascicles due to small blood vessel diseases.

For more information about this subject, see *Cecil Textbook of*

Table 23–49 ■ GUILLAIN-BARRÉ (GBS) SYNDROME AND RELATED IMMUNE-MEDIATED NEUROPATHIES

DISORDER	TYPE	CLINICAL CHARACTERISTICS	PATHOPHYSIOLOGY	TREATMENT
Guillain-Barré syndrome	Acute inflammatory demyelinating polyneuropathy	Prominent or predominant motor involvement of acute onset	Demyelination, lymphocytic infiltration	Plasmapheresis; intravenous immunoglobulin (IVIg); corticosteroids alone ineffective
	Fisher syndrome	Ataxia, ophthalmoparesis, and areflexia of acute onset	Antibodies against the ganglioside G_{Qlb}	(Probably) plasmapheresis or IVIg
	Axonal GBS	Motor-sensory or pure motor forms	Noninflammatory axonal degeneration predominates; strongly associated with antecedent *Campylobacter jejuni* infection	(Probably) plasmapheresis or IVIg
Chronic inflammatory demyelinating polyneuropathy		Slower onset of weakness and sensory loss; may be recurrent	Widespread demyelination with remyelination, secondary axonal loss; may occur in association with monoclonal gammopathy	Corticosteroids, plasmapheresis, IVIg
Multifocal motor neuropathy		Stepwise involvement of individual nerves; nearly pure motor involvement	Focal demyelination of motor fibers	IVIg or cytotoxic agents (corticosteroids and plasmapheresis ineffective)

Medicine, 21st edition. Philadelphia, W.B. Saunders Company, 2000. Chapter 499, Immune-Mediated Neuropathies, pages 2193 to 2196.

Hereditary Neuropathies

Heritable neuropathies rank among the most prevalent inherited neurologic diseases.

Charcot-Marie-Tooth disease identifies a group of heritable disorders of peripheral nerves that share clinical features but differ in their pathologic changes and specific genetic abnormalities. All forms of Charcot-Marie-Tooth disease tend to occur in the second to fourth decades with insidiously evolving footdrop. Most patients enjoy a nearly full spectrum of activity and they have a normal lifespan. The footdrop can be relieved by appropriate bracing of the ankle.

Amyloid neuropathies are caused by extracellular deposition of the fibrillary protein amyloid in peripheral nerve and sensory and autonomic ganglia, as well as around blood vessels in nerves and other tissues. The outstanding abnormalities affect the small sensory and autonomic fibers. This leads to loss of the ability to perceive mechanical and thermal injury and tissue damage. As a result, painless injuries present a major hazard of this disorder, and no definitive treatment is available other than education in prevention of injury to anesthetic limbs.

For more information about this subject, see *Cecil Textbook of Medicine,* 21st edition. Philadelphia, W.B. Saunders Company, 2000. Chapter 500, Hereditary Neuropathies, pages 2196 to 2197.

Metabolic Neuropathies

Diabetes is the most frequent cause of peripheral neuropathy worldwide (Table 23–50). The diagnosis of diabetic polyneuropathy is straightforward in established diabetics with a typical clinical picture. Electrodiagnostic studies, usually unnecessary, document neuropathy, and spinal fluid protein is frequently moderately elevated. In general, the diagnosis of diabetic neuropathy can comfortably be made only in the setting of long-standing diabetes, usually insulin-requiring.

Diabetes also can cause a variety of mononeuropathies and mul-

Table 23–50 ■ DIABETIC NEUROPATHIES

Diabetic Polyneuropathies

Rapidly reversible physiologic dysfunction associated with hyperglycemia
Symmetrical polyneuropathy
  Sensorimotor neuropathy
  "Small-fiber" neuropathy, with autonomic dysfunction, reduced pain sensibility, spontaneous burning pain

Diabetic Mononeuropathies and Plexopathies

Diabetic 3rd nerve palsy
Diabetic 4th nerve palsy
Diabetic truncal neuropathy
Diabetic lumbosacral plexopathy (proximal diabetic neuropathy)

tiple mononeuropathies. They probably represent vascular insufficiency or infarction in nerve.

For more information about this subject, see *Cecil Textbook of Medicine,* 21st edition. Philadelphia, W.B. Saunders Company, 2000. Chapter 501, Metabolic Neuropathies, pages 2197 to 2198.

Toxic Neuropathies

A wide array of environmental, occupational, recreational, and pharmaceutical agents can produce peripheral nerve disease (Table 23–51). Persons with pre-existing nerve disease may be unusually susceptible to neurotoxins.

For more information about this subject, see *Cecil Textbook of Medicine,* 21st edition. Philadelphia, W.B. Saunders Company, 2000. Chapter 502, Toxic Neuropathies, pages 2198 to 2199.

Entrapment and Compressive Neuropathies

The most frequently encountered entrapment and compressive neuropathies are median nerve compression at the wrist within the carpal tunnel (*carpal tunnel syndrome*); median nerve compression in the upper forearm; ulnar nerve compression in the hand (*cubital tunnel syndrome*), wrist, or at the elbow (*tardy ulnar nerve palsy*); tibial nerve compression behind the medial malleolus (*tarsal tunnel syndrome*); and peroneal nerve compression over the lateral fibular head. Unilateral facial paralysis of acute onset frequently occurs on an idiopathic basis (Bell's palsy). Trigeminal neuralgia is a recurring pain syndrome in which episodes of abrupt stabbing pain involve the second or third divisions of the trigeminal nerve.

Table 23–51 ■ INDUSTRIAL AND ENVIRONMENTAL NEUROTOXINS

Metals
Arsenic
Lead
Mercury
Thallium
Substance Abuse
Alcohol
Glue (hexacarbons) inhalation
Nitrous oxide inhalation
Industrial Poisons
Acrylamide
Carbon disulfide
Cyanide (chronic)
Dichlorophenoxyacetic acid
Dimethylaminopropionitrile
Ethylene oxide
Hexacarbon (n-hexane) (glue sniffer, occupational exposure to solvents, glues, or glue thinner)
Organophosphorus esters (triorthocresyl phosphate, leptophos, mipafox, trichlorphon)
Polychlorinated biphenyls
Tetrachlorbiphenyl
Trichloroethylene (trigeminal neuropathy)

For more information about this subject, see *Cecil Textbook of Medicine,* 21st edition. Philadelphia, W.B. Saunders Company, 2000. Chapter 504, Entrapment and Compressive Neuropathies, page 2200.

DISEASES OF MUSCLE (MYOPATHIES)

General Approach to Muscle Diseases

Myopathies can be broadly classified into hereditary and acquired disorders (Table 23–52). Clinical findings differentiating between muscle and nerve disease are presented in Table 23–53.

For more information about this subject, see *Cecil Textbook of Medicine,* 21st edition. Philadelphia, W.B. Saunders Company, 2000. Chapter 505, General Approach to Muscle Diseases, pages 2201 to 2206.

Muscular Dystrophies and Myopathies

Muscular dystrophies are inherited myopathies characterized by progressive muscle weakness and degeneration and subsequent replacement by fibrous and fatty connective tissue. Historically, muscular dystrophies were categorized by their distribution of weakness, age of onset, and inheritance pattern. Advances in the molecular understanding of the muscular dystrophies have defined the genetic mutation and abnormal gene product for many of these disorders.

Congenital myopathies are distinguished from dystrophies in three respects. First, these disorders have characteristic morphologic alterations demonstrated on light and electron microscopy. Second, as the name implies, congenital myopathies usually present at birth with hypotonia and subsequent delayed motor development. Finally, most congenital myopathies are relatively non-progressive with more benign outcomes than occur in the muscular dystrophies.

Metabolic myopathies include (1) glucose and/or glycogen metabolism disorders; (2) lipid metabolism disorders; and (3) mitochondrial disorders. A fourth group involving the utilization of adenine nucleotides is more controversial.

For more information about this subject, see *Cecil Textbook of Medicine,* 21st edition. Philadelphia, W.B. Saunders Company,

Table 23–52 ■ CLASSIFICATION OF MYOPATHIES

Hereditary
Muscular dystrophies
Congenital myopathies
Myotonias and channelopathies
Metabolic myopathies
Mitochondrial myopathies
Acquired
Inflammatory myopathies
Endocrine myopathies
Myopathies associated with systemic illness
Drug-induced/toxic myopathies

Table 23–53 ■ CLINICAL FINDINGS DIFFERENTIATING MUSCLE FROM NERVE DISEASE

	MYOPATHY	ANTERIOR HORN CELL DISEASE	PERIPHERAL NEUROPATHY	NEUROMUSCULAR JUNCTION DISEASE
Distribution	Usually proximal, symmetrical	Distal, asymmetrical, and bulbar	Distal, symmetrical	Extraocular, bulbar, proximal limb
Atrophy	Slight early, marked late	Marked early	Moderate	Absent
Fasciculations	Absent	Frequent	Sometimes present	Absent
Reflexes	Lost late	Variable, can be hyperreflexic	Lost early	Normal
Pain	Diffuse in myositis	Absent	Variable, distal when present	Absent
Cramps	Rare	Frequent	Occasional	Absent
Sensory loss	Absent	Absent	Usually present	Absent
Serum creatine kinase	Usually elevated	Occasionally slightly elevated	Normal	Normal

23

2000. Chapter 506, Muscular Dystropies; Chapter 507, Morphologically Distinct Congenital Myopathies; and Chapter 508, Metabolic Myopathies, pages 2206 to 2214.

Channelopathies (Non-Dystrophic Myotonias and Periodic Paralyses)

The non-dystrophic myotonias and the periodic paralyses are caused by mutations of various ion channels in muscle (Table 23–54).

For more information about this subject, see *Cecil Textbook of Medicine,* 21st edition. Philadelphia, W.B. Saunders Company, 2000. Chapter 509, Channelopathies (Non-Dystrophic Myotonias and Periodic Paralyses), pages 2214 to 2216.

Inflammatory Myopathies

Inflammatory myopathies include a heterogeneous group of acquired, non-hereditary disorders (Table 23–55) that are character-

Table 23–54 ■ CHANNELOPATHIES AND RELATED DISORDERS

DISORDER	CLINICAL FEATURES	PATTERN OF INHERITANCE
Chloride channelopathies		
Myotonia congenita		
Thomsen's disease	Myotonia	Autosomal dominant
Becker type	Myotonia and weakness	Autosomal recessive
Sodium channelopathies		
Paramyotonia congenita	Paramyotonia	Autosomal dominant
Hyperkalemic periodic paralysis	Periodic paralysis with myotonia and paramyotonia	Autosomal dominant
Potassium-aggravated myotonias		
Myotonia fluctuans	Myotonia	Autosomal dominant
Myotonia permanens	Myotonia	Autosomal dominant
Acetazolamide-responsive myotonia	Myotonia	Autosomal dominant
Calcium channelopathies		
Hypokalemic periodic paralysis	Periodic paralysis	Autosomal dominant
Schwartz-Jampel syndrome (chondrodystrophic myotonia)	Myotonia; dysmorphic	Autosomal dominant
Rippling muscle disease	Muscle mounding/ stiffness	Autosomal dominant
Anderson's syndrome	Periodic paralysis, cardiac arrhythmia, distinctive facies	Autosomal dominant
Brodie's disease	Delayed relaxation, no EMG myotonia	Autosomal dominant
Malignant hyperthermia	Anesthetic-induced delayed relaxation	Autosomal dominant

EMG = electromyogram.

Table 23–55 ■ CLASSIFICATION OF INFLAMMATORY MYOPATHIES

Idiopathic

Polymyositis
Dermatomyositis
Inclusion body myositis
Overlap syndromes with other connective tissue disease
(scleroderma, systemic lupus erythematosus, mixed connective tissue disease, Sjögren's syndrome, rheumatoid arthritis, polyarteritis nodosa)
Sarcoidosis and other granulomatous myositis
Behçet's syndrome
Inflammatory myopathies and eosinophila
Eosinophilic polymyositis
Diffuse fasciitis with eosinophilia
Focal myositis
Myositis ossificans

Infections

Bacterial: *Staphylococcus aureus,* streptococci, *Escherichia coli, Yersinia* spp., *Legionella* spp., gas gangrene *(Clostridium perfringens),* leprous myositis, Lyme disease *(Borrelia burgdorferi)*
Viral: acute myositis following influenza or other viral infections (adenovirus, coxsackievirus, echovirus, parainfluenza virus, Epstein-Barr virus, arbovirus, cytomegalovirus), retrovirus-related myopathies (HIV, HTLV-1), hepatitis B and C
Parasitic: trichinosis *(Trichinella spiralis),* toxoplasmosis *(Toxoplasma gondii),* cysticercosis, sarcosporidiosis, trypanosomiasis *(Taenia solium)*
Fungal: *Candida, Cryptococcus,* sporotrichosis, actinomycosis, histoplasmosis

HIV = human immunodeficiency virus; HTLV-1 = human T-cell lymphotropic virus type 1.

ized by muscle weakness and inflammation indicated by muscle biopsy.

For more information about this subject, see *Cecil Textbook of Medicine,* 21st edition. Philadelphia, W.B. Saunders Company, 2000. Chapter 510, Inflammatory and Other Myopathies, pages 2216 to 2221.

DISORDERS OF NEUROMUSCULAR TRANSMISSION

Disorders of neuromuscular transmission can be acquired or inherited and are associated with abnormal weakness and fatigability on exertion (Table 23–56).

MYASTHENIA GRAVIS. Myasthenia gravis is an acquired autoimmune disorder in which pathogenic autoantibodies induce acetylcholine receptor (AChR) deficiency at the motor end-plate.

Myasthenia gravis can involve either the external ocular muscles selectively or the general voluntary muscle system. The symptoms may fluctuate from hour to hour, from day to day, or over longer periods. They are provoked or worsened by exertion, exposure to extremes of temperature, viral or other infections, menses, and excitement.

Table 23–56 ■ CLASSIFICATION OF DISORDERS OF NEUROMUSCULAR TRANSMISSION

Autoimmune
Myasthenia gravis
Lambert-Eaton myasthenic syndrome (LEMS)
Congenital
Pre-synaptic defects
Defect in ACh resynthesis or packaging*
Paucity of synaptic vesicles and reduced quantal release*
Synaptic defect
Congenital end-plate AChE deficiency*,†
Post-synaptic defects: increased response to ACh
Slow channel syndromes‡
Post-synaptic defects: decreased response to ACh
Low-affinity fast channel syndromes*,§
Mode-switching kinetics of AChR*,§
AChR deficiency without kinetic abnormality*
Partially characterized syndromes
Congenital myasthenic syndrome resembling LEMS‖
Familial limb girdle myasthenia*
Benign CMS with facial malformations*
Toxic
Botulism
Drug-induced
Organophosphate intoxication

ACh = acetylcholine; AChE = acetylcholinesterase; AChR = acetylcholine receptor; CMS = congenital myasthenic syndrome.
*Autosomal recessive inheritance.
†Mutations in collagenic tail subunit of end-plate AChE.
‡Dominant inheritance.
§Mutations in AChR subunit genes.
‖Autosomal recessive inheritance suspected.

Initially, the symptoms are purely ocular in 40%, are generalized in 40%, involve only the extremities in 10%, and only the bulbar or bulbar and eye muscles in another 10%.

Two thirds of patients with MG have thymic hyperplasia and 10 to 15% have thymoma.

ANTICHOLINESTERASE TESTS. Edrophonium given IV acts within a few seconds, and its effects last for a few minutes. Edrophonium 1 to 2 mg IV is injected over 15 seconds. If no response occurs within 30 seconds, an additional 8 to 9 mg is injected. The evaluation of the response requires objective assessment of one or more signs, such as degree of ptosis, range of ocular movements, and force of the handgrip.

SEROLOGIC TESTS. The usual AChR antibody test measures the binding of antibody to AChR.

LAMBERT-EATON MYASTHENIC SYNDROME. This is an acquired autoimmune disease in which pathogenic autoantibodies cause a deficiency of voltage-sensitive calcium channels at the motor nerve terminal. Among patients above 40 years of age, 70% of men and 30% of women have an associated carcinoma, usually a small cell carcinoma of the lung. The syndrome may pre-date tumor detection by up to 3 years.

For more information about this subject, see *Cecil Textbook of Medicine,* 21st edition. Philadelphia, W.B. Saunders Company, 2000. Chapter 511, Disorders of Neuromuscular Transmission, pages 2221 to 2223.

CHAPTER 24

EYE, EAR, NOSE, AND THROAT DISEASES

DISEASES OF THE VISUAL SYSTEM

Exogenous Infections

Anterior blepharitis primarily involves the eyelash follicles, which are located within the anterior lamella of the eyelid. *Staphylococcus aureus* is the most common infectious agent. Patients are advised to clean the eyelids and eyelashes rigorously using a cotton-tipped applicator or washcloth daily. Ophthalmic antibiotic ointment (bacitracin or erythromycin) is more effective than eye drops for treating the lid margin.

The inflammation of *meibomianitis* localizes to the posterior lamella. Treatment requires daily eyelid hygiene. Warm, dilute solutions of baby shampoo and a clean washcloth may be used to massage the eyelid margin.

Acute, focal infection of a meibomian or Zeis gland is called a *hordeolum.* Commonly termed a "stye," a hordeolum may be painful and may produce blepharoptosis when it occurs in the upper lid. Hordeola usually respond to warm compresses over a period of days, whereas pre-septal cellulitis requires systemic antibiotics.

Chalazion describes a chronically inspissated meibomian gland. Conservative treatment involves warm soaks with or without antibiotic ointment. Incision and curettage is usually reserved for very large lesions or those persisting more than 1 month.

Clinical signs of *pre-septal cellulitis* are limited to external soft tissues. Decreased visual acuity, relative afferent pupillary defect, limited ocular motility, and pronounced chemosis herald post-septal involvement. In the presence of orbital signs, computed tomographic (CT) scans of the orbit and sinuses should be obtained. If untreated, *orbital cellulitis* may extend intracranially. Pre-septal cellulitis is treated with oral antibiotics in an outpatient setting. First-generation cephalosporins are generally effective.

Acute dacryocystitis produces pain, redness, and swelling of the lacrimal sac. Initial treatment with oral antibiotics may quell any acute inflammation, but definitive treatment usually requires dacryocystorhinostomy with intubation of the nasolacrimal system.

Conjunctivitis is a frequent complaint in which patients experience redness, itching, and foreign body sensation, with discharge ranging from watery to hyperpurulent. It must be differentiated from a corneal abrasion and other causes of a red, painful eye (Table 24–1). The great majority of cases are caused by viral

For more information about this subject, see in *Cecil Textbook of Medicine,* 21st edition. Philadelphia, W.B. Saunders Company, 2000. Part XXVI: Ear, Eye, Nose, and Throat Diseases, pages 2224 to 2262.

Table 24–1 ■ DIFFERENTIAL DIAGNOSIS OF COMMON CAUSES OF INFLAMED EYE*

FEATURE	ACUTE CONJUNCTIVITIS	ACUTE IRITIS†	ACUTE GLAUCOMA‡	CORNEAL TRAUMA OR INFECTION
Incidence	Extremely common	Common	Uncommon	Common
Discharge	Moderate to copious	None	None	Watery or purulent
Vision	No effect on vision	Slightly blurred	Markedly blurred	Usually blurred
Pain	None	Moderate	Severe	Moderate to severe
Conjunctival injection	Diffuse; more toward fornices	Mainly circumcorneal	Mainly circumcorneal	Mainly circumcorneal
Cornea	Clear	Usually clear	Steamy	Change in clarity related to cause
Pupil size	Normal	Small	Moderately dilated and fixed	Normal or small
Pupillary light response	Normal	Poor	None	Normal
Intraocular pressure	Normal	Normal	Elevated	Normal
Smear	Causative organisms	No organisms	No organisms	Organisms found only in corneal ulcers due to infection

* Other less common causes of red eyes include endophthalmitis, foreign body, episcleritis, and scleritis.
† Acute anterior uveitis.
‡ Angle-closure glaucoma.

infections. Patients diagnosed with viral conjunctivitis should be isolated from other patients. There may be copious watery discharge. Cool compresses may be used. Antibiotic solutions and ointments are not required, and topical corticosteroids are contraindicated. Bacterial conjunctivitis represents fewer than 5% of all cases. Moderate purulent discharge is seen. The disease is usually self-limited but responds well to broad-spectrum antibiotic solutions, including gentamicin and Polytrim (polymyxin B and trimethoprim). Hyperacute purulent conjunctivitis caused by *Neisseria gonorrhoeae* is transmitted through sexual contact. Third-generation cephalosporins may be given intramuscularly or intravenously.

Adult inclusion conjunctivitis is produced through sexual transmission of *Chlamydia trachomatis*. Systemic treatment with erythromycin or azithromycin is required. *Allergic conjunctivitis* is commonly associated with atopy, hay fever, and allergic rhinitis. Supportive treatment includes cool compresses and topical vasoconstrictors or antihistamines such as naphazoline or levocabastine.

Keratitis caused by herpes simplex virus usually represents secondary ocular infection. Treatment with topical corticosteroids reduces the risk of permanent corneal opacification. Prophylactic topical antiviral agents (e.g., trifluridine) are given during treatment with corticosteroids.

Bacterial keratitis may present as a minor peripheral corneal opacity or a large central suppurative ulcer. Symptoms include pain, redness, photophobia, and decreased vision. Empiric treatment with topical fluoroquinolones is reasonable. More severe cases require hospital admission.

Endophthalmitis, or inflammation of the intraocular cavity, may be exogenous or endogenous and infectious or sterile. The primary symptom is decreased vision. Prognosis is variable and depends on the specific pathogen.

Idiopathic Inflammatory and Autoimmune Conditions

Keratoconjunctivitis sicca, commonly called dry eye syndrome, results from deficiency of any of the tear film layers. Symptoms include gritty, foreign body sensations, burning, photophobia, and decreased visual acuity. Artificial tears and lubricating ointments at night are the mainstays of treatment.

Episcleritis is inflammation immediately underlying the conjunctiva. Pain, if present, is mild. Topical non-steroidal anti-inflammatory medications (NSAIDs) such as flurbiprofen or diclofenac may hasten resolution.

Scleritis frequently presents as severe pain and redness. Treatment may require topical or oral NSAIDs or corticosteroids.

Patients with *iritis* complain of pain, photophobia, and blurred vision. Greater than 50% of cases are unrelated to systemic disease. Initial episodes are usually treated with prednisolone acetate and cycloplegic drugs. Repeat episodes require systemic evaluation for autoimmune and infectious causes.

Neoplastic Diseases

Malignant melanoma of the conjunctiva may arise de novo, from nevi, or in areas of *primary acquired melanosis* (PAM). In cases without metastases, treatment is controversial and may involve focal radiation, laser ablation, excision, or enucleation.

Metastatic ocular disease and systemic neoplastic proliferations involving the eye are far more common than primary ocular malignancy. Choroidal metastases are seen most commonly with adenocarcinoma of the breast in women; primary lung tumors are the leading cause in men.

Degenerative Diseases

Cataract, or opacification of the crystalline lens, is the leading cause of blindness in the world and the leading cause of visual loss in Americans older than age 40 years. Cataract extraction is very successful.

Glaucoma consists of elevated intraocular tension, atrophic cupping of the optic nerve head, and characteristic visual field loss. Normal-tension glaucoma has been described. *Primary open-angle glaucoma,* the most common glaucoma, occurs in 15% of people older than age 80. The anterior chamber angle anatomy appears normal, but aqueous outflow is reduced. Progressive visual field loss begins in the periphery and occurs insidiously. Topical β-blockers, carbonic anhydrase inhibitors, miotics, and prostaglandins may be additive in their effects. *Angle-closure glaucoma* constitutes an ophthalmic emergency. Patients present with a red, painful eye. Nausea and vomiting are common. The pupil is usually fixed in a mid-dilated position, and the cornea appears cloudy due to pressure-driven edema. Emergent treatment requires topical administration of a β-adrenergic antagonist, an α-adrenergic agonist, and carbonic anhydrase inhibitors. Definitive treatment requires peripheral iridotomy, usually performed with a laser after the initial crisis is resolved.

Retinitis pigmentosa (RP) is a group of photoreceptor dystrophies in which damage to rods predominates. Nyctalopia (night blindness) and gradual, progressive loss of peripheral vision are invariably present. Although the appearance of the fundus varies greatly, signs include attenuation of retinal vessels, waxy pallor of the optic disk, and "bone spicule" pigmentation of the peripheral fundus. Approximately 35% of RP cases show autosomal recessive transmission, about one fifth are autosomal dominant, about 10% are X-linked recessive, and about 35% are sporadic. There is no current treatment for RP.

Age-related macular degeneration is an idiopathic atrophy of the photoreceptors and retinal pigmented epithelium. There is no known treatment for non-neovascular age-related macular degeneration.

Retinal detachment, or separation of the neurosensory retina from the retinal pigmented epithelium, is most commonly associated with severe, proliferative diabetic retinopathy or follows non-diabetic vitreous hemorrhage. Symptoms include acute decrease in acuity, photopsia (flashing lights), and floaters. Greater than 90% of cases demonstrated red blood cells in the vitreous (Shafer's sign). Acute, symptomatic cases must be repaired. Patients with vitreous hemorrhage should adhere to strict bed rest. Asymptomatic or chronic detachments may be observed in some cases.

Pingueculae are yellowish elevations of the interpalpebral conjunctiva in which the substantia propria demonstrates elastotic degeneration: ultraviolet radiation–damaged fibroblasts produce altered collagen. Lesions encroaching on the nasal or temporal cornea and demonstrating identical histopathologic findings are known as *pterygia.*

Infarction of the optic nerve head is called *anterior ischemic optic neuropathy.* Many cases are related to vasculitides, whereas others are non-arteritic (idiopathic). Patients present with acute, painless, unilateral loss of vision. Risk factors include hypertension and diabetes mellitus.

Common Ophthalmic Manifestations of Systemic Diseases

Nerve fiber layer infarcts seen clinically as "cotton-wool" spots are the most common ocular manifestation of the *acquired immune deficiency syndrome* (AIDS). *Cytomegalovirus retinitis* may present as subacute unilateral visual loss or vitreous floaters in immunocompromised patients. Intravenous gancyclovir or foscarnet is the mainstay of treatment. Herpes zoster and herpes simplex viruses may produce fulminating necrosis of the retina, *progressive outer retinal necrosis,* in patients with AIDS.

Ocular *toxoplasmosis* may represent reactivation of congenital disease or be acquired after birth. Symptoms include reduced vision and floaters. Treatment requires systemic combination of pyrimethamine, clindamycin, sulfonamides, prednisone, and folinic acid.

Graves' ophthalmopathy may be seen in hyperthyroid, euthyroid, or hypothyroid individuals. Inflammation of the extraocular muscles and orbital fat causes proptosis, corneal exposure, and limited ocular motility. Patients may present with pain, decreased vision, and vascular congestion. Active inflammation may be treated with systemic corticosteroids or external beam irradiation in conjunction with aggressive topical lubrication. Emergent surgical decompression may be required.

Sarcoidosis is a common cause of intraocular inflammation and chronic uveitis. Sarcoid may also involve the optic nerve, cranial nerves, and lacrimal glands. Anterior uveitis is treated topically with prednisolone. Posterior uveitis and neurologic manifestations require systemic corticosteroids.

Uveitis accompanies many autoimmune diseases, and there is often no correlation between ocular and systemic inflammatory activity. *Ankylosing spondylitis* causes acute, recurrent anterior uveitis. Anterior uveitis or conjunctivitis is seen in nearly all patients with *Reiter's syndrome.* Two to 12 per cent of patients with *inflammatory bowel disease* develop anterior uveitis, which is also commonly found in patients with *psoriatic arthritis.* Treatment with topical corticosteroids is usually sufficient to control the ocular disease.

Diabetic retinopathy leads to microaneurysm formation, exudation, capillary obliteration, and neovascularization. Non-proliferative disease, also called background diabetic retinopathy, manifests as microaneurysms, intraretinal hemorrhages, subretinal exudation, venous bleeding, and intraretinal vascular abnormalities. Macular edema, the most frequent cause of visual loss, is common in this stage. Macular edema meeting the criteria of the Early Treatment Diabetic Retinopathy Study is treated with focal laser photocoagulation. Retinal ischemia is thought to be the primary stimulus to proliferative diabetic retinopathy. Neovascularization at the optic disk or elsewhere may lead to vitreous hemorrhage and acute loss of vision. Proliferative disease meeting the criteria set forth in the Diabetic Retinopathy Study is treated with panretinal laser photocoagulation.

Accumulation of copper in the posterior cornea may aid in the diagnosis of *Wilson's hepatolenticular degeneration.* The characteristic Kayser-Fleischer ring fades after treatment.

Chronic *hypertension* produces arterial narrowing, nicking at arteriovenous crossings, nerve fiber layer infarcts, and intraretinal hemorrhages. Moderately sclerosed arterioles demonstrate "copper wiring," whereas severely sclerosed vessels show "silver wiring." Acute hypertension may produce optic nerve edema and serous retinal detachments.

Hypertension may also be implicated in retinal vascular occlusions. *Central retinal vein occlusion* produces dilated tortuous vessels in all quadrants, as well as variable degrees of retinal hemorrhage. Neovascularization of the iris or retina usually occurs 3 months after the initial insult. Panretinal photocoagulation should be deferred until neovascularization is detected.

In contrast to venous occlusive disease, *central retinal artery occlusion* is not generally associated with systemic hypertension. Emboli result most commonly from carotid stenosis. Amaurosis fugax, or transient unilateral visual loss, may precede frank occlusion and warrants urgent carotid evaluation. Fundus examination reveals a characteristic "cherry-red spot" that reflects diffuse opacification of the infarcting macula contrasted to the hyperpigmented fovea. *Branch retinal artery occlusion* may go unnoticed by the patient despite a permanent visual *scotoma* (visual field defect).

Temporal arteritis is an important cause of visual loss among the elderly. Symptoms include sudden, unilateral loss of vision. Headache, jaw claudication, scalp tenderness, weight loss, and malaise are common. Visual loss may result from arteritis or associated central retinal artery occlusion. Systemic corticosteroids should be initiated as soon as the diagnosis is suspected, and temporal artery biopsy should be performed within 7 days after beginning treatment.

Orbital involvement in *Wegener's granulomatosis* usually indicates extension from nasal or sinus mucosa and may produce proptosis. Retinal involvement in *polyarteritis nodosa* is usually limited to the small vessels, although central retinal artery occlusion can occur. Cranial nerve palsies are not uncommon. The occlusive vasculitis of *Behçet's disease* produces retinal vasculitis and iridocyclitis. Topical corticosteroids are used to treat anterior disease, whereas systemic corticosteroids and cytotoxic agents may be required for posterior disease.

Ocular Effects of Systemic Medications

Many systemic medications have ocular effects (Table 24–2). *β-Adrenergic antagonists* may cause bronchospasm or bradycardia. *Carbonic anhydrase inhibitors* may be administered topically and do not seem to carry the risk of central nervous system effects and aplastic anemia seen with systemic administration.

Table 24–2 ■ SYSTEMIC MEDICATIONS WITH OCULAR EFFECTS

AGENT	EFFECT
Chloroquine	Dyschromatopsia, visual field defects
Hydroxychloroquine	Dyschromatopsia, visual field defects
Thioridazine	Blurred vision
Chlorpromazine	Blurred vision
Digoxin	Yellow vision
Ethambutol	Optic neuritis
Amiodarone	Corneal whirls, pigmentary retinopathy
Corticosteroids	Glaucoma, cataract
Plaquenil	Pigmentary maculopathy
Tamoxifen	Retinopathy
Neuroleptics	Nystagmus
Compazine	Oculogyric crisis
Vitamin A	Pseudotumor cerebri

Visual Fields

What each eye "sees" is termed its *visual field* (Fig. 24–1). A quick screen of the visual fields can be made by having the patient fixate on the examiner's nose and identify the number of fingers flashed in each of the four visual field quadrants.

Common Causes of Visual Loss

Sudden visual loss is commonly due to circulatory conditions or trauma (Table 24–3). Retinal tears and detachments give rise to unilateral distortions of the visual image seen as sudden angulations or curves of objects containing straight lines (metamorphopsia). Hemorrhages into the vitreous humor or infections or inflammatory lesions of the retina can produce scotomata that resemble those resulting from primary disease of the central visual pathway.

Acute or subacute monocular vision loss due to optic nerve disease is most commonly produced by demyelinating disorders, vascular obstruction, or neoplasm. The common causes of transient monocular vision loss and their differential features are listed in Table 24–4.

Common Causes of Pupillary Abnormalities

With so-called benign pupillary dilation or physiologic anisocoria, there is a long-standing difference in the size of the two pupils with normal reflex reactions; the disparity remains constant during constriction and dilation. Adie's tonic pupil is a medium-to-large (3 to 6 mm) pupil that constricts little or not at all to light and very slowly to accommodation, but constricts with the instillation of dilute pilocarpine (0.125%) (Fig. 24–2). The condition usually affects one eye and carries no serious implications. Interruption of the emerging third cranial nerve in the ventral midbrain or along the proximal part of its course produces a dilated pupil 6 to 7 mm in diameter. Important causes of compression of the third nerve in this region are aneurysms, neoplasia, and brain herniation.

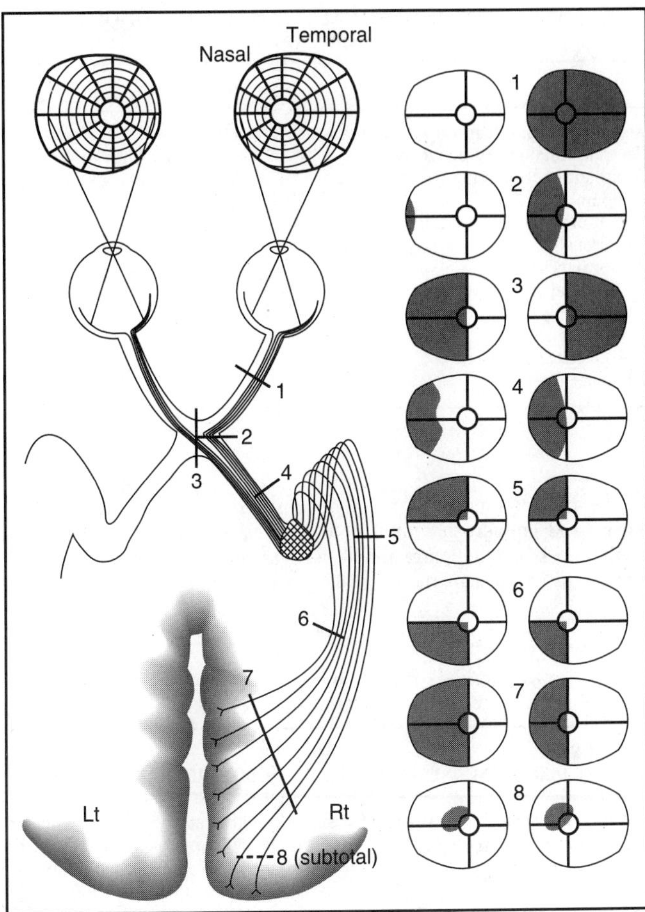

FIGURE 24–1 ■ Visual fields that accompany damage to the visual pathways. 1. Optic nerve: Unilateral amaurosis. 2. Lateral optic chiasm: Grossly incongruous, incomplete (contralateral) homonymous hemianopia. 3. Central optic chiasm: Bitemporal hemianopia. 4. Optic tract: Incongruous, incomplete homonymous hemianopia. 5. Temporal (Meyer's) loop of optic radiation: Congruous partial or complete (contralateral) homonymous superior quadrantanopia. 6. Parietal (superior) projection of the optic radiation: Congruous partial or complete homonymous inferior quadrantanopia. 7. Complete parieto-occipital interruption of optic radiation: Complete congruous homonymous hemianopia with psychophysical shift of foveal point often sparing central vision, giving "macular sparing." 8. Incomplete damage to visual cortex: Congruous homonymous scotomas, usually encroaching at least acutely on central vision.

Table 24–3 ■ DIFFERENTIAL DIAGNOSIS OF SUDDEN VISUAL LOSS

UNILATERAL	BILATERAL
Amaurosis fugax (carotid artery stenosis)	Eclampsia
Central retinal artery occlusion	Cavernous sinus thrombosis
Occipital lobe infarct	Vertebrobasilar infarct
Temporal arteritis	Trauma
Non-arteritic anterior ischemic optic neuropathy	
Hemorrhage	
Preretinal (high altitude, Valsalva's maneuver)	
Vitreous	
Aqueous (hyphema)	
Trauma	

The most common lesions producing Horner's syndrome (miosis, ptosis, and anhydrosis) involve the ascending second-order neuron in the neck or the extracranial postganglionic neuron; malignant tumors in the apex of the lung are most common. Dissection of the

Table 24–4 ■ COMMON CAUSES OF TRANSIENT MONOCULAR VISION LOSS

CATEGORY (TYPICAL DURATION)	CAUSES	DIFFERENTIAL FEATURES
Thromboembolism (1–5 min)	Atherosclerosis	Other atherosclerotic vascular disease, associated crossed hemiparesis, angiography (carotid atheromata)
	Cardiac	Valvular disease, mural thrombi, atrial fibrillation, recent myocardial infarction
	Blood dyscrasia	Blood tests positive for sickle cell anemia, macroglobulinemia, multiple myeloma, polycythemia, etc.
Vasospasm (5–30 min)	Migraine	Ipsilateral headache, other classic aura, and family history
Vascular compression (few seconds)	Increased intracranial pressure	Precipitated by position change, Valsalva's maneuver, or pressure waves
	Tumor	Associated slowly progressive monocular visual loss
Vasculitis (1–5 min)	Temporal arteritis	Associated headache, polymyalgia rheumatica, palpable temporal artery, elevated sedimentation rate

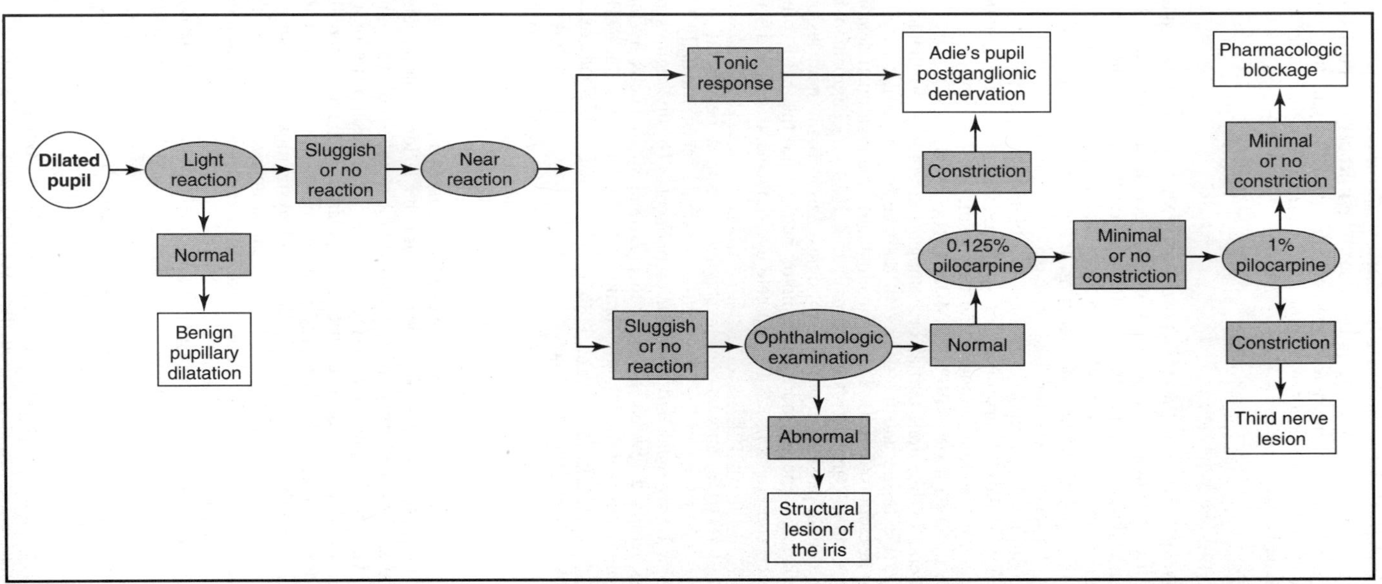

FIGURE 24–2 ■ Use of pilocarpine to help differentiate among different causes of a dilated pupil.

carotid artery is another serious cause. Argyll-Robertson pupils are small (1 to 2 mm), unequal, irregular, and fixed to light; they constrict minimally to accommodation. Their principal cause is tertiary neurosyphilis.

Abnormal Eye Movements

STRABISMUS (OCULAR MISALIGNMENT). An acquired skew deviation (vertical displacement of the ocular axes) indicates a lesion within the otolith-ocular pathways (usually the brain stem). Common causes of orbital restrictive disease include dysthyroid ophthalmopathy, orbital pseudotumor, trauma, and orbital mass lesions. Variable strabismus that increases with fatigue suggests myasthenia gravis. Common causes of an isolated third nerve palsy in an adult include aneurysm, small vessel occlusive disease (including diabetes mellitus), trauma, and neoplasm.

INTERNUCLEAR OPHTHALMOPLEGIA (INO). INO may be unilateral or bilateral, partial or complete, depending on the location of the lesion and the degree of damage to the medial longitudinal fasciculus (MLF). Demyelinating and small vascular lesions are the most common cause of unilateral INO unaccompanied by other ocular palsies or brain stem signs. Larger brain stem lesions that damage one or more oculomotor nuclei plus the MLF often produce combinations of disconjugate eye movements coupled with nuclear oculomotor palsies.

NYSTAGMUS. Spontaneous nystagmus due to a peripheral vestibular lesion (i.e., in the labyrinth or vestibular nerve) usually has combined horizontal and torsional components. The nystagmus resolves within a few days. Acquired persistent spontaneous nystagmus indicates a lesion in the brain stem and/or cerebellum. The latter is often purely vertical, horizontal, or torsional. Spontaneous downbeat nystagmus is commonly seen with lesions of the cerebellum or cervicomedullary junction. Gaze-evoked nystagmus is always in the direction of gaze and is usually present with and without fixation. It is most commonly produced by ingestion of drugs such as phenobarbital, phenytoin, alcohol, and diazepam. Asymmetrical horizontal gaze-evoked nystagmus indicates a structural brain stem or cerebellar lesion with the lesion usually being on the side of the larger-amplitude nystagmus. Rebound nystagmus is a type of gaze-evoked nystagmus that either disappears or reverses direction as the eccentric gaze position is held. When the eyes are returned to the primary position, nystagmus occurs in the direction of the return saccade. Rebound nystagmus occurs in patients with cerebellar atrophy and focal structural lesions of the cerebellum. Disconjugate gaze-evoked nystagmus most commonly results from lesions of the MLF.

OTHER OCULAR OSCILLATIONS. Ocular bobbing consists of a fast conjugate downward eye movement followed by a slow return to the primary position. The phenomenon accompanies severe displacement or destruction of the pons or, less often, metabolic central nervous systems (CNS) depression. Opsoclonus consists of rapid, chaotic, conjugate, repetitive, saccadic eye movements (dancing eyes). Opsoclonus accompanies cerebellar dysfunction.

For more information about this subject, see *Cecil Textbook of*

Medicine, 21st edition. Philadelphia, W.B. Saunders Company, 2000. Chapter 512, Diseases of the Visual System; and Chapter 513, Neuro-Ophthalmology, pages 2224 to 2241.

DISEASES OF THE MOUTH AND SALIVARY GLANDS

Painful short-term ulcerations are usually caused by mechanical trauma, immunologic mechanisms, and bacterial or viral infections (Table 24–5). Aphthous ulcers, which are idiopathic recurrent ulcers, afflict about 20 % of the population and are found on all areas of the oral mucosa. Lesions clinically identical to minor aphthous ulcers occur in Behçet's syndrome. Several mucocutaneous diseases can cause chronic multifocal oral mucosal lesions composed of ill-defined areas of erythema and ulceration (Table 24–6).

The term *leukoplakia* applies to a white plaque that does not rub off and whose appearance does not indicate another disease. On long-term follow-up, 2 to 6% of these lesions will undergo malignant transformation into squamous cell carcinoma.

Solitary red macules or plaques (*erythroplakia*) are less common in the mouth than white lesions but should be viewed with concern because they may exhibit microscopic dysplasia or represent carcinoma in situ.

Brown or gray-black macules on the oral mucosa are relatively common and may be caused by localized increase in melanin production, proliferation of melanin-producing cells, or deposition of local or systemically distributed pigmented substances (Table 24–7).

Oral Soft Tissue Tumors

The most common oral soft tissue tumors are small, pedunculated masses of hyperplastic fibrous connective tissue covered by normal-appearing mucosa (Table 24–8). Generalized enlargement of the gingiva (gingival hyperplasia) may be caused by chronic administration of phenytoin, cyclosporine, and many of the calcium channel blocking drugs (e.g., diltiazem, verapamil, or nifedipine).

Salivary Gland Diseases

Patients with enlargement of a major or minor salivary gland usually present a diagnostic challenge (Table 24–9). Unilateral major salivary gland enlargement that is markedly painful or tender to palpation and has a purulent exudate or nothing expressible from the duct suggests bacterial sialadenitis. Any exudate should be cultured, and initial treatment should be oral cephalexin or dicloxacillin. The salivary component of Sjögren's syndrome should be diagnosed from a labial salivary gland biopsy specimen containing at least five glands. The very common symptom of dry mouth (xerostomia) is most often a side effect of chronically administered drugs (Table 24–10).

For more information about this subject, see *Cecil Textbook of Medicine,* 21st edition. Philadelphia, W.B. Saunders Company, 2000. Chapter 514, Diseases of the Mouth and Salivary Glands, pages 2242 to 2246.

Table 24–5 ■ ORAL MUCOSAL ULCERS

TYPE/DISEASE	CLINICAL FEATURES
Insidious Onset, Chronic	
Multiple or bilateral	Shallow ulcers on mucosa, skin, or both
Pemphigus vulgaris	Begin as short-duration blisters
Mucous membrane pemphigoid	Begin as short-duration blisters
Lichen planus	Bilaterally symmetrical lesions (associated with hyperkeratoses and/or erythema)
Lupus erythematosus	Asymmetrical lesions, with or without systemic lupus (associated with hyperkeratoses and/or erythema)
Drug reaction	Variable lesions; appropriate history of drug use
Epidermolysis bullosa	Begin as blisters; lifelong history
Solitary	Indurated or cratered ulcers
Squamous cell carcinoma	Most common on tongue, oropharynx, lip, mouth floor
Adenocarcinomas, various	Most common on palate, cheeks, mouth floor
Tuberculosis	Usually painful
Actinomycosis	Often associated with draining sinus
Deep mycoses (particularly histoplasmosis, coccidioidomycosis)	Associated with systemic infection
Midline granuloma	Associated with necrosis, may perforate palate
Acute Onset, Often Self-Limiting	
Clusters	Usually small and shallow ulcers; history of blisters
Primary herpes simplex	Any oral mucosal site, associated with fever, malaise
Recurrent herpes simplex	Only on gingiva, hard palate, or lip (keratinized mucosa)
Varicella-zoster	Unilateral lesions along neural distribution
Herpangina	Usually on oropharynx
Measles (rubeola)	Precedes skin rash; associated with fever, malaise
Solitary or multiple (without clustering)	Variable, usually without history of blisters
Traumatic ulcers	Usually solitary; history of trauma
Recurrent aphthae	Circular, often multiple, only on nonkeratinized mucosa
Behçet's syndrome	Oral lesions similar to recurrent aphthae
Erythema multiforme	Multiple lesions, often involve lower labial mucosa; can be recurrent or chronic
Drug reaction	Appropriate history of drug use
Necrotizing sialometaplasia	Usually on palate
Primary syphilis	Solitary, indurated, painless, any site
Gonorrhea	Painful, surrounded by erythema, any site

Table 24–6 ■ WHITE AND RED ORAL MUCOSAL LESIONS

White Lesions (Plaques)

Squamous cell carcinoma (early)
Frictional keratosis
Leukoplakia (idiopathic)
Smokeless tobacco–associated lesions
Nicotine stomatitis (palate)
Lichen planus (reticular and plaque types)
Pseudomembranous candidiasis (thrush)
Hyperplastic candidiasis (candidal leukoplakia)
Hairy leukoplakia (HIV-associated; usually on lateral tongue)
Geographic tongue
Mucous patch or condyloma latum of secondary syphilis
Pseudomembrane-covered ulcers

Red Lesions (Macular, Maculopapular)

Squamous cell carcinoma (early)
Erythroplakia (epithelial dysplasia)
Erythematous (atrophic) candidiasis
Median rhomboid glossitis
Mucocutaneous diseases
Angular cheilitis
Telangiectasias and purpuras
Kaposi's sarcoma (blue-to-purple color)

HIV = human immunodeficiency virus.

SINUSES, MOUTH, NOSE, AND UPPER AIRWAY DISEASES

Sinusitis

A mucopurulent discharge and a painful face suggest *sinusitis,* an inflammation of the lining of the paranasal sinuses. Most cases occur as a complication of the common cold or other upper respira-

Table 24–7 ■ PIGMENTATIONS OF THE ORAL MUCOSA (BROWN OR GRAY-BLACK IN COLOR)

Increased Melanin Production (Flat Lesions)

Oral melanotic macule
Ephelis (vermilion border)
Systemic diseases: Addison's disease, von Recklinghausen's disease of skin, Albright's syndrome, Peutz-Jeghers syndrome

Proliferation of Melanin-Producing Cells (Flat or Raised Lesions)

Pigmented cellular nevi (benign and premalignant types)
Atypical melanocytic hyperplasia, melanoma in situ, radial growth phase of melanoma
Malignant melanoma

Non-Melanin Pigmentation

Amalgam tattoo
Focal deposition of systemically distributed metal (lead, bismuth, mercury, others) usually at sites of chronic inflammation
Systemically administered drugs (chloroquine, minocycline, ketoconazole, cyclophosphamide)

Table 24–8 ■ ORAL SOFT TISSUE TUMORS

Connective Tissue Hyperplasia (Normal-Appearing Overlying Mucosa)

Irritation fibroma
Denture-associated hyperplasia
Palatal papillomatosis
Generalized gingival hyperplasia
  Drug-induced (phenytoin, nifedipine, cyclosporine)
  Hereditary

Reactive Hyperplasia (Erythematous Overlying Mucosa)

Pyogenic granuloma/pregnancy tumor
Peripheral giant cell granuloma
Inflammatory gingival hyperplasia
Hyperplastic lingual tonsil

Epithelial Masses (Usually Irregular White Surface)

Papilloma/oral wart
Squamous cell carcinoma
Verrucous carcinoma
Focal epithelial hyperplasia (Heck's disease)
Condyloma acuminatum (veneral wart)
Keratoacanthoma (on lips)

Salivary Duct Obstruction (Minor Salivary Glands)

Mucocele/ranula (usually fluctuant)
Salivary stone (sialolith)

Subepithelial Neoplasms

Primary connective tissue or salivary gland tumors
Metastatic lesions (especially in the mandible)
Lymphoma (especially in the palate or posterior mandible)
Focal or generalized leukemic infiltrates in the gingiva (especially with acute monocytic leukemia)

Table 24–9 ■ CAUSES OF SALIVARY GLAND ENLARGEMENT

Usually Unilateral

Benign or malignant salivary gland neoplasms (>20 different histopathologic types)
Bacterial infection
Chronic sialadenitis (single gland)

Usually Bilateral and Associated with Salivary Hypofunction

Viral infection (mumps, cytomegalovirus, influenza, coxsackie A)
Sjögren's syndrome (benign lymphoepithelial lesion)
Chronic granulomatous diseases (sarcoidosis, tuberculosis, leprosy)
Recurrent parotitis of childhood
Human immunodeficiency virus infection/AIDS

Bilaterally Symmetrical, Soft, Nontender, Parotid Only

Sialadenosis (asymptomatic parotid enlargment), idiopathic or associated with:

Diabetes mellitus	Chronic pancreatitis
Hyperlipoproteinemia	Acromegaly
Hepatic cirrhosis	Gonadal hypofunction
Anorexia/bulimia	Phenylbutazone use

Table 24–10 ■ CAUSES OF DECREASED SALIVARY SECRETION

Temporary
Effects of short-term drug use (e.g., antihistamines)
Virus infections (e.g., mumps)
Dehydration
Psychogenic causes (fear, depression)
Chronic
Effects of chronically administered drugs (especially antidepressants, MAO inhibitors, neuroleptics, parasympatholytics, some combinations of drugs for treating hypertension)
Systemic Diseases (with or without Gland Enlargement)
Sjögren's syndrome
Granulomatous diseases (sarcoidosis, tuberculosis, leprosy)
Amyloidosis
HIV infection
Diabetes mellitus (uncontrolled)
Graft-versus-host disease
Depression
Therapeutic radiation to the head and neck
Absent or malformed glands (rare)

MAO = monoamine oxidase; HIV = human immunodeficiency virus.

tory tract infections, with occasional presentations due to extension of a periodontal infection under the maxillary sinus. Normal light transmission to the frontal sinus from the supraorbital ridge or to the maxillary sinus through the hard palate excludes sinusitis. A coronal CT image with bone window settings is the preferred test. Sinus aspiration and endoscopic sinuscopy may be necessary to recover organisms or to effect drainage. Surgical interventions are indicated for treatment failure, suppurative complications, diagnosis of nosocomial infection, and fever of unknown origin with sinus opacification.

The course of acute sinusitis is 3 to 4 weeks because of the anatomic difficulties in drainage. Decongestants improve nasal obstruction and may improve sinus drainage. Oral antibiotics are often prescribed. Fungal sinusitis is uncommon and presents with a chronic course. Maxillary antrum tumors produce a unilateral bloody nasal discharge that can be confused with sinusitis.

Jaw Pain

Pain in the lower jaw without swelling is commonly due to dental caries, periodontal disease, or temporomandibular dysfunction (otomandibular syndrome). Trigeminal neuralgia presents with a unilateral dull pain. Pain from cardiac angina also may be referred to the jaw and can be mistaken for periodontal disease.

Hoarseness

The most common cause of an acute onset of hoarseness is a bacterial or viral infection. Inhaled irritants (smoke or fumes) and overuse of the larynx present similarly. Stridor suggests more than

Table 24–11 ■ COMMON CAUSES OF LOSS OF TASTE AND SMELL

	TASTE	SMELL
Local	Radiation therapy	Allergic rhinitis, sinusitis, nasal polyposis, upper respiratory infection
Systemic	Cancer, renal failure, hepatic failure, nutritional deficiency (vitamin B_3, zinc), Cushing's syndrome, hypothyroidism, diabetes mellitus, infection (viral), drugs (antirheumatic and antiproliferative)	Renal failure, hepatic failure, nutritional deficiency (vitamin B_{12}, Cushing's syndrome, hypothyroidism, diabetes mellitus, infection (viral hepatitis, influenza), drugs (nasal sprays, antibiotics)
Neurologic	Bell's palsy, familial dysautonomia, multiple sclerosis	Head trauma, multiple sclerosis, Parkinson's disease, frontal tumor

edema and inflammation of the vocal folds and warrants evaluation for extrinsic or intrinsic airway encroachment.

Hoarseness persisting 2 weeks or more should be investigated by directly examining the laryngeal structures. Chronic hoarseness can result from benign and malignant processes, including gastroesophageal reflux, laryngeal carcinoma or polyps, arthritis, hypothyroidism, goiter, and infections (tuberculosis, syphilis, and histoplasmosis). Hoarseness following endotracheal intubation is common but should resolve within 3 to 5 days.

Smell and Taste

Disorders of taste and smell can be divided into local, systemic, and neurologic (Table 24–11).

Upper Airway Obstruction

Presenting symptoms of pharyngeal or laryngeal obstruction are air hunger and stridor at rest or on exertion. Direct examination may precipitate complete airway closure and should be performed in a controlled setting like an emergency department.

Table 24–12 ■ OTITIS MEDIA

TYPE	MECHANISMS	TREATMENT
Acute	*Streptococcus pneumoniae* and *Haemophilus influenzae;* rarely *Staphylococcus aureus, Streptococcus pyogenes, Proteus, Pseudomonas*	Oral antibiotics
Serous	Failure to clear fluid (Starling effect)	Antihistamines and decongestants
Chronic	Persistent eustachian tube obstruction (rarely tuberculosis)	Drainage tubes ± all of the above

Causes of acute obstruction include bacterial epiglottitis, trauma, angioneurotic edema, allergic reactions, and foreign body aspiration. Chronic obstruction can be a presenting feature of neoplastic disease (squamous cell carcinoma being the most common), cricoarytenoid arthritis, vocal cord polyps, bilateral vocal cord paralysis, goiter, and neurofibromatosis.

For more information about this subject, see *Cecil Textbook of Medicine,* 21st edition. Philadelphia, W.B. Saunders Company, 2000. Chapter 515, Upper Airway Diseases; and Chapter 516, Smell and Taste, pages 2246 to 2250,

EAR DISEASE, HEARING, AND EQUILIBRIUM

Otitis

Otitis media (Table 24–12) may occur at any age; however, the most frequent presentation is under age 10 years. The spectrum of organisms in immunocompromised hosts includes fungal infections (*Aspergillus* and *Candida*).

External otitis is characterized by severe pain, edema, and discharge along the auditory meatus. The ear and the tragus are painful to the touch. Treatment with topical broad-spectrum antibiotics combined with topical corticosteroids, so-called otic drops, resolves symptoms and results in cure in 3 to 5 days.

Hearing Loss

The logic for identifying common causes of hearing loss is shown in Figure 24–3. The most common cause of conductive hearing loss is impacted cerumen. The most common serious cause of conductive hearing loss is inflammation of the middle ear, otitis media.

Acute unilateral deafness usually has a cochlear basis. Bacterial or viral infections of the labyrinth, head trauma with fracture or hemorrhage into the cochlea, or vascular occlusion of a terminal branch of the anterior inferior cerebellar artery all can extensively damage the cochlea and its hair cells.

Subacute relapsing cochlear deafness occurs with Meniere's disease, a condition associated with fluctuating hearing loss and tinnitus, recurrent episodes of abrupt and often severe vertigo, and a sensation of fullness or pressure in the ear. The gradual, progressive, bilateral hearing loss commonly associated with advancing age is called presbycusis. Central hearing loss is unilateral only if it results from damage to the pontine cochlear nuclei on one side of the brain stem due to conditions such as ischemic infarction, multiple sclerosis, or, rarely, neoplasm or hematoma.

Tinnitus

The evaluation of common causes of tinnitus (Fig. 24–4) begins with a careful history to identify common offending drugs. Subjective tinnitus can arise from sites anywhere in the auditory system. Audiometric and brain stem–evoked response testing can help distinguish among lesions involving the conducting apparatus, the cochlea, and the auditory nerve. Tinnitus without observable deafness appears sporadically and for variable lengths of time in many persons without other evidence of an ongoing pathologic process.

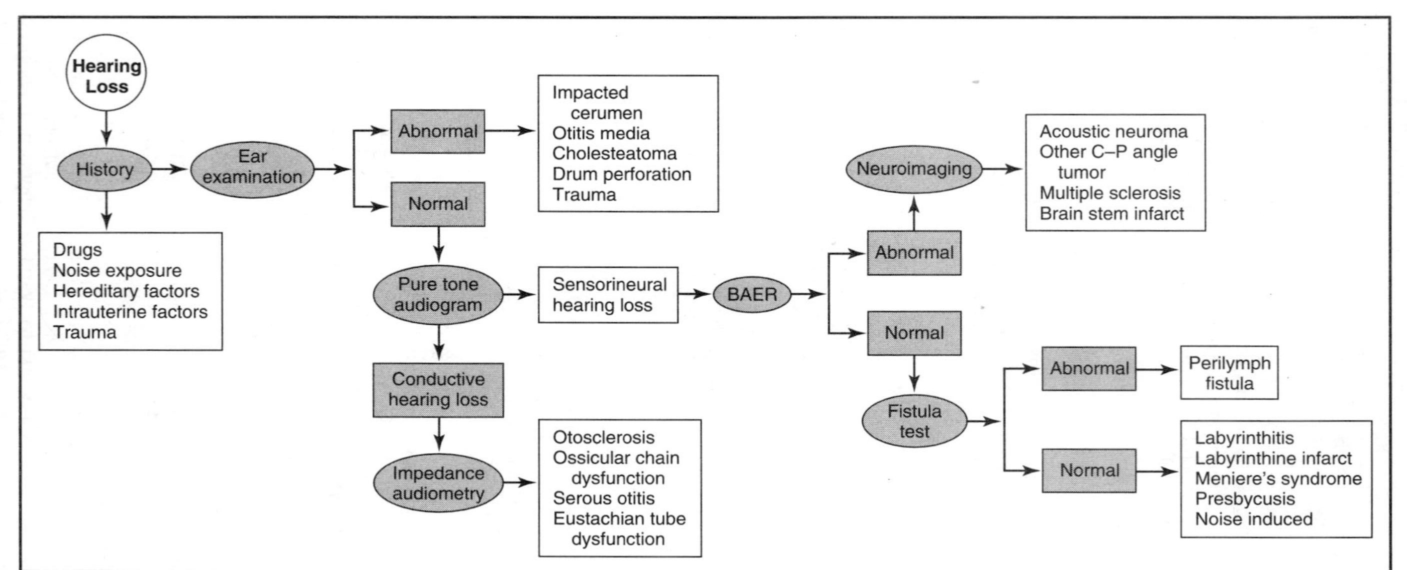

FIGURE 24–3 ■ Evaluation of hearing loss. BAER = brain stem auditory evoked response; C-P = cerebellopontine.

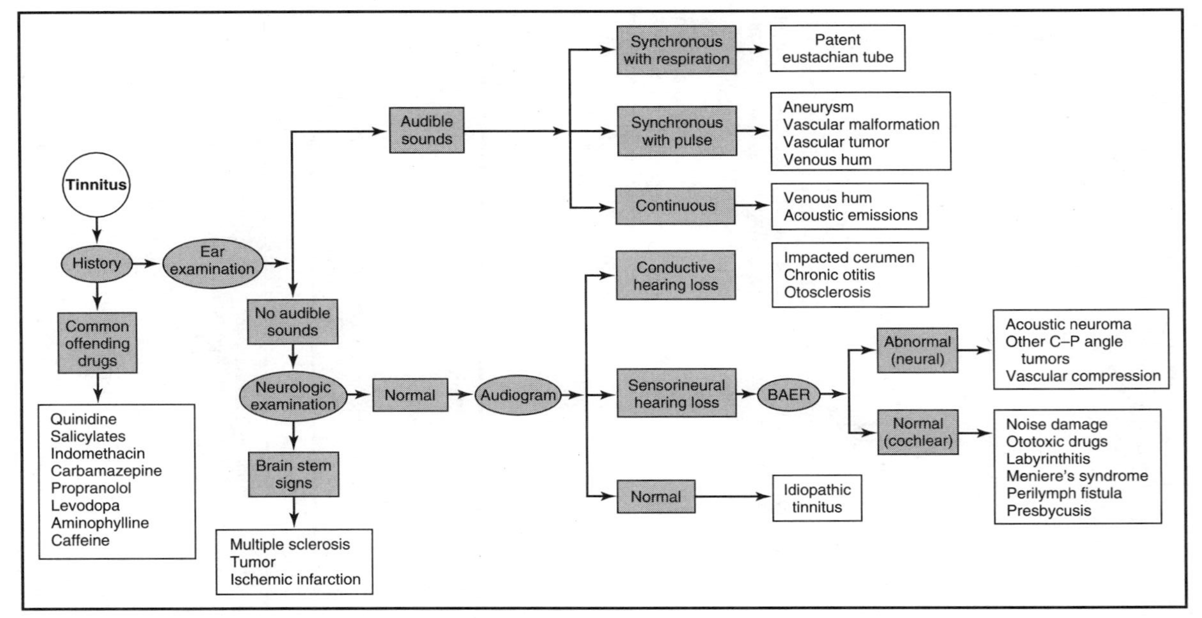

FIGURE 24–4 ■ Evaluation of tinnitus.

24

Evaluating the "Dizzy" Patient

In evaluating the "dizzy" patient the history is key because it determines the type of dizziness (vertigo, lightheadedness, feelings of dissociation, disequilibrium), associated symptoms (neurologic, audiologic, cardiac, psychiatric), precipitating factors (position change, trauma, stress, drug ingestion), and predisposing illness (systemic viral infection, cardiac disease, cerebrovascular disease) (Table 24–13). The examination should include complete neurologic, head and neck, and cardiac assessments. When vertigo is present without focal neurologic symptoms or signs, audiometry and electronystagmography aid in localizing the lesion to the labyrinth or eighth cranial nerve.

Common Causes of Vertigo

Physiologic vertigo includes common disorders such as motion sickness, space sickness, and height vertigo (Fig. 24–5). In these conditions, vertigo (defined as an illusion of movement) is minimal or absent while autonomic symptoms predominate. One of the most common clinical neurologic syndromes at any age is the acute onset of vertigo, nausea, and vomiting lasting for several days and not associated with auditory or neurologic symptoms (acute labyrinthitis).

Benign positional vertigo (BPV) is by far the most common cause of vertigo. Patients with this condition develop brief episodes of vertigo (<1 minute) with position change, typically when turning over in bed, getting in and out of bed, bending over and straightening up, or extending the neck to look up. BPV can result from head injury, viral labyrinthitis, and vascular occlusion, or it may occur as an isolated symptom (in about 50% of cases). The diagnosis rests on finding characteristic fatigable paroxysmal positional nystagmus after a rapid change from the sitting to the head-hanging position. BPV results from free-floating calcium carbonate

Table 24–13 ■ DISTINGUISHING BETWEEN VESTIBULAR AND NON-VESTIBULAR TYPES OF DIZZINESS

	VESTIBULAR	NON-VESTIBULAR
Common descriptive terms	Spinning (environment moves), merry-go-round, drunkenness, tilting, motion sickness, off balance	Lightheadedness, floating, dissociation from body, swimming, giddiness, spinning inside (environment stationary)
Course	Episodic	Constant
Common precipitating factors	Head movements, position change	Stress, hyperventilation, cardiac arrhythmia
Common associated symptoms	Nausea, vomiting, unsteadiness, tinnitus, hearing loss, impaired vision, oscillopsia	Perspiration, pallor, paresthesias, palpitations, syncope, difficulty concentrating, tension headache

From Baloh RW, Honrubia V: Clinical Neurophysiology of the Vestibular System, 2nd ed. Philadelphia, FA Davis, 1990.

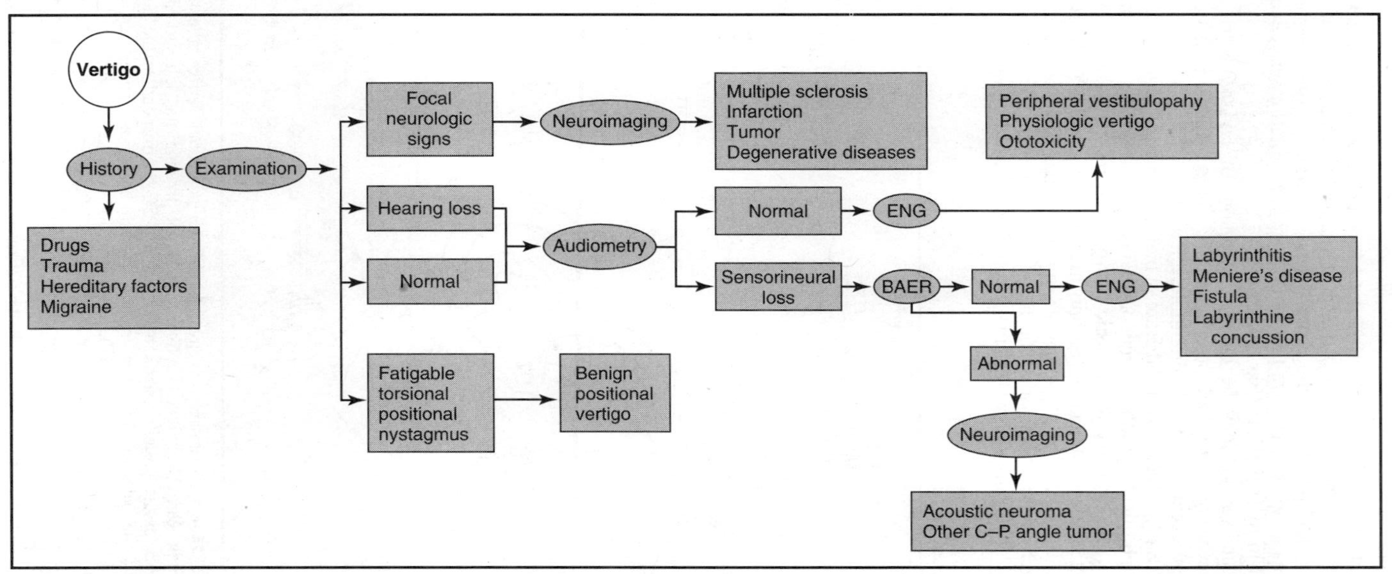

FIGURE 24–5 ■ Evaluation of vertigo. ENG = electronystagmography.

crystals (normally attached to the utricular macule) that inadvertently enter the long arm of the posterior semicircular canal. If the history and physical findings are typical, a simple bedside positioning maneuver can remove the debris from the posterior semicircular canal in most patients (Fig. 24–6).

Acute vertigo may be the first symptom of *multiple sclerosis*. However, only a small percentage of young patients with acute vertigo eventually develop multiple sclerosis.

TREATMENT. Specific therapies include antibiotics for bacterial or syphilitic labyrinthitis, anticoagulants for vertebrobasilar insufficiency, and surgery for acoustic neuroma. In most cases, however, symptomatic treatment is the only treatment available. Antivertiginous drugs such as phenergan 25 mg four times daily or diazepam 5 mg four times daily may be helpful. Prochlorperazine suppositories (25 mg) may stop vomiting. In more chronic vertiginous disor-

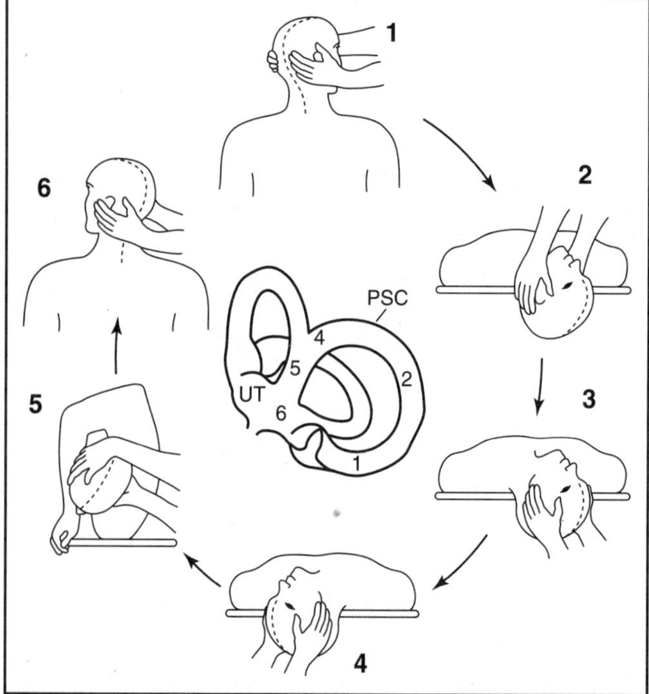

FIGURE 24–6 ■ Treatment maneuver for benign positional vertigo affecting the right ear. The procedure is reversed for treating the left ear. The numbers in the posterior semicircular canal (PSC) correspond to the position of the calcium carbonate crystals in each head position as they are moved toward the utricle (UT). Each position change is performed as rapidly as possible to accelerate the particles. Positions 2 and 3 are the same except that the therapist has moved from the front to the back of the patient to continue the maneuver easily. The entire sequence should be repeated until no nystagmus is elicited. (Courtesy of Carol A. Foster, MD. University of Colorado School of Medicine.)

ders when the patient is trying to carry on normal activity, less sedating antivertiginous medications such as meclizine 25 mg four times daily or transdermal scopolamine 0.5 mg every 3 days may provide relief.

For more information about this subject, see *Cecil Textbook of Medicine,* 21st edition. Philadelphia, W.B. Saunders Company, 2000. Chapter 517, Hearing and Equilibrium, pages 2250 to 2257.

HEAD AND NECK CANCER

Head and neck cancers are staged according to the American Joint Committee on Cancer (AJCC) staging system using a T (primary tumor size), N (regional node), M (distant metastasis) classification system (Table 24–14). Over 90% of head and neck cancers are primary squamous cell carcinomas of the upper aerodigestive tract. Seventy-five per cent of head and neck cancer patients have a history of both tobacco and alcohol use.

Presenting symptoms are related to the site of tumor origin. Tumors in the larynx or hypopharynx can cause hoarseness, dysphagia, odynophagia, stridor, and otalgia (ear pain referred from the pharynx by means of the glossopharyngeal nerve). An ill-fitting denture, non-healing "mouth sores," oral pain, or slurred speech may reflect an oral cavity tumor. Epistaxis, nasal obstruction, or headaches may be due to a paranasal sinus tumor. Unilateral serous otitis media in an adult is a nasopharyngeal neoplasm until proved otherwise. Early lesions can be as innocuous as an area of erythroplakia or, less often, leukoplakia. Other symptoms of head and neck cancers include trismus and cranial nerve palsies. Patients whose presenting complaint is an incidentally noted neck mass tend not to do as well because survival of those with nodal metastases at the time of diagnosis is half that of patients with stage I or II disease.

Head and neck squamous cell carcinoma spreads first through lymphatics to regional lymph nodes. Distant systemic metastases occur most often in lung and bone, although liver, skin, brain, and other tissues also can be affected. Systemic metastases virtually never occur in the absence of regional lymphadenopathy. Hypercalcemia is seen in up to 25% of patients in far-advanced stages of the disease.

For staging purposes and because of the incidence of concurrent second primary lesions, a thorough endoscopic examination of the entire upper aerodigestive tract is indicated for all patients newly diagnosed with head and neck squamous cell carcinoma. Radiologic staging, usually with contrast medium–enhanced CT or magnetic resonance imaging (MRI), helps assess the size, extent, and surgical resectability of a primary tumor. Excisional biopsy of a neck node is virtually never indicated because fine-needle biopsy can give reliable results and because violation of the lymphatics may invite seeding of the neck with cancer.

Either surgery or irradiation can be used as the primary treatment modality for stage I and stage II squamous cell carcinoma in most anatomic locations, but irradiation is the first choice of treatment for nasopharyngeal carcinoma. Stage III and IV tumors are treated with both surgery and irradiation. Postoperative irradiation should start within 4 to 6 weeks after the surgical procedure.

Table 24–14 ■ AMERICAN JOINT COMMITTEE ON CANCER (AJCC) STAGING FOR HEAD AND NECK SQUAMOUS CELL CARCINOMA

	LARYNX	ORAL CAVITY	OROPHARYNX	HYPOPHARYNX
Tis	Carcinoma in situ	Carcinoma in situ	Carcinoma in situ	Carcinoma in situ
T1	Tumor limited to one subsite of the larynx	Tumor ≤ 2 cm	Tumor ≤ 2 cm	Tumor ≤ 2 cm, limited to 1 subsite of the hypopharynx
T2	Tumor involving more than one subsite and/or impaired vocal cord mobility	Tumor > 2 cm and ≤4 cm	Tumor > 2 cm and ≤4 cm	Tumor > 2 cm and ≤4 cm, involving more than 1 subsite
T3	Paralyzed vocal cord; involvement of pre-epiglottic or post-cricoid areas (supraglottic primary)	Tumor > 4 cm	Tumor > 4 cm	Tumor > 4 cm, involving more than 1 subsite; paralyzed vocal cord
T4	Extension outside the larynx; cartilage invasion	Extension to soft tissues or bone outside the oral cavity	Invasion of adjacent bone or muscle	Invasion of adjacent bone/muscle cartilage

N0 No cervical lymph nodes positive
N1 Single ipsilateral lymph node ≤3 cm
N2a Single ipsilateral lymph node >3 cm and ≤6 cm
N2b Multiple ipsilateral lymph nodes, each ≤6 cm
N2c Bilateral or contralateral lymph nodes, each ≤6 cm
N3 Single or multiple lymph nodes >6 cm

M0 No distant metastasis
M1 Distant metastasis present
Mx Distant metastasis cannot be assessed

Stage	T	N	M
Stage I	T1	N0	M0
Stage II	T2	N0	M0
Stage III	T3	N0	M0
	T1–3	N1	M0
Stage IV	T4	N0–1	M0
	Any T	N2–3	M0
	Any T	Any N	M1

Side effects of surgical treatment for head and neck squamous cell carcinoma include impairment of function (swallowing, speech) due to loss of tissue and structures, and cosmetic defects. Short-term effects from irradiation include mucositis and skin desquamation. The most disabling long-term side effect is xerostomia resulting from permanent damage to the major and minor salivary glands.

Chemotherapy is currently used for palliation in recurrent, inoperable, or widely metastatic head and neck squamous cell carcinoma. Cisplatin-based multiagent regimens have responses equivalent or superior to methotrexate.

Second primary squamous cell carcinomas are the most common cause of death in patients previously treated for early-stage head and neck squamous cell carcinoma. The development of second primary tumors can be reduced by vitamin A derivatives, the retinoids.

Nodal metastasis at the time of diagnosis is the single most important prognostic factor and is associated with about a 50% reduction in 5-year survival compared with stage I and II disease (Table 24–15)

Non–Squamous Cell Head and Neck Cancer

Only 25 to 30% of salivary gland neoplasms are malignant, and over 50% of these malignancies occur in the parotid gland. Acinic cell carcinoma and low-grade mucoepidermoid carcinoma are considered low-grade tumors, whereas adenocarcinoma, adenoid cystic carcinoma, squamous cell carcinoma, carcinoma expleomorphic adenoma, high-grade mucoepidermoid carcinoma, and undifferentiated carcinoma are, histologically, high-grade tumors.

Cancer of the paranasal sinuses constitutes only 3% of all upper aerodigestive tract malignancies. Of these, over half are squamous cell carcinomas. Adenocarcinoma, the second most common histologic type, is found most often in the ethmoidal sinuses.

Ten per cent of lymphomas present in the head and neck. Over half of these originate in the lymphatic tissues of Waldeyer's ring (palatine tonsils, base of tongue, nasopharynx). Presenting symptoms are similar to those of squamous cell carcinoma. Sarcomas involving the head and neck are rare.

Paragangliomas arise from neural crest cells located at the carotid body, the vagal body, and the jugulotympanic region and are called carotid body tumors, glomus vagales, glomus jugulares, and

Table 24–15 ■ FIVE-YEAR DISEASE-FREE SURVIVAL, HEAD AND NECK SQUAMOUS CELL CARCINOMA, SELECTED SITES

	STAGE I	STAGE II	STAGE III	STAGE IV
Floor of mouth	68%	55%	28%	9%
Tonsil	>92%	71%	41%	21%
Base of tongue	82%	62%	48%	29%
Hypopharynx	59%	47%	28%	7%
Supraglottis	83%	67%	50%	25%
Glottis	>95%	80%	65%	45%

glomus tympanicum (limited to the middle ear). Approximately 10% are hormonally active.

For more information about this subject, see *Cecil Textbook of Medicine,* 21st edition. Philadelphia, W.B. Saunders Company, 2000. Chapter 518, Head and Neck Cancer, pages 2257 to 2262.

CHAPTER 25

SKIN DISEASES

STRUCTURE AND FUNCTION OF SKIN

The epidermis is a continuously renewing multilayered organ that constantly differentiates. The stratified structure contains two main zones of cells (keratinocytes): an inner region of viable cells known as the stratum germinativum and an outer layer of anucleate cells known as the stratum corneum, or horny layer.

The differentiation of the epidermal cells involves the formation of fibrous proteins known as keratin. New keratinocytes require about 14 days to evolve into stratum granulosum cells and another 14 days to reach the surface of the stratum corneum and be shed.

Melanocytes synthesize brown, red, and yellow melanin pigments that give the skin its distinctive coloration. Two kinds of melanin are recognized: eumelanin (brown-black biochrome) and phaeomelanin (yellow-red biochrome which contains large quantities of cysteine). Melanin serves as an excellent screen against the untoward effects of solar ultraviolet (UV) radiation, such as aging and wrinkling of the skin and the development of cutaneous neoplasms. Negroid skin contains the same number of melanocytes as white skin, but the pigmentation is more intense as a result of the synthesis of more melanin. Accordingly, black skin is much less likely to form skin cancers, and it ages more slowly than white skin.

Langerhans' cells, derived from bone marrow, contain surface receptors for immunoglobulins. Langerhans' cells thus play a central role in delayed hypersensitivity reactions of the skin (allergic contact dermatitis).

Beneath the epidermis lies the principal mass of the skin, the dermis, which is a tough, resilient tissue with viscoelastic properties. It consists of a three-dimensional matrix of loose connective tissue composed of fibrous proteins (collagen and elastin) embedded in an amorphous ground substance (glycosaminoglycans).

The structures situated at the interface between the epidermis and dermis constitute an anatomic functional unit of complex membranes and lamellae that together serve to support the epidermis, weld the epidermis to the dermis, and act as a filter to the transfer of materials and inflammatory or neoplastic cells across the junction zone. A variety of inherited mechanobullous diseases (epidermolysis bullosa), as well as autoimmune bullous diseases (pemphigoid, herpes gestationis, bullous systemic lupus erythematosus), involve separation and bullous formation at various levels of the dermoepidermal junction. A variety of inflammatory diseases often

For more information about this subject, see in *Cecil Textbook of Medicine,* 21st edition. Philadelphia, W.B. Saunders Company, 2000. Part XXVII: Skin Diseases, pages 2263 to 2298.

characterized by bullous reactions seem to be mediated by immunoreactants, including IgG, IgA, and IgM, and complement deposition along the dermoepidermal junctional area (Table 25–1).

Two to three million eccrine sweat glands distributed over all parts of the body surface participate in thermoregulation by producing hypotonic sweat that evaporates during heat or emotional stress. Apocrine sweat glands in the axillae, circumanal and perineal areas, external auditory canals, and areolae of the breasts secrete viscid, milky material which accounts for axillary odor when bacteria degrade the secretion.

Hair units are found over the entire skin surface except on the palms, soles, and glans penis. Hair follicles consist of a shaft surrounded by an epithelial sheath continuous with the epidermis, the sebaceous gland, and the arrector pili smooth muscle. Hair follicles are formed in early embryonic life and do not develop after birth. Hair growth consists of recurring cycles of growth, regression, and resting. In the adult scalp, 85% of the hairs are in a growth state, 14% in a resting state, and 1% in regression.

Most sebaceous glands adjoin a hair follicle, although some open

Table 25–1 ■ IMMUNOFLUORESCENT CUTANEOUS FINDINGS IN IMMUNOLOGICALLY MEDIATED SKIN DISEASE

DISEASES	BIOPSY FINDINGS OF DIRECT IMMUNOFLUORESCENCE IMMUNOREACTANTS (DIF)
Bullous Diseases	
Pemphigus (all forms)	Deposits of IgG in intercellular areas between keratinocytes
Bullous pemphigoid	IgG and/or complement (C) in BMZ
Cicatricial pemphigoid	IgG and/or C in BMZ
Herpes gestationis	Complement in BMZ—occasionally IgG
Dermatitis herpetiformis	IgA and C in dermal papillae (granular deposits)
Epidermolysis bullosa acquisita	IgG, C3 in BMZ
Linear IgA bullous dermatosis in childhood	IgA and complement in linear deposition in BMZ
Connective Tissue Diseases	
Bullous systemic LE	IgG, IgM, and complement in BMZ in involved and normal skin—linear homogeneous
Discoid LE	IgG, other Ig, and C in lesional skin at BMZ
Systemic LE	IgG band at BMZ in normal skin (over 90% in sun-exposed areas)
Systemic sclerosis	Nucleolar IgG
MCTD	IgG/IgM in BMZ in some patients; nuclear IgG in epidermis
Dermatomyositis	Negative

BMZ = basement membrane zone; LE = lupus erythematosus; MCTD = mixed connective tissue disease; Ig = immunoglobulin(s).

directly on the skin surface. The sebaceous glands and certain hair follicles are androgen-dependent target organs.

The stratum corneum normally harbors a number of aerobic and anaerobic resident organisms. Breaks in the stratum corneum, poor hygiene, and excessive humidity with maceration (especially in intertriginous areas) all contribute to cutaneous infections such as impetigo, erysipelas, folliculitis, furunculosis, and ecthyma.

Itch is mediated by cutaneous nerves (Tables 25–2 and 25–3). Generalized itching in the absence of primary skin disease (pruritus) may be an important sign of internal disease.

For more information about this subject, see *Cecil Textbook of Medicine,* 21st edition. Philadelphia, W.B. Saunders Company, 2000. Chapter 519, Structure and Function of Skin, pages 2263 to 2268.

AN APPROACH TO DIAGNOSING SKIN DISEASES

The entire skin should be examined for primary and secondary skin lesions (Fig. 25–1) that allow the examiner to place the patient in one of nine diagnostic groups (Tables 25–4 and 25–5). Of great importance is the distribution of the skin disease, because many conditions have typical patterns or affect specific regions. An important clue lies in the shape of the individual lesions and the arrangement of several lesions in relation to each other. A linear arrangement of lesions may indicate a contact reaction to an exogenous substance. *Zosteriform* refers to lesions arranged along the cutaneous distribution of a spinal dermatome. *Annular* lesions are round to oval with an area of central clearing; annular macules are observed in drug eruptions, secondary syphilis, and lupus erythematosus. *Target* lesions are a special type of annular lesion in which an erythematous annular macule or papule develops a second red ring or a purplish papule or vesicle in the center; target lesions are seen in erythema multiforme. *Arciform* lesions form partial circles or arcs and may be seen in dermatophyte infections.

Vesicular lesions with central delling or depression are suggestive of viral cutaneous infection. Dry, lichenified lesions suggest a chronic state, whereas wet, weeping, macerated lesions suggest acute reactions. Redness caused by dilation of superficial blood vessels blanches with pressure, whereas erythema caused by extravasated blood, as occurs in petechiae and purpuric lesions, does not blanch.

Gram stain for bacteria and bacteriologic cultures is important when the primary lesion is a pustule or furuncle or appears to be impetigo. The presence of mycelia may be ascertained by applying 10% potassium hydroxide (KOH) to scale or exudative material scraped from suspected lesions. Dermatophyte hyphae appear as long, branching, refractile, walled structures; *Candida* organisms appear as shorter, linear hyphae in association with budding yeast forms; tinea versicolor is seen as round yeast forms. The microscopic examination of cells from the base of vesicles reveals the presence of giant epithelial cells and multinucleated giant cells in herpes simplex, herpes zoster, and varicella.

Clinical indications for biopsy include lesions thought to be malignant; lesions that fail to heal, increase in size, bleed easily, or

Table 25–2 ■ SKIN DISEASES ASSOCIATED WITH ITCHING

Xerosis (dry skin)
Insect infestations (scabies, pediculosis, insect bites)
Dermatitis (atopic, contact, nummular), including poison ivy contact
Drugs (opiates, aspirin, quinidine)
Lichen planus
Urticaria
Dermatitis herpetiformis (burning itch)
Sunburn
Fiberglass dermatitis
Seborrheic dermatitis

ulcerate spontaneously; tumors or growths of uncertain nature; and many inflammatory conditions, especially those for which the diagnosis is uncertain.

For more information about this subject, see *Cecil Textbook of Medicine,* 21st edition. Philadelphia, W.B. Saunders Company, 2000. Chapter 520, Examination of the Skin and an Approach to Diagnosing Skin Diseases, pages 2269 to 2272.

Table 25–3 ■ PRURITUS ASSOCIATED WITH SYSTEMIC DISEASE

Uremia
Obstructive biliary disease
- Primary biliary cirrhosis
- Cholestatic hepatitis secondary to drugs
- Intrahepatic cholestasis of pregnancy
- Extrahepatic biliary obstruction

Hematologic and myeloproliferative disorders
- Lymphoma, including Hodgkin's disease
- Mycosis fungoides
- Polycythemia vera
- Iron deficiency anemia

Endocrine disorders
- Thyrotoxicosis
- Hypothyroidism
- Diabetes
- Carcinoid

Visceral malignancies
- Breast, stomach, lung

Psychiatric disorders
- Stress
- Delusions of parasitosis

Neurologic disorders
- Multiple sclerosis (paroxysmal itching)
- Notalgia paresthetica—local itch of back, medial shaft scapula (local neuropathy)

Brain abscess
Central nervous system infarct

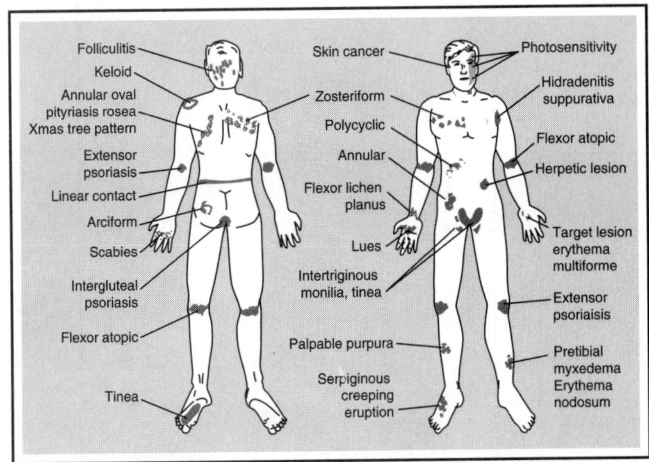

FIGURE 25–1 ■ Configurational and regional diagnostic aids for the diagnosis of primary and secondary skin lesions.

Table 25–4 ■ THE LANGUAGE OF DERMATOLOGY

Primary Skin Lesions

Macule—circumscribed flat change in skin color (e.g., cafe au lait spot)

Papule—solid elevated area with top; can be flat, pointed, or rounded (e.g., acne)

Plaque—evolves from a confluence of papules leading to flat-topped, circumscribed elevations (e.g., psoriasis)

Scale—desiccated, thin plates of cornified epidermal cells that result from altered keratinization (e.g., ichthyosis)

Wheal—circumscribed, flat-topped, firm elevation of skin with a well-demarcated, palpable margin; results from tense edema in papillary dermis (e.g., urticaria)

Nodule—large, solid, deep-seated, raised mass in dermal or subcutaneous tissues; usually >1 cm (e.g., erythema nodosum)

Vesicle/bulla—circumscribed, elevated lesion containing clear serous or hemorrhagic fluid; vesicles are <1 cm, bullae are >1 cm (e.g., herpes simplex and pemphigus vulgaris)

Pustule—a vesicle containing purulent exudate (e.g., folliculitis)

Atrophy—loss of epidermal or dermal tissue with some depression of skin surface and substance; epidermal atrophy leads to fine wrinkling of the skin surface (e.g., lichen sclerosis et atrophicus)

Secondary Skin Lesions

Lichenification—dry, leathery thickening of the skin with exaggerated skin markings (e.g., chronic eczema)

Scar—an area where fibrosis of the dermis or subcutaneous tissues results from an antecedent destructive process and replaces normal skin (e.g., healing wound)

Erosion—a moist, circumscribed, often depressed area that reflects loss of partial or full-thickness epidermis (e.g., ruptured bulla)

Fissure—a deep linear split in the skin extending through the epidermis (e.g., eczema)

Crust—dried exudate of serum, blood, sebum, or purulent material on the surface of the skin (e.g., acute eczema)

Telangiectasia—dilated, small blood vessels in the skin (e.g., discoid lupus erythematosus and necrobiosis lipoidica diabeticorum)

Table 25–5 ■ MAJOR GROUPS OF DERMATOLOGIC DISEASES BASED ON THE CLINICAL MORPHOLOGY OF THE SKIN CONDITION

GROUP	CLINICAL MORPHOLOGY	EXAMPLES OF DISEASES IN THE GROUP
Eczema or dermatitis	Macules (erythema), papules, vesicles, lichenification, fine scaling, excoriations, crusting	Contact dermatitis, atopic dermatitis, stasis dermatitis, photodermatitis, scabies, dermatophytoses, exfoliative dermatitis, candidiasis
Maculopapular eruptions	Macules, erythema, papules	Viral exanthems, drug reactions, verruca vulgaris, Kawasaki syndrome, vasculitic and purpuric eruptions
Papulosquamous dermatoses	Papules, plaques, erythema with unique scales	Psoriasis, Reiter's syndrome, pityriasis rosea, lichen planus, seborrheic dermatitis, ichthyosis, secondary syphilis, mycosis fungoides, parapsoriasis
Vesiculobullous diseases	Vesicles, bullae, erythema	Herpes simplex and zoster, hand-foot-and-mouth disease, insect bites, bullous impetigo, scalded skin syndrome, pemphigus, pemphigoid, dermatitis herpetiformis, porphyria cutanea tarda, erythema multiforme
Pustular diseases	Pustules, cysts, erythema	Acne vulgaris and rosacea, pustular psoriasis, folliculitis, gonococcemia
Urticaria, persistent figurate erythemas, cellulitis	Wheals and figurate, raised erythema; scaling	Urticaria, erythema annulare centrifugum, erysipelas, necrotizing fasciitis
Nodular lesions	Nodules and tumors, some associated with erosions and ulceration	Benign and malignant tumors—basal cell cancer, squamous cell cancer, rheumatoid nodules, xanthomas
Telangiectasia, atrophic, scarring, ulcerative diseases	Atrophic, sclerotic telangiectasia and ulcerative changes	Connective tissue diseases, radiation dermatitis, lichen sclerosus et atrophicus, vascular insufficiency (arterial and venous), pyoderma gangrenosum
Hypermelanosis and hypomelanosis	Increased and decreased melanin deposition in skin	Acanthosis nigricans, cafe au lait spots, vitiligo, tuberous sclerosis, xeroderma pigmentosum, chloasma, freckles

PRINCIPLES OF THERAPY

Removal of debris, such as excessive scale, hyperkeratoses, crusts, and infection, is crucial. Topical and systemic medications, dressings, and other treatments can alter skin temperature and blood flow and thus favorably affect the metabolism of the skin.

A bath is useful when the area of involvement is too large to apply compresses. Cool baths constrict vessels and usually soothe pruritus.

Wet compresses, especially with frequent changes, provide gentle débridement of crusts, scales, and cutaneous debris. If the compresses are permitted to dry (wet to dry compresses) and become adherent, the débriding effect is increased but there may be further damage to the skin. Dried-out dressings should be remoistened to facilitate removal. Dry dressings protect the skin from dirt and irritants and can be used to apply medications, prevent scratching and rubbing by the patient or from clothing and sheets, and keep dirt away.

The medication most commonly added to baths and dressings is aluminum acetate, which coagulates bacterial and serum protein. As a 5% preparation it is known as Burow's solution, and it must be further diluted for use.

Topical Medications

Powders promote dryness. *Lotions* are suspensions of insoluble powders in water. *Creams* are emulsions of oil in water. *Ointments* consist of oils with variably smaller amounts of water added in suspension; they have a pleasant lubricating effect on dry or diseased skin, but they give a greasy feeling to the skin and clothing.

Topical corticosteroids provide effective local anti-inflammatory and antipruritic effects. They cause immediate and profound cutaneous vasoconstriction (Table 25–6). Intermediate-potency corticosteroids are useful in most dermatologic conditions (Table 25–7). *Intralesional corticosteroids* are used to shrink inflammatory acne cysts and hypertrophic scars and keloids.

Topical antibiotics help suppress bacteria in erosions or superfi-

Table 25–6 ■ POTENCY RANKING OF SOME COMMONLY USED TOPICAL CORTICOSTEROIDS

POTENCY	GENERIC NAME
Most potent	Clobetasol propionate cream and ointment 0.5%, halobetasol propionate cream and ointment 0.5%, betamethasone dipropionate cream and ointment 0.5%, halcinonide cream and ointment 0.1%, fluocinonide ointment 0.5%
Intermediate potency	Triamcinolone acetonide 0.1%, betamethasone valorate cream 0.1%, amcinonide cream 0.17%
Low potency	Hydrocortisone cream and ointment 2.5% and 1.0%, desonide cream and ointment 0.5%, locoid ointment 0.1%, dexamethasone sodium phosphate cream 0.1%

Table 25–7 ■ GUIDELINES FOR SELECTING TOPICAL CORTICOSTEROIDS

LOCATION OR TYPE OF LESION	SUGGESTED POTENCY OF CORTICOSTEROID	SUGGESTED VEHICLE
Areas of Body		
Trunk, arms, legs	Intermediate or low	Ointment or cream
Palms, soles	Intermediate or high	Ointment
Scalp	Intermediate or low	Lotion, gel, aerosol
Intertriginous areas	Low	Cream, lotion
Face	Low	Cream, lotion
Area around eyes	Low	Cream or ophthalmic preparation
Ears	Intermediate or low	Cream, gel, or lotion
Types of Lesion		
Dry, scaling, fissuring, lichenified lesion	Intermediate	Ointment
Thickened, hyperkeratotic skin patches	High	Ointment
Oozing, weeping lesions	Intermediate	Lotion, cream
Ulcerative lesions	Do not use topical corticosteroids	

cial infections and occasionally in chronic leg ulcers. Silver sulfadiazine preparations are particularly useful as an adjunct to currently accepted principles of burn wound care. Commonly used topical antibiotics are bacitracin, neomycin, clindamycin phosphate, erythromycin, and tetracycline hydrochloride. Mupirocin, a new topical antibiotic ointment, is particularly useful in treating staphylococcal and streptococcal infections of the skin. *Topical retinoids* include tretinoin (Retin-A), adapalene (Differin), and tazarotene (Tazorac) and are used primarily to treat comedonal acne vulgaris.

Topical antifungal agents include clotrimazole, econazole, and miconazole creams and lotions, commonly used twice daily. No topical preparations are useful against nail infections. Ketoconazole is a broad-spectrum imidazole antifungal agent highly effective against dermatophytes, *Candida,* and tinea versicolor.

Sunscreens are rated by their sun protective factor (SPF), which ranges from 3 to 50. No sunscreen enhances tanning. Most sunscreens are less effective in blocking UVA (320 to 400 nm) than UVB (290 to 320 nm), but newer broad-spectrum products also contain benzophenones or anthranilate compounds and protect against both UVA and UVB.

Systemic Therapy

Antihistamines ameliorate or halt histamine-mediated disorders such as urticaria, angioedema, and allergic rhinitis. Antihistamines also suppress non–histamine-induced itching by soporific side effects.

Systemic corticosteroids are used in patients severely ill with life-threatening diseases known to be responsive to corticosteroids (anaphylactic reactions, extensive erythema multiforme, acute exfoliative dermatitis, pemphigus vulgaris) daily. They are also used in patients with acute and severe but self-limited conditions such as widespread poison ivy dermatitis, extensive sunburn, and acute generalized urticaria of known cause. Corticosteroids are also used for chronic dermatologic conditions that, because of periodic exacerbations, intermittently require low doses (15 to 20 mg) of prednisone together with supportive topical therapy. Examples include flares of chronic atopic dermatitis, pemphigoid, and some connective tissue disease.

Three primary types of systemic antifungal agents are commonly used to treat dermatologic disease: (1) griseofulvin, (2) terbinafine (Lamisil), and (3) oral azoles, including ketoconazole, fluconazole, and itraconazole. Griseofulvin is active against dermatophytes but not against tinea versicolor or *Candida.* The entire nail must grow out with griseofulvin incorporated into it before the tinea at the distal end of the nail is affected. Terbinafine is active against dermatophytes, but its efficacy against *Candida* has not been fully studied. Indications include fungal infection of the body, scalp, or nails. Ketoconazole is effective against tinea versicolor and *Candida.* The role of itraconazole and fluconazole in treating superficial fungal infections remains uncertain.

Erythromycin and tetracyclines can control acne vulgaris and acne rosacea. Isotretinoin has also proved to be especially useful in severe cystic acne.

Penicillins, cephalosporins, and erythromycins are commonly used to treat cutaneous bacterial infections. Trimethoprim-sulfamethoxazole is used for pyodermas in patients allergic to penicillin or caused by methicillin-resistant *Staphylococcus aureus.*

Sulfone and sulfonamides are used most often to control dermatitis herpetiformis. Intramuscular gold has been useful in the treatment of autoimmune bullous disease, particularly pemphigus vulgaris, with remissions of 21 months or longer. Dapsone is most commonly used to treat leprosy but is also useful in treating cutaneous vasculitis, pyoderma gangrenosum, bullous forms of systemic lupus erythematosus, and brown recluse spider bites. Chloroquine, hydroxychloroquine, and quinacrine benefit patients with cutaneous lupus erythematosus, polymorphic light eruption, solar urticaria, and porphyria cutanea tarda.

When psoriasis is generalized, severe, and life-ruining, it may be treated with modest doses of methotrexate, azathioprine, or hydroxyurea. UV phototherapy is used primarily to treat psoriasis and vitiligo but may also help patients with nummular and atopic eczema, pityriasis rosea, the pruritus of uremia, and mycosis fungoides.

For more information about this subject, see *Cecil Textbook of Medicine,* 21st edition. Philadelphia, W.B. Saunders Company, 2000. Chapter 521, Principles of Therapy [of the Skin], pages 2272 to 2276.

SKIN DISEASES OF GENERAL IMPORTANCE

Eczematous Diseases

Eczematous dermatitis is an inflammatory response of the skin to multiple exogenous and endogenous agents (Table 25–8). Eczemas can be acute, with marked spongiosis causing red papules and

Table 25-8 ■ TYPES OF ECZEMA

Contact dermatitis
Photodermatitis
Atopic dermatitis
Stasis dermatitis
Nummular eczematous dermatitis
Lichen simplex chronicus
Seborrheic dermatitis
Xerotic eczema and eczema craquelé
Hand eczema
Exfoliative dermatitis (erythroderma)
Drug reactions
Infectious eczematoid dermatitis
Non-specific eczematous dermatitis
Fungal infections of the skin mimicking eczema

vesicles with oozing, weeping, and crusting; or they may be chronic, with redness, scaling, fissuring, and especially lichenification.

Irritant contact dermatitis is produced by substances that simply irritate or have a direct toxic effect on the skin. Allergic contact dermatitis is a delayed-type hypersensitivity reaction that occurs in response to a wide variety of allergens commonly found in the environment.

A variety of skin reactions, termed *photosensitivity reactions,* may occur in response to exposure to UV radiation. Photoallergic dermatitis is immunologic.

Atopic dermatitis, a chronic, eczematous condition of the skin, is often associated with a personal or family history of asthma, allergic rhinitis, and/or atopic eczema. Pruritus is prominent. The treatment of atopic dermatitis is the same as for other eczematous eruptions and includes topical steroids, emollients, and systemic antihistamines.

Stasis dermatitis is an eczematous eruption that occurs on the lower legs secondary to peripheral venous insufficiency. These conditions trigger an inflammatory, brawny, edematous, red, and hyperpigmented petechial scaling or weeping reaction, usually around the medial malleolus or distal one third of the lower leg.

Nummular eczematous dermatitis is defined by recurrent coin-shaped patches predominantly on the extensor surfaces of the arms and legs, less often on the trunk. Topical steroids, 3% crude coal tar, and UV light help control persistent eczema.

Lichen simplex chronicus, also known as *neurodermatitis,* is a chronic, pruritic, lichenified eczematous eruption that results from constant scratching. Topical steroids and oral antihistamines may be helpful.

Seborrheic dermatitis is characterized by erythematous, eczematous patches with yellow, greasy scales localized to hairy areas and regions of the skin with high concentrations of sebaceous glands. Antiseborrheic shampoos containing tar, sulfur, salicylic acid, selenium sulfide, or pyrithione zinc provide the most useful treatment. Topical or oral ketoconazole helps in some patients.

Total-body cutaneous erythema, edema, scaling, and fissuring (exfoliative dermatitis or erythroderma) may occur as an idiopathic entity without preceding dermatologic or systemic disease, or it may result from a variety of cutaneous (atopic or contact dermatitis, psoriasis, seborrheic dermatitis, autosensitization, pityriasis rubra pilaris) or systemic disorders (mycosis fungoides, lymphomas, leukemias) or constitute a reaction to drugs (antibiotics, barbiturates, antiepileptic agents, gold). Increased heat loss may lead to decreased core temperature, shivering, and swings in temperature; in older people with underlying cardiac disease, high-output heart failure may ensue. Oral steroids reduce the cutaneous inflammation.

Fungal infections, including dermatophytosis, candidiasis, and tinea versicolor, may be confused with eczema. Three general dermatophytes cause these infections: *Trichophyton, Microsporum,* and *Epidermophyton* species. KOH preparations and cultures for fungi should be performed. Infections of the feet appear in three forms: (1) interdigital maceration, scaling, and fissuring; (2) diffuse, dry scaling and mild erythema of the plantar surface, often extending onto the sides of the feet in a moccasin distribution, occasionally associated with dry scaling of one palm; (3) vesiculopustular lesions on the insteps of the feet. Involvement of the nails, onychomycosis, often accompanies hand and foot dermatophytosis. If the dermatophytic or candidal glabrous skin infection is localized, econazole, miconazole, clotrimazole, ciclopirox, or terbinafine creams, ointments, and lotions are effective when applied two to three times a day for 3 to 4 weeks.

Tinea versicolor, a common superficial fungus infection, is identified by scaling, red-to-brown or white oval patches over the neck, trunk, and upper arms. Tinea versicolor also responds to common antifungal agents, but selenium sulfide, the 2% antidandruff shampoo, is less expensive and also effective.

Scalp, nail, or follicular (as evidenced by pustular lesions) involvement or widespread, resistant fungal infections may require systemic agents. Newer fungicidal agents such as terbinafine 250 mg/day for 2 weeks (body), 6 weeks (scalp or fingernails), or 12 weeks (toenails), as well as fungistatic azoles such as itraconazole, are effective, but potential medication reactions require laboratory monitoring.

Maculopapular Skin Diseases

A diverse group of cutaneous and systemic conditions are characterized by widespread erythematous macules and papules (Table 25–9). Because many viral exanthems are maculopapular, this group of skin diseases is often termed *morbilliform,* or measles-like. Erythema infectiosum (fifth disease) is an alarming-appearing red, slapped-cheek rash over the face with reticulate maculopapular lesions on the extremities that clear in 3 to 6 days; mucous membranes are sometimes involved.

Toxic shock syndrome is a serious condition arising from toxins elaborated by *S. aureus* or streptococcal infections, often in menstruating women using tampons but also in patients with post-surgical infections. The rash is an erythematous, macular, diffuse eruption that blanches readily with pressure followed by desquamation of the affected skin, in association with fever, strawberry tongue, hypotension, vomiting, and renal insufficiency.

Non-palpable purpuras include thrombocytopenic conditions, se-

Table 25–9 ■ MACULOPAPULAR SKIN DISEASES

- Viral exanthems
  - Measles (rubeola)
  - Rubella
  - Exanthem subitum (roseola infantum)
  - Erythema infectiosum (fifth disease)
  - Verruca vulgaris
  - Molluscum contagiosum
- Scarlatiniform eruptions
  - Scarlet fever
  - Kawasaki syndrome
  - Toxic shock syndrome
- Drug reactions
- Purpuric maculopapular skin lesions
  - Non-palpable purpuras
    - Actinic (senile) purpura
    - Meningococcemia
    - Gonococcemia
    - Rocky Mountain spotted fever
    - Infectious endocarditis
  - Palpable purpuras
    - Vasculitis (see Table 25–10)
    - Sepsis
    - Cryoglobulinemia
    - Drug reactions
    - Carcinomas

nile or actinic purpura, hypergammaglobulinemic conditions, blood clotting abnormalities, Schamberg's disease, and disseminated intravascular coagulation. Actinic (senile) purpura, which is a common problem in older people, is the result of increased vessel fragility from connective tissue damage to the dermis. Schamberg's disease, or pigmented purpuric dermatitis, is an idiopathic capillaritis that causes petechial lesions of the lower legs (occasionally the arms and trunk) in association with hyperpigmentation. A variety of infectious diseases cause cutaneous petechiae, purpura, or ecchymoses, including meningococcemia, disseminated gonococcemia, Rocky Mountain spotted fever, and infective endocarditis.

Palpable purpuras include vasculitis and necrotizing angiitis, in which there is segmental inflammation in the blood vessel wall with accumulation of neutrophils and fibrinoid necrosis. Papules with purpura result from extravasation of blood from the damaged vessels (Table 25–10).

Necrotizing leukocytoclastic vasculitis can occur in a variety of settings, including sepsis; connective tissue disease, especially systemic lupus erythematosus and rheumatoid arthritis; cryoglobulinemia, especially with hepatitis C; drug reactions; and, occasionally, underlying carcinomas, lymphomas, or leukemias. Hypocomplementemic vasculitis is characterized by urticaria-like lesions, arthritis, facial and laryngeal edema, and low serum complement level. Necrotizing cutaneous vasculitis may occur with hepatitis B or hepatitis C, after intestinal bypass surgery for morbid obesity, or in patients with jejunal diverticula or other gastrointestinal conditions characterized by bacterial overgrowth.

If the vasculitis is idiopathic and cutaneous, the skin responds to

Table 25–10 ■ TYPES OF VASCULITIS AND ASSOCIATED SKIN LESIONS

TYPE OF VASCULITIS	TYPE OF SKIN LESION
Leukocytoclastic or hypersensitivity angiitis: Henoch-Schönlein purpura, cryoglobulinemia, hypocomplementemic vasculitis	Purpuric papules, hemorrhagic bullae, cutaneous infarcts
Rheumatic vasculitis: systemic lupus erythematosus; rheumatoid vasculitis	Purpuric papules; ulcerative nodules; splinter hemorrhages; periungual telangiectasia and infarcts
Granulomatous vasculitis	
Churg-Strauss syndrome	Erythematous, purpuric, and ulcerated nodules, plaques, and purpura
Wegener's granulomatosis	Ulcerative nodules; peripheral gangrene
Periarteritis: classic type limited to skin and muscle	Deep subcutaneous nodules with ulceration; livedo reticularis; ecchymoses
Giant cell arteritis: temporal arteritis, polymyalgia rheumatica, Takayasu's disease	Skin necrosis over scalp

prednisone 60 to 80 mg/day or dapsone 100 to 150 mg/day. Systemic vasculitides may require prednisone and cyclophosphamide 2 mg/kg/day.

Papulosquamous Skin Diseases

Papulosquamous conditions include those that are both papular (even if only mildly elevated) and squamous or scaly (hyperkeratotic).

PSORIASIS. Psoriasis is the prototypical papulosquamous condition, characterized by well-demarcated erythematous papules and plaques with silvery scale. The pathogenesis is unknown, but there is an increased prevalence of psoriasis in individuals with human leukocyte antigens (HLAs) HLA-Bw17, -B13, and -Bw37.

Classically, lesions of psoriasis are distributed symmetrically over areas of bony prominence such as elbows and knees. Frequently they may also be found periumbilically, in the intergluteal cleft, or even on the glans of the penis. The palms and soles can be symmetrically involved with well-circumscribed plaques or even diffuse erythema with scale. Nail involvement occurs in up to 50% of cases and can be a diagnostic clue.

When the individual silvery scales are plucked from psoriatic plaques, tiny pinpoint capillary bleeding may be seen (Auspitz's sign). Another helpful diagnostic sign is Koebner's phenomenon, in which trauma to the skin induces new skin lesions.

There are several common variants of psoriasis: guttate psoriasis, in which numerous small papular lesions with silvery scaling evolve suddenly over the body; inverse psoriasis, in which plaques evolve in intertriginous areas and thus lack the typical silver scale because of maceration and moisture; and pustular psoriasis, a form of the disease in which superficial pustules may stud typical plaques, be confined to the palms and soles, or be associated with a generalized erythematous skin condition associated with fever and leukocytosis. Erythrodermic psoriasis with generalized erythema and scale covering the entire body may occur secondary to overvigorous therapy, a generalized Koebner phenomenon, a superimposed drug reaction, or withdrawal from oral corticosteroids.

At times, Reiter's syndrome may be confused with psoriasis. The skin lesions of the two disorders are indistinguishable clinically and histologically. Reiter's syndrome is suggested by asymptomatic erosions on the tongue and buccal mucosa, urethritis, iritis or conjunctivitis, arthritis, and occasionally diarrhea.

Intermediate- or strong-potency topical steroids may be used once or twice a day. Topical tar or anthralin preparations can be used and even compounded with topical steroids. UVB with tar or UVA with oral psoralens (PUVA) can provide excellent relief. Calcipotriene (Dovonex) when used twice a day as an ointment or cream is a "steroid-sparing" topical form of vitamin D that may be as effective as medium-potency steroids. Topical tazarotene is the first topical retinoid to treat psoriasis.

Systemic therapy should be considered only in recalcitrant disease. Antimetabolites or antimitotic agents, including methrotrexate, azathioprine, and hydroxyurea, are the most commonly used. Etretinate, a retinoid, is particularly useful in pustular and erythrodermic forms of psoriasis; it is being replaced by its active metabolite, acitretin.

PITYRIASIS ROSEA. Oval or round, tannish-pink or salmon-colored, scaling papules and plaques appear rapidly over the trunk, neck, upper arm, and legs. The generalized eruption is preceded by a single lesion. The lesions follow skin cleavage lines, in a pattern likened to a Christmas tree. Itching can be quite prominent but is not invariable. The condition resolves spontaneously in 1 to 2 months. Recurrences are extremely rare. Topical corticosteroids and antihistamines may relieve itching and decrease erythema.

LICHEN PLANUS. Lichen planus, an idiopathic, pruritic, inflammatory condition of the skin, is included in the papulosquamous group of disease because the primary lesion is a unique papule. The papules are flat-topped (planus) and polygonal in configuration and have a lilac or purple hue. Typical locations are the ankles, wrists, mouth, and genitalia. There may be only a few papules or innumerable ones in a generalized distribution. Mucous membranes are commonly involved. The cause of lichen planus is not known, but as many as 20 to 30% of patients have hepatitis C. Certain drugs, such as thiazides, phenothiazines, gold, quinidine, and antimalarials, can cause lichen planus–like, generalized eruptions. Topical steroids, particularly ultrapotent steroids for short periods (2 to 3 weeks), can be very helpful. Sometimes UV light is useful to control pruritus.

Vesiculobullous Diseases

Vesicles and bullae, when intact, are readily recognized primary skin lesions (Table 25–11). Biopsy of early vesicles or blisters is imperative in diagnosis.

Bullous impetigo, a subcorneal infection of the skin with staphylococcal and/or streptococcal organisms, causes large, fragile, clear, or cloudy bullae that form thin, honey-yellow crusts and a delicate

Table 25–11 ■ VESICULOBULLOUS DISEASES

Intraepidermal vesiculobullous diseases
Bullous impetigo
Staphylococcal scalded skin syndrome
Toxic epidermal necrolysis
Herpes simplex
Varicella (herpes zoster)
Pemphigus diseases
Pemphigus vulgaris
Pemphigus vegetans
Pemphigus foliaceus
Pemphigus erythematosus
Familial benign pemphigus
Dermal-epidermal vesiculobullous diseases
Bullous pemphigoid
Herpes gestationis
Cicatricial pemphigoid
Dermatitis herpetiformis
Erythema multiforme (Stevens-Johnson syndrome)
Porphyria cutanea tarda
Bullous disease of renal disease
Bullous disease in diabetes
Epidermolysis bullosa
Epidermolysis bullosa acquisita

collarette-like remnant of blister roof after the blisters rupture. *Toxic epidermal necrolysis* occurs in adults, often secondary to drugs (e.g., ampicillin, allopurinol) and occasionally to *Staphylococcus* infections in an immunosuppressed patient. Because of the extensive destruction of the epidermis and barrier stratum corneum layer, toxic epidermal necrolysis is often fatal and, when extensive, should be treated as a widespread burn.

Pemphigus diseases cause blistering in the epidermis by virtue of the process of acantholysis. The superficial bullae evolve just above the basal layer, rupture readily, and leave denuded, bleeding, weeping, and crusted erosions over the body that do not heal. The oral mucosa is almost always involved. Lesions occur anywhere but often in pressure and friction areas. A skin biopsy of early vesicles should be obtained. Immunofluorescence shows deposits of immunoglobulins (usually IgG) and/or C3 in the intercellular spaces around keratinocytes. Antibodies to the intercellular areas of the epidermis are found in the serum. High doses of systemic steroids (prednisone 100 to 200 mg/day over prolonged periods) usually control the disease. Methotrexate and other cytotoxic agents are useful as steroid-sparing agents.

In *bullous pemphigoid,* which is an autoimmune disorder of the elderly, tense, large blisters occur on normal or erythematous skin, often in the groin, axillae, and flexural areas. Healing usually occurs without scarring. Itching may be severe or absent. Skin biopsy displays a subepidermal blister, and direct immunofluorescence reveals deposition of IgG and complement directed against an antigen in the lamina lucida. The prognosis is good, and the disease usually subsides after months or years. Widespread bullae require therapy with oral prednisone 40 to 60 mg/day and occasionally with immunosuppressive agents. Large doses of erythromycin or tetracycline 2 g/day can occasionally control the disease.

Another subepidermal blistering disease, *herpes gestationis,* is a rare autoimmune condition that occurs during pregnancy and the postpartum period. Skin biopsy findings are indistinguishable by light microscopy from those of bullous pemphigoid, and examination of perilesional skin by direct immunofluorescence reveals C3 and less often an IgG linear band just below the epidermis. Most patients require oral prednisone 20 to 60 mg/day throughout pregnancy with intermittent tapering.

Erythema multiforme is an immunologic reaction in the skin and mucous membranes often mediated by circulating immune complexes that evolve in response to a number of antigenic stimuli (infections, drugs, connective tissue disease). When the mucous membranes of the mouth and eye are involved, the condition is called *Stevens-Johnson syndrome.* Target lesions are diagnostic. In one half of cases, no cause is found for the reaction, but drugs (penicillins, barbiturates, phenytoin, and sulfonamides) and infections (herpes simplex, streptococcal infections, *Mycoplasma pneumoniae*) should be considered in all cases. Recurrent herpes simplex infection is the most common cause of recurrent erythema multiforme. Stopping suspected drugs is imperative. The value of systemic steroids in erythema multiforme and Stevens-Johnson syndrome is controversial.

Dermatitis herpetiformis is associated with immunologic deposition of IgA in dermal papillae. The disease is associated with intense burning and itching. There is a high incidence of associated celiac sprue. *Epidermolysis bullosa* presents with tense blisters that erode and scar; severe forms may involve the mouth and esophagus.

Pustular Diseases of the Skin

Acne, the most common pustular condition of the skin, is an inflammatory disorder affecting pilosebaceous units primarily over the face and upper trunk. Therapy is usually successful in controlling the disease until the patient outgrows this condition. Topical agents, such as benzoyl peroxide and topical vitamin A preparations (e.g., tazarotene, adapalene), remove comedones and are particularly effective. Topical and oral antibiotics (tetracycline and erythromycin) are indicated in patients with inflammatory papules and pustules. Oral 13-*cis*-retinoic acid (isotretinoin, Accutane), which reduces sebaceous gland size and sebum production, should be used primarily for severe cystic acne because in high daily doses it produces undesirable side effects and can be teratogenic. Spironolactone, the potassium-sparing diuretic, has antiandrogenic properties that have made it a useful adjunctive therapy in doses of 100 to 200 mg/day.

Rosacea is a chronic inflammatory disorder affecting the blood vessels and pilosebaceous units of the face in middle-aged persons. Patients with rosacea have papules and pustules superimposed on diffuse erythema and telangiectasia over the central portion of the face. Rosacea can usually be differentiated from adult acne by the lack of comedones and the prominent vascular component. Rosacea and the eye complications usually respond well to tetracycline and/

or oral metronidazole. Topical antibiotics (metronidazole, MetroGel, Noritate) can be helpful alone or in combination with low-potency topical steroids.

Folliculitis, an *S. aureus* infection of the hair follicle, appears as pustules with a red rim with hair emanating from the center of the pustule. Folliculitis typically occurs in hairy regions. The key to diagnosis is finding a central hair in the pustule. Systemic antibiotics such as erythromycin or dicloxacillin usually clear extensive infections; topical antiseptic cleansers such as povidone-iodine or chlorhexidine can resolve mild folliculitis.

Candidiasis appears as beefy-red patches in intertriginous, moist areas characteristically surrounded by satellite pustules. *Dermatophytes* can, at times, infect hair follicles and result in pustules, particularly in the beard (tinea barbae) and scalp (kerions).

A variety of septicemias, including gonococcemia, staphylococcal septicemia, and *Candida* septicemia, cause pustular lesions associated with purpura. Paronychia, a painful red swelling in the periungual regions of the finger, may also drain pus.

Urticaria, Persistent Figurate Erythemas, and Cellulitis

Urticaria, persistent figurate erythemas, and cellulitis are skin lesions of disparate appearance and origin. The common feature is a raised, edematous, red plaque with a sharply demarcated border (Table 25–12).

Urticaria appears as wheals, which are transient erythematous and edematous swellings of the dermis caused by a local increase

Table 25–12 ■ URTICARIA, PERSISTENT FIGURATE ERYTHEMAS, AND CELLULITIS

- Urticarial reactions
  - Drugs
  - Viral infections
  - Sinus and tooth infections
  - Systemic parasites
  - Pollens
  - Injections (blood products and vaccinations)
  - Light (solar urticaria)
  - Cold (cold urticaria)
  - Heat or exercise (cholinergic urticaria)
  - Pressure or rubbing of the skin (dermatographism)
- Urticaria-like skin lesions
  - Erythema multiforme
  - Juvenile rheumatoid arthritis
  - Erythema marginatum
  - Urticaria pigmentosa (mastocytosis)
- Figurate erythemas
  - Persistent figurate erythema
  - Erythema repens
  - Erythema annulare centrifugum
  - Erythema chronicum migrans
- Cellulitis
  - Group A streptococcus
  - *Staphylococcus aureus*
- Necrotizing fasciitis

in permeability of capillaries and small venules. Urticarial reactions are immunologically mediated by such allergens as infections (viral hepatitis, sinus and tooth infections), infestations (systemic parasites), drugs, pollens, and injections (blood products, vaccinations). Physical modalities, including light (solar urticaria), cold (cold urticaria), heat or exercise (cholinergic urticaria), or pressure or rubbing of the skin (dermatographism), also cause hives.

Hives are transient; any given lesion persists less than 24 hours. Hives covering large areas and producing deep tissue swelling are termed *angioedema.* This condition can involve the tongue and throat and impinge upon the airway.

If the cause of the urticaria cannot be found or avoided, symptomatic control is achieved with antihistamines or oral steroids. Acute angioedema or laryngeal edema requires rapid systemic treatment with epinephrine and diphenhydramine.

Nodules and Tumors

Skin nodules and tumors (Table 25–13) can be classified as pigmented or non-pigmented, dermal or epidermal, benign or malignant. Benign lesions tend to be small, symmetrical, and well circumscribed. Malignant lesions, conversely, tend to be larger, asymmetrical, and poorly circumscribed (Table 25–14).

Basal cell carcinomas, the most common type of skin cancer, arise from the basal layer of the epidermis. They may present as nodular, superficial, sclerosing (morpheaform), or pigmented forms. A nodular basal cell carcinoma is classically a pearly papule with telangiectasias, a rolled and waxy border, and occasional "rodent ulcer" central ulceration. As with many malignant skin lesions, patients will commonly complain that these lesions fail to heal. Controlled cryotherapy, curettage and desiccation, scalpel excision, and fractional radiation all achieve a cure rate of greater than 90%. Mohs' micrographic surgery, which uses serial excisions guided by frozen section histologic examination, should be considered for larger lesions, lesions that may be recurrent, lesions on the central face or preauricular area, or in cases where tissue sparing is a concern.

Squamous cell carcinomas are malignant neoplasms of keratinocytic differentiation. They are less common than basal cell cancers but may be much more aggressive, occasionally metastasize, and even lead to death. Lesions are commonly found on sun-exposed skin. Usually they are firm, erythematous plaques or nodules with hyperkeratosis that sometimes can be quite dramatic, but they may be smooth or verrucous. Any lesion suspected to be squamous cell carcinoma should undergo biopsy. Treatment is excision or curettage and desiccation. Solar keratoses may be treated with liquid nitrogen or topical 5-fluorouracil.

Seborrheic keratoses, which are benign neoplasms of epidermal differentiation, appear on the face and trunk in middle age. These 2-mm to 5-cm, elevated, tan-to-brown or occasionally black, round-to-oval lesions give a verrucous, velvety, "stuck-on" appearance. No therapy is necessary unless they are of cosmetic concern, and then liquid nitrogen cryotherapy or curettage is effective.

Nevi, or *moles,* are benign accumulations of pigment-forming melanocytes. Nevi may be congenital or acquired, and most appear

Table 25–13 ■ NODULES AND TUMORS OF THE SKIN

- Non-pigmented nodules—benign
  - Warts
  - Sebaceous hyperplasia
  - Solar (actinic) keratoses—perhaps pre-malignant
  - Syringomas
  - Follicular cysts
  - Lipomas
  - Neurofibromas
- Non-pigmented nodules—malignant
  - Basal cell carcinoma
    - Nodular
    - Superficial
    - Sclerosing
    - Pigmented
  - Squamous cell carcinoma
    - Bowen's disease
  - Keratoacanthoma—possibly malignant
- Pigmented nodules—benign
  - Seborrheic keratoses
  - Dermatofibromas
  - Nevi (moles)
    - Junctional nevi
    - Compound nevi
    - Intradermal nevi
- Pigmented nodules—malignant
  - Malignant melanoma
    - Lentigo maligna melanoma
    - Superficial spreading melanoma
    - Nodular melanoma
    - Acral lentiginous melanoma
- Tumors and nodules of the hands
  - Heberden's nodes (osteoarthritis)
  - Rheumatoid nodules (rheumatoid arthritis)
  - Granuloma annulare
  - Multicentric reticulohistiocytosis
  - Tophi (gout)
  - Knuckle pads
  - Gottron's papules (dermatomyositis)
- Vascular tumors of the skin
  - Hemangiomas
    - Nevus flammeus
    - Strawberry hemangiomas
    - Cavernous hemangiomas
  - Pyogenic granuloma
  - Kaposi's sarcoma
- Inflammatory nodules of the skin
  - Erythema nodosum
  - Subcutaneous fat necrosis
- Nodules associated with metabolic diseases
  - Xanthomas
  - Xanthelasma
  - Tophi (gout)

Table 25–14 ■ CLINICAL FEATURES HELPFUL IN DISTINGUISHING BENIGN FROM MALIGNANT TUMORS

CLINICAL FEATURES	BENIGN	MALIGNANT
Configuration	Symmetrical sharp borders	Asymmetrical irregular borders
Rate of growth	Slow	Slow or rapid
Friability	No friability	Often friable
Bleeding or ulceration	Seldom bleed or ulcerate	Often bleed and ulcerate
Consistency	Firm or soft	Usually firm to hard
Color	Uniform color and pigmentation	Irregularity of color and pigmentation

by 35 years of age. *Junctional nevi* are macular, are light to dark brown, and are called junctional because the melanocytes are located at the dermoepidermal junction. *Compound nevi* are brown to dark brown and have flatter areas, which correspond to a junctional component, as well as a palpable portion. *Intradermal nevi* evolve from compound nevi and are usually sessile flesh-colored-to-brown papules. Benign nevi are usually less than 6 mm in diameter, uniform in color, and symmetrical, with smooth borders. Any symptomatic nevi or nevi that change raise the question of melanoma.

Malignant melanoma is the cutaneous neoplasm of melanocytes. Melanomas generally have features of asymmetry, irregular borders, variegated color, and diameter greater than 6 mm (Table 25–15). Suspicious lesions should be strongly considered for biopsy. *Lentigo maligna melanoma* is a melanoma on the head and neck arising in a pre-existing melanoma in situ. *Superficial spreading melanoma* may occur on any area of the body, with irregularly pigmented papules, nodules, and notched borders. Up to one third of melanomas may arise from existing nevi, so that a change in size, shape, and color or itching of a pigmented lesion (a common symptom in melanomas) should be carefully investigated. Any suspicious pigmented lesion must undergo biopsy, preferably by excision.

Table 25–15 ■ THE ABCD'S OF MALIGNANT MELANOMA

A = Asymmetry of the lesion is due to irregular, random growth of the malignant cells associated with irregular surface topography and papules and nodules.

B = Borders of the tumors are irregular with notching and pigment "spilling" out beyond the edges.

C = Color variegation consists of browns, blacks, blues, and even shades of red and white. The variations in color represent different depths of invasion of pigment cells along with inflammatory reaction and immunologic response to the malignant cells.

D = Diameter or size of melanomas tends to be >6 mm before they are recognized.

Hemangiomas, benign proliferations of dermal vessels, appear at or soon after birth as red, blue, or purple, flat, papular, or nodular lesions. Large lesions located in strategic locations (around the eye and mouth) may require systemic steroids to try to shrink these tumors. Ordinarily hemangiomas require no therapy.

Kaposi's sarcoma is a neoplasm of multifocal origin that presents as red-purple to blue-brown macules, plaques, and nodules of the skin and other organs. The cutaneous lesions may be firm or compressible, solitary or numerous, and may even appear initially as a dusky stain, especially about the toes. Kaposi's sarcoma is found in patients who are immunosuppressed by human immunodeficiency virus infection.

Erythema nodosum, an inflammatory reaction in subcutaneous fat, represents a hypersensitivity response to a number of antigenic stimuli. Well-localized, multiple, tender, red, deep nodules, 1 to 5 cm in size, usually develop bilaterally over the pre-tibial areas. They eventually involute, leaving yellow-purple bruises. Although no cause can be found in many patients, the following factors have been identified: drugs (especially oral contraceptives), pregnancy, inflammatory bowel disease, sarcoidosis, streptococcal infection, *Yersinia* enterocolitis, deep fungus infections, and tuberculosis. If the cause cannot be identified and eliminated, symptomatic therapy with aspirin, non-steroidal anti-inflammatory medications, potassium iodide, or short courses of systemic steroids may be useful.

Subcutaneous fat necrosis is a condition in which tender, red nodules occur on the lower legs and thighs in patients with pancreatitis or pancreatic carcinoma. Skin biopsy provides diagnostic findings.

Xanthomas are focal collections of lipid-containing histiocytes in the dermis and tendon sheaths. Xanthomas often arise in association with inherited hyperlipoproteinemias.

Atrophic Skin Conditions with Scarring, Induration, Ulceration, and Telangiectasias

Connective tissue diseases are the most common conditions that lead to the spectrum of cutaneous changes in atrophic skin conditions (Table 25–16).

Primary skin ulcers are caused by a wide variety of conditions. Ulcers of the extremities are frequently associated with vascular disease and diabetes mellitus. Ulceration of digits associated with a purplish-red color with dependency and pallor when the extremity is elevated suggests arteriosclerotic peripheral vascular disease. Brawny edema, brown discoloration, and dermatitis over the lower legs in association with ulcers around the malleoli are seen with venous insufficiency. Sickle cell anemia causes ulcerations in the lower third of the leg.

An unusual and dramatic ulcerative condition, *pyoderma gangrenosum,* often begins as an inflammatory nodule or pustule resembling a furuncle that breaks down, ulcerates, and gradually enlarges peripherally. These lesions, which typically evolve on the lower legs, are postulated to represent a Shwartzman-like hypersensitivity reaction to a number of underlying internal conditions, including chronic ulcerative colitis or Crohn's disease, rheumatoid arthritis,

Table 25–16 ■ ATROPHIC SKIN CONDITIONS WITH SCARRING, INDURATION, ULCERATION, AND TELANGIECTASIAS

Scarring
Lupus erythematosus
Dermatomyositis
Radiation
Dermal indurations (sclerosis)
Scleroderma
Lichen sclerosus et atrophicus
Myxedema
Cutaneous ulcers
Arterial insufficiency
Venous insufficiency
Sickle cell anemia
Neurotrophic ulcers
Pyoderma gangrenosum
Ecthyma gangrenosum (*Pseudomonas* spp.)
Genital ulcers
Herpes simplex
Syphilis
Chancroid
Lymphogranuloma venereum
Granuloma inguinale
Behçet's syndrome
Self-inflicted

dysproteinemias, and occasionally leukemia or lymphoma. In over one half of the cases, no cause is identified. *Ecthyma gangrenosum* is characterized by ulcerative lesions, often in the body folds (anogenital and axillary areas), in immunosuppressed patients with *Pseudomonas septicemia.*

Hyper- and Hypopigmentation of Skin Diseases

Hyper- and hypomelanoses can be subdivided into localized or generalized (total-body) alterations of pigmentation (Table 25–17). *Freckles (ephelides),* which are light–brown-red macules found in sun-exposed areas, are caused by increased melanin production in normal numbers of melanocytes. *Lentigines* are also hyperpigmented macules, but they occur because of increased numbers of melanocytes in the basal layer of the epidermis. Actinic lentigines are acquired in middle age and are related to sun damage over the face, arms, and dorsum of the hands. Actinic lentigines are sometimes difficult to distinguish from early lentigo maligna on the face, but actinic lentigines have no malignant potential.

Melasma (chloasma) of the face usually affects women; the melanocytes produce more melanin than normal in response to hormonal factors (during pregnancy or while on birth control pills) in association with UV radiation. This type of pigmentation occurs symmetrically over the malar eminences, forehead, and upper lip.

Diffuse brown hyperpigmentation is a feature of *Addison's disease.* A similar diffuse hyperpigmentation is seen following adrenalectomy, as well as in patients with pancreatic and lung carcinomas. The generalized hypermelanosis results from overproduction

Table 25–17 ■ HYPERPIGMENTATION AND HYPOPIGMENTATION

Localized hyperpigmentation
- Freckles (ephelides)
- Lentigines
- Melasma (chloasma)
- Post-inflammatory hyperpigmentation
- Cafe au lait spots
- Xeroderma pigmentosum

Generalized hyperpigmentation
- Excessive melanocyte-stimulating hormone or adrenocorticotropic hormone (ACTH)
  - Addison's disease
  - Cushing's disease after bilateral adrenalectomy
  - Ectopic ACTH
  - Small cell carcinoma of the lung
  - Pancreatic carcinoma
- Scleroderma
- Systemic lupus erythematosus
- Hyperthyroidism
- Medications
- Arsenicals
- Hemochromatosis
- Biliary cirrhosis

Localized hypopigmentary changes
- Vitiligo
- Piebaldism
- Tuberous sclerosis
- Pityriasis alba
- Chemicals, principally phenol derivatives

Generalized hypopigmentation
- Albinism

of either melanocyte-stimulating hormone or adrenocorticotropic hormone, both of which share common amino acid sequences.

Hyperpigmentation occurs with cyclophosphamide, busulfan, daunorubicin, and doxorubicin administration. Bleomycin can produce a distinctive linear "flagellate" pattern of hyperpigmentation. Antimalarials can cause a patchy slate-gray pigmentary alteration confined to cartilaginous structures. Amiodarone can also cause hyperpigmentation on the face.

Inorganic trivalent arsenicals (found in insecticides and contaminated water) may also produce a generalized brown pigmentation, but in this instance the hypermelanosis is studded with small, scattered, depigmented macules and punctate keratoses on the palms and soles. *Hemochromatosis* causes a metallic gray-brown generalized hyperpigmentation. Similarly, brown generalized hyperpigmentation, which is accentuated in exposed areas in association with pruritus, jaundice, and xanthoma, is typical of *biliary cirrhosis.*

Vitiligo, a circumscribed hypomelanosis of progressively enlarging amelanotic macules in a symmetrical distribution around body orifices and over body prominences, is familial in 36% of cases. Although most patients are healthy, there is an increased association with certain autoimmune conditions such as thyroiditis, hyperthyroidism, Addison's disease, pernicious anemia, and diabetes mellitus. Treatment is usually ineffective.

Disorders of the Nails

In 10% of *lichen planus* patients, accentuated longitudinal nail ridging occurs with pterygium formation resulting from destructive focal scarring of the matrix. Early treatment with oral steroids is indicated. *Atopic eczema* and other eczematous entities may cause pitting, transverse striations, and onycholysis. Nail changes in *psoriasis* involve fingernails more frequently than toenails. *Onychomycosis,* or fungal infections of the nail, may be caused by dermatophyte (tinea unguium) or candidal infections. Terbinafine, itraconazole, griseofulvin, and ketoconazole are effective therapies.

Paronychia, or painful, red swelling of the nail fold, can be either acute or chronic. Acute paronychia typically results from bacterial infection, whereas *Candida albicans* usually underlies chronic infection.

Splinter hemorrhages result from the extravasation of blood from longitudinally oriented vessels of the nail bed. Although often thought to be associated with bacterial endocarditis, they are much more commonly associated with trauma. *Clubbing of the nails* (increased bilateral curvature of the nails with enlargement of the soft connective tissue of the distal phalanges resulting in the flattening of the obtuse angle formed by the proximal end of the nail and the digit) occurs most often with bronchiectasis, lung abscess, and pulmonary neoplasms. Cardiovascular disease and chronic gastrointestinal diseases (ulcerative colitis, sprue) are also associated with clubbing. Clubbing accompanied by bone pain and proliferative periostitis is termed *hypertrophic osteoarthropathy.* Azidothymidine (zidovudine, AZT) can cause black or blue discoloration of the nail plate in a longitudinal, horizontal, or diffuse pattern. *Yellow nail syndrome* exhibits yellow thickening of the nails with absence of the lunula and variable degrees of onycholysis accompanying pulmonary conditions such as bronchiectasis, pleural effusion, and chronic obstructive pulmonary disease. The most important malignant tumor involving the nails is melanoma, which appears as a pigmented area at the base of the nail or as a longitudinal pigmented streak in the nail.

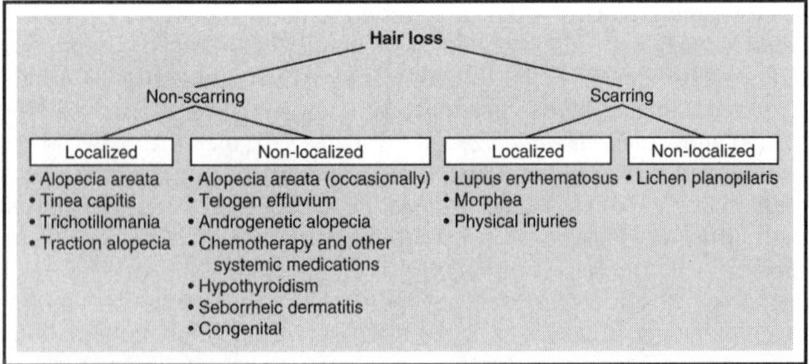

FIGURE 25–2 ■ An approach to the diagnosis of the cause of alopecia.

Hair Loss (Alopecia) (Fig. 25–2)

Alopecia areata is a fairly common form of alopecia that is almost always localized to discrete patches of alopecia on the scalp. Alopecia areata may have an autoimmune cause as it is occasionally associated with Hashimoto's thyroiditis as well as other thyroid gland dysfunction. It can also be found in patients with pernicious anemia. Most patients with alopecia areata localized to the scalp have a very good prognosis. Hair usually regrows within a few months. Topical or intralesional steroids and PUVA have variable results.

Tinea capitis can be confused with alopecia areata. Griseofulvin is the drug of choice to treat tinea capitis.

Androgenetic alopecia can occur in both males and females. Treatment of androgenetic alopecia may include topical minoxidil and surgical procedures to transplant hairs into areas of thinning. Recently, finasteride (Propecia) has been released as a treatment for androgenetic alopecia in men.

Hirsutism (Excessive Hair Growth)

Certain drugs may increase hair growth. Androgenic or steroidal medications, such as anabolic steroids, corticosteroids, and contraceptives, may cause increased hair growth in the beard, chest, and groin areas. Drugs such as phenytoin, phenothiazines, cyclosporine, and minoxidil cause excess hair growth in both men and women anywhere on the body.

Any woman with hirsutism and accompanying virilization should be tested for excess cortisol and androgen production. In general, virilization is a sign of markedly elevated androgen levels derived from the adrenal glands or ovaries, especially adrenogenital syndrome, congenital adrenal hyperplasia, Cushing's disease or syndrome, Stein-Leventhal syndrome (polycystic ovarian syndrome), and occasionally malignant adrenal or ovarian tumors.

Simple or *idiopathic hirsutism* denotes hirsutism in women in whom a specific diagnosis cannot be made and who have a normal or slightly elevated adrenal or ovarian androgen level. Such patients have been treated successfully with cyclically administered birth control pills.

Cutaneous Drug Reactions

Any drug can potentially produce a rash, and over-the-counter preparations should be considered when defining drug reactions (Table 25–18). Most drug eruptions resolve in 1 to 2 weeks after withdrawal of the drug, but some take months to clear.

For more information about this subject, see *Cecil Textbook of Medicine,* 21st edition. Philadelphia, W.B. Saunders Company, 2000. Chapter 522, Skin Diseases of General Importance, pages 2276 to 2298.

Table 25–18 ■ CUTANEOUS DRUG REACTIONS

TYPE OF SKIN REACTION	DRUGS LIKELY TO CAUSE SKIN REACTION
Eczematous (allergic contact reaction)	Antihistamines, neomycin, formaldehyde, sulfonamides
Photodermatitis	
Phototoxic	Chlorpromazine, psoralens, demeclocycline, doxycycline
Photoallergic	Promethazine, griseofulvin, chlorothiazide, hypoglycemic drugs
Exfoliative dermatitis	Carbamazepine, hydantoins, nitrofurantoin, isoniazid, gold, allopurinol, phenothiazines
Maculopapular eruption (exanthematous)	Penicillin, sulfonamides, hypoglycemic drugs, phenothiazines, allopurinol, phenytoin, quinine, gold salts, captopril, meprobamate
Papulosquamous reactions	
Psoriasiform, lichen planus, pityriasis rosea–like	β-blockers, lithium (psoriasiform); thiazides, gold, phenothiazines, quinidine, antimalarials (lichen planus–like); gold (PR-like); others—dapsone, ethambutol, furosemide
Vesiculobullous reactions	Azapropazone, captopril, clonidine, furosemide, gold, psoralens, barbiturates, phenytoin, hydrochlorothiazide, penicillamine
Toxic epidermal necrolysis	Acetazolamine, allopurinol, barbiturates, carbamazepines, gold, hydantoin, nitrofurantoin, pentazocine, tetracycline, quinidine
Pustular—acneiform reactions	Androgen hormones, corticosteroids, iodides, bromides, hydantoin, lithium
Urticaria and erythemas	
Urticaria	May occur with anaphylaxis: penicillin, xenogenic sera, cephalosporins, sulfonamides, barbiturates, hydralazine, phenylbutazone, hydantoin, quinidine, contrast media
Erythema multiforme	Sulfonamides, hydantoin, barbiturates, penicillin, carbamazepines, allopurinol, amikacin, phenothiazides
Nodular lesions	
Erythema nodosum	Birth control pills, sulfonamides, diuretics, gold, clonidine, propranolol, furosemide, opiates, penicillin
Vasculitis reaction	Allopurinol, barbiturates, carbamazepine, chlorothiazide, cimetidine, gold, indomethacin, hydantoin, piperazine, sulfonamides
Telangiectatic and LE reactions	Procainamide, hydralazine, phenytoin, penicillamine, trimethadione, methyldopa, carbamazepine, griseofulvin, nalidixic acid, oral contraceptives, propranolol
Pigmentary reaction	Anticonvulsants, antimalarials, antitumor agents (bleomycin, busulfan, cyclophosphamide, doxorubicin, melphalan), oral contraceptives, corticotropin, tetracyclines, phenothiazines, amiodarone
Other cutaneous reactions	
Fixed drug reaction	Phenolphthalein, barbiturates, gold, sulfonamides, meprobamate, penicillin, tetracyclines, analgesics
Alopecia	Alkylating agents, antimetabolites, heparin, coumarin, hydantoin, isotretinoin, gold, nitrofurantoin, propranolol, colchicine, allopurinol
Hypertrichosis	Anabolic agents, diazoxide, minoxidil, phenytoin

LE = lupus erythematosus; PR = pityriasis rosea.

INDEX

Note: Page numbers in *italics* refer to illustrations; page numbers followed by t refer to tables.

B

D